HANDBOOK OF PERCEPTION

Volume IV

Hearing

ADVISORY EDITORIAL BOARD

This is Volume IV of

HANDBOOK OF PERCEPTION

EDITORS: *Edward C. Carterette and Morton P. Friedman*

Contents of the other books in this series appear at the end of this volume.

HANDBOOK OF PERCEPTION

VOLUME IV

Hearing

EDITED BY

Edward C. Carterette and Morton P. Friedman

Department of Psychology
University of California
Los Angeles, California

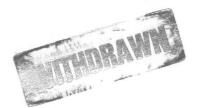

ACADEMIC PRESS   New York   San Francisco   London   1978

A Subsidiary of Harcourt Brace Jovanovich, Publishers

ACADEMIC PRESS, INC.
111 Fifth Avenue, New York, New York 10003

United Kingdom Edition published by
ACADEMIC PRESS, INC. (LONDON) LTD.
24/28 Oval Road, London NW1 7DX

Library of Congress Cataloging in Publication Data

Main entry under title:

Hearing.

(Handbook of perception ; v. 4)
Includes bibliographies.
1. Hearing.   2. Hearing disorders.   I. Carterette,
Edward C.   II. Friedman, Morton P.
QP461.H38   612'.85   78−8994
ISBN 0−12−161904−4 (v. 4)

PRINTED IN THE UNITED STATES OF AMERICA

CONTENTS

PART II.   MEASUREMENT, BIOPHYSICS OF THE COCHLEA, AND NEURAL CODING

Chapter 3.   Measurement of the Auditory Stimulus

Barry Leshowitz

Chapter 4.   Biophysics of the Cochlea

Peter Dallos

Chapter 5.   The Neural Code

I. C. Whitfield

PART III.   ANALYZING MECHANISMS OF FREQUENCY, INTENSITY, TIME, AND PERIOD

Chapter 6.   Loudness

Bertram Scharf

Chapter 7.   Frequency and Periodicity Analysis

Jan O. Nordmark

Chapter 8.   Masking: Experimental and Theoretical Aspects of Simultaneous, Forward, Backward, and Central Masking

J. J. Zwislocki

PART IV.   BINAURAL AND SPATIAL HEARING

PART V.   PSYCHOLOGY OF MUSIC

Chapter 12.   Musical Acoustics

Jean-Claude Risset

PART VI.   STRESS, TRAUMA, AND PATHOLOGY

Chapter 13.   Effects of Hearing Impairment on the Auditory System

Donald D. Dirks

Chapter 14.   Effects of Noise on People

J. D. Miller

Chapter 15. General Psychological and Sociological Effects of Noise

J. D. Miller

Chapter 16. General Physiological Effects of Noise

J. D. Miller

LIST OF CONTRIBUTORS

Numbers in parentheses indicate the pages on which the authors' contributions begin.

EDWARD C. CARTERETTE (3), Department of Psychology, University of California, Los Angeles, California 90024

H. STEVEN COLBURN (365, 467), Department of Electrical Engineering and Research Laboratory of Electronics, Massachusetts Institute of Technology, Cambridge, Massachusetts 02139

PETER DALLOS (125), Departments of Communicative Disorders (Audiology) and Electrical Engineering, Northwestern University, Evanston, Illinois 60201

DONALD D. DIRKS (567), Department of Surgery, Head, and Neck, UCLA School of Medicine, Los Angeles, California

NATHANIEL I. DURLACH (365, 467), Department of Electrical Engineering and Research Laboratory of Electronics, Massachusetts Institute of Technology, Cambridge, Massachusetts 02139

DAVID M. GREEN (337), Department of Psychology and Social Relations, Harvard University, Cambridge, Massachusetts 02138

BARRY LESHOWITZ (83), Department of Psychology, Arizona State University, Tempe, Arizona 85281

J. D. MILLER (609, 641, 677), Central Institute for the Deaf, St. Louis, Missouri 63110

JAN O. NORDMARK (243), Division of Physiological Acoustics, Department of Physiology II, Karolinska Institutet, S-104 01 Stockholm 60, Sweden

ROY D. PATTERSON (337), Medical Research Council Applied Psychology Unit, Cambridge CB2 2EF, England

JEAN-CLAUDE RISSET (521), Institut de Recherche et Coordination Acoustique/Musique, Centre Georges-Pompidou, F-75004 Paris, France

BERTRAM SCHARF* (187), Department of Psychology, Northeastern University, Boston, Massachusetts 02115

EARL D. SCHUBERT (41), Hearing and Speech Sciences, Stanford University School of Medicine, Stanford, California 94305

I. C. WHITFIELD (163), Neurocommunications Research Unit, The Medical School, Birmingham B15 2TJ, England

J. J. ZWISLOCKI (283), Institute for Sensory Research, Syracuse University, Syracuse, New York 13210

* Present address: Laboratoire de Mécanique et d'Acoustique, 31, chemin Joseph-Aiguier, 13 274 Marseille, France.

FOREWORD

The problem of perception is one of understanding the way in which the organism transforms, organizes, and structures information arising from the world in sense data or memory. With this definition of perception in mind, the aims of this treatise are to bring together essential aspects of the very large, diverse, and widely scattered literature on human perception and to give a précis of the state of knowledge in every area of perception. It is aimed at the psychologist in particular and at the natural scientist in general. A given topic is covered in a comprehensive survey in which fundamental facts and concepts are presented and important leads to journals and monographs of the specialized literature are provided. Perception is considered in its broadest sense. Therefore, the work will treat a wide range of experimental and theoretical work.

This ten-volume treatise is divided into two sections. Section One deals with the fundamentals of perceptual systems. It is comprised of six volumes covering (1) historical and philosophical roots of perception, (2) psychophysical judgment and measurement, (3) the biology of perceptual systems, (4) hearing, (5) seeing, and (6) which is divided into two books (A) tasting and smelling and (B) feeling and hurting.

Section Two, comprising four volumes, will cover the perceiving organism, taking up the wider view and generally ignoring specialty boundaries. The major areas include (7) language and speech, (8) perceptual coding of space, time, and objects, including sensory memory systems and the relations between verbal and perceptual codes, (9) perceptual processing mechanisms, such as attention, search, selection, pattern recognition, and perceptual learning, (10) perceptual ecology, which considers the perceiving organism in cultural context, and so includes aesthetics, art, music, architecture, cinema, gastronomy, perfumery, and the special perceptual worlds of the blind and of the deaf.

The "Handbook of Perception" should serve as a basic source and reference work for all in the arts or sciences, indeed for all who are interested in human perception.

EDWARD C. CARTERETTE
MORTON P. FRIEDMAN

PREFACE

Eastern and Western acoustical science developed independently in adapting concepts having common origins in Mesopotamia. Usually attributed to the Pythagoreans, the theoretical basis of music was probably a discovery of the Babylonians. This ancient discovery, that sublengths of a given stretched string fix musical intervals, has the hallmark of all work in hearing, which is the intertwining of physics, physiology, and psychology.

Part I of this volume reviews the history of research on hearing. Chapter 1 (Carterette) takes us from the antiquity of acoustics and traces the physical and mathematical developments out of which auditory facts and theories sprang. Auditory perception, physiology, and theory are followed up to about 1940, though a particular aspect, the work on analysis synthesis and perception of speech, is traced up to about 1960. It has been nearly four decades since E. G. Boring's fairly complete coverage in his 1942 *Sensation and Perception in the History of Experimental Psychology*. Beginning where Boring left off, Schubert (Chapter 2) traces the main threads of structure and function as they figure in "the search for a more complete understanding of the auditory process as a channel of sensory information."

Part II deals with measurement, biophysics of the cochlea, and neural coding. We deduce underlying mechanisms of the processing of acoustic information by means of an analysis of the way in which a subject's response is related to the stimulus. Thus, a precise description of the auditory stimulus is a *sine qua non*. Leshowitz (Chapter 3) reviews the physical and mathematical basis for measuring the sound stimulus and introduces linear (time-invariant) filtering systems and the representation of coherent and random signals. This brief treatment of signal processing is useful at once in understanding Dallos's comprehensive summary (Chapter 4) of the biophysics of the cochlea, "the most highly developed and complex mechanoreceptor system" of animals. A succinct anatomy of the cochlea is followed by a systems analysis of gross and fine patterns of cochlear mechanics. As Dallos says, we have a good understanding of the nature, purpose, and operation of the basilar membrane, but the actual function of the well-studied receptor potentials in stimulus transduction has never been established with certainty. ''An even more general question is whether or not these potentials actively (causally) participate in the initiation of neural responses in the auditory nerve . . . , and we simply do not have a convincing solution to the problem.'' Nonetheless, Dallos covers fully what is known about the properties of these cochlear potentials. In his compact chapter on the neural code, Whitfield starts at the auditory nerve with the observation that auditory information is coded by (1) the presence or absence of spike activity in a given fiber, (2) the mean number of spikes in a unit of time, and (3) the temporal relationship between successive impulses in a fiber or group of fibers. With only these three coding ''axioms,'' Whitfield lays out the coding which underlies the pitch of simple and complex tones, two-tone inhibition, and critical bands. There is, finally, a brief discussion of the factors in temporal coding and localization; certain experimental findings imply that within the cochlear nucleus some cells process place information of intensity and frequency whereas other cells process the temporal aspects of transient signals.

Four chapters make up Part III: *Analyzing Mechanisms of Frequency, Intensity, Time, and Period*. Loudness, given a thorough treatment by Scharf in Chapter 6, is the *subjective* intensity of a sound, which means that ''a sentient listener, human or animal, must respond to the sound.'' The intensity of a sound is the major determinant of loudness but a sound's spectral and temporal features are also important as are other, background, sounds and the interaction of these with the state of the listener. Scharf's discussion of these stimulus variables and the listener is followed by discussions of physiological aspects, models, and meaning of loudness. A definitive characterization of loudness remains elusive. Yet, as Scharf makes clear, loudness has an important role in auditory pathology and in the measurement and control of environmental noise.

Chapter 7, on frequency and periodicity analysis, is based on explicit recognition of the limited resolving power of the ear, a distinction between the proximal and distal stimulus, and concern for the constraints on auditory research resulting from the use of Fourier mathematics. Nordmark gives a review and a critique of the attempts to solve the classical central problems—selectivity of the ear, beats and other interactions, periodicity pitch, the gestalt concept of a tonal complex—and manages also to relate the psychological and physiological findings and models.

When one sound makes another difficult or impossible to hear, masking has occurred. Zwislocki (Chapter 8) limits his coverage of the vast domain of masking to monaural, simultaneous, forward, and backward masking. But he also gives what is perhaps the first systematic review of ''some aspects of central masking that occur when the masker is introduced to one ear, the test sound to the other, and acoustic leakage between the two ears is prevented.'' Certain of the experimental results of Chapter 8 (Section II) are singled out for psychophysical theorizing with inquiry into both psychophysical and psychophysiological relationships. The inquiry into masking embraces problems of signal-to-noise ratio, the loudness function, auditory frequency analysis, the relationship between monaural and central masking, and associated neural activity. Zwislocki concludes, "On the basis of experimental evidence and mathematical derivations, it is shown that central masking tells us more about the mechanisms of hearing than does monaural masking."

Masking shows that frequency analysis has failed and the data of masking experiments aid in quantifying the limits of frequency analysis. Patterson and Green (Chapter 9) have selected from the empirical findings of 50 years of modern masking studies and "attempt to relate a subset of the data to theory about the hearing mechanism, and particularly to current thinking about frequency analysis." These data are treated by a signal-to-noise ratio analysis, that is, by means of a critical band or auditory filter concept in which statistical fluctuations are ignored.

In Part IV, *Binaural and Spatial Hearing,* it is proved that two ears *are* better than one. In their large and profusely illustrated Chapter 10 on "Binaural Phenomena," Durlach and Colburn review the wide variety of binaural hearing phenomena. They do not cover dichotic listening (selective attention) research or applications of binaural research but focus on basic results most likely to illuminate the operations of the ear. They deal with interaural difference, that most central feature of binaural perception (Section II), perceptual attributes of the binaural image (Section III), and the sensitivity of the binaural system (Section IV).

"Binaural Phenomena" provides a rich background for the survey of "Models of Binaural Interaction" (Chapter 11). In Chapter 11 Colburn and Durlach treat models built to explain the perception of interaural differences. They restrict themselves mostly to models that are based on the analysis of the two stimulus waveforms and that are well formed enough to make quantitative psychoacoustic predictions. Five classes of models are covered and an overview is given of their similarities and differences: (1) count comparators, (2) interaural-difference detectors, (3) noise suppressors (e.g., by equalization and cancellation), (4) cross correlators, and (5) discriminators of auditory-nerve firing patterns.

Being a composer, performer, aesthetician, and expert in musical computation, J. C. Risset is well placed to review "Musical Acoustics" (Chapter 12 and Part V). His view is that many of the results of psychoacoustics must be qualified because they are based on simple stimuli, whereas musical structures are time-varying tonal complexes. With this reservation Risset reviews the classical topics of music as related to hearing and perception: pitch, duration, rhythm, timbre, preference, and musical aptitude tests. The discussion of musical instruments shows that only recently have precise analyses of transient musical sounds become possible. Even so, early instrument makers intuitively grasped the relationships among music, listener, and physical acoustics, as the relative perfection of sixteenth century violins attests. Following a note on musical reproduction, Risset ends with brief but authoritative discussions of electronic music and computer composition.

Stress, Trauma, and Pathology, Part VI, begins with Dirks' chapter on the effects of hearing impairment. Of the two major classes of hearing impairment, one, loss of auditory sensitivity, is usually a disorder of the peripheral auditory system. The other, dysacusis, is usually associated with a sensorineural disorder, and often with no loss of sensitivity, though speech may be hard to understand. Dirks reviews the basis of modern audiometric tests and their use in diagnosing whether a disorder is peripheral or central and the locus of its probable cause: external or middle ear, cochlea, VIIIth nerve, brainstem, or auditory cortex. The final section covers the difficult problem of defining a handicapping hearing loss and assessing its effect, often profound, on an individual's life.

The three final chapters, all written by James D. Miller, review what is known up to the early 1970s about the actions of environmental noise on people. Miller observes in Chapter 14, "Effects of Noise on People," that the secular adaptation of evolution has not prepared men or animals for the hazards of the incessant noise of the modern world. He reviews the causes and extent of temporary and permanent damage to hearing wrought by environmental sounds, with considerable attention to the attendant decline of our ability to hear and understand speech.

In Chapter 15, Miller takes up the more general psychological and sociological effects of noise, such as interference with sleep, annoyance, and disruption of social activities, and the degree to which the disturbance to sleep "may constitute a hazard to one's physical and mental health." He also reviews the methods of measuring the dimensions of auditory experience (e.g., loudness and perceived noisiness), and data on annoyance and community response to noise, and how to measure and predict these. The brief section on noise and performance, acoustical privacy, anxiety, stress, and mental disorders tells us that noise has many deleterious psychological and social effects. But there is no evidence that aircraft noise causes mental disorders although there may be more admissions to psychiatric hospitals from areas subjected to high levels of aircraft noise than from areas subjected to lower levels of aircraft noise.

Chapter 16 very briefly reviews transient physiological effects of noise with an eye toward their possible persistence and relates them to neuroendocrine stress theory (Selye). Does exposure to noise cause or increase susceptibility to disease? There are suggestions and suspicions, but Miller says that "the only conclusively established effect of noise on health is that of noise-induced hearing loss."

Financial support has come in part from The National Institute of Mental Health (Grant MH-07809), The Ford Motor Company, and The Regents of The University of California.

Editors of Academic Press both in New York and in San Francisco have been enormously helpful in smoothing our way.

Part I

History of Research on Hearing

Chapter 1

SOME HISTORICAL NOTES ON RESEARCH IN HEARING

EDWARD C. CARTERETTE

I. INTRODUCTION: FROM THE MONOCHORD TO ELECTROACOUSTICS

A. Early Acoustics, West and East

Acoustics, broadly defined to cover the nature of sound, was one of the earliest fields in the West or the East to be treated by exact measurement.

HANDBOOK OF PERCEPTION, VOL. IV

The approach of the ancient Greeks was analytical and that of the ancient Chinese, correlative (Needham, 1962). For the Pythagoreans, sound embodied number that was the basis of the musical note, as it was for the Chinese. To the Chinese, sound also was a form of activity bound to the pneumatic concept of *chhi*—fragrant steam of the cooking pot—having many meanings, for example, vapor, air, breath, vital principal. *Chhi* rose from earth in prayers to one's ancestors, as a synthesis of sound, color, and flavor. And from heaven, *chhi* was sent down, mixing as wind (thunder), rain (rainbows), and seasonal growth (herbs).

Sound was connected with motion and impulse very early in acoustical theory of the Greeks, who grasped the importance of air and other media in transmitting impulses (Aristotle, *De Audibilibis*). However, as Needham points out, the acoustics of the ancient Chinese philosophers was consonant with their notion of a universal continuum in which action at a distance resulted from transmitted waves. They conceived of *chhi* somewhat as we would matter, in a form between rarefied gas and radiant energy. The literary tradition of the scholars in China was sharply distinct from the oral tradition of the craftsmen who were expert in acoustics and music. Nonetheless it has become clear from the remarkable work of Needham and his associates (Needham, 1962) that the Chinese were asking questions parallel to those of the Greeks.*

Although Eastern and Western acoustical science developed independently in adapting concepts having common origins in Mesopotamia, there are two possible points of interaction, both of them musical. The first concerns the theoretical basis of music, the second the equally tempered scale.

According to Needham (1962, pp. 176–183) the controversy about whether the Greek Pythagoras or the Chinese Ling Lun invented the theoretical basis of music would be resolved if each of them drew upon an earlier discovery due to the Babylonians. The Babylonian discovery is hypothetical but the surviving evidence suggests that this was the truth. In any case the fundamental observation (usually attributed to Pythagoras) was that if one takes the one-half, two-thirds, and three-quarter lengths of a given string, one obtains its octave, fifth, and fourth, respectively.

"The princely gift" to mankind of Chu Tsai Yü (1584) "was the discovery of the mathematical means of tempering the scale in equal intervals, a system of such fundamental utility that people in all Western countries today take it for granted and are unaware of its existence [Needham, 1962, p. 220]." The player can move fluidly from one key to another because the octave has been divided up into 12 intervals so that the successor of any note has a frequency $2^{1/12}$ times that of the note next below it in frequency. Needham gives the

---

* Sound pervaded Chinese science. Bronze bells were cast anciently (fourteenth century B.C. or before) and their complex tuning was based on a bamboo tube whose pitch, *Huang-chung*, was standardized by its length (20.574 cm). By the fifth century A.D. distance, weight and capacity were based on the *Huang-chung* pipe which was itself defined by its capacity of 1200 grains of millet!

honor of the first formulation of the equally tempered scale to China, from whence, although not proven, it almost certainly got to the West.

Sometime in the sixth or fifth century B.C., Pythagoras or his followers showed experimentally that there was a relationship between the lengths of vibrating strings and their heard pitches (see Fig. 1). Theon of Smyrna in the second century A.D. says that Pythagoras "investigated these ratios (the fourth, the fifth, the octave, and so on) on the basis of the length and thickness of strings and also on the basis of the tension obtained by turning the pegs, or by the more familiar method of suspending weights from the strings [Cohen & Drabkin, 1948, p. 295]."

Archytas (fourth century A.D.) said that no sound can exist "without the striking of bodies against one another [Clagett, 1955, p. 73]." High-pitched sound arose from a swift motion, and low-pitched sound from a slow motion. Aristotle saw that a sound source was in some kind of continuous relation to hearing when he said ". . . it is air which causes hearing, when being one and continuous it is set in motion. . . . That, then, is resonant which is capable of exciting motion in a mass of air continuously one as far as the ear. And because the ear is in air, when the external air is set in motion, the air within the ear moves [*On the Soul,* translated by Hicks, Chapter 2, p. 8]." Aristotle, in *De Audibilibus* (probably written by Strato or some other in the Lyceum, says Clagett, 1955, p. 73) is even more explicit: "For when the nearest portion of it is struck by the breath which comes into contact with it, the air is at once driven forcibly on, thrusting in like manner the adjoining air, so that sound travels unaltered in quality as far as the disturbance of the air manages to reach."

We should note that Aristotle did more than generalize the notions of the Pythagoreans. Even if he was wrong in his suppositions that the whole air mass advanced, he apparently realized that the propagation of sound involved variations in density.

Boethius (Lindsay, 1973) in the fifth century A.D. even stated a primitive wave theory including reflections of waves. And, well before Boethius, the Roman architect Vitruvius (first century A.D.) postulated a qualitative theory of the wave nature of sound by pointing out the analogy between the propagation of ripples on the surface of shallow water and the propagation of sound in air. The two ideas were not fused in an effective way until Galileo Galilei: "Waves are produced by the vibrations of a sonorous body, which spread through the air, bringing to the tympanum of the ear a stimulus which the mind interprets as sound [*Dialogues Concerning Two New Sciences,* 1683]."

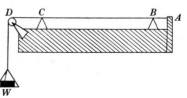

FIG. 1. The monochord. The weight *W* keeps the string in tension and the bridges *B* and *C* limit the vibration of the total range *AD* to the range *BC*, so that range and tension are both under control. [From J. H. Jeans (1937), *Science and Music.* Copyright 1937 by Cambridge University Press.]

Neither did the Chinese neglect the psychology of audition. In the seventh century, the idea was held that hearing may be likened to striking a drum with a drumstick. Sounds struck the ear drumskin, but the actual hearing (perceiving) of the sound was considered a matter of responding to it. Like Galileo's, this is an essentially modern view.

B. Velocity, Frequency, and Pitch

Descartes' fellow student Marin Mersenne (1588–1648) may have been the first to measure the velocity of sound in air; he found it to be 450 m sec^{-1}. His result was improved upon shortly after 1650 by two distinguished groups. The one, from the Italian *Accademia del Cimento* (Florence), obtained 350 m sec^{-1} and the other, from the *Académie de Sciences* (Paris), found 357 m sec^{-1}. A modern value is 344 m sec^{-1}, at 20°C. These early scientists timed the difference between seeing the flash of a cannon and hearing its sound. Although the speed of light was assumed infinite, the correction to be made for finite speed would have been negligible since the velocity of light is about 10^6 times that of sound! Newton computed a theoretical velocity of 298 m sec^{-1}. Mersenne, in an interesting way, found a less disparate result (316 m sec^{-1}). First he noted that it took him exactly 1 sec to shout *Benidicam Dominum*. He then found a distance from a wall such that a shout was tail-to-head to the echo. Thus he heard *BENIDICAM-DOMINUMbenidicamdominum* when he was 158 m from the wall.

It is not difficult to see that these apparently large discrepancies could easily arise from reaction time errors and the fact that air temperature has a great influence. The velocity of sound is approximately 331.45 + .61°C m sec^{-1}. Thus Bianconi in 1740 found winter speeds slower by 22 m sec^{-1} than summer speeds, corresponding to a thermometer difference of 36°C (Boring, 1942, p. 322). Incidentally, Colladon (1893) in 1826 clocked the average velocity of sound in the water of Lake Geneva as 1435 m sec^{-1}, at 8°C.

Galileo noticed that a chisel scraping a brass plate gave off a high-pitched sound and that it left a serrated track of parallel scratches. Stretched strings in the ratio 3 : 2 (the fifth) vibrated sympathetically when the chisel left 45 scratches for the higher pitch and 30 scratches for the lower pitch over tracks of equal length. Boring (1942) says this was "from the psychologist's point of view, the great acoustic event of the seventeenth century . . . [p. 322]." Perhaps, but it was Galileo's pupil Mersenne who, in 1636, demonstrated the law connecting the length l of a string with the period τ of its vibration, $\tau = 2l(\rho/T)^{1/2}$, where ρ is the density and T the tension, and first determined the actual rate of vibration of a known musical note.*

* The fundamental principle of the monochord is that for a given string and a given tension, the time varies as the length. Lord Rayleigh (1894) believed the principle to be understood by the Greeks, citing Thomas Young who said Aristotle ". . . knew that a pipe or a chord of double length produced a sound of which the vibrations occupied a double time; and that the properties of concords depended on the proportions of times occupied by the vibrations of the separate sounds [Vol. I, p. 404]."

The relation between frequency of vibration and pitch was first clearly quantified by a Frenchman, Joseph Sauveur (1701). By sounding together two organ pipes whose fundamentals were set by ear to an interval of a semitone ($f_1/f_2 = {}^{15}/_{16}$), he heard a beating tone of 6 beats sec^{-1}. Assuming the beat frequency to be $f_2 - f_1$, solving the two independent linear equations gives $f_2 = 96$ Hz, $f_1 = 90$ Hz.

C. Linear Systems and Fourier's Theorem

1. LINEARITY

Sauveur noted that a stretched string vibrated so that there were *nodes*, points where the string never moved, and *loops*, where the string motion was most violent. He grasped that the number and position of the nodes were related as the integers to the basic string frequency and length, and called the pitch of the lowest tone *fundamental*, and the pitches of the multiples *harmonics*. He made the important observation that a vibrating string can sound its various notes simultaneously. Daniel Bernoulli showed that the vibrations of a taut string (without mass but loaded with finite masses at particular points) would always be broken up into as many periodic vibrations as there are such points. This is the famous *superposition* principle which, as Euler (1753) saw, implied that the equation of motion of this string is *linear*.

2. "A REMARK OF FOURIER'S"

There was controversy during this period among the eminent mathematicians Euler, d'Alembert, Bernoulli, and Lagrange about the analytic representation of any arbitrary function as an infinite series of sines and cosines. Nearly 50 years later, "a remark of Fourier's threw new light on this subject; a new epoch in the development of this part of mathematics began . . . [Birkhoff, 1973, p. 19; the controversy is discussed on pp. 15–19]." Fourier (1807, 1822), looking for a solution to the problem of heat transfer in a disk, observed that for a function $f(x)$ given by certain trigonometric series, there was a way to determine the coefficients that was valid even if the function $f(x)$ is arbitrary.* Fourier's theorem says, in short, that every curve however obtained can be composed by superposing a sufficient number of simple harmonic curves. The original paper of 1807 has been published (for the first time!) in Grattan-Guinness (1972).

---

* Fourier (1807) observed that in the trigonometric series

$$f(x)a_0/2 + a_1 \cos x + a_2 \cos 2x + \cdots + b_1 \sin x + b_2 \sin 2x + \cdots,$$

the coefficients can be determined by the formulas

$$a_n = 1/\pi \int_{-\pi}^{\pi} f(x) \cos nx \, dx, \qquad b_n = 1/\pi \int_{-\pi}^{\pi} f(x) \sin nx \, dx.$$

3. MATHEMATICAL ACOUSTICS AND MODELS OF VIBRATIONS

In the eighteenth century, many problems of acoustical physics were tackled and solved by mathematicians. The acoustical aspects are reviewed by Lindsay (1973) and the mathematical aspects in Birkhoff (1973). Thus, Lagrange (1867) in 1759 predicted theoretically the harmonics of open and closed pipes, something Euler (1926) had done even earlier (in 1727). Robert Hooke (1676) gave a solution to the simplest case of a linear rod or bar: "*Ut tensio sic vis;* That is, the Power of any Spring is in the same proportion with the Tension thereof." Sophie Germain (Lindsay, 1973) provided in 1815 a mathematical theory of the vibrations of plates using experimental work of E. F. F. Chladni (1802). A more accurate theory was that of G. R. Kirchhoff in 1850; and S. D. Poisson gets credit for the theory of vibrations of flexible membranes such as drumheads. Electrical oscillations were discovered in the middle of the nineteenth century, but no one knew how to use them for driving practical mechanical systems. In 1880, the Curie brothers described piezoelectric crystals that generated currents when deformed or were deformed by currents, but it was not until the invention of the electronic valve (vacuum tube) nearly 40 years later that wide-band frequency generation and reception became practical.

4. ELECTROACOUSTICS

Electrical oscillators and amplifiers drove out the tuning fork as a standard, whereupon the mathematical theories of vibrations could be applied in the real world by means of microphones and loudspeakers. Acoustics was transformed into electroacoustics. Selective historical reviews of development, early in the twentieth century to about 1940, are given on electroacoustics by Hilliard (1977) and on acoustical measurement and instrumentation by Miller (1977). These two papers survey a wide array of electroacoustic transducers. Miller points up the significance of Wente's 1917 condenser microphone for absolute calibration of acoustical measurements. The device had only one resonance, located an octave above its working band, and served as an artificial ear as well as a free-field microphone from the outset. The famous Western Electric 1-A and 2-A audiometers that served as standards for so many decades are described in Fletcher (1929) and so are many of their early devices such as the Phonodeik, phonautograph, and Mader's harmonic analyzer.

II. FREQUENCY AND INTENSITY LIMITS OF THE EAR

In order to determine precisely the frequency limits of the ear, the French physicist Savart (1830) remarked that previous works of certain celebrated physicists were inexact and that with respect to limits "acoustics has made no real progress since the time of Sauveur [p. 203]." Using fans and rotating wheels of his own invention, Savart put the minimum audible frequency at 8 Hz, the maximum at 24 kHz. Other lower limits ranged from 16 to 32 Hz, as reported by Biot (1808), Koenig (1899), and Helmholtz (1865) but this range of three octaves for a lower limit meant little when sound pressure level (SPL) and subject differences were unknown. Wien (1903) obtained an audibility curve using a telephone receiver, and fixed absolute intensity thresholds for frequencies between 50 Hz and 12 kHz. Maximal sensitivity near 2200 Hz was 10^8 times that at 50 Hz!

The first modern result was given by Wegel (1922) at the Bell Telephone Laboratories (see Fig. 2). The auditory sensation area was mapped out for frequencies (20 Hz to 20 kHz) between the threshold of audibility and the threshold of feeling. The absolute threshold was well below .001 dyne cm^{-2} at 2200 Hz. Wien's results were surely in error but the lesson is clear:

1. The upper and lower limits of audibility of pitch depend entirely upon the intensities at which the measurements are made.
2. The ear is a very sensitive device that rivals the eye.

The differential threshold for pitch was also beset with differences due to instrument and method. For example, Luft (1888) found .25 Hz and Vance (1914) found 1.80 Hz, but using an electrical oscillator Shower and Biddulph found 2.60 Hz.

Differential sensitivity for intensity only became important after Fechner's (1860) reports on Weber's law. Renz and Wolf (1856) asked subjects to detect changes in the loudness of a ticking watch as its distance was varied.

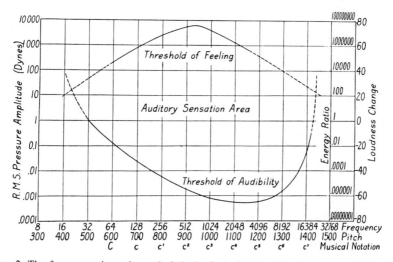

FIG. 2. The frequency–intensity and pitch–loudness limits of the human ear. [After Wegel, from Fletcher (1923).]

Threshold at 75% correct judgments was found at an intensity ratio of about 1000/870, a difference of 13%. By dropping lead balls on an iron plate (about 1880, reported by Boring, 1942), Nörr found the 75% differential threshold to be about 5% of stimulus intensity. Note that these workers were using noise. They all tended to verify Weber's law, that $\Delta I/I$ is constant at about 10% more or less independent of intensity I. The first good modern determination was due to Riesz (1928), who used an electronic valve amplifier. For intensities of about 55 dB SPL, Riesz found $\Delta I/I$ to be about 10% but rising exponentially to 70% at 10 dB.

Beyond beats, described by Sauveur (1701) and mentioned above, in 1701 Tartini (1754) discovered the difference tone of two primaries and used it in tuning strings. Others in between gave partial descriptions of beats and difference tones, but it was Helmholtz (1865) who discovered *summation* tones of two primaries and verified difference tones of higher order. These two classes he called *combination* tones and gave the physical conditions of origin (nonlinearity) and the relevant mathematical equations. Helmholtz explained subjective beats by his resonance–place theory of hearing as a failure of Ohm's acoustical law and understood quite well that combination tones arise from nonlinear distortion.

III. TIMBRE, FUSION, NOISE, AND MASKING

Two instruments or two voices giving the same note sound similar but are not confused at all. Helmholtz (1865) was, in 1859, the first to see that *timbre,* or Klangfarbe, was defined by the patterns of partials of a musical note, that is, by frequency, amplitude, and combination of different frequencies. His theory of vowel color was based on this principle and still stands (see also Section IX).

Both Helmholtz and Rayleigh understood that a physically pure tone was made impure by the nonlinearity of the ear. But neither made clear that these distortions, now called *aural harmonics,* were not necessarily combination tones. Clarification was due to Wegel and Lane who in 1924 generated two frequencies in the ear simultaneously and by use of an exploring tone found many resultant frequencies, including the second and third harmonics of the two generators which were not difference or summation tones.

Stumpf (1890) believed that tones interpenetrated and fused so that the total percept was different from the concurrent presence of the components. This once important notion disappeared as introspection waned after 1915 and because there was no evidence for it.

Over 100 years ago Helmholtz described the tonality of noises in a way that implied continuity from tone to noise. He first held, but later discarded, the belief that tones and noise had different organs. This duplicity theory of noise and tone disappeared for want of evidence. Ohm's acoustical law, in Helmholtz's hands, kept the tone preeminent in psychoacoustics, but the strong conclusion that noise is a complex fusion of tones grew when electrical oscillators, noise generators, and amplifiers made experiments with the continuum feasible. Thus, in 1938 Fletcher's studies on the masking of tones by noise were based on the principle that thermal (white) noise contains all frequencies at equal amplitudes (Fletcher, 1938a,b).

The classic 1924 paper of Wegel and Lane on tonal masking shows beautifully how the precision of control by electroacoustics gave new, definitive results. Among other features, Fig. 3 shows that a fixed frequency f_1 masks $f_2 = f_1 + \Delta f$ such that smaller Δf leads to greater masking. However, masking is lessened in the region where f_1 and f_2 beat together. And aural harmonics cause the masking function to repeat itself at harmonics of f_1.

IV. AUDITORY LOCALIZATION

A. The Reign of Binaural Intensity Differences

Venturi between 1796 and 1801 (Gulick, 1971, p. 181) hypothesized that the difference in sound intensity at the two ears was the basis of localization. He carried out free-field tests using brief flute tones on normal and unilaterally deaf listeners. His hypothesis explained median-plane confusions and why his deaf listeners could not localize.

By denying that tones had extent, the nineteenth-century psychologists doubted that a true auditory space existed (Boring, 1942, p. 381). How, they asked, are nonspatial tones spatially placed? How is auditory space built up from other sensations? This doubt kept them from pursuing the recognized

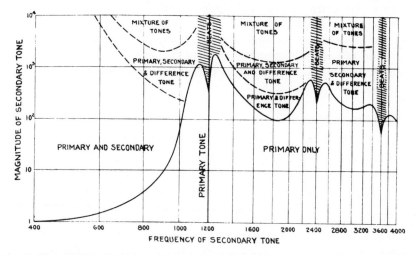

FIG. 3. The sensation caused by two tones. [From Wegel and Lane (1924), Auditory masking of one pure tone by another and its possible relation to the dynamics of the inner ear, *Physical Review*, **23**, 266–285.]

fact that the distance between the ears was a basis for localization. And, even though auditory theory mapped pitch onto cochlear place, a spatial pattern did not appear in introspection. Localization of sound was built from experience said the empiricists, pointing out how visual cues assisted.

E. H. Weber (1848) recognized that left–right was the primary auditory dimension. Rayleigh (1877) showed by experiment that *(a)* voices are better localized than tones; *(b)* high tones are better localized than low tones; *(c)* the binaural ratio of intensities at the two ears is crucial for localization; *(d)* right and left are not confused; and *(e)* symmetrically located front and back sources are confused. These results amount to an intensity theory of localization that was supported by Thompson's (1879) experiments with the pseudophone, a pair of acoustical ear trumpets that could be pointed in any direction. Other workers added details between then and 1934 when Steinberg and Snow quantified precisely the effect of the head's shadow on the binaural ratio of intensities at different frequencies (Fig. 4).

B. Phase Differences Rear Their Heads

The phase theory of localization begun by Thompson and proposed by Rayleigh in 1907 was based on the movement within the head of two low-frequency beating tones (tuning forks) dichotically presented over tubes. Wilson and Myers (1908) led the sound of one tuning fork separately to each ear over tubes of adjustable length, showing clearly that low tones were localized on the side of leading phase within variations of half a wavelength. It was not clear whether localization was governed by intensity differences for tones of middle and high frequency or by phase differences for tones of low frequency. The open-air free-field study of Stevens and Newman (1934) was definitive in showing that low tones are localizable. For low tones dichotic phase works, whereas for high tones dichotic intensity works. Errors of localization fall off on either side of a maximum near 3000 Hz where the wavelength, 11.5 cm, is on the order of half the distance between the ears.

C. Phase versus Time

Phase is hard to see as such in complex sounds. In 1908 Mallock said that localization could be based on binaural time differences, a view supported by Aggazotti in 1911. What was the least binaural time delay? Klemm (1920) reported 2 μsec, whereas von Hornbostel and Wertheimer (1920) found a 30-μsec threshold, with no uncertainty at about 600 μsec. However Klemm showed that time and intensity could be traded off and felt that the *time* hypothesis should be reduced to an intensity hypothesis *(a)* in view of the astonishingly brief delays, and *(b)* given that successive sounds in one ear had to be separated by 2 msec before being heard as a pair.

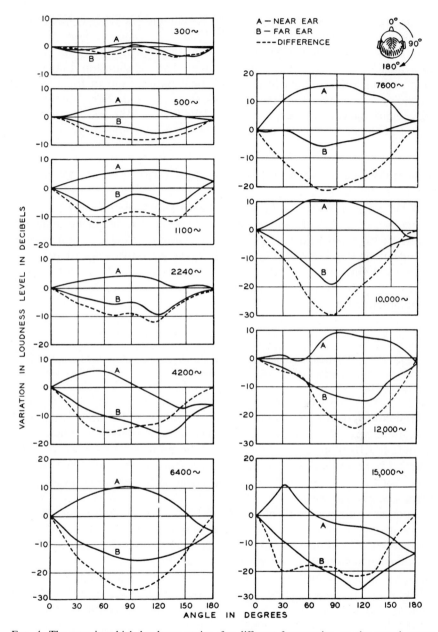

FIG. 4. The way in which loudness varies, for different frequencies, as the sound source moves from 0 to 180° azimuth. [From Steinberg and Snow (1934), with permission of Bell Laboratories.]

The problem of successivity also led Kreidl and Gatscher (1923) to reject the time hypothesis. Boring (1942) in 1926 ". . . showed how phase and time could be the physiological equivalent of intensity [p. 390]," a wrong equivalence by recent electrophysiology. The relationship between the number and kind of cues in the acoustical pattern and in the underlying physiology is more complex than was then realized. For example, head movement figures in source location (Wallach, 1940) and there is more recent evidence that the fine structure of the pinnae are subtly involved.

V. FREQUENCY ANALYSIS AND PERIODICITY DETECTION

If the ear is a frequency analyzer, then it should be possible to hear the harmonics of a periodic sound separately. With care it can be done. Mersenne (1636) could hear f_0, $2f_0$, . . . , $7f_0$. Ohm (1843) gave the first correct statement of this notion: A tone of frequency f will be heard only if the complex sound contains $\sin(2\pi ft + \theta)$ as a component. This, *Ohm's acoustical law,* was the basis of Helmholtz's theory of tonal perception and Helmholtz amplified it:

> Every motion of the air, which corresponds to a composite mass of musical tones, is, according to Ohm's law, capable of being analyzed into a sum of simple pendular vibrations, and to each such simple vibration corresponds a simple tone, sensible to the ear, and having pitch determined by the periodic time of the corresponding motion of the air [1865, p. 33].

Helmholtz could hear, by directed attention, up to $17f_0$ and Stumpf (1890) thought he heard $27f_0$. Other ways to identify the partials of a complex sound include localization, direct judgment of the number of partials, or judging whether a probe heard afterward was present in the prior tonal complex. Most such studies show the resolving power of the ear to be poor, belying Ohm's acoustical law.

Another complication is that the sound of a musical instrument is heard as unity, having a single pitch with timbre due to the harmonics which are themselves almost never heard. This apparent failure of the ear as a sharply tuned analyzer implies that pitch is based on periodicity rather than frequency. (The frequency–periodicity issues are taken up in detail in Chapter 2.) Yet, a frequency analysis seems demanded to account for the hearing of component tones, combination tones, loudness summation, timbre, or the relation between the roughness and frequency separation of beating tones.

The truth is probably that pitch is discerned by means of both frequency analysis and periodicity mechanisms. Based on an historical review and important new work of his own, Plomp (1966, 1976) concludes that *(a)* the ear processes sounds in two successive stages—a peripheral analysis followed by a central synthesis; *(b)* the frequency analyzing power of the ear is limited by the critical bandwidth, and only the first five to eight harmonics give separate peaks in the auditory pattern; *(c)* the ear is inherently nonlinear and combination tones have real effects; *(d)* the suppression of one tone by another enhances contrast, perhaps subtly, in the frequency domain.

VI. ATTRIBUTES, SCALES, AND PSYCHOPHYSICS

We must brush on this vast topic because hearing has always been centrally involved. Boring (1942, pp. 375–381) surveys the problem of attributes of tone between Külpe in 1893 and S. S. Stevens in 1934, and identifies seven important proposals for the attributes of tone sensations, that is, for independently variable aspects. The possible attributes were *pitch, loudness, volume, density, brightness, vocality,* and *tonality.* Pitch and loudness were admitted by all but the rest were equivocal. Today, many workers would accept pitch, loudness, volume, and density as tonal attributes. We now examine "attributes" as parameters or dimensions using pattern recognition and multidimensional scaling methods (see Chapter 2).

The problem of tonal scales goes back to Fechner, ". . . who assumed that all j.n.d. (just noticeable differences) are equal and, on the basis of Weber's law, built up a scale of intensities (Fechner's law by counting the j.n.d.) from the absolute threshold up to the intensity being measured [Boring, 1942, pp. 350–351]." The major objections were that *(a)* sensations have no magnitudes, so can not be measured; *(b)* Weber's law was only an approximation; and *(c)* jnd's are not constant over the stimulus range. This third objection suggests that sensory distances be measured directly.

An early direct ratio–scaling procedure, the production of loudnesses which were some fixed fraction or multiple of a standard, led to the original *sone* scale of loudness. One sone was the loudness of a binaural tone of 1000 Hz heard at 40 dB above its threshold. An analogous interval scale of equal-sense distances was also created for pitch by the method of fractionation (and on very little data!) by Stevens, Volkmann, and Newman (1937; also Stevens & Volkmann, 1940). The pitch unit is the *mel,* with 1000 Hz being set to 1000 mels. In crude fashion, the mel scale follows the cochlear map of pitch.

These scales were peripheral to sensory psychology until Stevens in 1955 began a flourishing enterprise with the direct ratio-scaling of loudness by the method of magnitude estimation which requires only that the subject give a numerical response to a stimulus. For many sensory dimensions the sensation magnitude ψ is a power function of the stimulus intensity, for example, $\psi = kI^\alpha$, where k and α are constants. In particular, for loudness, $L = kI^{.67}$, where I is intensity in decibels sound pressure level (that is, dB SPL, where the reference pressure is .0002 dyne cm^{-2}). In words, loudness grows in proportion to the .67 power of sound pressure. Magnitude estimation is easy, fast, and said to be versatile. For a critique and an alternative method, see Anderson in Volume 2 of this *Handbook* (1974).

Psychophysics, and especially psychoacoustics, has been enormously influenced by the development of signal detection theory and, to a considerable degree, by multidimensional scaling methods. These topics are too recent for this historical survey, but are treated by Schubert in Chapter 2 of this volume. For a brief history of signal detection theory and its roots in psychophysics and scaling see Green and Swets (1966, Chapter 5).

VII. THE NEW PHYSIOLOGY OF HEARING

What Boring (1942) called "The New Physiology of Hearing" was born in electrophysiology and electroacoustics and gave new facts and theories, the decade 1930–1940 being especially fruitful. We look briefly at four topics: the cochlear response, action potentials, localization of pitch, and cochlear dynamics.

A. Cochlear Response

The brain's response to stimulation of the eye by light was recorded by the English physician Caton in 1875. He used electrodes placed directly on the surface of the brain. In the same way, brain potentials were obtained in response to very loud sounds in 1890 by Beck and in 1891 by Danilevsky. Attempts were made to record the electrical response of the auditory nerve (Beauregard & Dupuy, 1896; Buijtendijk, 1910) over a range of frequencies, but the very small deflections kept them from showing more than that they probably obtained action currents.

By means of the string galvanometer* Buijtendijk (1910) had recorded deflections from the auditory nerve in response to intense sounds. Recording from the brainstem of cats, using a single-stage electronic valve amplifier and the string galvanometer, Forbes, Miller, and O'Connor (1927) got an inconclusive hint that nerve fibers might carry the frequency code of a sound stimulus. The clicks of a ratchet noisemaker were followed up to about 220 Hz, but results with pure tones were equivocal.

An absolutely fundamental effect was observed by Wever and Bray in 1930. They set out to test the telephone theory of Rutherford (1886) against

---

* The string galvanometer was invented by Einthoven in 1903 and had a brief but important life until it was supplanted by the cathode-ray oscillograph. If a wire in a magnetic field carries current, it will undergo movement. This principle was realized by making the string of a thin metal coated quartz fiber. The string was illuminated by a strong light so that its deflections could be traced on photographic paper.

the frequency-analyzer theory of Helmholtz. Wever and Bray listened over earphones to the amplified potentials from an electrode placed on the cat's auditory nerve and were startled to hear their own speech over the cat's ear. Pure tones from 100 to 5000 Hz also gave audible responses. Artifacts were ruled out and they concluded that this "microphonic" sound (now called *cochlear microphonic* or simply *microphonic*) was of biological origin because it waned and waxed as the blood supply did, disappearing with the death of the animal.

They considered but rejected the hypothesis that the microphonic arose in the cochlea, favoring rather a neural origin. In 1931, E. D. (later Lord) Adrian put forth the hypothesis rejected by Wever and Bray, that the microphonic arose from some mechanical interaction of tissues of the inner ear, but soon reversed the view because the effect disappeared when the auditory nerve was cocainized, thus implying a true neural origin (Adrian, Bronk, & Phillips, 1931).

B. Action Potentials

Hallowell Davis and L. J. Saul showed in 1931 and 1932 that both groups had rejected the correct hypothesis. The cochlear microphonic did not arise from nerve fibers, because it had no apparent threshold and followed the stimulating frequency perfectly even at rates nearly a hundred times greater than the highest frequency of a single fiber (about 180 sec^{-1}) and about 20 times greater than the fastest rate for a bundle of many fibers (about 800 sec^{-1}). The technically brilliant device of Davis and Saul was the use of a coaxial electrode to isolate the cochlear microphonic from auditory nerve potentials. What all the others had seen was the summation of these two kinds of potentials. (Later, in 1949, Davis and his colleagues made another great advance by using differential electrodes to cancel the large action potential, thereby revealing the cochlear microphonic alone.)

Even now the origin of the microphonic is not truly understood; its most likely site is the intracellular potentials of the hair cells. Despite this, the cochlear potential has been an exceedingly important tool in auditory physiology. It could be fairly said that its role in hearing has been analogous to that of the bubble chamber in nuclear physics.

How could the auditory nerve follow frequencies whose periods were some 100 times shorter than the refractory period of a single neuron? Wever and Bray's (1930) explanation was the volley theory: At stimulus periods below the refractory period, a neuron fires once at each cycle, but, as the stimulus period shortens, a given neuron fires on only the second or the third, or the nth cycle. Groups, or platoons, of neurons fire in different phases or volleys. The coaxial electrode of Davis and Saul made possible a test of the volley theory (Fig. 5) and its verification.

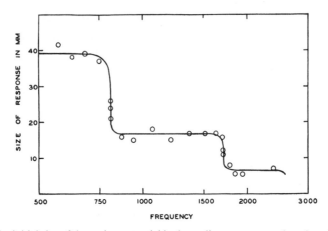

Fig. 5. The initial size of the action potential in the auditory nerve as a function of frequency. Above 800–1000 Hz, the frequency at which individual fibers can follow, every other cycle is followed, hence the abrupt drop at about 900 Hz. At about 1800 Hz, twice the critical frequency, each fiber responds only to every third cycle. [From Stevens and Davis (1936), with permission of the Acoustical Society of America.]

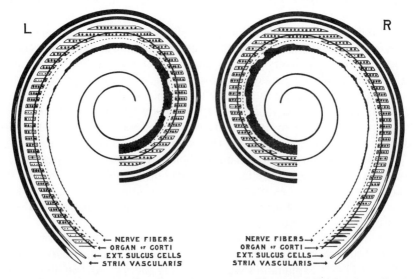

Fig. 6. The spiral reconstruction charts of these two cochleas are similar but the audiogram of L shows an abrupt high-tone loss, that of R shows gradual high-tone loss. Healthy inner and outer hair cells are shown as large black dots, impairment by a small or absent dot. The three long, solid black bars represent healthy tissue and the degree of atrophy by the ratio of white to black. [From Crowe, Guild, and Polvogt (1934), Observations on the pathology of hightone deafness, *Bulletin of the Johns Hopkins Hospital*, **54**, 315–379.]

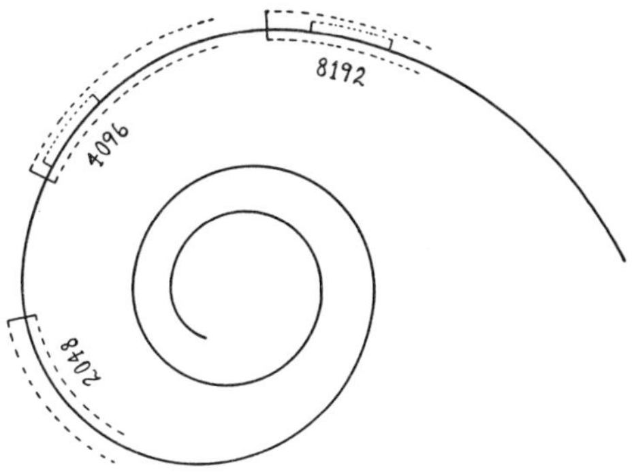

FIG. 7. Tone localization for three frequencies based on the method of Fig. 6. Based on eight cases of abrupt high-tone loss and extensive atrophy of the organ of Corti. [From Crowe, Guild, and Polvogt (1934), Observations on the pathology of hightone deafness, *Bulletin of the Johns Hopkins Hospital*, **54**, 315–379.]

C. Localization of Pitch in the Cochlea

If pitch and place in the cochlear are correlated, then behavioral and cochlear responses ought to be associated with localized damage dysfunction, or interference along the cochlear partition.

Long exposure to intense impure tones led to large regions of degeneration in the organ of Corti, but the effect of lower tones was toward the apex, and of higher tones toward the base (Yoshii, 1909). Histological damage by intense pure tones or noise bursts was widespread with a tendency to be maximal near the second turn of the cochlea, as reported in Kemp's (1935) review of stimulation deafness. But from audiograms of human subjects mapped, postmortem, against cochlear degeneration, Crowe, Guild, and Polvogt in 1934 found degeneration to high frequencies in the basal turn always and to low frequencies beyond the first turn. They localized degeneration for 8192, 4096, and 2048 Hz (see Figs. 6 and 7). Culler (1935) obtained a very consistent map by exploring the cochlear outside for the point of maximal response. Stevens, Davis, and Lurie (1935) scaled the basilar membrane for frequency by boring tiny holes in the cochlear wall and then finding the locus of minimal cochlear response. Fletcher (1938b) localized pitch on the cochlea by inference from the masking of tones by thermal noise (see Fig. 8).

D. Cochlear Dynamics

Wegel and Lane (1924) had modeled the Helmholtzian ear by a bank of tuned, independent, electrical resonators connected in parallel. But these studies of localization showed clearly that the spread of excitation along the cochlea is great and so the assumption of independence is wrong. Thus, later workers were compelled to consider the cochlea as a tube with elastic walls, in short, as a complete hydrodynamic system.

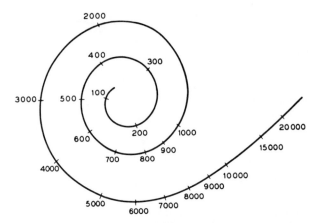

Fɪɢ. 8. Frequency sensitivity along the basiliar membrane. The plot was obtained by theoreti-
cal considerations from *(a)* the masked thresholds of pure tones in wide-band noise and *(b)*
Steinberg's estimate of distances along the basilar membrane which *(c)* were in turn based on
Guild's count of the number of ganglion cells. [From Fletcher (1938b), with permission of the
National Academy of Sciences.]

VIII. AUDITORY THEORY

A. From the Greeks to Du Verney

The beginnings of auditory theory are summarized well by Wever (1949) so
that the briefest sketch will do here. As was mentioned before, the Greeks
had some primitive notions about the conduction of sound in media. Em-
pedocles (fifth century B.C.) had an elementary anatomy of the external and
middle ear, and knew of the ear drumskin and the air-filled tympanic cavity.
Sensation, based on the principle of resemblances, required that the emana-
tions of material objects meet a substance of like nature for a percept to
occur. The "implanted" tympanic air was the proper substance for hearing.
Later (175 A.D.), Galen divided the bundles of nerves running from brain to
internal auditory meatus into the two branches we know as the auditory and
facial nerves. It is likely that he knew nothing about the inner ear.

Vesalius (1543) gave an accurate description of, and named, the malleus
and incus. The tiny, elusive stapes, the round and the oval windows were
discovered by Ingrassia (1546) (cited by Wever, 1949), but Fallopius (1561)
gave the details of form and articulation. Eustachius (1564) described well
the tensor tympani muscle, also suggesting its function, and the Eustachian
tube, but Varolius (1591) was the first to describe correctly the stapedius muscle. Coiter's *De auditus instrumento* (1566) opposed the implanted-air hypothesis in the first book dealing specifically and systematically with the ear.

The first resonance theory was due to Bauhin (1601), who believed that the
dimensions and shapes of the various cavities of the ear work as selective
resonators. From newer knowledge, Willis (1672) gave an improved version

of the theory with "an account of sound transmission that is remarkable for its time [Wever, 1949, p. 11]."

Nearly modern in form was Du Verney's (1683) theory of the peripheral analysis of sound by resonance. He saw clearly the form of the basilar membrane, his drawing of the cochlea (Fig. 9) being the first to show it. He localized low tones at the base, and high tones at the apex, a sensible view, given his belief that the bony spiral lamina was the true receptive apparatus.

B. Du Verney to Compound Microscope to Retzius to Held

After Du Verney there were refinements, until Cotugno (1760) transferred the role of receptive apparatus to the membraneous lamina. And because the lamina grows wider as it rises in the cochlea, he put high pitches at the base, low pitches at the apex. The inner ear was compared to a stringed keyboard instrument (cembalo). This was the way things stood until the modern period of auditory research began with Helmholtz (1857).

The compound microscope was perfected around 1830, which made possible a description of the finer structures of the cochlea. Reissner (1851) discovered the membrane, named after him, that partitions the scala vestibuli. Corti's (1851) landmark anatomical studies of the cochlea showed the then unknown features: the rods of Corti, the hair cells, and the tectorial membrane. His viewing point, down onto the organ of Corti, was a distorted flat projection, but Deiters (1860) saw the rods in their true perspective, and also the relation between hair cells and reticular membrane (Figs.

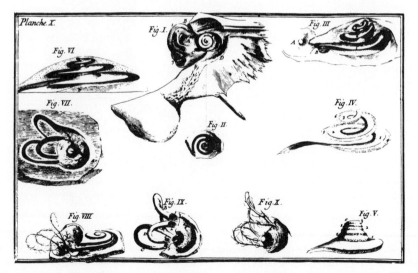

FIG. 9. Du Verney clearly saw the spiral form of the cochlea. [Plate X from Du Verney (1683). By courtesy of the Historical Division, Biomedical Library, University of California, Los Angeles.]

10 and 11). Deiters also discovered other supporting cells, as did several contemporary anatomists.

It remained to map the routes of the auditory nerve fibers. Schultze (1858) worked out many true connections; Nuel (1872) followed the spiral fibers for some way but lost them when they turned in radially. Retzius (1884) traced their outward course, and saw their endings on the hair cells. Held (1897) worked out more details. Now, finally, the hair cells were seen as the true sensory elements and the other cells as accessory.

From this new structural knowledge sprang new interest in auditory function and in Du Verney's hypothesis of a peripheral resonance analyzer.

C. Helmholtz's Resonance–Place Theory of Hearing

The great Helmholtz stated the first modern theory of hearing (1863), drawing upon the newest and best sources of physiological acoustics, anatomy—that of Corti (1851) in particular—the doctrine of specific nerve energies, and Ohm's acoustical law as it transmuted Fourier's theorem. The cochlea was assumed to be an array of spatially tuned analyzers, responsive to higher frequencies at the base and lower frequencies toward the apex.

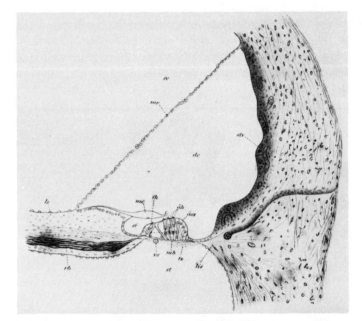

FIG. 10. The position of the organ of Corti on the basilar membrane *(mb)* in the scala media. Above Reissner's membrane *(mv)* lies the scala vestibuli *(sv)*. Other prominent features are the scala tympani *(st)*, inner *(ih)* and outer *(äh)* hair cells, tectorial membrane *(mc)*, spiral ligament *(lis)* and stria vascularis *(stv)*. [From Retzius (1884), Fig. 1, Tafel XXXV. By courtesy of the Historical Division, Biomedical Library, University of California, Los Angeles.]

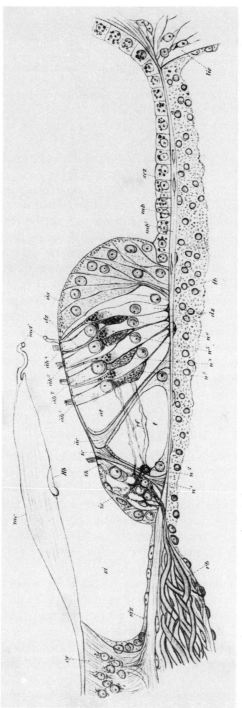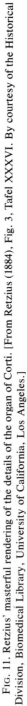

FIG. 11. Retzius' masterful rendering of the details of the organ of Corti. [From Retzius (1884), Fig. 3, Tafel XXXVI. By courtesy of the Historical Division, Biomedical Library, University of California, Los Angeles.]

Helmholtz seized first on Corti's rods as the resonators, then later on the transverse fibers of the basilar membrane, which were graded over its 30 mm extent, varying from about 40 mm at its base to 500 mm at its tip. The presumed mode of action was selective vibrations of the transverse fibers that were transmitted to the hair cells via the rods of Corti. Although Helmholtz dealt with the obvious major issues—the degree of coupling between resonators and the tuning, number, and selectivity, and damping of resonators—as more became known, the limitations imposed by the anatomical and physiological facts became more apparent.

Critics attacked many features of this resonance–place theory, for example, stretched strings in the cochlea was a far-fetched idea; there were not enough resonators; being damped, the resonators should respond to a broad band of frequencies, hence a single pitch should not be heard. "Thereupon appeared Gray's principle of maximum stimulation to give the theory a new significance [Wever, 1949, p. 110]." Gray's principle is that only the relative maximal stimulation on the basilar membrane gives rise to pitch, neighboring stimulation either summating or contrasting with the maximum. In any case, critics had developed alternative theories (often without regard to the complicated dynamics at issue) based on resonance patterns, frequency followed by the whole membrane, standing waves, and traveling waves. Boring (1942) mentions 21 theories in all and Wever (1949) devotes a monograph to comparing their assumptions, operation, and explanatory power.

D. Békésy: Cochlear Dynamics and Fluid Mechanics

Békésy (1960) noted in some informal experiments in 1928 that if the vibration frequency were high enough, any object having internal elasticity would show traveling waves in response to a touch by a tuning fork. He could see no physical reason why the basilar membrane should not have traveling waves when set into motion by an alternating pressure, for the basilar membrane was a gelatinous mass embedded in fluid. Figure 12 is a schematic diagram of the inner ear showing the basilar membrane on which the hair cells are located.

In his clearly formulated program of research, he set out to measure the elasticity and friction of the basilar membrane. First he had to measure and map all the vibration amplitudes and phases for sinusoidal motions of the stapes footplate. Then he had to find the physical constants that were responsible for the patterns. With these values, a mechanical model could be built. If the model showed the right patterns, then one could try a mathematical approach.

By a series of brilliant and aesthetically pleasing experiments, Békésy was able to show that traveling waves did exist along the human basilar membrane and, as Fig. 13 shows, eddies were formed in the surrounding fluid.

To see the vibration patterns, Békésy invented new techniques of mi-

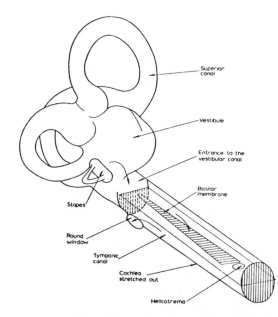

FIG. 12. Schematic drawing of the middle and inner ear. The cochlea is shown uncoiled into a straight tube. The arrows show the displacement of the fluid for an inward movement of the eardrum. [After von Békésy.]

crodissection, stimulation, and recording. At high magnification, using stroboscopic illumination, he observed the vibration pattern. He found (see Fig. 13) that movements of the stapes footplate evoke a wave complex in the basilar membrane, which travels from the stiffer basal part to the more flexible part in the apex of the cochlea. The crest of the largest wave first increases, then quickly decreases. The position of the maximal amplitude was found to be dependent on the frequency of the stimulating sound waves in such a way that the highest crest of the traveling wave appears near the apex of the cochlea for low-frequency tones and near its base for high frequencies (see Fig. 14).

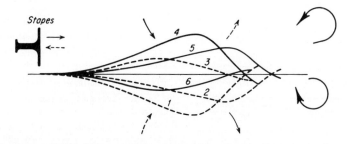

FIG. 13. The relationship of the motion of the stapes to that of the traveling wave. [From *Experiments in Hearing* by G. von Békésy (1960). Copyright 1960 by McGraw-Hill. Used with permission of the McGraw-Hill Book Company.]

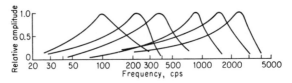

F<small>IG</small>. 14. Plots of the relative amplitude of the basilar membrane response as a function of frequency. [From *Experiments in Hearing* by G. von Békésy (1960). Copyright 1960 by McGraw-Hill. Used with permission of the McGraw-Hill Book Company.]

It was now possible to decide which of the four major rival theories was the correct one (see Fig. 15): *(a)* the resonance theory of Helmholtz, *(b)* the telephone theory, which assumes that the cochlear partition moves up and down as one unit, *(c)* the traveling wave theory, and *(d)* Ewald's standing-wave theory. But Békésy made the decision in a surprising way. It turned out that it was possible to go continuously from one theory to the other merely by changing the numerical value of one parameter, namely, the volume elasticity. Thus, all these apparently contradictory theories belong to one large family. This may be seen in Fig. 16, which shows the different types of deformation produced in a rubber membrane, depending on the thickness and the lateral stress of the membrane.

Between the seventeenth century (Du Verney, 1683) and the middle of the twentieth century, many serious attempts were made to give partial or complete analytical treatments of cochlear dynamics. Among those since Helmholtz's tuned-element theory of 1857, Wever (1949) compares some nine place theorists and six frequency theorists. Following Békésy's work of 1928 and after, some headway was made with mathematical solutions, and Zwislocki (1953) reviewed the mechanical theories of cochlear dynamics at that time, including his own (Zwislocki, 1948). In Chapter 2 of this volume, Schubert covers very recent developments. For a comprehensive review of the physiology and biophysics of cochlear mechanisms, see Dallos (1973).

Békésy also asked how the hair cells are stimulated. With a thin needle,

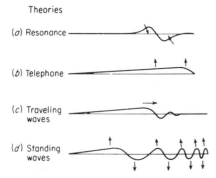

F<small>IG</small>. 15. Showing how the four major, different hearing theories form one family of vibration patterns differing only in the stiffness of the membrane. [From *Experiments in Hearing* by G. von Békésy (1960). Copyright 1960 by McGraw-Hill. Used with permission of the McGraw-Hill Book Company.]

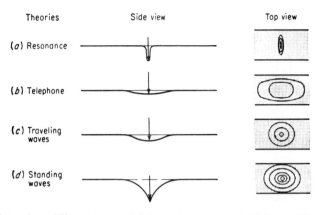

Fig. 16. Shows how different types of deformation are produced in a rubber membrane, according to the thickness and the lateral stress of the membrane. [From *Experiments in Hearing* by G. von Békésy (1960). Copyright 1960 by McGraw-Hill. Used with permission of the McGraw-Hill Book Company.]

the point of which touched the basilar membrane, different parts of the membrane could be set in vibration in various directions. The needle's point worked both as a stimulus and as an electrode for recording the electrical potentials from the receptor cells. It was found that a local pressure on the basilar membrane is transformed into strong shearing forces that act on the hair cells in different degrees (see Fig. 16).

IX. HEARING, PERCEIVING, ANALYZING, AND SYNTHESIZING SPEECH

A. Introduction

Practically nothing is known about the origin of language itself. We do know quite a lot about attempts to describe, understand, and use language as grammar and speech. Vitruvius, writing about the time of Augustus, pays a good deal of attention to the acoustics of the theatre. He devotes a brief chapter to the use of sounding vessels in the theater as acoustical amplifiers and gives details for building and tuning them. A less ingenious use of the principle of resonance is Vitruvius' explanation for the pitch of the human voice. He placed on the circle of the Earth a line rising upward at an angle from the South Pole (Fig. 17). Dropping perpendicular chords from this line made a figure somewhat like a harp or lyre. Since the short chords toward the south were associated with high pitch, he reasoned that the southern peoples should have voices of high pitch. The long chords to the north explained the low pitched voices of the Scandanavians and Germanic peoples. The Greeks lived in the lands under the chords of intermediate length and so had voices of middle pitch.

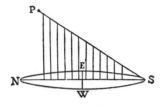

FIG. 17. Vitruvius explains the geographical distribution of fundamental voice pitch in terms of the Greek musical instrument, the *sambuca*.

B. Early Speaking Machines

Long before the mechanisms of the Cartesian corpuscular philosophy, the Greeks, the Arabs, the Indians, and the Chinese pressed into use all the basic mechanical principles they knew for the purpose of amusing persons of rank. Some of the toys they made were elaborate automata and imitated the sounds of birds, animals, musicians, human speech, and singing.

In the seventeenth century the English physicist Robert Hooke attempted the synthesis of musical and vocal sounds with a toothed wheel; Hooke's wheel is often called Savart's wheel. It was an objective frequency standard but never got much use because the tuning fork was invented in 1711.

The first true speaking machine was built about 1780 by the Hungarian Wolfgang Ritter von Kempelen. Prior to his machine, the force of mechanistic philosophy was seen in many speculative accounts of the mechanism of speech. For example, in 1668, the English Bishop John Wilkins in *An Essay Towards a Real Character and a Philosophical Language* gave a surprisingly advanced account of vocal tract dynamics and codified it in an alphabet of physiological symbols. In 1779 the Imperial Academy of St. Petersburg offered its annual prize to whoever could explain and instrument the physiological differences in five vowel sounds, /a/, /e/, /i/, /o/, /u/. Christian Gottlieb Kratzenstein (1782) won the prize with five tubes each in a rough match to the size and shape taken by the vocal tract in uttering one of the sounds (Fig. 18). The /i/ tube was blown directly, the other four were activated by a vibrating, free reed.

Von Kempelen's speaking machine was begun a decade before Kratzen-

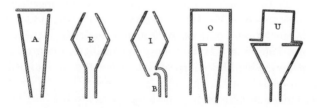

FIG. 18. The schema of Kratzenstein's five vowel synthesizers. [After Dudley and Tarnoczy (1950), from Young's *Natural Philosophy* (1845), with permission of the Acoustical Society of America.]

stein won his prize. Von Kempelen classified vowels by the degree of mouth opening and construction of the oral cavity by the tongue. The vowel /u/ is most closed, /o/, /i/, /e/, respectively, less so to the most open /a/. (This is the diffuse–compact axis of the linguist.) The series /i e a o u/ goes from least to most "tongue channel opening" or "acute to grave," to use linguistic terminology. He varied properties of glottal frequency, tongue position, nasality, teeth, lip position, manner of production, and cavity size. Using von Kempelen's description, Sir Charles Wheatstone built a model of much smaller dimensions than the one originally made by von Kempelen and exhibited it in Dublin at the 1835 meeting of the British Association for the Advancement of Science. In a way much like a modern engineer, von Kempelen conceived of speech production as the imposition of modulations upon a carrier. The carrier was periodic or noisy, a vibrating reed or air passing through a constriction, respectively.

C. Acoustical Analysis and Synthesis of Speech

Wheatstone found that a resonator produces a whole family of resonances, not just one. Then Helmholtz showed that vowels resulted from the excitation of a resonator (for whose behavior he gave a mathematical theory), the vocal cavity, by a periodic source of fixed frequency, the glottal pulse. In order to test his theory of *Klangfarbe* (timbre) Helmholtz used tuning forks to build up tones of different timbre by combining simple tones (Fig. 19). He imitated human vowel sounds because they resembled steady musical tones. The theory assumes that the vocal tract is a resonator in which different overtones will be selectively intensified according to the shape of the resonator. It follows that changing the position of the mouth will give different vowel sounds from the same fundamental; that is, from the note produced by the glottal pulse.

As resonators, Helmholtz used little glass bulbs with two openings, one of which could be inserted into the ear. With these resonators he was able to demonstrate as well as verify the accuracy of his theory of the vowels and to show that difference of phase made no difference to timbre. The formants determined by this method were astonishingly accurate.

There is a parallel history of the acoustical analysis of consonants, beginning about 1870. The activity was considerable, but the results were meager owing largely to the lack of proper equipment. Early Fourier analysis of sounds was hopeful but led to nothing.

The last large-scale study of speech sounds using the most advanced acoustical equipment available was begun in 1913 by the psychologist Stumpf. His book *Die Sprachlaute* was already obsolete when published in 1926, both because of his approach and because Harvey Fletcher published his fundamental *Speech and Hearing* in 1929. Fletcher worked as an engineer, but more important, he used electrical equipment, microphones, amplifiers,

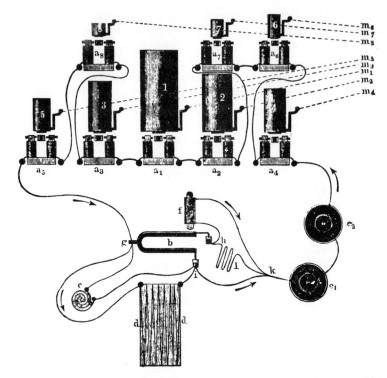

FIG. 19. Helmholtz's apparatus for performing the experiments on the composition of the vowels. Figures 1–8 are the resonators, and below them their tuning forks activated by the electromagnets a_1–a_8. Electromagnet f activates the interrupting fork b which constitutes an electronic switch since the prongs on b dip in and out of mercury baths and control the current of the batteries e_1 and e_2. There is also a parallel shunt—the condenser c and resistance d. [From Helmholtz (1865); English edition, *On the Sensations of Tone*, published by Dover, 1954. Copyright 1954 by Dover Publications, Inc.]

and telephone headsets. The valve amplifier control grid developed by De Forest in 1907 had made possible the modern era of research in speech and hearing. The oscillograph and cathode ray oscilloscope replaced the string galvanometer of Einthoven.

D. Automatic Analysis and Synthesis of Speech

By 1930, devices had been made for the automatic analysis of the frequencies of sound. Coupled with the phonograph, the study of connected speech was possible. The analysis of short segments could be used to calculate the sequence of Fourier spectra and so represent the speech signal according to its frequency components over time. Selective recombining of coded spectra by means of parallel bandpass filters was used in Homer Dudley's (1939) invention of the Vocoder for analysis–synthesis telephony. The spectrum synthesizer part made its debut as the speaking machine Voder at the 1939 World's Fair in New York. Principles established by Dudley's invention set the stage for deeper inquiries into the efficient representation of speech signals (Flanagan & Rabiner, 1973). These principles were embodied in the sound spectrograph (Fig. 20), a device that became commercially available shortly after 1941 when Koenig, Dunn, and Lacy (1946) described its operation and construction according to the method proposed by Potter in 1930 (Potter, Kopp, & Green, 1947).

The sound spectrograph has been the fundamental tool in quantitative studies of speech perception, its three-dimensional representation of frequency, intensity, and time having proved felicitous. Very soon after the development of the sonagraph, there arose the notion of abstracting or cartooning the features of the spectrogram. A device called the "Pattern Playback" (Cooper, Liberman, & Borst, 1951) emits harmonically modulated light beams that are reflected to photocells from different loca-

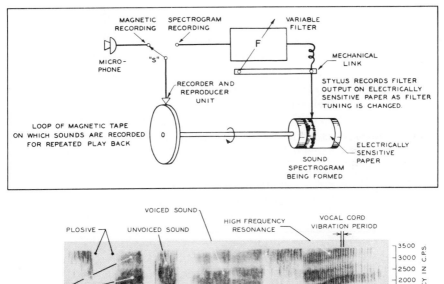

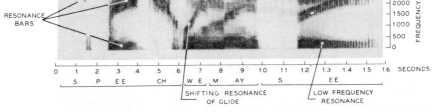

FIG. 20. *Top:* Diagram of the sound spectrograph showing how the analysis of a repeated speech sample is recorded line by line. *Bottom:* Sound spectrogram of the words */speech we may see/*. The wide-band analyzing filter (300 Hz) emphasizes vocal resonances. [From Potter, Kopp, and Green (1947), *Visible Speech.* Copyright 1947 by Van Nostrand. The top is Fig. 4, p. 10, and the bottom is Fig. 6, p. 12.]

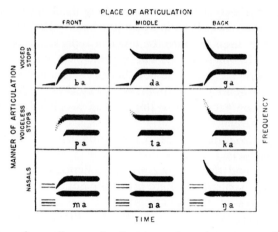

FIG. 21. Patterns of acoustic cues for the stop and nasal consonants. [From Liberman, Ingemann, Lisker, Delattre, and Cooper (1959), with permission of the Acoustical Society of America.]

tions on hand-painted cartoons of sound spectrographic patterns. The varying photocell currents when summed and amplified drive a loudspeaker. Note that this is a Fourier synthesis, since the final waveform is the sum of 50 components each specified by frequency, amplitude, and phase. This method of speech analysis and synthesis was used by the workers at The Haskins Laboratories in their pioneering and fundamental work on the distinctive acoustic cues for speech perception (see Figs. 21 and 22).

A major departure that led to a deeper grasp of the acoustics of speech was based on wave-equation and transmission-line methods, as in the work of Dunn (1950). If the vocal tract is treated as a series of cylindrical sections to represent acoustic lines, transmission-line theory can be used to find the

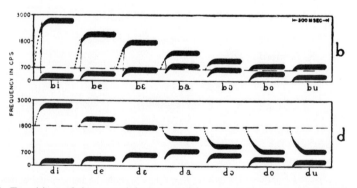

FIG. 22. Transitions of the second formant which are heard as /b/ and /d/ before various vowels. [From Liberman, Ingemann, Lisker, Delattre, and Cooper (1959), with permission of the Acoustical Society of America.]

resonances. On this analogy Dunn based an "Electrical Vocal Tract" that produced acceptable vowels. Stevens, Kasowski, and Fant (1953) used transmission-line theory in their more detailed electrical analogs of the vocal and nasal tracts.

Another approach to speech synthesis models the vocal tract from the glottis to the lips in terms of frequency–transmission properties. Such analogs of speech production are called terminal-analog or formant synthesizers. Vocal-tract transmission properties can be modeled by cascades of resonators with independent control of formant frequency and bandwidth. The basic theoretical work of Fant (1960), Flanagan (1957), and Lawrence (1953) led to the construction of analog synthesizers in many countries.

A very great advance was in controlling synthesizers by digital computer, which avoids the problems of interactive circuits made up of electronic analog elements. In fact, by 1963, a synthesizer was completely simulated in digital hardware and ran in real time (Flanagan, Coker, & Bird, 1963). Swift developments in speech analysis and synthesis came with the rediscovery of the fast Fourier transform and the theory of digital signal processing. It became possible to synthesize connected, contextual speech automatically by means of rules obtained from speech perception work in linguistics, phonetics, and psychology. These developments and parallel ones concerned with computer voice response are traced in the papers collected by Flanagan and Rabiner (1973).

Digital signal theory and digital hardware drove the search for efficient and accurate methods, one of which, predictive coding, has yielded remarkable results. The method of linear prediction models the speech waveform as the output of an all-pole digital predictor which is excited by glottal pulses and pseudorandom noise. Predictor coefficients that vary over time are obtained by solving sets of (linear) equations under constraints to minimize the error between the original and synthesized speech samples. Atal and Hanauer (1971) give the basic theory with applications. Markel and Gray (1976) survey the methods, and their history, of linear prediction of speech.

E. Hearing and Understanding Speech

The most incredible perceptual–motor ability of man is speaking and understanding speech. In a review of research on the speech code, one major finding was that the hoped-for invariance between the acoustic waveform and the phoneme did not exist: ". . . many phonemes are encoded so that a single acoustic cue carries information in parallel about successive phoneme segments. . . . [Also] cues vary greatly with context, and there are, in these cases, no commutable acoustic segments of phonemic size. Phoneme perception therefore requires a special decoder [Liberman, Cooper, Shankweiler, & Studdert-Kennedy, 1967, p. 43]." They propose that decoders for consonants are more complex than those for vowels. The work preceding this conclusion was begun nearly 20 years before at the Haskins Laboratory (Cooper, 1950; Cooper, Delattre, Liberman, Borst, & Gerstman, 1952) using the sonagraph and synthetic speech generated by the Pattern Playback from hand-drawn spectrograms. This enormously influential work identified the acoustic features of those cues that are sufficient and important for the perception of nearly all the segmental phonemes.

As an example, Fig. 21 taken from Liberman, Ingemann, Lisker, Delattre, and Cooper (1959) shows some of the acoustic cues. For the stop and nasal consonants, in any column the sounds have the same *place* of articulation, as signaled by the same second-format transitions (upper bar of a pair); whereas in any row, the *manner* of articulation is the same, as signaled by the same first-format transitions (lower bar of a pair). Figure 22 shows that the second-formant transitions for /b/ (or /d/) before various vowels are strikingly different, yet the /b/ in /bi/ and /ba/ are perceived the same.

Other important cues have been revealed such as the delay of voicing between consonant and vowel, coarticulation, and the relative timing of articulators (jaws, lips, and tongue). The speech motor commands have been found to be more invariant with phonemes than the acoustic signals which, when coupled with the notion of special decoders, naturally led some, as Liberman, Cooper, Harris, and MacNeilage (1962), to the theory that speech is perceived by reference to production. Closely related is K. N. Stevens's (1960) analysis-by-synthesis model of speech perception.

Research in speech perception has grown at an astonishing rate, spurred by computers, digital filtering, and developmental psychology, as well as by the great driving force of communication technology. We cannot survey the current work but merely point to several useful reviews. Darwin, in Volume 7 of this *Handbook* (1976), has reviewed speech perception. Several useful collections of papers are, for acoustic phonetics, Lehiste (1967); for speech synthesis, Flanagan and Rabiner (1973); invaluable are the wide-ranging *Status Reports on Speech* of The Haskins Laboratories (New Haven, Connecticut) and the *Quarterly Progress and Status Report* of the Royal Institute of Technology's Speech Transmission Laboratory (Stockholm, Sweden).

References

Adrian, E. D., Bronk, D. W., & Phillips, G. The nervous origin of the Wever and Bray effect. *Journal of Physiology*, 1931, **73**, 2–3.

Aggazzotti, A. Sul più piccolo intervale di tempo percettibile nei processi psichici, *Archivio de Fisiologia*, 1911, **9**, 523–574.

Aristotle. *De audibilibus*. 811al-b3,803b18-804a8. Translation of T. Loveday and E. S. Forster (Oxford, 1913). In Cohen and Drabkin, pp. 289–290.

Aristotle. *On the soul*. II. 8. Translation of R. D. Hicks. In Cohen and Drabkin, pp. 288–289.

Atal, B. S. & Hanauer, Suzanne L. Speech analysis and synthesis by linear prediction of the speech wave. *Journal of the Acoustical Society of America*, 1971, **50**, 637–655.

Bauhin, Caspar. *Theatrum anatomicum*. Francofurti at Moenum, 1605.

Beauregard, H., & Dupuy, E. Sur la variation électrique (courant d'action) determinée de la nerf acoutique par la son. *Archiv. International Laryngologica, otol.* 1896, **9**, 383–386.

Beck, A. Die Bestimmung der Localisation der Gehirn und Rückermarkfunctionen vermittelst der electrischen Erscheinungen. *Centralblatt für Physiologie*, 1890, 473–476.

Békésy, G. von. A new audiometer. *Acta Oto-Larynologica*, 1947, **35**, 411–422.

Békésy, G. von. *Experiments in hearing.* New York: McGraw-Hill, 1960. (Includes a complete author's bibliography to all of Békésy's own work in German and English, 83 papers in all between 1928 and 1958.)

Biot, J. B. *Annales de Chimie et de Physique*, 1808, **13**, 5ff.

Birkhoff, G. *A source book in classical analysis.* Cambridge: Harvard University Press, 1973.

Boethius (Anicius Manlius Saverinus). Concerning the principles of music. Translation by R. Bruce Lindsay from *De institutione musicae*. Leipzig: G. Friedrich, 1867. Sections 1, 3, 8, 9, 10, 11.

Boring, E. G. Auditory theory with special reference to intensity, volume, and localization. *American Journal of Psychology*, 1926, **37**, 157–158.

Boring, E. G. *History of sensation and perception in experimental psychology.* New York: Appleton-Century Crofts, 1942.

Buijtendijk, F. J. J. On the negative variation of the nervus acusticus caused by sound. *Akad. Wettensch Amsterdam, Proc. Sect. Sci.*, 1910, **13**, 649–652.

Caton, R. The electric currents of the brain. *British Medical Journal*, 1875, **2**, 278.

Chiba, T., & Kajiyama, M. The vowel, its nature and structure. Tokyo: Tokyo–Kaiseikan Publishing Co., 1941.

Chladni, E. F. F. *Die akustik.* Leipzig: Breitkopf & Hartel, 1802.

Clagett, M. *Greek science in antiquity.* New York: Abelard-Schuman, Inc., 1955.

Cohen, M. R., & I. E. Drabkin. *A source book in Greek science.* New York: McGraw-Hill, 1948.

Coiter, Volcher. *De auditus instrumento,* in *Externarum et internarum principalium humani corporis,* partium tabulae, Noribergae, 1573, pp. 88–105. (First appeared separately, 1566.)

Colladon, J.-D. *Souvenirs et mémoires: Autobiographie de J.-Daniel Colladon.* Geneva: Aubert-Schuchardt, 1893. (Exerpt translated by R. Bruce Lindsay, 1974, pp. 195–201.)

Cooper, F. S., Delattre, P. C., Liberman, A. M., Borst, J. M., & Gerstman, L. J. Some experiments on the perception of synthetic speech sounds. *Journal of the Acoustical Society of America*, 1952, **24**, 597–606.

Cooper, F. S., Liberman, A. M., & Borst, J. M. The interconversion of audible and visible patterns as a basis for research in the perception of speech. *Proceedings of the National Academy of Sciences*, 1951, **37**, 318–325.

Corti, Alphonse, Recherches sur l'organe de l'ouïe des mammifères. *Zeits. f. wiss. Zool.*, 1851, **3**, 109–169.

Crowe, S. J., Guild, S. R., & Polvogt, L. M. Observations on the pathology of hightone deafness. *Bulletin of The John Hopkins Hospital*, 1934, **54**, 315–379.

Culler, E. A. Symposium: is there localization in the cochlea for low tones? *Annals of Otology, Rhinology and Laryngology*, 1935, **44**, 807–813.

Curie, P., & Curie, J. *Comptès Rendus*, 1880, **91**, 294ff, 383ff.

Dallos, P. *The auditory periphery.* New York: Academic Press, 1973.

Danilevsky, Y. V. Zur Frage über die elektromotorische Vorgánge im Gehirn als Ausdruck seines Tätigkeitzustandes. *Centralblatt für Physiologie*, 1891, **5**, 1–4.

Darwin, C. Speech Perception, Ch. 6 in Carterette, E. C., & Friedman, M. P., Vol. 7 *(Language and Speech), Handbook of perception.* New York: Academic Press, 1976.

Davis, H. & Saul, L. J. Electrical phenomena of the auditory mechanism. *Transactions of the American Otological Society*, 1932, **22**, 137–145.

Deiters, Otto. Untersuchungen über die Lamina spiralis membranacea, Bonn, 1860.

Dudley, H., Riesz, R. R., & Watkins, S. A. A synthetic speaker. *Journal of the Franklin Institute*, 1939, **227**, 739–764.

Dudley, H., & Tarnoczy, T. H. The speaking machine of Wolfgang von Kempelen. *Journal of the Acoustical Society of America*, 1950, **22**, 151–166.

Dunn, H. K. The calculation of vowel resonances and an electrical vocal tract. *Journal of the Acoustical Society of America*, 1950, **22**, 740–753.

Du Verney, J. G. *Traité de l'organe de l'ouie*. Paris: E. Michallet, 1683. (English translation of 2nd edition, 1748.)

Euler, L. Remarques sur les mémoires précédents de M. Bernoulli. Berlin: Royal Academy, 1753, pp. 1–196.

Euler, L. Dissertatio physica de sono. *Leonhardi opera omnia*. III. Leipzig: Teubner, 1926, Vol. 1, pp. 182–198. Translated from the Latin by R. Bruce Lindsay, 1973.

Eustachius, Bartholomaeus. *Opuscula anatomica*. Venetiis, 1564, 148–164.

Fallopius, Gabriel. *Observationes anatomicae*, ad Petrum Mannam, Venetiis, 1561.

Fant, G. *Acoustic theory of speech production*. s'Gravenhage: Mouton & Co., 1960.

Fechner, G. T. *Elemente der psychophysik*. Leipzig: Breitkopf & Hartel, 1860. (English translation of Vol. I by H. E. Adler, edited by D. H. Howes & E. G. Boring, New York: Holt, Rinehart & Winston, 1966).

Flanagan, J. L. Note on the design of ''terminal-analog'' speech synthesizers, *Journal of the Acoustical Society of America*, 1957, **29**, 306–310.

Flanagan, J. L. *Speech analysis, synthesis, and perception*. New York: Springer Verlag, 1972, 2nd edition.

Flanagan, J. L., Coker, C. H., & Bird, C. M. Digital computer simulation of formantvocoder speech synthesizer. Paper, Audio Engineering Society Meeting, 1963.

Flanagan, J. L., & Rabiner, L. R. (Eds.). *Speech synthesis*. Stroudsburg (Pennsylvania): Dowden, Hutchinson, & Ross, 1973.

Fletcher, H. Physical measurements of audition and their bearing on the theory of hearing. *Journal of the Franklin Institute*, 1923, **196**, 289–326.

Fletcher, H. *Speech and hearing*. New York: Van Nostrand, 1929.

Fletcher, H. Loudness, masking and their relation to the hearing process and the problem of noise measurement. *Journal of the Acoustical Society of America*, 1938, **9**, 275–293. (a)

Fletcher, H. The mechanism of hearing as revealed through experiment on the masking effect of thermal noise. *Proceedings of the National Academy of Sciences*, 1938, **24**, 265–274. (b)

Forbes, A., Miller, R. H., & O'Connor, J. Electric responses to acoustic stimuli in the decerebrate animal. *American Journal of Physiology*, 1927, **80**, 363–380.

Fourier, J. B. J. *La théorie analytique de la chaleur*. Paris: F. Didot, 1822. (The text of the original seminal paper of 1807 has been published for the first time in I. Grattan-Guinness, 1972.)

Galen, Claudius (sic) *Opera omnia*, medicorum Graecorum opera quae exstant, ed. by D. C. G. Kühn, Lipsiae, 1822, II, 837ff; III, 644ff.

Galilei, Galileo. *Dialogues concerning two new sciences*, (1638), translated by H. Crew and A. DeSalvio. Evanston: Northwestern University Press, 1939, pp. 95–108.

Grattan-Guinness, I. *Joseph Fourier 1768–1830*. Cambridge: MIT Press, 1972.

Green, D. M., & Swets, J. A. *Signal detection theory and psychophysics*. New York: Wiley, 1966.

Held, H. Zur Kenntniss der peripheren Gehörleitung, *Archiv. f. Anat. Physiol., Anat. Abt.*, 1897, 350–360.

Helmholtz, H. L. F. von. *Die Lehre von den Tonempfindungen als physiologische Grundlage für die Theorie der Musik*, Braunschweig: Viewig & Son, 1865, (2nd ed.), *On the sensations of tone*, New York: Dover, 1954. (Reprinting of the 2nd English edition, 1885).

Hilliard, J. K. Electroacoustics to 1940. *Journal of the Acoustical Society of America*, 1977, **61**, 267–273.

Hooke, R. A description of helioscopes and some other instruments, 1676. Reprinted in R. T. Gunther, *Early Science in Oxford*. London: Oxford University Press, 1931, Vol. 8, pp. 119–152.

Hornbostel, E. M. von, & Wertheimer, M. Ueber die Warnehmung der Schallrichten, *S B Preussichen Akadamischen Wissenschaften*, 1920, **15**, 388–396.

Jeans, J. H. *Science and music*. Cambridge: Cambridge University Press, 1937.

Kemp, E. H. A critical review of experiments on the problem of stimulation deafness. *Psychological Bulletin*, 1935, **32**, 335–342.

Kempelen, W. de. *La mécanisme de la parole suivi de la description d'une machine parlante*, 1791.

Kirchhoff, G. R. Ueber das Gleichgewicht und die Bewegung einer elastischen Scheibe. *Crelle's Journal*, 1850, **40**, 51ff.

Klemm, O. Über den Einfluss des binauralen Zeitunterscheides auf die Lokalisation, *Archiv fuer (die Gesamte) Psychologie*, 1920, **69**, 117–146.

Koenig, K. R. *Annalen Physik*, 1899, **69**, 626ff, 721ff.

Koenig, W., Dunn, H. K., & Lacy, L. Y. The sound spectrograph. *Journal of the Acoustical Society of America*, 1946, **18**, 19–49.

Koenigsberger, L. *Hermann von Helmholtz*. Oxford: The Clarendon Press, 1906. (Reprinted by Dover Publications, New York, 1965.)

Kratzenstein, Christian Gottlieb. Sur la naissance de la formation des voyelles. *Journale de Physique*, 1782, **21**, 358–380.

Kreidl, A., & Gatscher, S. Ueber die dichotische Zeitschwell. *Pflügers Arch. ges., Archiv fuer die Gesamte Physiologie des Menchen und der Tiere*, 1923, **200**, 366–373.

Lagrange, J. L. Recherche sur la nature et la propagation du son. *Ouevres de Lagrange*. Paris: Gauthier-Villars, 1867, Vol. I, p. 39ff.

Lawrence, W. The synthesis of speech from signals which have a low information rate. In Jackson, W. (Ed.), *Communication theory*. London: Butterworth, 1953, pp. 460–469.

Lehiste, I. (Ed.), *Readings in acoustic phoentics*. Cambridge: MIT Press, 1967.

Liberman, A. M., Cooper, F. S., Harris, K. S., & MacNeilage, P. F. A motor theory of speech perception. *Proceedings of the speech communication seminar*. Stockholm: Royal Institute of Technology, 1962, vol. 2.

Liberman, A. M., Cooper, F. S., Shankweiler, D. P., & Studdert-Kennedy, M. Perception of the speech code. *Psychological Review*, 1967, **74**, 431–461.

Liberman, A. M., Ingemann, F., Lisker, L., Delattre, P. C., & Cooper, F. S. Minimal rules for synthesizing speech. *Journal of the Acoustical Society of America*, 1959, **31**, 1490–1499.

Lindsay, R. Bruce (Ed.). *Acoustics: historical and philosophical development*. Stroudsburg, Pennsylvania: Dowden, Hutchinson and Ross: 1973.

Luft, E. Ueber die Unterscheidsempfindlichkeit für Tonhöhen. *Philosoplische Studien*. (Wundt), 1888, **4**, 511–540.

Mallock, A. Note on the sensibility of the ear to the direction of explosive sound. *Proceedings of the Royal Society* (London) Series A, 1908, **80**, 110–112.

Markel, J. D., & Gray, A. H., Jr. *Linear prediction of speech*. Heidelberg and New York: Springer Verlag, 1976.

Mersenne, M. *Harmonic universelle*. Paris: S. Cramoisy, 1636.

Mersenne, M. *Traitez de la nature des sons et des mouvement de toutes sorte de corps*. Paris: S. Cramoisy, 1636, p. 214, Bk. 3.

Miller, H. B. Acoustical measurements and instruments. *Journal of the Acoustical Society of America*, 1977, **61**, 274–282.

Needham, J. *Science and civilization in China*. (Vol. 4 Physics and physical technology. Part I: Physics.) Cambridge: Cambridge University Press, 1962.

Newton, I. *Mathematical principles of natural philosophy*. Translated by Andrew Motte (1729), New York: D. Adee, 1848, pp. 356–357.

Nuel, J. P. Beitrag zur Kenntniss de Säugethierschnecke, *Archiv. f. mikr. Anat.* 1872, **8**, 200–215.

Ohm, G. S. Ueber die Definition des Tones, nebst daran geknüpfter Theorie der sirene und ähnlicher tonbildener Vorrichtungen. *Annalen der Physik und Chemie*, 1843, **135**, 497–565.

Plomp, R. *Experiments on tone perception*. Soesterberg, Netherlands: Institute for Perception RVO-TNO, 1966.

Plomp, R. *Aspects of tone sensations*. New York: Academic Press, 1976.

Poisson, S. D. Sur l'integration de quelques équations linéaires aux difference partielles. *Mémoires de l'Académie Royale des Sciences de l'Institut de France, Année 1817*, 1820, **3**, 121ff.

Potter, R. K., Kopp, G. A., & Green, H. C. *Visible speech*. New York: Van Nostrand, 1947.

Pythagoreans. See Cohen and Drabkin (1948), p. 298.

Rayleigh (J. W. Strutt, Lord Rayleigh). *Theory of sound*. London: Macmillan, 1877 (2d ed., revised, 1894). Reprinted by Dover, New York.

Reissner, Ernest. (1) *De auris internae formatione*, Dorpat (Livonia), 1851. (2) Zur Kenntniss der Schnecke im Gehörorgan der Säugethiere.

Renz, T., & Wolf, A. Versuche über die unterscheiderung differenter schallstärken, *Archiv für Physiologische Heilkunde*. 1856, **15**, 185–193.

Retzius, G. *Das Gehörorgan der Wirbeltiere*. Vol. II. *Das Gehörorgan der Reptilien, der Vögel und der Säugethiere*. Stockholm: Samson and Wallin, 1884.

Riesz, R. R. Differential intensity sensitivity of the ear for pure tones. *Physical Review*, 1928, **31**, 867–875.

Rutherford, W. A. A new theory of hearing. *Journal of Anatomy and Physiology*. 1886, **21**, 166–168.

Sabine, H. J. Building acoustics in America, 1920–1940. *Journal of the Acoustical Society of America*, 1977, **61**, 255–263.

Sauveur, J. System général des intervales du son. *Mémoires de l'Académie Royale des Sciences*. (France), 1701 (pp. 297–300, 347–354, translated to English by R. Bruce Lindsay, 1973, pp. 88–94).

Savart, F. *Poggendorff's Annalen Physik*, 1830, **20**, 290ff.

Schultze, Max. Ueber die Endigungsweise des Hörnerven im labyrinth. *Arch. f. Anat. Physiol. wiss. Med.*, 1858, 343–381.

Shankland, R. S. Architectural acoustics in America to 1930. *Journal of the Acoustical Society of America*, 1977, **61**, 250–254.

Steinberg, J. C., & Snow, W. B. Physical factors in auditory perspective. *Bell System Technical Journal*, 1934, **13**, 245–258.

Stevens, K. N. Toward a model for speech recognition. *Journal of the Acoustical Society of America*, 1960, **32**, pp. 47–55.

Stevens, K. N., Kasowski, S., & Fant, C. G. M. An electrical analog of the vocal tract. *Journal of the Acoustical Society of America*, 1953, **25**, 734–742.

Stevens, S. S. The measurement of loudness. *Journal of the Acoustical Society of America*, 1955, **27**, 815–829.

Stevens, S. S., & Davis, H. Psychophysiological acoustics: Pitch and loudness. *Journal of the Acoustical Society of America*, 1936, **8**, 1–15.

Stevens, S. S., & Davis, H. *Hearing*. New York: Wiley, 1938.

Stevens, S. S., Davis, H., & Lurie, M. The localization of pitch perception on the basilar membrane. *Journal of General Psychology*, 1935, **13**, 297–315.

Stevens, S. S., & Newman, E. B. The localization of pure tones. *Proceedings of the National Academy of Sciences*, 1934, **20**, 593–596.

Stevens, S. S., & Volkmann, J. The relation of pitch to frequency. *American Journal of Psychology*, 1940, **53**, 329–353.

Stevens, S. S., Volkmann, J., & Newman, E. B. The relation of pitch to frequency. *American Journal of Psychology*, 1937, **8**, 185–190.

Stumpf, C. *Tonpsychologie*. Leipzig: S. Hirzel, 1890.

Stumpf, C. *Die Sprachlaute*. Berlin: Springer Verlag, 1926.

Tartini, G. *Trattato di musica secondo la vera scienza dell'armonia*. Padua: G. Manfré, 1754.

Thompson, S. P. The pseudophone. *Philosophical Magazine*, 1879, **8**, 385–390.

Vance, T. F. Variations in pitch discrimination within the tonal range. *Psychological Monographs*, 1914, **16**, 115–149.

Varolius, Constantius. *Anatomiae sive de resolutione corporis humani*, libri IIII, Francofurti, 1591.

Venturi, J. B. cited in Gulick, W. L. *Hearing: Physiology and psychophysics*. New York: Oxford University Press, 1971.

Vesalius, Andreas. *De humani corporis fabrica*, libri septum, Basileae, 1543.

Vitruvius (Marcus Vitruvius Pollio). *Ten books on architecture, Book VI*. New York: Dover, 1960 (Reprint of the first edition of the English translation by Morris Hicky Morgan, originally published by the Harvard University Press in 1914).

Wallach, H. The role of head movements and vestibular cues in sound localization. *Journal of Experimental Psychology*, 1940, **27**, 339–368.

Weber, E. H. Ueber die Umständ durch welche man geleitet wird manche Empfindungen auf aüssere Objecte zu beziehen. *Berichte Ueber die Verhandlungen der Koeniglichen Saechsischen Gesellschaft der Wissenschaften (Mathematisch-Physische Klasse)*, 1848, **2**, 226–237.

Wegel, R. L. The physical examination of hearing and binaural aids for the deaf. *Proceedings of the National Academy of Sciences*, 1922, **8**, 155–160.

Wegel, R. L., & Lane, C. E. Auditory masking of one pure tone by another and its possible relation to the dynamics of the inner ear. *Physical Review*, 1924, **23**, 266–285.

Wever, E. G. *Theory of hearing*. New York: Wiley, 1949.

Wever, E. G., & Bray, C. W. The nature of the acoustic response; the relation between sound frequency and frequency of impulses in the auditory nerve. *Journal of Experimental Psychology*, 1930, **13**, 373–387.

Wheatstone, C. *Scientific papers of Sir Charles Wheatstone*. London: (for Physical Society of London) Taylor & Francis, 1879.

Wien, M. Ueber die Empfindlichkeit des menschlichen Ohres für Töne verschiedener Höhe. *Archiv fuer die Gesamte Physiologie des Menchen und der Tiere*, 1903, **97**, 1–57.

Wilkins, John (Bishop). An essay towards a real character and a philosophical language, 1668.

Willis, R. On vowel sounds and on reed organ pipes. *Transactions of the Cambridge Philosophical Society*, 1829, **3**, 231–268.

Willis, Thomae. *De anima brutorum*, Londini, 1672, 189–202.

Wilson, H. A., & Myers, C. S. The influence of binaural phase difference in the localization of sound. *British Journal of Psychology*, 1908, 363–385.

Yoshii, U. Experimentelle Untersuchungen ueber die Schadigung des Gehörorgans durch Schalleinwirkung. *Zeitschrift für Ohrenheilkrankheit*, 1909, **58**, 201–251.

Zwislocki, J. Theorie der Schneckenmechanik. *Acta Oto-Laryngologica*, 1948, Suppl. 72.

Zwislocki, J. Review of recent mechanical theories of cochlear dynamics. *Journal of the Acoustical Society of America*, 1953, **25**, 743–751.

Chapter 2

HISTORY OF RESEARCH ON HEARING

EARL D. SCHUBERT

I. INTRODUCTION

As has been repeatedly stated, one is never very safe when attempting any evaluative account of recent events—it is difficult to be a good historian in one's own field in one's own time. On the other hand, in a very defensible sense, the older the events being chronicled, the less the usefulness of the recital from the standpoint of heuristic assessment of the present and accurate foreshadowing of the future in an area of scholarly pursuit. An intrinsic part of the problem is that the topics of interest still are subject to differences of opinion, and any writer is unlikely to be completely objective. In this brief treatise, where I have recognized my own biases on rereading, they have been softened, or at least better disguised. Where unrecognized biases remain, perhaps they will serve to stir up a productive counterstatement.

Certain aspects of research in audition have been treated historically from time to time, either in connection with specific experimental reports or incidental to the expounding of some point of auditory theory. However, the last relatively complete history of the study of audition is contained in Boring's

Sensation and Perception in the History of Experimental Psychology published in 1942—a very useful overview of progress in the understanding of audition up to a few decades ago. The considerably briefer account presented here begins where Boring leaves off and traces a few threads of study and interest that have colored the search for a more complete understanding of the auditory process as a channel of sensory information.

Because the emphasis of this book is on perception, many actively investigated facets of auditory operation, such as its neurophysiology and electrophysiology, have been introduced only as they impinge on that emphasis. On occasion, however, reference is made to works that cover much more adequately at least some aspects not thoroughly treated here. Also, in the interest of some reduction in redundancy, topics that are treated elsewhere within this book itself have been deemphasized to a certain extent in this recital of the history of the area. The topics that have been assigned chapters not only are the important topics in audition, but presumably—since these emphases do not change capriciously—have been areas of study for some time. Thus, it follows that the recital of history as formulated here must be supplemented by the accounts throughout the book to meet any requisites for full coverage.

The study of audition, viewed from the outside, may seem narrow and highly specialized, but the problem confronting researchers in audition has been quite the reverse. They very early discover that the study of audition is necessarily a multidisciplinary affair. Researchers in the field cannot avoid some contact with neurophysiology, since what little we know of the output of the cochlea implies that the system relies heavily on a very complex neural network presumably evolved to process what is, if not the most complex then at least the most difficult, sensory input—a consequence of the fact that the input signal is inherently fleeting and is the most rapidly moving sequence the organism must process in real time. In addition, there is little evidence that in man any great reduction of detail occurs ahead of the neural input; therefore, a similar complication is presented by the interfacing of these complicated signals with the periphery of the neural network. Chapter 4 of the present volume makes it eminently clear that understanding the electrophysiology of the cochlea requires more knowledge than one acquires through a brief sortie into the area.

With regard to the physical signal itself, a wealth of unsolved acoustic problems support the contention that many aspects of acoustics stubbornly refuse to be translated from the realm of art to science: Yet the researcher in audition cannot ignore completely the need for specifying naturally occurring signals as accurately as possible. Fortunately, this challenge has aroused the interest of a large corps of scholars, including psychologists, mechanical and electrical engineers, biologists, and an occasional physicist, along with those audiologists and otologists who are concerned with the problems for sometimes more practical reasons.

It is relevant that, in an inquiry potentially as broad as the search for complete understanding of a channel of sensory information, many factors have combined to determine which problems have been the focus of attack and which appear in retrospect to have been neglected. When examining the course of research work in audition over the past three decades, several such influencing factors should be kept in mind—some of them rather obvious, others more subtle. First is the rapidly increasing availability of electronic aids to signal programming. In the early part of the period to be examined, the devices for production and control of the signals desired in the laboratory were so inferior to the system being studied that, from the vantage point of the present, one marvels that any enduring progress was made. This factor is directly related to another that weighed heavily in determining who chose to work on research in audition. At the time Boring (1942) wrote his assessment of the research in audition, much of the relevant work was being done in the realm of psychology and primarily in academic departments of psychology. Shortly following that, however, and especially just after World War II a number of influences combined to reduce the emphasis on audition in the academic field of psychology. Possibly the main reason for this is that by the end of World War II auditory research had evolved into a highly instrumented and, therefore, rather expensive undertaking. Substantial support for both research and training came primarily from agencies concerned with research to be applied to remedial procedures in hearing, thus shifting some auditory research into the field of clinical audiology—much too strongly applications oriented for the psychological climate of the time.

A second and undoubtedly related reason is that during the period just after the Second World War, a great deal of auditory research was necessarily concerned with physical aspects of the signal and with the physics and physiology of the auditory system rather than being intrinsically involved with its perceptual responses. This was a source of frustration to many psychology students, who resented the need to spend so much time mastering the physics required to understand the signal and the peripheral mechanism before concentrating on the psychologically interesting aspects of research in audition.

There is no certain way to assess accurately the effect of this preoccupation with nonpsychological aspects—certainly most experimental psychologists interested in the study of audition found it difficult or impossible to ignore the physical and physiological aspects—but it may well be that some of the waning of interest in the study of audition inside psychology departments can be attributed to the necessity for concern with such problems. Most psychologists prefer to concentrate on areas related to an organism's *use* of a sense organ rather than with physics and mechanics of the organ per se.

In the introduction to his book, *The Human Senses,* Geldard (1972) depicts the gradual shift away from the study of sensation toward the study of behavior, and the concomitant transformation of a large portion of those researchers in sensation from sensory generalist to sensory specialist. This specialization has closed psychology department doors to some of the researchers in audition—their places now being in various other departments.

Whatever the interacting influences may have been, audition has been emphasized less and less in psychology courses; and in the past few decades, this has had a definite effect on the types of workers in auditory research and therefore on methods and emphases. Recognition of this state of affairs should not obscure the fact that noteworthy contributions to auditory research are still being made by psychologists interested in the auditory channel as a special source of sensory information and as an important area of the study of perception.

As usual, it is risky to suggest cause and effect, but it appears to be true that with the movement of auditory research out of psychology, the *perception* of signals became, to a distressing degree, only a tool for assessing the mechanics of operation of the system, and not the primary object of study by students of audition.

To return briefly to the first point, the plan of this chapter is to describe the course of progress on each of the problems that have been the center of attention of research workers in audition. For any highly specialized field of inquiry, the history of research is primarily a discussion of the unsolved and partially solved problems in the area. Certainly this appears to be a useful way to examine the history of research in audition. No attempt is made to acknowledge the influence or lack of influence of a particular contributor during the period, except as it bears heavily on one of the central problems. It is difficult to find fault with this method of proceeding if one is convinced that work of value is its own sufficient reward, and convinced also that a fortunate state of affairs exists when an area of scientific endeavor emerges from the vulnerable stage where the credibility of a finding is weighted by knowledge of its source.

II. PINNA

Literally the most visible of the auditory components whose function might be of interest to the psychologist are the pinnae. Intriguing from the psychological point of view is the assertion that front–back confusions in localization of sounds are at least partially eliminated by the presence of the pinna. This was apparently first noted by Lord Rayleigh and reported in 1907, and has been confirmed informally innumerable times since. Much more recently, Roffler and Butler (1968) demonstrated that the pinna is involved in the judgment of the height of the source of sound. But the most dramatic claim for the function of this appurtenance is the assertion by D. W. Batteau (1968) that the pinna could actually be the chief element in auditory localization.

Batteau postulated that the pinna acts as a small array of discrete reflecting elements, with the total transit time per reflection depending on the direction of the incident sound. If such were the case, then a number of procedures by which the ear could systematize the relative delays are conceivable—e.g., a correlation of the sound in the ear with a delayed version of itself, involving a mechanical or a neural tapped delay line. Each time the correlation delay corresponds to the delay introduced by a reflecting element of the pinna, a peak in the correlation function is registered. To implement such an operation requires either a buffer memory in which to store the signal while correlating it with delayed versions of itself, or else a pair of delay lines with different propagation velocities, so that the waves in the two delay lines scan past each other with a constantly varying relative delay. Licklider's (1951a) mechanism for temporal processing of pitch phenomena, and Jeffress's (1948) scheme for binaural processing resemble the former; Batteau favored the latter mechanism, suggesting that the cochlea acts as a delay line for a pressure wave, as well as for the cochlear traveling wave.

If the pinna did function as a small number of discrete reflecting elements, the sound just in front of the eardrum, in response to a very short impulse of incident sound, would consist of a series of short pulses, each pulse delayed by an amount related to the position of the element that originated the reflection. This series of pulses would be the impulse response of the pinna, changing systematically with each change of the angle of incidence of the source wave. One of the most interesting claims made by Batteau was that people actually localize more accurately when listening with a replica of their own pinnae on a dummy head than with a smooth (convolutionless) model of their pinnae or with a pair modeled from a different individual.

This was confirmed by Freedman (1968) in a somewhat more systematic investigation than Batteau had attempted. A suitable comparison is achieved only through quite difficult experimentation and as finer points are pursued in the study of auditory processing we may still not have heard the final word on this interesting but admittedly rather obscure point.

III. MIDDLE EAR

One might suppose that the function of the middle ear would have been long ago described very simply, and would therefore have ceased to be a matter of more than passing notice for scholars interested primarily in the auditory system as a sensory input. This is not so however. There still appears to be some question whether the adequacy of the middle ear as an impedance-matching device should be judged on how well it approaches the impedance match needed to transfer energy optimally from an air medium to a water medium. The middle ear is undoubtedly an impedance-matching device. Straightforward theoretical analysis and many empirical mea-

surements have corroborated this during the past few decades. But throughout the period, there has been disagreement about the appropriateness of
insisting that the energy transfer is optimal only if the middle ear compen-
sates for an air-to-water mismatch.

The originally attractive notion was that the auditory system first served
marine organisms, and that, therefore, the middle ear of mammals evolved
to match the impedance of the more recently imposed air medium to the
water surround in which the mechanism first operated. Relevant to the complexity of this point is van Bergeijk's (1964) description of the evolution of
vertebrate hearing, which furnishes persuasive evidence that this particular
evolutionary transition was not a simple conversion of the same mechanism
for a slightly modified function.

Whatever the appropriate view may be of the total evolutionary sequence,
descriptions of the function of the middle ear were plagued with an ambiguity
about which aspect of the fluid response was the adequate physical stimulus
for hearing. If the adequate event in the fluid of the cochlea *were* a compressional wave, the stapes would have to be considered the source of such a
wave, which would spread through the tissue, fluid, and bone relatively
unimpeded since there is little change in density; and it is very difficult to
envision such a pressure wave being attenuated to the extent indicated by
measurements at the locus of the opposite cochlea. In fact, Hallpike and
Scott as early as 1940, when discussing this same problem, pointed out that if
one considers the stapes to be the source of a pressure wave in a homogeneous medium, the distance to the near cochlea would be about 2.8 mm and
that to the far cochlea about 80 mm, making the maximum drop between ears
about 30 dB. Fletcher (1929) appears to have held the question open in his
early work, *Speech and Hearing*, although since he had already estimated the
difference in level between the ears to be 60 dB for monaural stimulation
(Fletcher, 1923) he must have been reluctant to postulate a compressional
wave as the adequate stimulus. But more is said of Fletcher's enigmatic role
shortly.

The problem was exacerbated by the fact that, during the early 1940s,
most psychologists who were students of audition laid their foundation of
auditory knowledge from the excellent and durable treatise by Stevens and
Davis (1938). On this particular point, these authors were unclear. They
suggest, for example, that the large area of the drum compared to the
footplate of the stapes "is an important advantage in passing from air as a
conducting medium to a fluid such as the endolymph [p. 259]." In their
continuing discussion they suggest (very wisely, it seems in retrospect)
"whether this [middle ear] match is exact or not, we do not know for we
have not determined the exact impedance of the inner ear [p. 260]."

It appears, on reexamination, that the problem should have been cleared
up after 1950, since Kostelijk (1950) pointed out in *Theories of Hearing*, in
describing the behavior of the round window,

A liquid, however, enclosed in the very elastic surrounding may be regarded as being practically incompressible with respect to pressure-variations affecting such a system. We may therefore assume that the elasticity of the inner ear system is set up by the compensatory areas and not by the compressibility of the fluid [p. 73].

Paradoxically, in discussing the action of the middle ear in the same treatise, Kostelijk begins with the exposition of the impedance ratio between an air medium and a water medium. Fortunately, he follows this immediately with the statement that "It has not been possible yet to determine the impedance of the inner ear experimentally, but it is probably much less than the impedance of water [p. 136]."

Only a few years after Kostelijk's book appeared, Fletcher (1952) presented an analysis of middle-ear function, based on Békésy's measurements, that indicated how different the transmission function of the middle ear actually is than it would be if the inner-ear impedance were nearly infinite. For those who would like to see a simple resolution of a simple problem it is unfortunate that Licklider's (1953) subsequent statement on the "ideal transformer" view of the middle ear was buried in a footnote. Licklider believed that ". . . Fletcher [here reference is made to Fletcher's 1952 analysis of inner-ear impedance] has demolished the old theory, well recounted only recently by Lawrence, that the drumskin and ossicles constitute an effective impedance matching transformer [p. 90]."

From the experimental psychologist's point of view, perhaps the most convincing demonstration that a compressional wave in the cochlea is not the adequate stimulus for hearing comes from Zwislocki's (1953b) measurement of as much as 90 dB of acoustic isolation between the two ears. These measurements convincingly inveigh against the efficacy of a compressional wave in the cochlea, considering that, as noted earlier, the density of the surrounding tissue and bone is very nearly the same as that of the fluids, and that the distance between the two cochleas is about 80 mm in man.

Furthermore, the relative phase in the farther ear was measured also by Zwislocki (1953b), and the travel time between ears indicates a slowly traveling flexural wave rather than a wave conducted from the stimulated ear by a pressure wave through a relatively homogeneous medium. Any compressional wave transmitted, then, must be even further down than the event that did constitute the adequate stimulus for hearing in the remote ear. This is a very important study, both for the imagination displayed in working out the method of psychoacoustic measurement and for its implication concerning the nature of mechanical transmission in the cochlea.

As hinted earlier, the puzzling performer in this drawn-out drama is Fletcher who starts out with the standard line in his 1929 book, *Speech and Hearing*: "This [middle ear] transformer action permits the sound waves due to speech to pass more readily from the air into the liquid [p. 116]." This sentence is footnoted as follows: "The impedance of the air is 43 and that of

the water is 144,000. The transformer ratio which will transform a maximum amount of power from one medium to the other is the square root of the ratio of impedances, or 58 [p.116].'' But even in 1929, Fletcher immediately followed that sentence with this reassuring insight: "However, the body of liquid in the ear is so small ['and', one might wish to add, 'so readily displaced'] that it probably moves bodily back and forth and is not compressed. Consequently, *the impedance at the oval window may be very different from that offered by the same area in a large body of water* [p. 116, italics added].''*
This is very helpful considering that it was followed some 20 years later by a comparison of transmission into the inner-ear impedance computed from Békésy's measurements contrasted with transmission into an infinite inner-ear impedance. What is puzzling is to find the same sentence and the same footnote in *Speech and Hearing in Communication* in 1953 with the ''impedance'' corrected to ''specific impedance'' and the value given at 41.5 rather than 43 (p. 111). One has to conclude that Fletcher did not really become interested in the problem until the 1952 treatment, and that the sentence in the later (1953) text was actually written before that time.

Wever and Lawrence, in their book *Physiological Acoustics* (1954) and elsewhere, were particularly active in promulgating this view that the adequacy of the middle ear should be judged by how closely it succeeded in matching the impedance of air to the impedance of water. What was never satisfactorily explained during this period of confusion was how it was possible to have a compressional wave in the fluid of the ear and still achieve the nearly 90 dB of isolation between the ears demonstrated by Zwislocki; or why it should be—if the task is to create an acoustical wave in a new medium—that when the round window was successfully blocked, and therefore for a given input pressure the amount of compression increased, hearing *loss* actually increased over most of the frequency range (Lawrence, 1958a; Tonndorf & Tabor, 1962). Indeed, in this regard, it is pertinent to ask why fixation of both windows causes *any* appreciable change in hearing level if the appropriate view is that acoustic energy—presumably in the form of a compressional wave—is being transferred to a new medium of the density of water. Von Gierke clearly expounded this aspect in 1958 with the statement that:

> This impedance of water or tissue is a well-known constant only if we have undisturbed propagation in an almost infinitely large medium. This is practically never the case for sound in tissue, and therefore, the impedances of the middle and inner ear do not so much depend on the acoustical constants of the tissue as they do upon the geometrical shape and the boundaries of the elements involved [p. 350].

---

*In analyzing the function of a moving-coil microphone, one would not likely concern himself with the impedance match between air and copper simply because the bulk of the moving element was composed of that material.

It is difficult to see, then, how transfer of energy from one *medium* to another could have been taken to mean something other than a compressional wave propagated in the new medium.

What rescued this impossible situation for most serious scholars in audition was the work beginning in the late 1950s by Zwislocki, Flanagan, Møller, and others, which indicated that the operation of the middle ear is best described by its transfer function; and one would suppose that, for those for whom transfer functions were not convincing, a description like the 1929 conjecture of Fletcher about bodily movement of the total parcel of fluid would suffice. The appropriate common-sense view would appear to be that the mechanical auditory system functions properly only to the extent that the release mechanism of the round-window route permits bodily movement of a small parcel of the fluid, and *minimizes* the transfer and of an acoustic compressional wave to the entire fluid of the head.

That the old theory was not exorcised however is evidenced by the reappearance of the comparison in a sophisticated authoritative description of the function of the middle ear (Møller, 1972), a rigorous application of the "ideal transformer" principle to the middle ear in Dallos's *The Auditory Periphery* (1973), and the restatement of the principle in what promises to be a fairly widely adopted beginning text in hearing, Gulick's *Hearing* (1971).

Dallos's book, *The Auditory Periphery,* which will undoubtedly be an invaluable reference for some time, is frustratingly unclear on this point. Dallos includes a section on the ideal transformer ratio of the middle ear, expounding very clearly the problem of transferring energy from an air medium to a water medium, and completely unperturbed by the problems just raised. He then goes on to derive from the best available evidence the transfer function, and arrives at the point where the best estimate of "the real cochlear impedance" is about 5600 dyn sec cm^{-3} (p. 113). Then why the "ideal" match would be to an impedance of 144,000 dyn sec cm^{-3} (p. 92 ff.) is indeed difficult to fathom.

Gulick (1971), following the presentation of a simple formula indicating the amount of energy transmitted from one medium to another, proceeds as follows:

> If aerial sound were to act directly upon fluids with properties like those of the internal ear, then 99.9% of the energy would be reflected and hence lost to the internal ear. It is obvious, therefore, that the direct effects of aerial sound upon the inner ear would be negligible. The basic problem is one of obtaining a mechanical advantage so that the energy of an aerial sound can be more effectively communicated to the inner ear. As an *acoustical transformer* the middle ear provides the solution to this problem [p. 33].

A. Middle Ear Muscles

As with the middle ear itself, the muscles might well have been put easily into proper perspective with the help of physiologists and a little physics.

The appeal, however, of an analogy with the iris muscles of the eye heightened the acceptance of an "accommodation theory" of their utility, even though it never was easy to envision such a mechanism acoustically. Beatty (1932) held the opinion that the muscles were very useful in animals but served little or no function in man. Woodworth (1938) clearly stated his opinion that they serve only as a protective device and assured his readers, following Stevens, Davis, and Lurie (1935), that the muscles serve only to act as a sort of protective equalizer that reduces the amplitude of the low tones more than the higher ones. Nevertheless, as recently as 1963 Jepsen lists five theories of middle-ear muscle function, all of which presumably were being seriously considered to one degree or another. In addition to the protection theory, these comprise the accommodation theory, "presupposing that the individual by an effort of the will should be able to select and follow certain sounds [Jepsen, 1963, p. 228]," the fixation theory, which held that the function of the muscles is to maintain the proper articulation of the bony chain over a large range of displacement and velocity amplitudes, a theory that the muscles controlled the labyrinthine pressure to optimize the mechanical performance of the ear, and finally one theory that assigned the muscles a role in the formation of overtones.

Although psychoacoustic measures of the acoustic effect of middle ear muscle contraction have been unpredictably difficult, such measures as we do have indicate that the view of Stevens *et al.* (1935) is essentially correct.

In the latest edition of *Modern Developments in Audiology* (Jerger, 1973)—the Jepsen list of theories appeared in the original version—the chapter on middle ear muscles has given way to a discussion of the usefulness of the muscle action in diagnosing defects in hearing.

IV. THE COCHLEA

Conjecture on the precise function of the cochlea constitutes a most interesting sequence in the study of audition. From the old *air internus* and the *camera acusticae* through the relatively unsophisticated early mechanical and hydraulic models to the frustratingly incomplete electrical and mathematical analogs of modern times, the search for an adequate parallel reveals a slow recognition of the bedeviling complexity of the input transducer to the auditory system. Actually, older drawings are commendably detailed, and many of the names assigned to small structures remind us of the skill of early anatomists. However, the pragmatic inclination of would-be theorists was to ignore specialized structures in an effort to arrive at a general description of the way the device operates. Even from the vantage point of later review this method appears defensible—the problem being that having successfully bypassed troublesome detail for the purposes of the moment, one tends to neglect it permanently rather than temporarily.

Actually it is true that even a simple biological transducer of the demonstrated sensitivity, reliability, and durability of the cochlea might require considerable intricacy just to perform faithfully only the straightforward task required by the old telephone theory; thus it is conceivable that much of the detail that now becomes clearer with better histological techniques and improved microscopes has little direct bearing on the job of mechano-electric transduction, but may have to do with keeping a sensitive biological instrument "in calibration."

Despite gratifying progress along a number of lines that converge on the problem, one of the early sources of argument continues to be a matter of active conjecture today—namely the extent to which the cochlea performs a preliminary analysis of the sound wave rather than simply transforming it to a neural analog. The early history of this protracted speculation is skillfully summarized in Wever's *Theory of Hearing*, published in 1949.

Certainly one of the most interesting of several attempts to settle the argument about whether the cochlea is an analyzer or simply a transducer is the experiment that produced the Wever–Bray phenomenon. Wever and Bray inserted a large (by modern standards) electrode into the eighth nerve of a cat just at its exit from the internal meatus. They led the signal from this electrode out through the wall of the electrically and acoustically isolated chamber containing the cat to an amplifying system in an adjoining room. The outcome of interest to them was the fact that sounds made in the isolated room in the presence of the cat's ear could be recognized through the loudspeaker from the amplified neural signal. It appeared the signal sent to the brain was a reasonable replica of the original sound—not the already coded spectral breakdown predicted by the place theory.

Looking back, one can conjecture that, ironically, the device they set out to analyze actually contributed to misleading them. One of their methods—if not the main one—was to listen from an adjoining room to the transduced output of a gross electrode on the eighth nerve while recognizable sounds were being fed into a cat's ear. Even today there is no instrumentation available that—operating in real time—will enhance the signal-to-noise ratio under noisy conditions as successfully as will the human ear. Any monitoring device other than the ear would in all likelihood have convinced them they had a rather unusable mixture of input waveform and (action potential) noise. In other words, the mixture of cochlear microphonic and action potential they must have been listening to from their pickup electrode on the nerve would have been construed as *mostly noise* by any analyzing device except the listening ear. One supposes it was primarily a recognition of sounds by the ear that encouraged them to believe they were hearing a fairly clear transmission of the original signal and to endorse the "telephone" theory of cochlear function.

It is by now a piece of familiar history that advancement in electronic and electrophysiological techniques has permitted the separation of cochlear microphonic and action potential, opening an entirely new avenue for explication of cochlear function. As a consequence we know a great deal about the process of acoustic-to-mechanical-to-electrical-to-neural transduction; and yet the question of sharpness of frequency resolution in the cochlea remains one of the central questions in auditory theory. Békésy's measurement of the amplitude response envelope of a point on the membrane and his tracing of damped response consistently indicated only a very limited frequency resolution by the membrane itself. Nearly concomitantly, early indications from the work on masking and Fletcher's (1940) further refinement on the frequency segment of the noise that interferes with a tone suggested some increase in resolution early in the analytic process. But Huggins and Licklider (1951) plotted as a function of frequency the bandwidths implied by mechanical resolution and by masking measurements (critical ratio) (see their Fig. 4), and demonstrated that the change in bandwidth with frequency for these two frequency-resolving mechanisms follows quite a different form in the two cases. One would not conclude from the form of the curves that the narrowing of the critical band was simply the continuation of the process begun by the mechanical resolution of the cochlea. Only a short time later in the *Handbook of Experimental Psychology*, Licklider (1951b), possibly influenced by Fletcher's display of the relation between the just noticeable difference in frequency (jnd) and the width of the masking band (1929, Fig. 169), pictured how many other kinds of auditory processing show the earmark of critical band filtering; and the question of how early in the process this narrowing occurs became more crucial. Similarly, the publication in 1957 by Zwicker, Flottorp, and Stevens of a series of experiments extended the variety of auditory contexts in which the critical band appeared; and the fact that such a wide range of auditory processing operations were affected made it seem more probable that this narrowing to approximately the width of one-third octave took place as far peripherally as the cochlea itself. For one reason and another the question of how much frequency resolution does take place in the cochlea has been a topic of spirited discussion, at least sporadically, ever since Helmholtz (Pumphrey & Gold, 1948) and is still a lively one.

In the last few years, new measurements of the cochlea utilizing the Mössbauer effect have been made independently by Johnstone and Boyle (1967) and by Rhode (1970). Some of Rhode's measurements, particularly, indicate a much sharper response than the original Békésy data, and, in some quarters at least, have raised the old question of narrow mechanical frequency resolution in the cochlea (Huxley, 1969; deBoer, 1967; Evans and Wilson, 1971; Kohllöffel, 1972). Each of the methods by which investigators have tried to measure the precise behavior of the cochlea has been beset with uncertainties. It would be gratifying to the psychologist if the definitive measurement could be accomplished psychoacoustically. Of course, deducing the behavior of the cochlea using responses from the output of the entire system, as psychoacoustics is constrained to do, seems on the face of it a method not likely to succeed; but in the hands of skillful investigators it has certainly been useful in validating other methods of measurement. Historically, one line of reasoning appears to be that perhaps the data from all measurements could be combined and the uncertainties resolved if we evaluated the measurements against reasonable analogs of the cochlea.

A. Cochlear Analogs

To a large degree, useful cochlear analogs begin with Békésy's adaptation of his early models to reflect the results of the measurement of cochlear properties that he reported in 1942. Békésy's own previous models and those of others belong to a different class, since there were no systematic measurements of the requisite properties to be modeled. Békésy's use of these models is commendable, in the sense that he attempted, at least to a limited degree, not simply to duplicate the skimpy amount then known of the established behavior of the cochlea with another device, but to use the analog to elicit some further predictions, such as the constancy of behavior of the membrane with large changes in the depth of the channels, and the effect of static pressure changes.

Fletcher's space–time theory of the operation of the cochlea profited greatly from the Békésy measurements. Fletcher first published the theory in 1930 without the benefit of direct measurement of cochlear behavior, but by the time of the publication of *Speech and Hearing in Communication* in 1953, he had incorporated the results of Békésy's observations along with several other measurements, and his calculated curves agreed with the Békésy data quite well. Zwislocki (1950) definitely assigned the impetus for his hydrodynamic theory to the measurements of Békésy.

Tonndorf (1957) essentially followed Békésy in his use of models and in the kind of model employed, seeking parallels with what Békésy's other versions of the cochlea had hinted and also with what was more or less firmly established by psychoacoustic investigations. Békésy (1955), on the other hand, gravitated toward the use of a model with which he could separate the cochlear and subsequent neural functions. He built a mechanical analog fashioned to contact the arm, thereby making use of the nerves of the skin to perform at least some of the functions supposedly normally the province of the auditory nerve.

Flanagan (1960) also used Békésy's measurements, but chose to evolve a more generalized mathematical model and to program it on the computer along with a very usable and very instructive visual display output. Siebert (1962) also took the Békésy data and incorporated them into a mathematical model. This is far from a complete list of the mechanical, electrical, and mathematical models generated during the period. A perusal of those available demonstrates that the Békésy measurements revolutionized the process of cochlear modeling, and that models have become a highly useful tool in our search for an understanding of the cochlea.

A remaining argument carried on during the past two decades, mostly rather dispassionately, centers on the appropriateness of viewing the cochlea as a transmission line as opposed to a continuous array of parallel resonators. The transmission line view postulates the existence of an actual traveling wave propagated by the membrane itself from the stapes to the helicotrema. On the parallel resonator view one gets the appearance of a traveling wave primarily because the gradually changing properties of the parallel resonators dictate that the stapes end simply responds more rapidly and the more distalward points progressively more slowly. At the present stage of development, for psychologists, and except for the importance of phase, the argument is a somewhat academic one. Békésy's phase measurements, as Siebert (1962) has pointed out, require considerable interpretation. However, in any event, they seem irreconcilable with the parallel resonator theory on which a phase difference greater than 2π would be extremely difficult to explain.

V. THE QUESTION OF NONLINEARITY

At times, particularly in audition, there has been some ambiguity about the nature of the sensory psychologist's concern with nonlinearity. Basically, all that need be required of a sensory input is that it be valid and reliable, in the sense that it codes *enough* detail to differentiate between relevant events in the environment, and that upon repetition the same external event elicits the same internal code. Thus, distortion, in the engineering sense, is not inherently evil so long as it does not violate those two simple requirements.* In some discussions of "nonlinear" responses of the ear this principle seems to have been forgotten. However, if one eventually aspires to describe a system completely, particularly if the system is as complex as the auditory system, it becomes necessary to ascertain at each level what form the signal has assumed; thus even forms of distortion that might accurately be claimed to be perceptually irrelevant may still be legitimate items for scrutiny.

Somewhere, of course, the auditory code ceases to be a straightforward analog of the external sound wave. How much of this recoding and possible loss of detail occurs prior to the cochleo–neural interface is a question of major importance.

In the early days of electronic instrumentation, the prevailing view was that the ear rather routinely exceeded its limits of linear operation. Evidence for difference tones, combination tones, and aural harmonics appeared

*If, to take a once-popular topic for an example, one has never heard speech without interband masking, then speech with interband masking effects somehow eliminated would presumably sound distorted to the observer.

throughout the literature. Stevens and Newman (1936) constructed, from this evidence, an operating characteristic for the ear at about the same time that Stuhlman (1937) derived a similar curve for the middle ear. The general view expressed by Stevens and Davis (1938) prevailed for some time subsequently: "Except at low sensation levels, the spectrum in the inner ear is vastly more complex than in the outer ear [p. 199]."

However, as early as 1951, Wever was asserting in the *Annual Review of Psychology* that at least the middle ear, contrary to previous belief, operates essentially linearly. Nevertheless, still stubbornly contributing to the notion that there were significant amounts of nonlinearity present somewhere in the system were the audibility of the fundamental when there should be no energy present at that frequency, the hearing of the difference tone under other circumstances (Tartini tones), and the beating of mistuned ratios (best beat measurements).

Now, regarding the "missing fundamental," Schouten had explained very clearly as early as 1938 that he could reinsert the fundamental frequency in the appropriate phase to cancel out whatever audible energy was present at the fundamental frequency, and that having accomplished this, he could differentiate the sound of the fundamental, as it was made to appear and disappear, from the sound of the "residue" pitch that remained. He pointed out that the apparent pitch of the complex remained the same with the fundamental canceled. It was possible to show, in the process, that the energy of the difference tone, resulting from adjacent harmonics, was rather far down (.5% of the second harmonic), so that actually this evidence for nonlinearity should not have been invoked so cavalierly in the ensuing years.

Schouten had also described in the same article how he could use the technique of cancellation to demonstrate convincingly the rather sizable error made by previous investigators—notably Békésy and Fletcher—in using the method of best beats to estimate the level of aural harmonics. Schouten's measurement showed that the level of the second harmonic decreased very rapidly with a decrease in the sound pressure level (SPL) of the primary, and was almost 30 dB down even when the primary was 100 dB SPL. He gave a most persuasive demonstration that the method of best beats is not suitable for estimating the level of aural harmonics. Yet the auditory literature of the decade following this publication contains a wealth of studies using the method of best beats for precisely this purpose. One is forced to conclude that the article, published in English but in the *Proceedings of the Netherlands Academy of Science*, simply did not come to the attention of most American scholars. None of the protagonists in the heated argument over the use of best beats in the late 1950s cited Schouten's work, and it was not until 1957 that Békésy (p. 500, footnote), reasoning from grounds other than the Schouten demonstration, indicated that he no longer placed any faith in best beats as a measure of aural harmonics.

It is pertinent to this point that for many scholars of audition Fletcher's rather impressive graph (Fig. 90 of *Speech and Hearing;* Figs. 76 & 77 of Stevens and Davis, 1938) of the level at which each of the second to fifth harmonics became audible as a distortion product served to prolong the conviction that harmonic distortion had been objectively measured and was a factor to be reckoned with even at moderate signal levels. The description was repeated and expanded in Fletcher's 1953 publication, apparently without benefit of knowledge of Schouten's experiment.

An otherwise compelling notion regarding nonlinearity pursued by Lawrence (1958b) and some of his coworkers is that a biological device required to operate over a large dynamic range would not show the normal evidence of overload, because its perceptual output is diminished. This rather extensive effort to establish a measure for degree of inner-ear dysfunction and perhaps even a predictor for ears more susceptible to exposure damage than average ran afoul of the same problem, namely that one may be responding to something different from harmonics when he listens for "best beats."

Convincingly successful measurement of the level of several aural harmonics was reported by Kameoka and Kuriyagawa (1966) using essentially vector addition at the same frequency as the suspected harmonic. Their results indicated that at levels of the primary tone of 80–90 dB SPL the second and third aural harmonics are about 20 dB further down than estimated by the best-beat method.

Clack, Erdreich, and Knighton (1972) independently employed a method resembling that of the Japanese workers over a much wider range of primary levels. The Clack *et al.* results indicate that the second harmonic component measured by this method behaves as a quadratic distortion product, and that at moderate signal levels the second harmonic is as much as 35–40 dB down.

If this finding were unchallenged we might conclude that harmonic distortion products show the ear to be operating essentially linearly up to levels of at least 75–80 dB SPL. However, both Nelson and Bilger (1974) and Lamoré (1977) have made similar measurements of the effects of second harmonic components and they do not corroborate the evidence for quadratic growth of the measured second harmonic. Instead, octave masking appears to interfere with the measurement, and the amount of second harmonic distortion is still not well established.

Two remaining pieces of evidence for preneural nonlinearity in the system remain. One of these is the cubic distortion product $2f_1 - f_h$ (where f_h and f_1 are the two primary tones) examined in a thoroughly sophisticated manner by J. L. Goldstein (1967). Goldstein interprets the behavior of the component as level of the primaries changes as evidence of an "essential nonlinearity" in the transfer characteristic of the mechano-electric part of the system. Its precipitous change in level with change in frequency separation of primaries is reminiscent of the low-frequency "skirt" of the mechanical amplitude envelope of the basilar membrane; as though, perhaps, it were being generated at the point of maximum response to the primaries and thus subject to the rapid impedance change of that point for progressively lower frequencies.

Hall (1972) has verified that fact that this distortion product and the difference tone can be within 30 dB or less of the primaries when the primaries are of low frequency and close spacing. However, when the auditory distortion products being measured are of lower frequency than the primaries, it is pertinent that what is reported is the SPL of an externally introduced tone needed to cancel the tone generated in the cochlea. To make an estimate of distortion to be compared with devices measured by other methods the differential loss in the transmission path for the two frequency regions should be taken into account. This is particularly applicable to Hall's reported levels of $f_2 - f_1$.

The other persistent nonlinearity has also been most admirably demonstrated (Deatherage, Bilger, & Eldredge, 1957; Deatherage, Davis, & Eldredge, 1957), particularly since it furnishes one of those enviable examples in which an auditory phenomenon has been explored in parallel with both psychoacoustic and neurophysiological procedures in the same laboratory complex. It appears psychoacoustically as "remote masking" and physiologically as low-frequency energy mirroring the amplitude envelope of a higher-frequency band of noise, with delay appropriate to indicate it is being generated mechanically at the point of maximum. Since its masking effect on other low frequencies can be detected only when the externally introduced energy approximates 70 dB SPL, the most reasonable conjecture is that it is comparable to the product cancelled by Schouten in his 1938 experiment. Otherwise, however, when the readout is psychoacoustic and the measurement has been by cancellation, with the physical controls carefully reported, such estimates as those by Schouten (1938), Clack *et al.* (1972), and Kameoka and Kuriyagawa (1966) support the view that for signals of moderate level the preneural transmission channel of the auditory system is one of acceptably low distortion.

VI. THRESHOLD AND DETECTION

Measurement of the sensitivity of the ear has always claimed a considerable amount of the attention of scholars in the field of hearing. Initially, at least, part of this interest undoubtedly stemmed from astonishment at the extreme limits of sensitivity of the ear in the mid-frequency range. This in turn was undoubtedly somewhat exaggerated through the notion that some sort of basic quantum was involved in the difference between perception of auditory signal versus silence. This latter feeling has fortunately been dispelled by the gradual realization that the neural input to the auditory system is essentially noisy in the sense that all primary auditory neurons exhibit a random firing rate, and, apparently, the existence of an auditory signal is recognized by a change in the pattern of this firing rate. Gradually, even before this characteristic of peripheral nerves had been recognized, the realization was growing that when one measures so-called absolute threshold one is actually only measuring the ability to detect a specified signal in the presence of some sort of ambient or physiological noise—at least this is true over the sensitive portion of the auditory frequency range. The fact of the matter is that much of the measurement of so-called thresholds even early in this period of auditory history was oriented toward verifying the *change* in sensitivity over the frequency range. And, as apparatus became available, part of the reason for preoccupation with the form of the curve had to do with the necessity for recognizing, through audiometric measurement, departures from normal—namely hearing losses. Part had to do also, however, with the recognition that by specifying the frequency response at this minimal level one stood to learn a great deal about how the system functions. Zwislocki's (1965) chapter in the *Handbook of Mathematical Psychology,* Volume 3, draws together much of the rationale contributing to this attempt to use auditory sensitivity data to further our understanding of how the mechanism operates.

It is interesting to note that as much as 25 pages of the now classic text by Stevens and Davis (1938) is occupied with methods and interpretation of the measurement of quiet threshold. It was probably as much as a decade after the publication of that text that the realization had grown nearly to its present strength that so-called absolute thresholds were simply a particular form of masked thresholds, but in 1953 and 1954 events occurred that must be considered a breakthrough in the manner of measurement and in the methods of thinking about detection of signal in noise. They came in the form of the exposition of the theory of signal detection in noise and had several easily enumerable benefits. Actually, in parallel with most such innovations, signal detection was not as radical a departure as some of its proponents were wont to claim. Treisman (1965; Treisman & Watts, 1966), along with several others (Green & McGill, 1970; Lee, 1969; Levitt, 1972), has skillfully detailed some of the resemblances between the new measurement and the old; but on the whole, there is no question but that the theory of signal detection has been of nearly inestimable value to auditory psychophysics in the last two decades. In addition to benefits directly traceable to the model, much good accrued from recasting old problems in a more systematic framework.

Possibly the most widespread of these benefits was the clarity with which the model described the probabilistic nature of detection of a signal in noise. As a side benefit to this it promoted much improvement in methods of measuring detectability of signals. It also rather cleanly separated the level of detection, i.e., the level at which detection occurred, from the influence of the criterion being adopted by the subject for a "signal" response, removing thereby much of the uncomfortable awkwardness about lack of control for, or even awareness of, the subject's criterion and its variability. One of its important emphases has been the insistence on generating detailed stable curves on a single individual rather than running the risk of averaging out some very important characteristics by lumping performance of various subjects. Finally it introduced a great many scholars in audition who had not thought previously about the problem to both the advantages and limitations of formal models.

A description of the theory itself and many of its interfacings with various aspects of audition are contained in an excellent text by Green and Swets (1966). They give a highly readable account of the similarities and differences between classical psychophysics and detection theory.

VII. LOUDNESS

Boring (1942) has already pointed out that formal attempts to formulate a scale of loudness lagged well behind a similar effort on the dimension of pitch, at least partly because it was comparatively late before instrumentation for suitable control of loudness or energy was available. Loudness is an easily identifiable auditory response, and loudness nearly always appears as a separate topic of discussion in texts and in general treatises of audition such as the early *Annual Reviews*. However, except for attempts to relate loudness to masking concepts it does not really intertwine with other aspects of auditory theory, as, for instance, concepts of frequency, spectrum, and time do. Wever, in his 1949 treatise, occupied himself primarily with the desirability of discovering the neural mechanism mediating loudness, which Békésy had suggested must be the perceptual concomitant of the number of impulses—a notion recently systematized by Luce and Green (1972). But in a number of ways, the history of the study of loudness shows that intensity changes are not simply and independently mapped onto a single stable perceptual loudness dimension. The present status of our understanding of this relation is recounted in Chapter 6.

Almost as a separate endeavor—and not solely prompted by psychological considerations—a number of studies were begun in the early 1930s attempting to formulate a scale of loudness primarily through the setting of subjective ratios of loudness with, as already suggested, the newly developed methods of controlling sound pressure levels.

From the beginning, one of Stevens's primary concerns was with proper procedures for scaling the psychological magnitude, loudness. As a consequence this early work on the evolving of a loudness scale is well covered in the 1938 publication of *Hearing: Its Physiology and Psychology,* by Stevens and Davis.

Historically, the concern with the proper form for a psychophysical scale for loudness has contributed to a running exchange of views. And although a form for the loudness scale has been adopted officially for some time, not everyone agrees that it is by any means universally applicable. In the animated exchange, Stevens has played a dominant role. Stevens's burden has been that in the history of scaling prothetic continua, the once-revered Fechner formulation is in error in assuming a constant size for the subjective jnd. It is this assumption of a constant size for the jnd unit that supports the rationale for the logarithmic form of the psychophysical function. Stevens placed great weight on the fact that his scale of loudness took the form of a power law, and that this could be shown to be the most useful model for several sensory prothetic continua. Certainly, Stevens and his followers have been successful both verbally and experimentally in demonstrating the appropriateness of the power function as the form of the scales of sensory magnitude, at least when magnitude implies a prothetic continuum. Support for this form of the scale as well as for validity of the scale in a very broad internal-consistency framework comes from the success of cross-modality matches, which have been demonstrated between vision, audition, strength of hand grip, electric shock and vibration. Stevens is aware, of course, "that validity is not something we can prove or disprove. Depending on how we conceive the problem, each of us may set highest value on a different measure or a different procedure [1959, p. 996]." This does, indeed, seem to be at the heart of the arguments about the loudness scale. But the question of basic interest to a sensory psychologist regarding the scale of loudness is the question whether one *can* formulate a generalizable loudness scale.

Is there a single generalizable loudness function? Stevens appears, at least, to be endorsing an affirmative answer in his insistence that what underlies his loudness scale is a property or behavior of the transducer itself. However, if each set of operations performed points toward a different shape of function, then the loudness response, no matter how intuitively simple it may appear, scarcely promises to yield reliable information about the basic intensity concomitants of the system. Garner's (1958) primary concern was that different forms of the direct methods for estimating loudness do give widely varying results. He has also pointed out, in answer to the objection about context effects in loudness experiments, that what permits context effects to operate strongly is precisely the fact that observers have little confidence in their judgments.

Warren (1958) advanced a more specific argument along the same line, contending that the scale one should expect to find is one that would mirror the effects of correlative sensory experiences with their physical concomitants. This was the burden of Warren's physical correlate theory (Warren, Sersen, & Pores, 1958) which suggests that in the main the loudness scale should be characterized by an exponent of .5 since most of the time we do our listening, and therefore our learning about changes in loudness, in only partially reverberant environments, which roughly obey the inverse square law.

The basic tenet that a psychological scale is defined by, and in general must be taken to be applicable to, only those operations performed to derive it has on occasion been subjugated by the desire to simplify the loudness scale. It is not too difficult to defend the thesis that one should not expect a particularly stable scale of loudness to be demonstrable. By the very nature of its task, the auditory system is most useful if it does not associate a given identifiable signal with a particular fixed loudness. Conversely, it is most adaptable if it learns about signals in everyday use irrespective of their loudnesses, and recognizes a signal no matter how variable its actual loudness or intensity may be from one time or one environment to another. Given that this is the situation in which the system works, it would seem natural that the reaction to loudness differences and loudness changes is very much a function of the listening context, and the probability of one generalizable loudness scale goes down accordingly. In view of this situation it is surprising that loudness scales and methods of computing loudness of complex sounds have enjoyed as much success as they have.

Actually, the physical correlate theory may be a little easier to attack simply because its label may be poorly chosen. On the positive side, it appears related to a rationale ably espoused by Gibson (1966), that one's sensory dimensions do not operate in isolation. In arguing against Warren's physical correlate view of loudness structuring, Stevens insists that its proponents are committing the stimulus error, specifically, in this case, *learning* to make judgments of differences in decibels. Stevens points out that he has asked acoustical engineers to judge apparent ratios of loudness and to estimate how many decibels there are between two stimuli. He suggests that they can *learn* to make judgments corresponding to the decibel scale, and hastens to add that at the same time they can also judge "how the sound really sounds to them." But this characterization only confounds the question further. On a related dimension, Pierce and David (1958) furnished a good example of a potentially different perceptual response to a supposedly similar set of stimuli by plotting on the usual graph portraying the mel scale the presumably learned equal-tempered musical scale. It turns out that the form of the (learned) musical scale is completely different from the form of the mel scale. Which one indicates how the pitch relations really are perceived may be an open question.

It is not easy to parallel the Pierce and David pitch comparison with one for the loudness gradations used in musical performance, using musicians, but Winckel (1967) raised some serious question about the universal application of methods for computing loudness. Winckel (p. 37 ff.) had some first-chair personnel of the Cleveland Symphony Orchestra produce individually a scale progression under instructions to keep the successive tones at equal loudness. Computing the loudness of the individual tones that resulted indicates they succeeded only poorly. Now if one considers that the supreme calibrated instrument for a subjective scale of loudness is the highly trained musician performing on his or her own instrument, it is not the musician's performance but the applicability of the computational procedure that is on trial.

In retrospect, at least Treisman (1964a,b) appears to have furnished oil for the troubled waters in that he did not seem to espouse strongly one side or the other, but has pointed out the inherent restrictions of scales (particularly loudness scales) as models, and the fruitlessness of searching for, or insisting upon, absolutes in the selection of an appropriate scale for loudness.

Although Stevens appears to recognize that everyday operations of loudness by the auditory system may indeed call for different loudness scales, his contention is that the most important of these is the one mirrored by his power function, which portrays something of the inherent characteristic of the sensory transducer.

A. Temporal Integration

Closely related to the concept of loudness, and possibly the source of a clue to the formulation of a loudness percept is the relation of loudness to the duration of very short signals.

Beginning with an experiment reported in 1947 by Garner and Miller, it has gradually become well established that the auditory system behaves as though it integrates the energy of a signal both for increasing minimum audibility of very weak signals and for increasing the loudness of stronger signals of short duration. Garner's original experiment was done partly to demonstrate a parallel with Crozier's statistical theory of visual sensitivity. Later, particularly with the work of Blodgett, Jeffress, and Taylor (1958), which indicated very nearly the same slope for the function relating duration to intensity required for minimally audible signals under different interaural conditions, the question that arose was whether the phenomenon was attributable to energy integration or to increased probability of detection with increasing duration. Using a double pulse with variable spacing, Zwislocki (1960) demonstrated that the integration hypothesis was the more defensible. This, he pointed out, is even more reasonable in view of the similar summing behavior of strong signals (summation of loudness), where the probabilistic consideration does not enter.

In one of its aspects, then, the auditory processor appears to behave like a simple integrator with a time constant around 200 msec. But this is at best a secondary aspect of auditory processing. Considering the much finer temporal grain of the minimal patterns that are preserved by the system (see Section IX) the complex multiple nature of processing has gradually become more apparent, and there is certainly no longer any temptation to refer to this sluggish operation as reflecting *the* time constant of the auditory system.

Occasionally such a simplified view of the system still seems to persist, as when Campbell and Counter (1968) proposed that at those frequencies for which the system integrates energy it could not also preserve pulses for periodicity pitch. In general, over the period described, enchantment with application of the law of parsimony has gradually given way to the recognition of the diversified parallel processing the system must do, and the efficacy of redundancy as an error-reducing attribute.

VIII. MASKING

The auditory system usually operates in an environment with more than one potential signal present, or with interfering noise competing with the signal. The success of the system as a sensory information input, then, is strongly dependent on its capability for resolving components that are simultaneously present. It follows that the degree to which it accomplishes this task and the conditions under which it fails furnish relevant clues for understanding more completely how the system functions.

Early scholars must have realized that the ability of a signal processor to separate signals in the environment is a central measure of its usefulness, but quantitative study of the phenomenon was scarcely feasible before the vacuum tube era. The history of masking, then, properly begins with Wegel and Lane (1924), who incidentally, point out that Mayer's earlier investigation in 1876 was necessarily only qualitative in nature.

Masking as a focus for experimental scrutiny has appeared frequently throughout the period under discussion here. The experimental data have been drawn together and interpreted in Chapter 8 and in two chapters of Tobias's (1972) *Foundations of Modern Auditory Theory*. These descriptions will not be paralleled here. It may suffice to point out briefly the implications of the changing and expanding view of the concept. During the few decades since Wegel and Lane, masking has suffered the usual degradation attributable to our tendency to definitional untidiness. The term was borrowed from visual concepts, and originally meant simply the failure to recognize the presence of one stimulus in the presence of a second one at a level normally adequate to elicit the first perception—a masking of the first by the second. Wegel and Lane (1924) included, on the first page of their fairly extensive report, a concise definition of the phenomenon. "If a minimum audible pressure of one tone is p_1 and the introduction of a second tone changes its minimum detectable value to p_2, the ratio p_2/p_1 is taken as the magnitude of the masking of the first tone by the second . . . [p. 266]." From this original concept, intended to quantify the failure of auditory spectral resolution, the category has grown to include temporal interference at either the same or different points in the spectrum and in either forward or reverse temporal order, along with combinations of this temporal aspect with signals in neighboring locations in the spectrum.

Furthermore, for good and sufficient experimental reasons, the response strategy most frequently employed has been to report only a change in the stimulus without regard to whether anything perceptually *identifiable* is present or absent. There is no certain indication that the distinction was noted in the Wegel and Lane measurements, but as an indication of the miscellaneous nature of the category it is remarkable that throughout the subsequent history of masking experiments seldom is any differentiation made between those instances where a recognizable percept was missing and those where simply *some* change was discernible. It is likely that data taken with the latter response strategy furnish the most stable estimates of the limits of resolution of the system, but the term had become less and less descriptive until an encouraging tendency to sort out the mixture gradually had its influence. It is now much more useful to recognize *operational* differences in detection, recognition, threshold shift, temporal resolution in the forward and backward direction, and spectral resolution; and only as these are being explored separately continue to be alert for the common element(s) that may eventually reliably indicate a common underlying operation. The original term *is* a very accurately descriptive one in clinical audiology, where the straightforward intent in the use of the second signal is to make certain that the perception of the first through an unwanted channel is masked out.

About the time of the publication of the critical-band work of Zwicker, Flottorp, and Stevens (1957) it appeared that a unifying concept was emerging, and for the two decades since then, the critical-band metric has been applied to many measures of signal resolution. It did serve, fortunately, to separate out some of the kinds of operations formerly lumped under the masking label.

An interesting thread running through the history of masking experimentation concerns the suitability of the filter model for explaining spectral resolution capabilities of the auditory system. Fletcher (1940) indirectly suggested the parallel, but actually he only implied the idea of an equivalent flat-topped steep-sided filter, confining his references to *bandwidth of the noise* implied by the ratio of tonal intensity to intensity-per-cycle of the noise which just masked the tone. Schafer, Gales, Shewmaker, and Thompson (1950) specifically proposed the usefulness of the filter model, saying "In this paper the selectivity characteristic of the ear is interpreted in terms of a simple 'filter,' a filter being a familiar device having frequency selective properties which are useful for discriminating signal from noise [p. 491]." Subsequent sporadic arguments about the width of the critical band appeared to be couched in terms that implied a filter-like device in the auditory system, yet the participants were sometimes less cognizant than Schafer *et al.* of the nature of any physiologically realizable filter. It is difficult to envision two engineers arguing for very long about the correct filter width if one of them had measured the half-power bandwidth and the other the effective width. Only for a limited class of filter would the two be equal. Yet this seems to be the nature of the discussion of the *correct* bandwidth of the implied auditory critical band. Fortunately, use of the filter model has now progressed beyond that stage.

IX. TIMING INFORMATION

Even from very early times it must have been intuitively apparent to scholars interested in the process of hearing that the primary form for conveying information about the environment to the hearing sense consists of temporal patterns. This is convincingly demonstrated by the necessity for preserving patterns of speech, rhythmic patterns, and the time sequences of other transient events that come to us in the form of sound. Viewed from the superior vantage point of the present, it is perplexing that it took so long to recognize that time is the primary dimension of audition. Probably, as in so many instances, it was the intensity of the argument over the nature of frequency analysis and the stature of the protagonists that kept this seemingly natural emphasis in the background for so long. What undoubtedly also had its effect is the vast difference between recognizing the role of time in ordering events that are obviously perceptually separate and recognizing its importance in processing what are, to other senses, microintervals of time. Recognition of the importance of timing patterns in audition grew along two seemingly independent but, as we shall see, closely related paths until the latter part of this last decade.

One of these paths leads to the emergence of a tonal percept when there are periodic maxima or similar repetitive epochs in the envelope of a signal waveform. At present, it borders the residue of Schouten, the time separation pitch of Nordmark (1963), Small and McClellan (1963) and others, the sweep pitch of Thurlow and Small (1955), the repetition pitch of Bilsen (1966) and Bassett and Eastmond (1964), and probably the binaural interaction pitch of Cramer and Huggins (1958), and Houtsma and Goldstein (1972).

Historically, Wever (1949) notes that Robert Smith, as early as 1749, reported the possibility that rapid temporal variation in the form of "beat tones" might be the source of additional tone perceptions. The beat-tone theory asserts that the same mechanism that gives rise to the sensation of beats in the presence of slow envelope variations when two tones are only slightly mistuned leads to a tonal sensation when the envelope variations are sufficiently rapid. Plomp (1966) has furnished an interesting account of the early arguments and the early experimentation on the general problem of the perception of combination tones. One can deduce from his report that Helmholtz was faced with a problem like the beat-tone theory as a result of Hällstrom's explanation of the perception of combination tones in 1832. Helmholtz chose, however, to attribute the phenomenon to distortion products, probably because he was convinced that the guiding principle in auditory analysis was Ohm's acoustic law. A number of otherwise troublesome perceptions could be accounted for by accepting the interpretation that certain consecutive partials in the spectrum were contributing to the combination tones, originating in the middle ear, the cochlea, or both, and that therefore physically present additional tones were being created.

A. Periodicity Pitch

But except for the preoccupation with demonstrations of distortion stemming from nonlinearity, the modern beginning for what has now become a vast literature on the auditory phenomenon called *periodicity pitch* probably would have been Fletcher's identification of the so-called "missing fundamental." Work at the Bell Telephone Laboratories prior to 1929 established the fact, probably noted earlier by musicians interested in such phenomena as Tartini tones, that the pitch of complex tones with several harmonic partials did not change when the fundamental, or, in fact, a number of the lower partials, was filtered out.

Fletcher may have faced the same choice as Helmholtz when he became aware that when certain complex sounds with low-frequency fundamentals decayed in level until the lower partials were below the threshold of hearing, the complex sounds still did not change in pitch. Fletcher had the advantage of having filters available, so he was able to recreate the phenomenon artificially and test its generality. In his report in the *Physical Review* in 1924, Fletcher gave a straightforward explanation of the effect by invoking nonlinear (difference tone) distortion. However, by the time he was writing *Speech and Hearing* (1929) he had evidently had second thoughts. In that work he says

It should be pointed out that the time pattern theory of hearing outlined in this book will also account for these experimental results on pitch and at the low intensities may be the main contributing factor. According to the nerve mechanism set forth in this theory the nervous discharge due to an impressed sinusoidal stimulus will always take place at the same phase of vibration, but not at every vibration. Consequently when the four tones having frequencies of 400, 500, 600, and 700 cycles per second act upon the ear, the impulses in the auditory nerve will be timed somewhat as follows. There will be certain fibres excited by the 400-cycle tone firing every 5th vibration, certain ones excited by the 600-cycle tone which will be firing every 6th vibration and certain ones from the 700-cycle tone which will be firing every 7th vibration. These discharges will all unite to form impulses in the auditory nerve having a time interval of .01 second. Similarly a number of combinations will unite to give an impulse at 1/2, 1/3, 1/4, 1/5, 1/6, and 1/7 of this interval. There will be discharges at other time intervals, but the number of fibres causing them will be considerably less than at the particular ones given above. It may be that the recognition of these time intervals by the brain aids in the recognition of pitch [pp. 253–254].

Stevens and Davis (1938)—definitely place theorists at the time of publication of their classic text—in reporting Fletcher's work briefly, make the rather uninterpretable statement that "Since the harmonics present in the note differ by a constant amount, namely, an amount equal to the frequency of the fundamental, the harmonics alone are sufficient to determine the pitch of the note [p. 99]."

One should not suppose that during this period early in the twentieth century frequency theories were completely out of favor. Boring's (1926) assessment went "I think that the case for a frequency theory is no weaker than the case for a resonance theory . . . [p. 177]," and Boring claimed at least partial credit for the fact that shortly thereafter Wever and Bray undertook what was certainly intended to be the critical experiment to settle the question (see Boring, 1942, p. 495).

However, it turns out that the definitive early work on periodicity pitch is the work of Schouten, discussed earlier in connection with auditory nonlinearity. Schouten succeeded in demonstrating that when he had introduced sufficient energy at the fundamental in the appropriate phase to cancel the comparatively small amount that was physically present, he no longer perceived a beat when he introduced a sinusoid tuned a few cycles away from the fundamental; yet he could hear a more sharply audible pitch whose audibility, if anything, appeared to increase when the energy of the fundamental frequency was canceled, and whose pitch appeared to him to be that of the fundamental. Still it was to be another 10 years before the complete ascendency of the place theory was challenged by serious presentations of a time basis for pitch by both Wever and Licklider. Davis, Silverman, and McAuliffe (1951), in their report of perception of a pitch definitely attributable to the rate at which they pulsed a filter rather than to the center frequency of the filter, *did* make at least a passing reference to the 1940 publication of Schouten in which he described the "residue." Davis *et al.* explained "We therefore do not regard pitch as a single attribute, but as a composite of 'buzz' (the correlate of physiological frequency) and 'body' (the correlate of physiological place or channel [p. 42]." And even at that point, there were mixed opinions about the propriety of entertaining the possibility of both mechanisms. Miller and Taylor's (1948) study on perception of repeated bursts of noise included matching the pitch of the recurrent noise bursts to that of a pure tone and a square wave. Newman, in discussing the outcome in the 1950 *Annual Review of Psychology* was apparently willing to extend the implication beyond interrupted noise, since he remarked that "The results lend support to the view that periodicity of response underlies the discrimination of tones with frequencies below 250 cycles [p. 57]." However, Garner, 2 years later, noting that duplex theories of pitch perception had been proposed by both Wever and Licklider, questioned the wisdom of such a move. He insisted there was no evidence that required it, and that postulating such a theory in addition to place violated the law of parsimony.

Schouten had left at least one puzzling demonstration unresolved. Why is the pitch of a complex of tones at 300, 500, 700, and 900 Hz the same as a 100

Hz tone rather than a 200 Hz tone? Ignoring some interesting but perceptually weak effects called the *first and second effects of pitch shift*, the pitch predicted by the "residue" hypothesis for such combinations of partials corresponds to the periods between envelope maxima, which in this instance would yield a pitch corresponding to 200 Hz rather than 100 Hz. Perhaps the answer is in the experiments of Flanagan and Guttman (1960), who demonstrated that with wide pulse spacing pitch may be assigned according to the period between pulses (irrespective of polarity) rather than repetition period of the waveform. Schouten's waveform, in fact, bears some resemblance to one of the Flanagan and Guttman waveforms, since removing the fundamental from a square wave moves the waveshape toward pulses of alternating polarity.

A separate line of evidence that timing intervals are preserved in auditory coding and can lead to a sensation other than pitch comes from the history of research in binaural hearing. As early as 1907, Lord Rayleigh reported the existence of a moving image when he listened to tones of slightly different frequencies in the two ears. Here is a clear instance of a timing pattern generating a percept not intuitively related to the time pattern, but rather to the perception of the position of the apparent source.

Later, with better control of the signal, it became clear that if the frequency difference between ears is increased, the perceived movement ceases, and binaural beating is heard instead. Wever (1949) traced the early reports of binaural beating and recounted the few experiments that were done, culminating at that point in the fact that two of his students (Loesch and Kapell) reported that, with enough practice, their subjects could follow the rotating image even when the periods of the tones involved were well under a millisecond. But the effort to utilize this rather straightforward binaural proof of the preservation of small time intervals in the neural code is best embodied in the systematic study by Licklider, Webster, and Hedlun (1950) shortly after the appearance of Wever's book. These investigators ascertained, more precisely than anyone previously, the upper frequency limit for which they could discern rapid interaural phase changes. They definitely considered the utility of their results to be in the demonstration of a possible limiting case in the preservation of timing information in neural coding. Their upper limit of about 1500 Hz is also roughly the same limit marked by the failure of the binaural system to benefit from the interaural differences between signal and noise waveforms. Another salient feature of such studies is the indication of a percept other than pitch attributable to the presence of a small time interval preserved in the neural code.

But prior to the Licklider *et al.* study, Miller and Taylor (1948) had separated, at least incompletely, the pitch response from other responses to their interrupted noise. On either side of the interruption rates for which pitch matches could be made were the lower and upper limits of the perception of intermittency.* Most closely related to the *upper* limit of the preservation of timing information is the report that their subjects found it possible to hear the difference between steady and interrupted noise until the interruption rate was as high as 2000 per second. A later study by Pollack (1969) is in at least rough agreement on this point, and G. G. Harris (1963) reports one subject who could make matches to interruption rates as high as 2000 per second.

At roughly the time of the Licklider *et al.* study, Klumpp and Eady (1956) were exploring, for a wider variety of signals, the limits of microtime-interval preservation by the binaural system. Their results, indicating the ability of the binaural system to respond to differences of the order of tens of microseconds, captured the imagination of a number of laboratories, and there were at least informal reports of the ability of individual observers to detect minimal lateralization of signals with interaural separations no greater than a few microseconds.

This form of temporal resolution should not be confused with maximum information rate for the auditory channel. Attempts at direct experimentation on this dimension have been impossible to interpret, and acceptable analytical estimates must await more complete models of the processing system. Liberman, Cooper, Shankweiler, and Studdert-Kennedy (1967) make the statement that

> Thirty sounds per second [phonemes] would overreach the temporal resolving power of the ear; discrete acoustic events at that rate would merge into an unanalyzable buzz; a listener might be able to tell from the pitch of the buzz how fast the speaker was talking, but he could hardly perceive what had been said [p. 432].

In support of the statement, Liberman *et al.* cite only the Miller and Taylor (1948) study on perception of repeated bursts in noise, so it is impossible to deduce what they consider to be the experimental antecedents of the statement.

Unfortunately, even at this time, the prevailing view of functional temporal auditory resolution is embodied in the oft-cited Hirsh (1959) study on temporal order. Some very enlightening relevant work by Patterson and Green (1970) is hidden in an appendix. The work has been independently corroborated and extended by Efron (1973).

Now we have a comparative (hard-earned) wealth of studies indicating the

---

*A number of investigators have been persuaded, as was Garner in 1952 (p. 101), that all judgments of changes in interruption rate of broad-band noise should be labeled judgments of intermittency rather than pitch. One part of the argument runs that there is nothing of the aura of musical pitch about these pitch judgments of interrupted noise. The demonstration by Burns and Viemeister (1976) that melodies generated by the proper sequence of interruption rates of broad-band noise can be recognized by observers, even when the interruption waveform is sinusoidal rather than abrupt, effectively nullifies that argument.

versatility of the auditory system in utilizing small time intervals, capped, even before the present volume, by a review of time-resolution capabilities in audition (Green, 1971).

X. BINAURAL PHENOMENA

Interest in the advantages of having two ears rather than one has a long history. It is natural that the location of sound sources should be the earliest object of investigation on this point. But anything resembling a study of the limits of what a number of authors have referred to as the exquisite time sensitivity of the two-eared system necessarily awaited the development of electronic timing controls. This work has been thoroughly covered in Chapters 10 and 11 and was also systematically described in A. W. Mills's (1972) chapter in *Foundations of Modern Auditory Theory*. A more recent line of inquiry deals with the possibility of using the two inputs in a competing fashion to deduce something about the processing of different complex signals in the two hemispheres of the brain. This aspect moves so quickly into areas of speech perception and processing that it will not be pursued here.

A third line of activity having to do with the function of the two ears is also methodically chronicled in Chapters 10 and 11 and is also drawn together in Tobias's (1972) *Foundations* collection, but its history is such that each observer's account emphasizes a different aspect and each may contribute to our complete comprehension of the phenomenon. This is the phenomenon of enhanced signal selection by the binaural system usually measured as a masking level difference between one- and two-eared listening.

Following a long history of interest in auditory localization, there was a sudden surge of interest in this other possible consequence of having two spaced auditory inputs. Hirsh (1948) measured binaural summation (and interaural inhibition), Licklider (1948) demonstrated an intelligibility gain for speech signals of opposite polarity in the two ears, and Koenig (1950) was struck by the subjectively different impression created by listening in a natural environment with one ear rather than two. Most of the studies of binaural enhancement of the speech signal explore the principles suggested by Licklider and Koenig. The small difference demonstrable for speech compared to its dramatic subjective impression, commonly dubbed *the cocktail party effect,* has been a source of consternation. At least a partial key is given by the work of Levitt and Rabiner (1967) who measured considerably greater binaural release from masking when *detection* of the speech is compared monaurally and binaurally than when *gain in intelligibility* is the criterion. Furthermore, the greatest *contrast* in the two measures occurred under the most generalizable listening condition, i.e., delay between the two ears rather than polarity reversal.

A brief analysis indicates, however, that it is really quite difficult to compare the tonal situation with speech. Even for a signal much simpler than speech, unexplained contrasts occur when the binaural system is operating. Stevens and Sobel (1937) reported that during listening to binaural beats the signal was louder when the signals were in phase; however, Egan (1965b) suggests an effective way to listen to the difference in the same two conditions (N_0S_0 and N_0S_π) using tones that differ slightly in frequency. It is well established in this paradigm that the tone is most audible during the antiphasic portion. Somewhere slightly above "threshold" there must be an interesting transition region. By implication, this simple demonstration ought to serve notice that release from masking for a multilevel signal like speech is not easily equated to tonal release.

In addition to demonstrating the same sort of binaural listening advantage, one of the most interesting things about the Hirsh (1948) work on summation for tones was the rather strange outcome when the tone was in only one ear and the noise in both. It led Hirsh to believe that under some conditions the binaural system actually partially inhibited the tonal signal the subject was listening for. It was a time of heightened awareness of the concept of inhibition in psychology, thus it seemed an attractive kind of explanation because it seems to exemplify a principle frequently encountered in sensory systems. Further than that, Hirsh thought he had experimental evidence for lessened audibility of the desired signal, and the short saga of that kind of interaural inhibition is of intrinsic historical interest. As he pointed out:

> The existence of interaural inhibition can be demonstrated very simply. With a fairly high level of noise in both earphones, a listener may set the level of low-frequency tone in one ear so that it is clearly audible but near threshold. Then when he brings the intensity of the tone in the other earphone up to the same level, the perception of tone disappears. Both intensities must be raised 5–8 dB above the monaural threshold in order for the tone to be heard binaurally [p. 210].

It was not until 1956 that a clear explanation emerged of this apparent binaural contretemps. Jeffress, Blodgett, Sandel, and Wood (1956) compared the whole repertoire of interaural tone-and-noise conditions necessary for demonstrating that the binaural system did not behave in this nonadaptive fashion.

In tracing the history of interaural signal inhibition, it is instructive to place the Jeffress *et al.* demonstration in juxtaposition with the Hirsh one: Following their statement that "all binaural stimulus conditions produce 'summation' . . . there is no binaural inhibition," they proceed as follows.

> This fact can be illustrated by the following demonstration. We start with both signal and noise presented to one earphone, say the left, and adjust the level of the signal which is occurring periodically, until it is a few decibels below threshold and we can no longer hear it. This is the monaural condition. Now as we bring the noise up in the right earphone we find that the signal becomes clearly audible. When the noise levels in the

two phones are equal we have Hirsh's "monaural" condition. Now we add the signal
gradually to the noise in the right earphone. By the time the level has reached that in
the left phone the signal has again become inaudible, and we have the homophasic
binaural condition [p. 417].

Had Hirsh begun with the noise in one phone, this form of binaural inhibition
might never have appeared.

Thus Jeffress *et al*. (1956) performed a real service in clearing up a troublesome point in the operation of the binaural signal selection mechanism.
However, both statements just quoted should be taken only in the context in
which they were made.

Although Hirsh was mistaken in the form taken by interaural inhibition he
was not as far wrong as correcting the detail made it seem. It is readily
apparent, though not easily quantifiable, that if one listens in the presence of
two sounds, either of which might, under given circumstances, be the signal
and the other the interfering noise, either of them can be made perceptually
stronger than the other more or less at will. To a degree this must also be true
of a signal in the interfering noise, and the process by which it is accomplished must in turn be some form of inhibition of the unwanted signal.
The fact that with certain waveform differences between ears this can be
accomplished binaurally to a greater degree than monaurally still leaves open
the possibility that what is being accomplished is inhibition of the interference rather than some form of direct enhancement of a wanted signal. The
superiority of N_0S_π over $N_\pi S_0$ may mean just that, since in either case the
periodicity of the signal is the same but the detail of the noise that effectively
interferes is different in the former case than the latter.

The other statement that all binaural conditions produce summation would
probably today read "all interaurally different conditions," and the possible
confusion has been largely dispelled by the same group from which the
statement emanated. Two aspects that deal with the relation of binaural to
monaural hearing are involved. The difference between monaural and
binaural threshold, i.e., under monotic and diotic signal conditions, has
concerned a number of investigators and until recently has been difficult to
interpret. Two studies dispel a great deal of the uncertainty. Egan (1965a)
performed some very careful measurements indicating that when the interfering noise is actually the same in the two ears, there is no difference in the
level of the noise required to keep a tone at the 80% detection level in the
N_mS_m and N_0S_0 conditions. This finding, combined with a brief but valuable
paper by Diercks and Jeffress (1962), clears up a great deal about the nature
of the measurement of detectability thresholds when ambient or physiological noises influence the measurement. In addition, Weston and Miller (1965)
show how persistently noise in the untested ear influences the measurement
of monaural thresholds. Unfortunately, this set of papers has not been
brought to the attention of many practicing audiologists.

This operation of the binaural system for signal enhancement, masking level difference, release from masking or whatever label is most appropriate has been the subject of lively activity for the last 15 years. Since the last three chapters of the *Foundations of Modern Auditory Theory*, Vol. II, are concerned with describing and interpreting this experimentation it will not be further treated here.

XI. AUDITORY THEORY

Over 15 years ago, Licklider (1959) began his exposition of what he called several "part theories" of hearing by asserting that "There is no systematic over-all theory of hearing [p. 42]." This state of affairs has not changed during the ensuing nearly two decades of fairly vigorous research activity. Consequently, it is difficult to say whether auditory theory has progressed, in the sense usually intended, during that time. Probably the reason the Licklider statement is still an accurate appraisal is that, to a greater degree than in 1959 when the statement was made, evidence continues to accumulate about how much must be subsumed under a complete theory of hearing.

With the exception of the Licklider work, most of the offerings that have used the title are attempts to explain the operation of the cochlea. This includes most of the theories listed in Wever's (1949) *Theory of Hearing;* and the book itself, despite its title, was not the promulgation of any encompassing theory of hearing. Kostelijk's (1950) book *Theories of Hearing* also made no pretense at covering events beyond the mechanical operation of the cochlea.

In 1956 a useful analysis of the "Current Theories of Hearing" was offered by Békésy. It was primarily a comparison of views of cochlear operation, and Békésy explained that the reason was that

> Theories of hearing are usually concerned only with answering the question, "How does the ear discriminate pitch?" Since we must know how the vibrations produced by a sound cue are distributed along the length of the basilar membrane before we can understand how pitch is discriminated, theories of hearing are basically theories concerning the vibration pattern of the basilar membrane and the sensory organs attached to it [p. 779].

There are some exceptions. A few scholars have ventured beyond the description of cochlear function. Fletcher's (1953) version of his space–time theory of hearing went beyond the cochlea in suggesting laws for describing the neural substrate of loudness and masking, but certainly the most firmly grounded aspect of his theory involves the cochlea. Wever's volley theory as stated in the final pages of *Physiological Acoustics* is actually an excellent general statement of one overall working principle of the auditory system. A provocative title, "Theory of Audio Information," identifies an article by

T. S. Korn (1969) that suggests a possible systems-analysis approach to a
principle of auditory processing, using "elementary messages of discrete
frequency" as the unit, but the author proposes to base his analysis on
dynamic masking behavior of the ear; and he asserts that the appropriate
masking data have not yet been gathered. Highly useful suggestions regarding the principles on which the system might be modeled are contained in
Siebert's (1968) article "Stimulus Transformations in the Peripheral Auditory System."

A most refreshing example of a perceptually oriented rule is found in some
work of W. H. Huggins. Huggins's (1953) discourse on "A Theory of Hearing" is mostly concerned with the method of frequency resolution in the
system, but he also presents one of the few unifying principles advanced
over these decades for the perception of meaningful sounds. His thesis is
that the system encodes the characteristic (resonant) frequencies and the
characteristic damping rates of the sound sources to which it responds.
Earlier, Huggins (1950) described the system-function principle specifically
for speech sounds and concluded by pointing out that:

> In effect, *the speaker's mouth is part of the listener's ear.* . . . From an operational
> point of view, it seems altogether possible that the "gestures" of the speaker's mouth
> are reconstructed within the ear and auditory pathways of the listerner's brain far more
> effectively than by the visual reading or tactile feeling of the speaker's lip motion by
> the deaf and blind listener [italics in original; p. 767].

Of Licklider's part theories, the most often cited is the theory of pitch
perception. It is probably quite correct to say that since the time Licklider
wrote, what has increased has been the realization that such restricted models promise, in general, to be more useful than a complete hearing theory.
This is an attitude apparently endorsed by Flanagan (1972) in raising the
question of the advisability of straining for an all-encompassing theory. Pon-
dering the status of hearing theory in the light of the history of auditory
research in the last two decades reveals that to a great extent it has been,
among other things, a period of learning the advisability of differentiating
between purely descriptive modeling and heuristic modeling, between
theories that simply organize or systematize and those that also generate
testable predictions. Even during recent years, the history of auditory research is so predominantly the story of a piecemeal search for observable
relations that we may not for some time even recognize the proper role of
theory in auditory perception.

At least during the 1960s and early 1970s we seem to have progressed into
a period of dynamic analysis of the system by the method of fabrication of a
specialized set of signals particularly generated to explore some specific
principle of operation. The genesis of this method is at least partly attributable to the advent of computerized signals, partly from increased identification of the important physical parameters of the signals available, and further

probably from a realization that analysis of the dynamic operation of the cochlea will not be possible by direct means even with further improvement of such viewing devices as the phase-contrast microscope. The method brings, however, a new frustration, namely the uncertainty about what transpires between the input and the eventual response, this frustration being heightened by the general dearth of quantifiable auditory responses. Eventually one may be able to explore atomistically a great deal of the area of audition using nothing but yes–no or same–different responses, but it seems more likely that without substantially increasing the response repertoire many areas of interest to scholars in psychology will simply remain unexplored. As a progressively greater number of the physical and neurophysiological concomitants of the perceptually discriminable events are identified and mapped, the complexity of the total analyzer becomes a little more awesome. No simple model should be expected to account for the total of auditory processing.

References

Bassett, I. G., & Eastmond, E. J. Measurement of pitch versus distance for sounds reflected from a flat surface. *Journal of the Acoustical Society of America,* 1964, **36,** 911–916.

Batteau, D. W. Role of the pinna in localization: theoretical and physiological consequences. In A. de Ruech & J. Knight (Eds.), *Hearing mechanisms in vertebrates.* Boston: Little, Brown, 1968.

Beatty, R. T. *Hearing in man and animals.* London: Bell, 1932.

Békésy, G. von. Über die Schwingungen den Schnickentrennwand beim Präparat und Ohrenmodell. *Akust. Zeits.,* 1942, 7, 173–186. [Published in English in *Jornal of the Acousitcal Society of America,* 1949, **21,** 233–245.]

Békésy, G. von. Current status of theories of hearing. *Science,* 1956, **123,** 799–783.

Békésy, G. von. Sensations on the skin similar to directional hearing, beats, and harmonics of the ear. *Journal of the Acoustical Society of America,* 1957, **29,** 489–501.

Bilsen, F. A. Repetition pitch: Monaural interaction of a sound with the same, but phase shifted sound. *Acustica,* 1966, **17,** 295–300.

Blodgett, H. C., Jeffress, L. A., & Taylor, R. W. Relation of masked threshold to signal-duration for various interaural phase-combinations. *American Journal of Psychology,* 1958, **71,** 382–290.

Boring, E. G. Auditory theory with special reference to intensity, volume and localization. *American Journal of Psychology,* 1926, 37, 157–188.

Boring, E. G. *Sensation and perception in the history of experimental psychology.* New York: Appleton, 1942.

Burns, E. F., & Viemeister, N. F. Nonspectral pitch. *Journal of the Acoustical Society of America,* 1976, **60,** 863–869.

Campbell, R. A., & Counter, S. A. Temporal integration and periodicity pitch. *Joournal of the Acoustical Society of America,* 1968, **45,** 691–693.

Clack, T. D., Erdreich, J., & Knighton, R. W. Aural harmonics: the monaural phase effects at 1500 Hz, 2000 Hz, and 2500 Hz observed in tone-on-tone masking when $f_1 = 1000$ Hz. *Journal of the Acoustical Society of America,* 1972, **52,** 536–541.

Cramer, E. M., & Huggins, W. H. Creation of pitch through binaural interaction. *Journal of the Acoustical Society of America,* 1958, **30,** 413–417.

Dallos, P. *The Auditory Periphery* New York: Academic Press, 1973.

Davis, H., Silverman, S. R., & McAuliffe, D. R. Some observations on pitch and frequency. *Journal of the Acoustical Society of America,* 1951, **23,** 40–42.

Deatherage, B. H., Bilger, R. C., & Eldredge, D. H. Remote masking in selected frequency regions. *Journal of the Acoustical Society of America,* 1957, **29,** 512–514.

Deatherage, B. H., Davis, H., & Eldredge, D. H. Physiological evidence for the masking of low frequency by high. *Journal of the Acoustical Society of America,* 1957, **29,** 132–137.

de Boer, E. Correlation studies applied to the frequency resolution of the cochlea. *Journal of Auditory Research,* 1967, **7,** 209–217.

Diercks, K. J., & Jeffress, L. A. Interaural phase and the absolute threshold for tone. *Journal of the Acoustical Society of America,* 1962, **34,** 981.

Durlach, N. I. Binaural signal detection: Equalization and cancellation theory. In J. V. Tobias (Ed.), *Foundations of modern auditory theory.* Vol. II. New York: Academic Press, 1972.

Efron, R. Conservation of temporal information by perceptual systems. *Perception and Psychophysics,* 1973, **14,** 518–530.

Egan, J. P. Demonstration of masking-level differences by binaural beats. *Journal of the Acoustical Society of America,* 1965, **37,** 1143–1144. (a)

Egan, J. P. Masking-level differences as a function of interaural disparities in intensity of signal and of noise. *Journal of the Acoustical Society of America,* 1965, **38,** 1043–1049. (b)

Evans, E. F. & Wilson, J. P. Frequency sharpening of the cochlea: The effective bandwidth of cochlear nerve fibers. *Proceedings of the Seventh International Congress on Acoustics, Budapest,* 1971, 453–456.

Flanagan, J. L. Models for approximating basilar membrane displacement—Part I. *Bell System Technical Journal,* 1960, **39,** 1163–1191.

Flanagan, J. L. Models for approximating basilar membrane displacement—Part II. *Bell System Technical Journal,* 1962, **41,** 959–1009.

Flanagan, J. L. Signal analysis in the auditory system. In E. E. David & P. B. Denes (Eds.), *Human communication: A unified view.* New York: McGraw Hill, 1972.

Flanagan, J. L., & Guttman, N. On the pitch of periodic pulses. *Journal of the Acoustical Society of America,* 1960, **32,** 1308–1319.

Fletcher, H. Physical measurements of audition and their bearing on the theory of hearing. *Bell System Technical Journal,* 1923, **2,** 145–182.

Fletcher, H. The physical criterion for determining the pitch of a musical tone. *Physical Review,* 1924, **23,** 427–437.

Fletcher, H. *Speech and hearing.* New York: Van Nostrand, 1929.

Fletcher, H. A space-time pattern theory of hearing. *Journal of the Acoustical Society of America,* 1930, **1,** 311–343.

Fletcher, H. Auditory patterns. *Reviews of Modern Physics,* 1940, **12,** 47–65.

Fletcher, H. Dynamics of the middle ear and its relation to the acuity of hearing. *Journal of the Acoustical Society of America,* 1952, **24,** 129–131.

Fletcher, H. *Speech and hearing in communication.* New York: Van Nostrand, 1953.

Freedman, S. J. (Ed.) The neuropsychology of spatially oriented behavior. Homewood, Illinois: Dorsey Press, 1968.

Garner, W. R. Hearing. *Annual Reviews of Psychology,* 1952, **3,** 85–104.

Garner, W. R. Advantages of a discriminability criterion for loudness scaling. *Journal of the Acoustical Society of America,* 1958, **30,** 1005–1012.

Garner, W. R., & Miller, G. A. The masked threshold of pure tones as a function of duration. *Journal of Experimental Psychology,* 1947, **34,** 293–303.

Geldard, F. A. *The human senses.* (2nd ed.) New York: Wiley, 1972.

Gibson, J. J. *The senses considered as perceptual systems.* Boston: Houghton, 1966.

Goldstein, J. L. Auditory nonlinearity. *Journal of the Acoustical Society of America,* 1967, **41,** 676–689.

Green, D. M. Temporal auditory acuity. *Psychological Review,* 1971, **78,** 540–551.

Green, D. M., & McGill, W. J. On the equivalence of detection probabilities and well-known statistical quantities. *Psychological Review*, 1970, **77**, 294–301.

Green, D. M., & Swets, J. A. Signal detection theory and psychophysics. New York: Wiley, 1966.

Gulick, W. L. *Hearing: Physiology and psychophysics.* New York: Oxford Univ. Press, 1971.

Hall, J. L. Auditory distortion products $f_2 - f_1$ and $2f_1 - f_2$. *Journal of the Acoustical Society of America*, 1972, **51**, 1863–1871.

Hallpike, C. S., & Scott, P. Observations on the function of the round window. *Journal of Physiology*, 1940, **99**, 76–82.

Harris, G. G. Periodicity perception using gated noise. *Journal of the Acoustical Society of America*, 1963, **35**, 1229–1233.

Hirsh, I. J. Binaural summation and interaural inhibition as a function of the level of masking noise. *American Journal of Psychology*, 1948, **61**, 205–213.

Hirsh, I. J. Auditory perception of temporal order. *Journal of the Acoustical Society of America*, 1959, **31**, 759–767.

Houtsma, A. J. M., & Goldstein, J. L. The central origin of the pitch of complex tones: Evidence from musical interval recognition. *Journal of the Acoustical Society of America*, 1972, **51**, 520–529.

Huggins, W. H. System function analysis of speech sounds. *Journal of the Acoustical Society of America*, 1950, **22**, 765–767.

Huggins, W. H. A theory of hearing. In W. Jackson (Ed.), *Communication theory*. London: Butterworths, 1953.

Huggins, W. H., & Licklider, J. C. R. Place mechanisms of auditory frequency analysis. *Journal of the Acoustical Society of America*, 1951, **23**, 290–299.

Huxley, A. F. Is resonance possible in the cochlea after all? *Nature*, 1969, **221**, 935–940.

Jeffress, L. A. A place theory of sound localization. *Journal of Comparative Physiology & Psychology*, 1948, **41**, 35–39.

Jeffress, L. A. Masking. In J. V. Tobias (Ed.), *Foundations of modern auditory theory*. Vol. I. New York: Academic Press, 1970.

Jeffress, L. A. Binaural signal detection: vector theory. In J. V. Tobias (Ed.), *Foundations of modern auditory theory*, Vol. II. New York: Academic Press, 1972.

Jeffress, L. A., Blodgett, H. C., Sandel, T. T., & Wood, C. L. III. Masking of tonal signals. *Journal of the Acoustical Society of America*, 1956, **28**, 416–426.

Jepsen, O. Middle-ear muscle reflexes in man. In J. Jerger (Ed.), *Modern developments in audiology*. New York: Academic Press, 1963.

Jerger, J. (Ed.) *Modern developments in audiology*. (2nd ed.) New York: Academic Press, 1973.

Johnstone, B. M., & Boyle, A. J. F. Basilar membrane vibration examined with the Mössbauer technique. *Science*, 1967, **158**, 389–390.

Kameoka, A., & Kuriyagawa, M. P.S.E. tracing method for subjective harmonics measurement and monaural phase effect on timbre. *Journal of the Acoustical Society of America*, 1966, **39**, 1263. Report of Central Research Laboratory, Tokyo Shibaura Electric Co., Komukai, Japan (1967).

Klumpp, R. G. & Eady, H. R. Some measurements of interaural time difference thresholds. *Journal of the Acoustical Society of America*, 1956, **28**, 859–860.

Koenig, W. Subjective effects in binaural hearing. *Journal of the Acoustical Society of America*, 1950, **22**, 61–62.

Kohllöffel, L. U. E. A study of basilar membrane vibrations. III. The basilar membrane frequency response curve in the living guinea pig. *Acustica*, 1972, **27**, 82–89.

Korn, T. S. Theory of audio information. *Acustica*, 1969, **22**, 336–344.

Kostelijk, P. J. *Theories of hearing.* Central National Council for Applied Scientific Research in the Netherlands, Section on Sound of the Research Committee for Sanitary Engineering T.N.O., Report No. 2. Leiden: Universitaire pers Leiden, 1950.

Lamoré, P. J. J. Pitch and masked threshold in relation to interaction phenomena in two-tone stimuli in general. *Acustica*, 1977, **37**, 249–257.

Lawrence, M. Process of sound conduction. *Laryngoscope*, 1958, **68**, 328–347. (a)

Lawrence, M. Audiometric manifestations of inner ear physiology: The aural overload test. *Transactions of the American Academy of Ophthalmology and Otolaryngology*, 1958, **62**, 104–109. (b)

Lee, W. Relationships between Thurstone category scaling and signal detection theory. *Psychological Bulletin*, 1969, **71**, 101–107.

Levitt, H. Decision theory, signal-detection theory and psychophysics. In E. E. David, Jr. & P. B. Denes (Eds.), *Human communication: A unified view*. New York: McGraw-Hill, 1972.

Levitt, H., & Rabiner, L. R. Binaural release from masking for speech and gain in intelligibility. *Journal of the Acoustical Society of America*, 1967, **42**, 601–608.

Liberman, A. M., Cooper, F. S., Shankweiler, D. P., & Studdert-Kennedy, M. Perception of the speech code. *Psychological Review*, 1967, **74**, 431–461.

Licklider, J. C. R. The influence of interaural phase relations upon the masking of speech by white noise. *Journal of the Acoustical Society of America*, 1948, **20**, 150–159.

Licklider, J. C. R. A duplex theory of pitch perception. *Experientia*, 1951, 7, 128–134. (a)

Licklider, J. C. R. Basic correlates of the auditory stimulus. In S. S. Stevens (Ed.), *Handbook of experimental psychology*. New York: Wiley, 1951. (b)

Licklider, J. C. R. Hearing. *Annual Reviews of Psychology*, 1953, **4**, 89–110.

Licklider, J. C. R. Three auditory theories. In S. Koch (Ed.), *Psychology, a study of a science*. New York: McGraw-Hill, 1959.

Licklider, J. C. R., Webster, J. C., & Hedlun, J. M. On the frequency limits of binaural beats. *Journal of the Acoustical Society of America*, 1950, **22**, 468–473.

Luce, R. D., & Green, D. M. A neural timing theory for response times and the psychophysics of intensity. *Psychological Review*, 1972, **79**, 14–57.

McClellan, M. E., & Small, A. M., Jr. Pitch perception of randomly triggered pulse pairs. *Journal of the Acoustical Society of America*, 1963, **35**, 1881–1882 (A).

Miller, G. A., & Taylor, W. G. The perception of repeated bursts of noise. *Journal of the Acoustical Society of America*, 1948, **20**, 171–182.

Mills, A. W. Auditory localization. In J. V. Tobias (Ed.), *Foundations of modern auditory theory*. Vol. II. New York: Academic Press, 1972.

Møller, A. R. Transfer function of the middle ear. *Journal of the Acoustical Society of America*, 1963, **35**, 1526–1534.

Møller, A. R. The middle ear. In J. V. Tobias (Ed.), *Foundations of modern auditory theory*. Vol. II. New York: Academic Press, 1972.

Munson, W. A. The growth of auditory sensation. *Journal of the Acoustical Society of America*, 1947, **19**, 584–591.

Nelson, D. A., & Bilger, R. C. Pure tone octave masking in normal hearing listeners. *Journal of Speech and Hearing Research*, 1974, **17**, 223–251.

Newman, E. B. Hearing. *Annual Reviews of Psychology*, 1950, **1**, 49–70.

Nordmark, J. Some analogies between pitch and laterlaization phenomena. *Journal of the Acoustical Society of America*, 1963, **35**, 1544–1547.

Patterson, J. H., & Green, D. M. Discrimination of transient signals having identical energy spectra. *Journal of the Acoustical Society of America*, 1970, **48**, 894–905.

Pierce, J. R., & David, E. E. *Man's world of sound*. Garden City, New York: Doubleday, 1958.

Plomp, R. *Experiments on tone perception*. Soesterberg, The Netherlands: Institute for Perception RVO-TNO, 1966.

Pollack, I. Periodicity pitch for interrupted white noise—fact or artifact? *Journal of the Acoustical Society of America*, **45**, 1969, 237–238 (L).

Pumphrey, R. J., & Gold, T. Phase memory of the ear: A proof of the resonance hypothesis. *Nature*, 1948, **161**, 640.

Rayleigh, Lord. On our perception of sound direction. *Philosophical Magazine, Sixth Series*, 1907, **13**, 214–232.

Rhode, W. S. Observations on the vibration of the basilar membrane in squirrel monkey using the Mössbauer technique. *Journal of the Acoustical Society of America*, 1970, **49**, 1218–1231.

Roffler, S. K., & Butler, R. A. Localization of tonal stimuli in the vertical plane. *Journal of the Acoustical Society of America*, 1968, **43**, 1260–1266.

Schafer, T. H., Gales, R. S., Shewmaker, C. A., & Thompson, P. O. The frequency selectivity of the ear as determined by masking experiments. *Journal of the Acoustical Society of America*, 1950, **22**, 490–496.

Scharf, B. Critical bands. In J. V. Tobias (Ed.), *Foundations of modern auditory theory, Vol. I*. New York: Academic Press, 1970.

Schouten, J. F. The perception of subjective tones. *Proceedings Kon. Ned AKAD Wetensch*, 1938, **41**, 1086–1093.

Schouten, J. F. The perception of pitch. *Phillips Technical Review*, 1940, **5**, 286–294.

Siebert, W. M. Models for the dynamic behavior of the cochlear partition. *M.I.T. Research Laboratory of Electronics, Quarterly Progress Report*, 1962, No. **64**, 242–258.

Siebert, W. M. Stimulus transformations in the peripheral auditory system. In P. A. Kolers & M. Eden (Eds.), *Recognizing patterns*. Cambridge, Massachusetts: M.I.T. Press, 1968.

Small, A. M., Jr., & McClellan, M. E. Pitch associated with time delay between two pulse trains. *Journal of the Acoustical Society of America*, 1963, **35**, 132–137.

Stevens, S. S. A scale for the measurement of a psychological magnitude: loudness. *Psychological Review*, 1936, **43**, 405–416.

Stevens, S. S. On the validity of the loudness scale. *Journal of the Acoustical Society of America*, 1959, **31**, 995–1003.

Stevens, S. S. Issues in psychophysical measurement. *Psychological Review*, 1971, **78**, 426–450.

Stevens, S. S., & Davis, H. *Hearing: Its psychology and physiology*. New York: Wiley, 1938.

Stevens, S. S., Davis, H., & Lurie, M. H. The localization of pitch perception on the basilar membrane. *Journal of General Psychology*, 1935, **13**, 296–315.

Stevens, S. S., & Newman, E. B. On the nature of aural harmonics. *Proceedings of the National Academy of Sciences*, 1936, **22**, 668–672.

Stevens, S. S., & Sobel, R. The central differentiation of synchronized action potentials in the auditory nerve. *American Journal of Psychology*, 1937, **119**, 409–410.

Stuhlman, O. The non-linear transmission characteristics of the auditory ossicles. *Journal of the Acoustical Society of America*, 1937, **9**, 119–128.

Thurlow, W. R., & Small, A. M., Jr. Pitch perception for certain periodic auditory stimuli. *Journal of the Acoustical Society of America*, 1955, **27**, 132–137.

Tobias, J. V. (Ed.) *Foundations of modern auditory theory*. Vol. II. New York: Academic Press, 1972.

Tonndorf, J. Fluid motion in cochlear models. *Journal of the Acoustical Society of America*, 1957, **29**, 558–568.

Tonndorf, J., & Tabor, J. R. Closure of the cochlear windows. *Annals of Otology, Rhinology & Laryngology*, 1962, **71**, 5–29.

Treisman, M. Sensory scaling and the psychophysical law. *Quarterly Journal of Experimental Psychology*, 1964, **16**, 11–22. (a)

Treisman, M. What do sensory scales measure? *Quarterly Journal of Experimental Psychology*, 1964, **16**, 387–391. (b)

Treisman, M. Signal detection theory and Crozier's law: derivation of a new sensory scaling procedure. *Journal of Mathematical Psychology*, 1965, **2**, 205–218.

Treisman, M., & Watts, T. R. Relation between signal detectability theory and the traditional procedures for measuring sensory thresholds: estimating d' from results given by the method of constant stimuli. *Psychological Bulletin*, 1966, **66**, 438–454.

van Bergeijk, W. A. The evolution of vertebrate hearing. In W. D. Neff (Ed.), *Contributions to Sensory Physiology*. Vol. 2. New York: Academic Press, 1964.

Von Gierke, H. Discussion on "process of sound conduction." *Laryngoscope*, 1958, **68**, 347–354.

Warren, R. M. A basis for judgments of sensory intensity. *American Journal of Psychology*, 1958, **71**, 675–687.

Warren, R., Sersen, E., & Pores, E. A basis for loudness-judgments. *American Journal of Psychology*, 1958, **71**, 700–709.

Wegel, R. L., & Lane, C. E. The auditory masking of one pure tone by another and its possible relation to the dynamics of the inner ear. *Physical Review*, 1924, **23**, 266–285.

Weston, P. B., & Miller, J. D. Use of noise to eliminate one ear from masking experiments. *Journal of the Acoustical Society of America*, 1965, **37**, 638–646.

Wever, E. G. *Theory of hearing*. New York: Wiley, 1949.

Wever, E. G. Hearing. *Annual Review of Psychology*, 1951, **2**, 65–78.

Wever, E. G., & Bray, C. W. The nature of acoustical response: The relation between the sound frequency and frequency of impulses in the auditory nerve. *Journal of Experimental Psychology*, 1930, **13**, 373–387.

Wever, G., & Lawrence, M. *Physiological acoustics*. Princeton: Princeton Univ. Press, 1954.

Winckel, F. *Music, sound and sensation, a modern exposition*. New York: Dover, 1967.

Woodworth, R. S. *Experimental Psychology*. New York: Holt, 1938.

Zwicker, E., Flottorp, G., & Stevens, S. S. Critical band width in loudness summation. *Journal of the Acoustical Society of America*, 1957, **29**, 548–557.

Zwislocki, J. Theory of the acoustical action of the cochlea. *Journal of the Acoustical Society of America*, 1950, **22**, 778–784.

Zwislocki, J. Review of recent mathematical theories of cochlear dynamics. *Journal of the Acoustical Society of America*, 1953, **25**, 743–751. (a)

Zwislocki, J. Acoustic attenuation between the ears. *Journal of the Acoustical Society of America*, 1953, **25**, 752–759. (b)

Zwislocki, J. Some impedance measurements on normal and pathological ears. *Journal of the Acoustical Society of America*, 1957, **29**, 1312–1317.

Zwislocki, J. Theory of temporal auditory summation. *Journal of the Acoustical Society of America*, 1960, **32**, 1046–1060.

Zwislocki, J. Analysis of some auditory characteristics. In R. D. Luce, R. R. Bush, & E. Galanter (Eds.), *Handbook of Mathematical Psychology*. Vol. 3. New York: Wiley, 1965. Pp. 1–97.

Part II

Measurement, Biophysics of the Cochlea, and Neural Coding

Chapter 3

MEASUREMENT OF THE AUDITORY STIMULUS *

BARRY LESHOWITZ

* This paper was supported in part by a grant from the National Institutes of Health. The author wishes to thank M. J. Penner, Gil Ricard, Patrick Zurek, Edward Cudahy, and W. Sisson for their helpful comments pertaining to an earlier draft of this paper. Thanks are also due to G. Jenkins, B. Garner, and H. Rubio for their assistance in preparation of the figures.

I. INTRODUCTION

In an auditory psychophysical experiment, the observer is typically asked to evaluate some aspect of a sound stimulus. The observer's task may be to detect the sound's presence, recognize some feature of the sound (e.g., pitch) or perhaps assess its loudness. From an analysis of the way in which behavioral responses are related to specific aspects of the stimulus, one attempts to deduce mechanisms underlying processing of acoustic information. Obviously, the analysis requires a precise description of the auditory stimulus.

The physical system underlying generation and propagation of sound can be described in terms of a source, a medium, and a receiver. Sound originates at the source as vibration (i.e., periodic motion) of a body. The motion of the body produces oscillations of pressure compression and expansion which are transmitted as sound waves through a medium. If the propagated sound is not absorbed or reflected, it travels in a straight line to the receiver. The receiver may be either an electroacoustic transducer, such as a microphone, or the physiological transducer within the ear.

II. HARMONIC MOTION

Sound energy is produced by the *periodic* motion (vibration) of a body. Motion is considered periodic if it repeats itself in some interval of time. In nature, one type of periodic motion is often observed. The movement of a pendulum, the up and down motion of a spring, and the oscillation of a tuning fork are all examples of simple *harmonic* motion. Harmonic motion can be represented graphically by a sinusoidal function, which describes the position of an oscillating particle over time. Harmonic motion is the most basic type of motion since all motion, no matter how complex, can be described as a sum of simple harmonic vibrations. Because harmonic motion is so important to an understanding of sound, we present below a more complete description.

A. An Example of Harmonic Oscillation: Mass on a Spring

An example of a physical system whose motion is harmonic is the mass on a spring shown in Fig. 1. When the mass is pulled to the right from its equilibrium or rest position at $x = 0$, a restoring force exists to pull it back. The force pulling the mass back to rest when the spring is stretched is proportional to the amount of stretch. That is,

$$F = -kx. \tag{1}$$

From elementary physics we know whenever the position of a body is al-

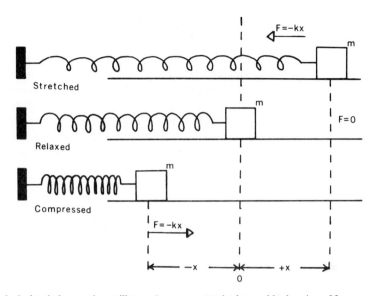

FIG. 1. A simple harmonic oscillator. A mass m attached to an ideal spring of force constant k moves over a frictionless surface.

tered a force must be exerted. Force is measured by determining the acceleration it imparts to the mass. That is,

$$F = ma, \qquad (2)$$

where a is acceleration of the mass m. Combining Eqs. (1) and (2), we arrive at the description of movement of a mass on a spring in terms of the equation:

$$-kx = ma,$$
$$d^2x/dt^2 + (k/m)x = 0, \qquad (3)$$

where the change in velocity with respect to time is acceleration or d^2x/dt^2.

Equation (3) is a differential equation since it gives a relation between the function $x(t)$ and its second time derivative $d^2x(t)/dt^2$. To solve the differential equation we must find a function whose second derivative is the negative of the function itself, except for a proportionality constant. From calculus we know that the cosine function satisfies this condition. For the movement of the particle, we can write the following tentative solution:

$$x(t) = A \cos(\omega_0 t + \theta) \qquad (4)$$

and

$$dx/dt^2 = -A \omega_0 \sin(\omega_0 t + \theta),$$
$$d^2x/dt = -A \omega_0^2 \cos(\omega_0 t + \theta). \qquad (5)$$

Substituting Eqs. (4) and (5) into Eq. (3) we obtain

$$-\omega_0^2 A \cos(\omega_0 t + \theta) = (-k/m)A \cos(\omega_0 t + \theta). \tag{6}$$

By observation, Eq. (6) is satisfied when $\omega_0^2 = k/m$. Thus, we have confirmed that Eq. (4) does indeed describe the motion of the mass on a spring, and, therefore, constitutes a solution of the simple harmonic oscillator.

Observe that the motion described by Eq. (4) depends on the parameters, A, θ, and ω_0. From inspection we can discern the physical significance of the various parameters. First, we observe that x repeats itself every $2\pi/\omega_0$ sec, since

$$x(t) = A \cos\{\omega_0[t + (2\pi/\omega_0)] + \theta\} = A \cos(\omega_0 t + \theta). \tag{7}$$

Therefore, the *period* of the motion, T (i.e., the time required to complete one complete oscillation), is equal to $2\pi/\omega_0$ and is given by

$$T = 2\pi/\omega_0 = 2\pi(m/k)^{1/2}. \tag{8}$$

Thus the period of oscillation is related to the mass m of the vibrating particle and the force constant k. The system's *natural frequency* of vibration, f_0, measured in hertz (Hz), is the number of complete oscillations per unit time and is given by

$$f_0 = 1/T = \omega_0/2\pi. \tag{9}$$

The quantity ω_0 is the *angular frequency* and its unit is radians per second. The constant A, is the *amplitude* of the motion, and is the maximum displacement from the equilibrium position. Finally, the constant θ is the *phase* constant and determines the position of the particle when $t = 0$.

Of note is the observation that the two primary auditory dimensions are associated with the parameters of the sinusoidal function. The repetition rate or frequency of vibration corresponds to pitch, the amplitude of vibration to

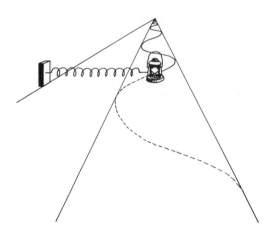

FIG. 2. The path tracing the movement of the mass (lantern) on a spring is etched on a light-sensitive plate that moves at a constant speed into the page away from the reader.

intensity or loudness. Other auditory sensations, such as timbre, brightness, and volume, are less well understood, but are probably related to the amplitude and phase of the harmonic components comprising the complex sound.

The description of the motion of a mass on a spring as a sinusoidal function can be confirmed in a simple demonstration. Suppose that a small beam of light is attached to the oscillating mass as shown in Fig. 2. In agreement with Eq. (4), a sinusoidal function is etched on the light-sensitive screen moving into the page away from the reader.

III. PROPAGATION OF SOUND*

The periodic motion of a mass on a spring is one example of harmonic motion. An example more relevant to a discussion of sound is the vibratory movement of a tuning fork. The to-and-fro movement of the tuning fork's prongs in response to an impulse is identical to the harmonic motion first described.

Sound waves are identical to mechanical oscillation, except that wave oscillation appears not only as a time oscillation at one place, but also as a propagation in space as well. This means that energy originating at the source as mechanical oscillation is propagated as sound waves. As an illustration of sound propagation, consider the sound waves created by movement of the tuning fork. When the prong moves to the right, the gas in front of the prong is compressed, and the pressure and density of the gas rise above their normal values. The compressed layer of gas moves forward compressing layers next to it. With movement of the prong to the left, pressure and density in the vicinity of the prong fall below normal, and rarefaction exists. The continuous to-and-fro vibration of the prong produces a *train* of compression and rarefaction that travels away from the source.

It is important to note that in the propagation of sound, individual vibrating molecules remain close to their equilibrium point and that motion of individual molecules is identical to the oscillation of the source. Thus, propagating sound waves can be represented as a series of successive chain reactions in which work (energy) produced by the initial displacement of the source is transferred from point to point, with each element oscillating about its equilibrium position. The displacement of an element about its rest position as a function of time as well as the displacement of elements along

---

* A basic discussion of the physics of sound is contained in Chapter 3 of Denes and Pinson's (1963) text, *The Speech Chain*. A somewhat more advanced presentation appears in Roederer's (1973) introductory text on psychophysics and music. General Radio's *Handbook of Noise Measurement* (Peterson & Gross, 1967) contains a great deal of practical information on instruments for measuring sound.

the direction of propagation at any given time is described by a single expression. This expression is termed the *wave equation* and is

$$y = f(x - vt), \tag{10}$$

where y gives the displacement of a particle at time t from its equilibrium position at x, the distance from the source. The velocity of the wave is v. For the particular case of harmonic oscillation we have

$$y = A \cos[(2\pi/\lambda) (x - vt)], \tag{11}$$

where the wavelength λ is the distance traveled by the sound wave in one period of oscillation T. That is,

$$\lambda = vT. \tag{12}$$

Thus, at some time t a given value of y repeats itself at $x + \lambda, x + 2\lambda$, etc. Figure 3 presents displacement of a particle from its equilibrium position as a function of the x-direction of propagation at some time t. Fixing t in this way provides a snapshot of the wave. If, on the other hand, we observe movement of a particle about its equilibrium position over time at some point x, we observe the sinusoidal motion described previously in connection with harmonic oscillation.

A. Standing Longitudinal Wave

The reflection of sound waves by barriers gives rise to *standing waves*. The phenomenon of standing waves is simply an example of interference between two waves—the incident wave and the reflected wave—traveling in opposite directions. At the barrier, the reflected wave is 180° out of phase with the incident wave, since the displacement of a particle at the barrier must be zero. Thus, at the barrier, a displacement node is created. For the case of tonal waveforms, the distance between adjacent nodes is one-half the wavelength of the sound. Thus perceptually, the presence of a standing wave gives rise to differences in loudness depending on the observer's position. Variations in loudness become rather large when the frequency of the sound corresponds to the *resonant* frequency of the enclosure. These natural modes of oscillation are determined by the physical dimensions of the enclosure and

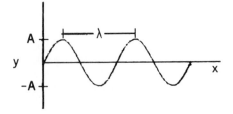

FIG. 3. Particle displacement at a fixed moment of time t as a function of distance from the tuning fork. The movement of the particle is sinusoidal having amplitude A and wavelength λ. Sound waves are *longitudinal* since motion of a particle is back and forth along the direction of propagation.

the speed of sound. For example, for standing longitudinal waves in a gas column closed at both ends resonance occurs at frequencies given by

$$f = (n/2l)v, \qquad n = 1, 2, 3, \ldots, \qquad (13)$$

where v is the speed of the wave and l is the length of the tube.

IV. MEASUREMENT OF SOUND INTENSITY*

Up to this point, we have described sound waves in terms of displacement of a particle from its equilibrium position. Obviously, large displacement amplitudes are associated with high-intensity wave motion. However, measurement of the intensity of the sound wave in terms of displacement amplitude is extremely difficult to carry out, since the actual displacement corresponding to audible sound is extremely small. For example, at absolute threshold for 1000-Hz tone, the displacement amplitude $(= 10^{-11}$ m) is smaller than the diameter of an atom. Consequently, the intensity of sound is usually measured in terms of the magnitude of *pressure* variations.

A. Pressure of Sound Waves

In order to relate displacement and pressure, we must rewrite the wave equation in terms of pressure variations. The change in pressure Δp caused by movement of a particle is proportional to the fractional change in volume of the gas. That is,

$$\Delta p = -B\Delta V/V, \qquad (14)$$

where the constant B called the bulk modulus of elasticity, is a property of the medium, and Δp represents the change from the undisturbed pressure p_0. Observe that increases in pressure are positive because there is a concomitant decrease in volume. Let A represent the cross-sectional area of a layer of gas, ΔX the thickness of the layer of gas at equilibrium (undisturbed pressure), and ΔY the amount by which the thickness changes during compression and rarefaction. Thus, rewriting Eq. (14) we have

$$\Delta p = -B\Delta V/V = -BA\,\Delta Y/A\,\Delta X. \qquad (15)$$

As $\Delta X \to 0$, we obtain, using partial derivative notation,

$$\Delta p = -B\delta Y/\delta X. \qquad (16)$$

When the variable t is constant, from Eq. (11) we obtain

$$\Delta p = BkA \sin(kx - \omega t), \qquad (17)$$

---

* The word *intensity* will be used initially as a generic term for magnitude or strength of sound. A more precise definition of intensity is developed in Section IV,D.

where $k = 2\pi/\lambda$. Thus, as was the case for displacement, pressure variation at each position x is also harmonic. However, the displacement wave is $90°$ out of phase with the pressure wave. Also note the pressure amplitude is proportional to the displacement amplitude.

B. Power in Sound Wave Motion

When measuring sound intensity, we are interested in specifying the effectiveness of a given sound as given by its ability to do work. More precisely, we would like to specify the rate at which work is done, which is the instantaneous *power* in the sound wave. The work done by a force on a particle is the product of the magnitude of the force F and the distance d through which the particle moves. We write this as

$$\omega = Fd. \tag{18}$$

1. INSTANTANEOUS POWER

The power delivered at an instant in time is called the *instantaneous power,* or more simply, *power,* and is

$$P = d\omega/dt. \tag{19}$$

In order to derive power we need to know the force F exerted at some position x at some time t. We have only to note that force divided by cross-sectional area is equal to pressure. Thus, from Eq. (16) we can write the force at some time t as

$$F = -lB\,\partial Y/\partial X, \tag{20}$$

where l is a proportionality constant. The incremental change in distance per unit time caused by the force and is $\partial Y/\partial t$. Thus, for instantaneous power we can write an equation analogous to Eq. (18):

$$P = -lB(\Delta Y/\Delta X)(\partial Y/\partial t). \tag{21}$$

Recall that the sound wave in terms of displacement is a simple cosine wave and is

$$y = A\,\cos(kx - \omega t). \tag{11}$$

From Eq. (20) we can write force as

$$F = -lB\,\delta Y/\delta X = lBkA\,\sin(kx - \omega t), \qquad t = \text{constant}. \tag{22}$$

Similarly,

$$\delta Y/\delta t = \omega A\,\sin(kx - \omega t), \qquad x = \text{constant}. \tag{23}$$

Hence, the instantaneous power expended by the force at x at time t, or the energy passing through x per unit time in the x-direction is

$$P = (BklA)(\omega A)\sin^2(kx - \omega t)$$
$$= Bkl\omega A^2 \sin^2(kx - \omega t). \tag{24}$$

Thus, the instantaneous power of a wave is proportional to the square of the displacement amplitude. We have already shown that displacement is proportional to pressure. Hence, the power of a wave is proportional to the square of pressure.

2. AVERAGE POWER

Notice also that the instantaneous power is not constant over time. Power is often taken to be the *average* over one period of motion. The *average power* $\bar{P}$ delivered is obtained by integrating the instantaneous power over one period T and is

$$\bar{P} = (1/T) \int_t^{t+T} P(t)\, dt. \tag{25}$$

Making use of the trigonometric identity that $\sin^2 x$ over one cycle is $T/2$, we obtain

$$\bar{P} = 1/2 A^2 l\omega Bk = 2\pi^2 A^2 l f^2 B/v, \tag{26}$$

since velocity v of sound is the product of frequency f and wavelength λ. Observe that average power is proportional to the amplitude of displacement squared. The quantity $A^2/2$ is called the *mean-square power,* the quantity $(A^2/2)^{1/2}$, the *root-mean-square power* or *rms.*

Observe, in Eq. (26), when power is expressed in terms of displacement, frequency appears explicit in the expression. However, from Eq. (17), we observe that pressure amplitude p is proportional to the product of displacement amplitude and frequency. Rewriting Eq. (26) as

$$\bar{P} = mp^2, \tag{27}$$

we observe the average power is proportional to the square of pressure. Hence, by measuring pressure changes, we can compare the intensity of sounds having different frequencies directly.

C. Decibel Scale

Ordinarily the power of sound is calibrated by measuring pressure changes. The pressure variations corresponding to audible sound are small but can be measured with a sensitive calibrated microphone. By calibrated we mean that a given voltage at the output of the microphone is linearly related to input sound pressure. A convenient unit for measuring pressure is the bar, where 1 bar is equal to 10^5 newton m^{-2}.

The common method for establishing sound pressure values at the ear is to measure the sound pressure in a small cavity, called the *coupler.* The standard 6-cm^3 coupler has been constructed so that it closely matches the volume of the human auditory canal and enclosed pinna. This volume closely simulates the compliance characteristics of the human ear. Considerable data on sound pressure measured in the standard coupler exist for the Telephonics TDH 39 earphone. We shall return to the analysis of the response of this earphone in Section V.

A logarithmic scale called the *decibel* scale is used to specify sound intensity. Decibels are defined in terms of a power ratio. If the power produced by a sound source is $\bar{P}_s$, its decibel rating is given by

$$\bar{P}_s \text{ (in dB)} = 10 \log(\bar{P}_s/\bar{P}_{ref}), \tag{28}$$

where the reference power is 10^{-16} W cm^{-2}. There are 10 decibels in a *bel*. As mentioned above, sound is usually measured in terms of pressure. If the sound pressure produced by a source is p_s, its sound pressure level (SPL) in decibels is

$$p_s \text{ (in dB)} = 20 \log(p_s/p_{ref}), \tag{29}$$

where the reference pressure p_{ref} in open air corresponding to 10^{-16} W cm^{-2} is .0002 μbar. (*Note:* 1 bar = 10^6 dyne cm^{-2}.)

D. Measurement of Sound Level

In actual laboratory practice we do not routinely measure pressure at the output of the earphones. Rather, rms power (voltage) at the input to the earphones is used to specify sound level. A typical measurement procedure can be illustrated with a simple example. Specifications for the TDH 39 earphone state that 1 V rms power corresponds to a sound level of 110 dB SPL measured in a standard 6-cm^3 coupler. This means, for example, that a .1 V rms reading corresponds to an output of 90 dB SPL for a 1000-Hz signal.

In general voltmeters are of three types: *true* rms meters; peak-amplitude meters, and average reading meters. For a sinusoidal waveform, there exists a simple relation between rms power, peak voltage, and average rectified voltage, namely, that rms power equals .7 × peak voltage of 1.1 × average rectified voltage. Thus, these meters are calibrated in terms of *equivalent rms* power. For nonsinusoidal waveforms (e.g., noise), rms power is not easily related to peak amplitude. A true rms meter is, therefore, required for accurate measurement. A true rms meter actually squares the input waveform with an analog square-law device in the manner described in Eq. (25). The output of such a device is the square root of the average power or rms power.

E. Intensity of a Point Source

Sound waves transmitted from a point source are three-dimensional waves. Consequently, we define the *intensity* of a sound wave as the average power transmitted across a unit area normal to the direction in which the wave is traveling. Now as distance d increases from the sound source, the wavefront expands so that

$$\bar{P} = 4\pi d_1^2 I_1 = 4\pi d_2^2 I_2 , \tag{30}$$

where I_1 and I_2 are the intensities in power per unit area at d_1 and d_2, respectively. Hence,

$$I_1/I_2 = d_2^2/d_1^2. \tag{31}$$

Thus, sound intensity varies inversely as the square of distance and pressure varies inversely as the distance from the source.

V. SYSTEM PERFORMANCE

Ordinarily, in a psychoacoustic experiment we employ an *electroacoustic* transducer as a sound source rather than a mechanical system. For example, if tonal stimuli are to be used as sound stimuli, it is a simple matter to lead a sinusoidally varying voltage to an earphone or loudspeaker. Sinusoidal variations of the magnetic fields of the electromagnet in the earphone gives rise to concomitant variations of displacement of the earphone cone. These changes in displacement (or pressure) as a function of time serve as the source of sound. Thus, the quality and strength of the sound stimulus is manipulated by altering the electrical waveform to the earphone.

Obviously it is important to know the degree to which the electroacoustical stimulus delivery system converts the electrical waveform into sound energy. This translation of electrical into acoustical energy can be assessed by determining the system's *amplitude* and *phase response.* An illustrative example is presented in the next section.

A. Amplitude Characteristic

The performance of a sound system is specified by the *system response,* which includes both the amplitude and phase characteristics. Suppose we are interested in determining the system response of the TDH 39 earphone. The usual procedure for measuring the amplitude characteristic is to present to the earphone a relatively high level voltage at various frequencies. For example, in the region of maximum sensitivity of the TDH 39 earphone, 1 V rms at 1000 Hz produces a sound pressure level of 110 dB re .0002 μbar. The amplitude response of a TDH 39 earphone is shown in Fig. 4, where sound pressure level (SPL) is plotted against frequency of the signal. As can be seen, the amplitude response is relatively flat for frequencies from 50 Hz to 4

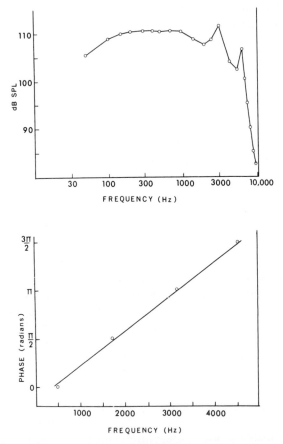

FIG. 4. Amplitude and phase response of the TDH 39 earphone. The acoustic output was measured for the earphone mounted in a standard 6-cm³ coupler with a condenser microphone. For the phase measurements, the sinusoidal signal applied to the earphone was compared with the acoustic output by means of Lissajous patterns. All measurements were made with sinusoids at 1.4 V peak amplitude.

kHz. Beyond 5 kHz and below 50 Hz the response rapidly falls off. At about 4 kHz, we observe a small resonance in the amplitude characteristic.

B. Phase Characteristic

In general, the phase characteristic of the earphone is not included as part of the earphone specification. The purported insensitivity of the ear to phase probably accounts for why the phse characteristic has not generally been reported. However, renewed interest in monaural discrimination of phase has emphasized the importance of considering the phase response of the sound delivery system. To obtain the phase response of an earphone, one merely notes the difference in phase between the electrical input to the earphone and the acoustic output. The phase difference can be measured by connecting the two signals to the horizontal and vertical amplifiers of an oscilloscope. In this mode, the oscilloscope becomes an x–y plotter, and the phase relationship of the two signals can be estimated from an examination of these plots, called Lissajous figures. Some examples are shown in Fig. 5. More precise measurements of phase require a phase meter.

The phase characteristic for the TDH 39 earphone is also shown in Fig. 4. It can be seen that the phase delay introduced by the phone is linearly related to frequency. A linear phase shift in the passband is desirable, since it represents a pure time delay of the auditory waveform. To demonstrate this

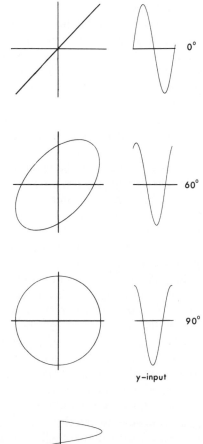

FIG. 5. Lissajous figures indicating phase relation of two signals of the same frequency. Figures are for patterns corresponding to phase differences of 0°, 60°, and 90°.

assertion, we note when phase delay (in radians) is linearly related to frequency, $\theta(f) = -k2\pi f$. For each frequency, we can express the time waveform as

$$s(t) = \sin(2\pi ft - k2\pi f)$$
$$= \sin[2\pi f(t - k)]. \tag{32}$$

Thus, each component is delayed by k seconds. When the auditory waveform is complex, consisting of many frequencies, all the components will be delayed by k seconds. Hence the entire complex waveform will be time delayed by k seconds. Phase shifts due to distance between the earphone and the microphone would be an example of a linear phase delay.

C. Harmonic Distortion

A final specification of the sound system relates to the generation of harmonic and intermodulation distortion. In general, at intense sound levels, acoustic systems behave nonlinearly and thus produce distortion tones not present in the input. (A description of a nonlinear system is presented in Section XI.) It is therefore necessary to measure the amount of distortion present in the acoustic signal and to judge whether that amount of distortion is within tolerable limits. A reasonable goal might be to keep harmonic distortion below 1% of the steady-state SPL. However, if the purpose of the psychophysical investigation is to measure internally generated distortion products, it might be necessary to adopt a more stringent requirement.

In order to measure the level of distortion at the coupler, the microphone output is led to a *wave analyzer*. The wave analyzer consists of a near-rectangular bandpass filter whose center frequency is continuously varied. The passband of the filter is adjustable; e.g., the bandwidths of the General Radio 1900 A wave analyzer filter are 3, 10, and 50 Hz. The output of the analyzer's filter across frequency provides a measure of the input's frequency content.

Suppose the input to the earphones is a complex sound consisting of two primary tones f_1 and f_2. The difference between the level of the primaries and the level of the distortion components provides a measure of harmonic distortion. The distortion is greatest at integral multiples of the primaries ($2f_1$, $2f_2$, $3f_1$, etc.) and at the sum and different frequencies ($nf_1 \pm mf_2$).

Great care should be exercised when specifying distortion on the basis of coupler measurements. This procedure may be unreliable, especially in animal experimentation, where the coupler may provide only a rough approximation to the external auditory canal. In animal preparations, for example, it is not unusual to obtain considerable under- and overestimations of the amount of distortion actually present in the sound field at the eardrum. A more complete treatment of problems in distortion measurement is provided by Dallos (1969).

VI. INTRODUCTION TO LINEAR FILTERS*

The *selectivity* with respect to the amplitude and phase of sinusoidal functions displayed by the earphone is the characteristic property of devices called *filters*. An understanding of filters is an absolutely essential requisite for both conducting and interpreting psychoacoustical research. It is for this reason that we next present in some detail the mathematical basis of linear filters.

A. Forced Oscillation: An Example of a Mechanical Filter

In describing harmonic oscillation of a mass on a spring, we assumed that no external forces act on the system. That is, we derived the movement of the mass in response to a momentary disturbance. Let us now derive the response of the mechanical system to an externally applied force. Suppose the force applied to the mass is the sinusoidal function.

$$f(t) = B \cos \omega t. \tag{33}$$

Intuitively, if the driving frequency ω is very different from the natural frequency ω_0, the system will hardly respond to the driving force. Obviously, only with great difficulty could a very large mass be driven at a very high frequency. Irrespective of the resultant amplitude, we guess that after the initial *transient* response has decayed, at *steady state* the time course of oscillation of the mass will follow the applied sinusoidally varying force. Hence,

$$x(t) = C \cos \omega t. \tag{34}$$

Adding the additional force $f(t)$ to Eq. (3) we obtain

$$m d^2 x/dt^2 = -kx + B \cos \omega t. \tag{35}$$

We solve for the resultant vibration by substituting Eq. (34) into Eq. (35) and obtain

$$-Cm\omega^2 \cos \omega t = -m\omega_0^2 C \cos \omega t + B \cos \omega t, \tag{36}$$

where $k = m\omega_0^2$. Dividing the quantity $\cos \omega t$ out of Eq. (36) we have

$$C = B/[m(\omega_0^2 - \omega^2)]. \tag{37}$$

---

* For those who are not familiar with linear systems and Fourier analysis, Chapters 21–25, Volume 1 of *The Feynman Lectures on Physics* (Feynman, Leighton, & Sands, 1963) are highly recommended. An excellent treatment of Fourier analysis and linear systems is presented in a programmed-learning format by Hsu (1967). This book begins with a basic mathematical background of Fourier analysis and ends with an up-to-date treatment of applications of Fourier analysis to various branches of science. The classic text by Papoulis (1962) is a more advanced presentation of applications of Fourier analysis.

Thus, our initial guessed solution does indeed constitute a solution when C is defined by Eq. (37). Inspection of Eq. (34) reveals that the movement of the mass in response to a sinusoidal driving force is also sinusoidal with frequency ω. The resultant amplitude is related to the difference between the frequency of the driving force ω and the natural frequency of the system ω_0. Amplitude of vibration plotted as a function of the frequency of the driving force is shown in Fig. 6. When ω is considerably different from ω_0, the denominator of Eq. (37) is large and displacement amplitude is small. As ω approaches ω_0, the amplitude approaches infinity. This selectivity for different frequencies displayed by the mechanical system is called *resonance* and is a property of all filters.

In addition to attenuating selectively the input amplitude, filters may introduce a time delay to the output. Observe in Eq. (37) when $\omega > \omega_0$, C is negative. This means that the applied force leads the output by one-half period. The phase shift at various frequencies is also shown in Fig. 6.

B. Forced Vibration with Damping

Up to this point, we have considered harmonic oscillation and forced vibration under conditions where frictional forces are negligible. In analyzing real mechanical systems, frictional forces cannot be neglected. Consider simple harmonic oscillation of the mass on a spring when friction is present. It is reasonable to assume that the amplitude of the return cycle will not be as

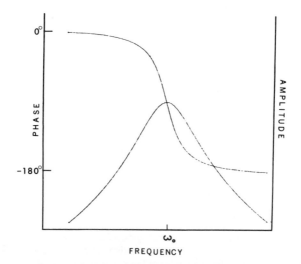

FIG. 6. Amplitude and phase response of the harmonic oscillator in response to forced vibration. Angular frequency of the applied force is plotted on the abscissa. The lag (in degrees) of the resultant movement is plotted on the left ordinate, the amplitude of vibration on the right ordinate.

large as the initial displacement. As a descriptive model, let us suppose that the magnitude of successive oscillations is reduced by a constant fraction. An equation that describes this *damped* oscillation is

$$x = \exp(-t/\lambda) \cos \omega_0. \tag{38}$$

The *time constant* λ is defined as the time required for an oscillation to decay $1/e$ ($e \cong 2.718$) of its initial amplitude. A large frictional force corresponds to a small time constant and rapid decay of oscillation. Such a system is said to be highly damped. Examples of damped oscillation are shown in Fig. 7.

Friction also affects the resonant properties of the system. As can be seen in Fig. 7, as frictional forces increase, the left-hand curves become more rounded. If we use as a measure of frequency selectivity, the half-amplitude points, as friction increases, the resonant curves become more broadly tuned.

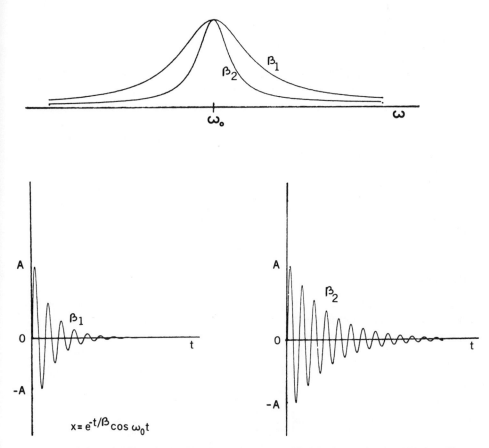

FIG. 7. Resonance curves (left) and damped cosine oscillations for two levels of friction. The time constant λ is inversely related to the passband of the resonance curves. Thus $\lambda_1 < \lambda_2$.

VII. THE LINEAR–TIME-INVARIANT SYSTEM

A. Introduction

The harmonic oscillator as represented by the mass on a spring is an illustration of a *system*. From a systems theory point of view, a system is any device that alters the properties of the input *signal*. The signal may be a deterministic function such as a cosine wave, or it may be a random signal that can only be described statistically. The relation between the input and output signal characterizes the system completely.

We represent the harmonic oscillator in Fig. 8 by a block and the input $f_i(t) = A \cos \omega t$ by an arrow into the system, the output $f_o(t) = B \cos \omega t + \theta$ by an arrow directed out of it. Symbolically we can express the output of the system as

$$L[f_i(t)] = f_o(t), \tag{39}$$

where L describes the relation between the input and output. Recall that for the case of the harmonic oscillator, the transformation of the input is a simple change in amplitude and phase. The harmonic oscillator is a member of a broad class of systems that are *linear* and *time-invariant*.

The linear–time-invariant (LTI) system is encountered not only in the laboratory but also in the various descriptions of the hearing mechanism. In attempts to describe auditory sensation, it has often been assumed that the relation between the psychophysical response and the auditory signal is both linear and time invariant. Because some knowledge of linear system theory is absolutely basic to an understanding of ordinary laboratory equipment as well as to an appreciation of much of what is happening today in physiological and psychological acoustics, a brief presentation of linear systems theory is presented in what follows.

B. Complex Numbers

In order to derive the input–output relation of an LTI system, a *complex* waveform is often employed as input to the system. One reason for using complex exponential notation is that algebraic manipulation involving exponentials is easier to handle than multiplication of trigonometric functions. Before we can evaluate the response of the LTI system, it is necessary to provide a brief discussion of complex numbers.

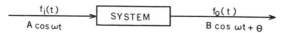

$$f_i(t) \qquad \boxed{\text{SYSTEM}} \qquad f_o(t)$$
$$A \cos \omega t \qquad\qquad\qquad B \cos \omega t + \theta$$

FIG. 8. Block diagram of a linear–time-invariant system.

A complex number consists of a *real* and an *imaginary* part and is expressed as

$$a = x + jy, \tag{40}$$

where x and y are the real and imaginary parts, respectively, and $j = (-1)^{1/2}$. The *complex exponential* is defined by the identity

$$re^{j\theta} = r \cos \theta + jr \sin \theta, \tag{41}$$

where $r \cos \theta$ and $r \sin \theta$ are the real and imaginary parts, respectively. In Fig. 9, $re^{j\theta}$ is represented as a point in the *complex plane*. The real part is plotted on the abscissa, the complex part on the ordinate.

As is the case for real forces, a complex exponential force has both magnitude and direction. To obtain the squared magnitude of a complex force, we multiply it by its complex conjugate. That is,

$$|a|^2 = aa^* = (x + jy)(x - jy),$$
$$|a| = \sqrt{aa^*}, \tag{42}$$

where a^* is the complex conjugate. The direction or phase of the complex force is the arctangent of the imaginary part divided by the real part of the complex number. From the preceding relations we calculate the magnitude and direction of the complex exponential as $|r|$ and θ, respectively. We express these quantities in *phasor* form as

$$R = |r|e^{j\theta}, \tag{43}$$

where $|r|$ is the magnitude, and θ the phase.

Now consider the complex exponential $re^{j\omega t}$. In phasor form we can express the function as

$$R = |r|e^{j\omega t}. \tag{44}$$

From examination of Fig. 9, it is seen that $re^{j\omega t}$ is a vector rotating about the origin. The position of the vector whose magnitude is r is a function of both time and angular frequency. The vector's projection on the real axis is the

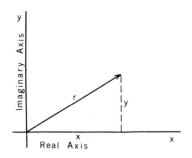

FIG. 9. The complex number, $re^{j\theta}$, represented in the complex plane. $r^2 = x^2 + y^2$; $x = r \cos \theta$; $y = r \sin \theta$; $\theta = \tan^{-1}(y/x)$.

real function $r \cos(\omega t)$, which is in agreement with the observation that the projection of circular motion is a sinusoidal function.

C. Response of an LTI System to a Complex Exponential Force

It must be emphasized that forces have no imaginary part in the physical world. Forces are always real. The trick will be to obtain solutions in terms of complex forces and to then compute the real part. If we apply the complex exponential of unit magnitude to the LTI system, we have

$$L[e^{j\omega t}] = f_o(t). \tag{45}$$

When a system is *time-invariant,* the response to a delayed input simply is a delayed output. The time-invariance property of the linear system can be expressed as

$$L[f_i(t + \tau)] = f_o(t + \tau). \tag{46}$$

Then Eq. (45) becomes

$$L[e^{j\omega(t+\tau)}] = f_o(t + \tau),$$
$$e^{j\omega\tau}L(e^{j\omega t}) = f_o(t + \tau), \tag{47}$$

since $e^{j\omega\tau}$ is a constant. Now let $t = 0$, and since τ is a dummy variable, from Eq. (45) we have

$$\begin{aligned} f_o(t) &= f_o(0)e^{j\omega t} \\ &= ke^{j\omega t}. \end{aligned} \tag{48}$$

Observe that the output is proportional to the input, where the proportionality constant k is complex and a function of ω. The complex constant k is called the system function and is denoted $H(j\omega)$. Expressing the system function $H(j\omega)$ in terms of its magnitude and phase, we have

$$H(j\omega) = |H(j\omega)|e^{j\theta(\omega)}. \tag{49}$$

The complex exponential, $e^{j\omega t}$, is called the *eigenfunction* of an LTI system, since, except for a change in phase and magnitude, the output function is identical to the input function. This assertion is illustrated in Fig. 10.

Now in actual practice, the response of an LTI system is obtained by measuring the response of the system to a real sinusoidal function. For example, earlier we obtained the frequency response of a filter (earphone) by noting the change in amplitude and phase of input sinusoids having different frequencies. We can, of course, confirm that this procedure is in agreement

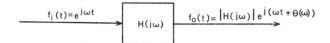

FIG. 10. Block diagram showing response of an LTI system to a complex exponential input.

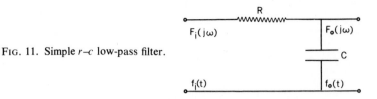

FIG. 11. Simple r–c low-pass filter.

with the present analysis of linear systems. Simply note that the real part of the input $e^{j\omega t}$ is cos ωt and the real part of the output $|H(j\omega)|$ $e^{j\omega t + \theta(\omega)}$ is $|H(j\omega)|\cos[\omega t + \theta(\omega)]$. That the observed steady-state output response of a filter is identical to the solution derived analytically lends support to the assertion that solutions in terms of complex exponentials are reasonable.

D. An Example of an LTI System: An r–c Low-Pass Filter

As an example of an LTI system, consider the electrical network shown in Fig. 11, consisting of the resistance–capacitance (r–c) circuit. The circuit can be analyzed as a simple voltage divider with resistances given by their *equivalent impedance*. The impedance of the capacitor is a function of frequency and is $1/j\omega c$. The system function can be written as

$$H(j\omega) = \frac{1/j\omega c}{r + 1/j\omega c} = \frac{1/rc}{j\omega + 1/rc}.$$ (50)

1. Amplitude Characteristic

The amplitude (magnitude) and phase characteristics of the filter's system function is simple to calculate by applying Eq. (42). The magnitude characteristic of the system is expressed analytically as

$$|H(j\omega)| = \left|\frac{1/rc}{j\omega + 1/rc}\right| = \left[\frac{(1/rc)^2}{(j\omega + 1/rc)(-j\omega + 1/rc)}\right]^{1/2}$$

$$= \left[\frac{\lambda^2}{\omega^2 + \lambda^2}\right]^{1/2},$$ (51)

where $\lambda = 1/rc$. It is convenient to plot the magnitude spectrum in terms of logarithmic units of decibels. Thus,

$$|H(j\omega)|_{dB} = 20 \log|H(j\omega)|$$
$$= 10 \log[\lambda^2/(2 + \lambda^2)].$$ (52)

A graphical representation of the magnitude spectrum is shown in Fig. 12. Observe that at the angular frequency $1/rc$ the amplitude is down 3 dB from its value at zero frequency. The frequency $1/rc$ is thus often used as the measure of the filter's bandwidth.

2. Phase Characteristic

The phase response of the filter is plotted linearly against the frequency scale in Fig. 12. Analytically the phase response is obtained by computing

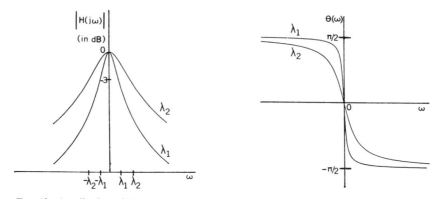

FIG. 12. Amplitude and phase response of the r–c filter shown in Fig. 11. Amplitude response (left figure) is plotted on a logarithmic (decibel) scale. Phase response (right figure) is plotted in π radians. The parameter is λ or $1/rc$. Note: $\lambda_1 < \lambda_2$.

the ratio of the imaginary to the real part of $H(j\omega)$. To obtain the real and imaginary parts of the system function $H(j\omega)$, we write Eq. (50) as

$$H(j\omega) = \frac{\lambda}{j\omega + \lambda} = \frac{(-j\omega + \lambda)\lambda}{(-j\omega + \lambda)(j\omega + \lambda)}$$
$$= \frac{-j\omega + \lambda^2}{\omega^2 + \lambda^2} .$$

Thus,

$$\mathrm{Re}[H(j\omega)] = \lambda^2/(\omega^2 + \lambda^2) ,$$
$$\mathrm{Im}[H(j\omega)] = -\omega/(\omega^2 + \lambda^2) ,$$
$$\theta(\omega) = \tan^{-1} -\omega/\lambda^2 . \tag{53}$$

VIII. MATHEMATICAL REPRESENTATION OF SIGNALS

A. Fourier Series and Discrete Spectra

The basic principle governing signal analysis was proposed by Fourier, who demonstrated that most functions can be represented mathematically as a sum of simple sinusoidal components having different frequencies. Each component in the set of sinusoidal functions has a characteristic amplitude and phase. This principle of Fourier analysis is applied first to the representation of *periodic* functions. A periodic function is any function for which $f(t) = f(t + T)$, where T is the period of the function. An example of a periodic function is the pulse train shown in Fig. 13.

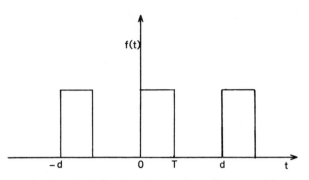

FIG. 13. An example of a periodic function. A pulse of amplitude A and duration T is repeated every d second.

1. TRIGONOMETRIC FOURIER SERIES

Fourier showed that a periodic function $f(t)$ with period T can be represented by the trigonometric Fourier series,

$$f(t) = C_0 + \sum_{n=1}^{\infty} C_n \cos(n\omega_0 t - \theta_n). \tag{54}$$

The function $f(t)$ consists of the sum of harmonically related sinusoidal components of frequency $\omega_n = n\omega_0 = 2\pi/T$. The first component in the sum ω_0 is called the fundamental, because it has the same period as $f(t)$. The numerical constants C_n, θ_n, give the magnitude and phase of each component and uniquely determine $f(t)$ in the frequency domain.

Taking advantage of the trigonometric identities depicted in Fig. 14, the trigonometric Fourier series can be rewritten as

$$f(t) = a_0/2 + \sum_{n=1}^{\infty} a_n \cos n\omega_0 t + b_n \sin n\omega_0 t, \tag{55}$$

where a_n and b_n are the Fourier coefficients.

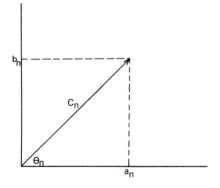

FIG. 14. Vector diagram relating two forms of the trigonometric Fourier series. $a_0 = 2C_0$; $a_n = C_n \cos \theta_n$; $b_n = C_n \sin \theta_n$; $\theta_n = \tan^{-1}(b_n/a_n)$.

The Fourier coefficients in Eq. (55) are derived by applying the *orthogonality property* of sine and cosine functions. From elementary calculus we obtain the following orthogonality relations:

$$\int_{-T/2}^{T/2} \sin n\omega_0 t \, \cos m\omega_0 t = 0,$$

$$\left.\begin{array}{c} \int_{-T/2}^{T/2} \cos n\omega_0 t \, \cos m\omega_0 t \\ \int_{-T/2}^{T/2} \sin n\omega_0 t \, \sin m\omega_0 t \end{array}\right\} = 0 \quad \text{if} \quad n \neq m, \quad T/2 \quad \text{if} \quad n = m, \tag{56}$$

where n and m are integers and $\omega_0 = 2\pi/T$. The Fourier coefficients can now be written as

$$a_n = 2/T \int_{-T/2}^{T/2} f(t) \, \cos n\omega_0 t \, dt, \tag{57}$$

$$b_n = 2/T \int_{-T/2}^{T/2} f(t) \, \sin n\omega_0 t \, dt. \tag{58}$$

It is easy to confirm that Eqs. (57) and (58) do indeed yield coefficients that satisfy Eq. (55). Simply multiply both sides of Eq. (55) by $\cos n\omega_0 t$ and take the average over one period T. As a result of the orthogonality relations in Eq. (56) all terms drop out except a_n. Passing $f(t)$ through integral Eqs. (57) and (58) yields the amplitude and phase of the sinusoidal components with which the function $f(t)$ can be synthesized.

2. CONVERGENCE OF THE FOURIER SERIES

The *convergence* of the Fourier series of $f(t)$ as the number of terms in the series increases is shown in Fig. 15. For the function in Fig. 15, we obtain the following Fourier series:

$$f(t) = 4\pi(\sin \omega_0 t + \tfrac{1}{3} \sin 3\omega_0 t + \tfrac{1}{5} \sin 5\omega_0 t + \cdots). \tag{59}$$

In Fig. 15, observe that as the number of terms increases, the resulting curves oscillate with increasing frequency and decreasing amplitude. Note that at the discontinuity of the time waveform the series approximation overshoots $f(t)$, even as the number of terms becomes large. This overshoot is called *Gibbs phenomenon*.

3. PARSEVAL'S THEOREM

The power in a wave is the average energy expended over time. Hence, for a periodic waveform, assuming a 1-Ω resistance,

$$\text{Power} = 1/T \int_{-T/2}^{T/2} f^2(t) \, dt$$

$$= 1/T \int_{-T/2}^{T/2} [a_0/2 + \sum_{n=1}^{\infty} a_n \cos n\omega_0 t + b_n \cos \omega_0 t]^2 \, dt. \tag{60}$$

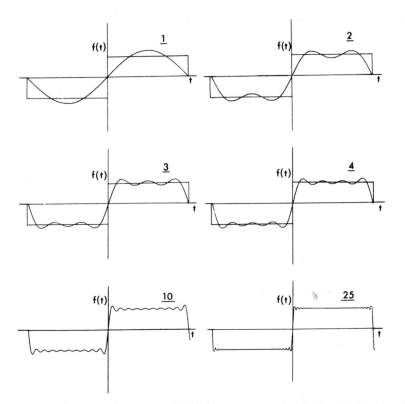

FIG. 15. Approximation of $f(t)$ by the finite Fourier series presented in Eq. (59). Each panel is labeled with respect to the number of terms used to approximate the function.

Because of the orthogonality property of sinusoidal functions, except for the squared terms, the integral of all cross-product terms of the type shown in Eq. (56) are zero. Then

$$1/T \int_{-T/2}^{T/2} f^2(t)\, dt = 1/T[Ta_0^2/4 + T/2(a_1^2 + a_2^2 + \cdots + b_1^2 + b_2^2 + \cdots)]$$

$$= a_0^2/4 + \tfrac{1}{2}\sum_{n=1}^{\infty} (a_n^2 + b_n^2). \tag{61}$$

Equation (61) is called *Parseval's theorem* and shows that the total power is the sum of the powers of all Fourier components. Taking advantage of the identities in Fig. 14, we have for the power of $f(t)$

$$1/T \int_{-T/2}^{T/2} f^2(t)\, dt = C_0^2 + \sum_{n=1}^{\infty} \left| \frac{C_n}{\sqrt{2}} \right|^2, \tag{62}$$

where $C_n/\sqrt{2}$ is the *root-mean-square power*.

B. Fourier Integral and Continuous Spectra

1. DEFINITION OF THE FOURIER TRANSFORM

Most waveforms encountered in the laboratory are *nonperiodic* functions. The Fourier representation of nonperiodic functions is called the Fourier integral. We define the Fourier integral or Fourier transform as

$$F(j\omega) = \int_{-\infty}^{\infty} f(t)e^{-j\omega t}\, dt. \tag{63}$$

Similarly, $f(t)$ is called the *inverse Fourier transform* and is

$$f(t) = (2\pi)^{-1} \int_{-\infty}^{\infty} F(j\omega)e^{j\omega t}\, d\omega. \tag{64}$$

Any nonperiodic function thus has two equivalent modes of representation: One function exists in the time domain, Eq. (64), and the other in the frequency domain, Eq. (63). Note that Eqs. (63) and (64) are analogous to Eqs. (58), (57), and (55) for the Fourier series representation.

The coefficient $F(j\omega)$ is complex and can be represented in *phasor form* as

$$F(j\omega) = |F(j\omega)| e^{j\theta(\omega)}. \tag{65}$$

Equation (64) then becomes

$$f(t) = (2\pi)^{-1} \int_{-\infty}^{\infty} |F(j\omega)| e^{j(\omega t+\theta(\omega))}\, d\omega. \tag{66}$$

The Fourier integral representation of $f(t)$ in Eq. (66) shows us that any function can be synthesized from a sum of complex exponentials of appropriate magnitude and phase spaced infinitesimally apart. We call the plots of $|F(j\omega)|$ and $\theta(\omega)$ versus ω the continuous *amplitude* and *phase* spectra of $f(t)$.

2. AN EXPLANATION OF NEGATIVE FREQUENCIES

Note that in Eq. (66) the summation includes both positive and negative frequency components. The notion of negative frequency may, at first inspection, seem somewhat strange. The conceptualization of a sinusoidal function as a rotating vector in the complex plane is especially helpful in understanding negative frequency. Suppose we want to employ a sinusoidal force, $a_n \cos n\omega_0 t$. Although it may seem absurd, let us suppose the force is actually complex. From Eq. (41), we can express the cosine function as the sum of two exponentials, $a_n/2(e^{jn\omega_0 t} + e^{-jn\omega_0 t})$. The cosine function, then, can be conceptualized in terms of two phasors of magnitude $a_n/2$ revolving about the origin at angular frequencies of $\pm n\omega_0$. Now in the real world, we can only experience the projection of the phasor on the real axis. From Fig. 9, it is seen that the real parts of the phasors representing positive and negative frequencies are $a_n/2 \cos n\omega_0 t$ and $a_n/2 \cos n\omega_0 t$, respectively. The real part of the nth harmonic is obtained by computing the sum of the projections of the nth positive and negative components on the real axis. Thus, for the nth harmonic we have $a_n \cos n\omega_0 t$, which is where we started before we introduced an imaginary part.

The presence of negative frequencies presents no special problem in the measurement of acoustic power. Since the functions we employ in the laboratory are always real, the magnitude of the nth positive harmonic is equal to the magnitude of the nth negative harmonic. Thus we need only sum the powers of those components in the positive frequency region.

3. COMPUTATION OF THE $\sin(x)/x$ SPECTRUM

To illustrate computation of the Fourier transform, let us find the Fourier transform of the rectangular pulse

$$f(t) = \begin{cases} A, & 0 \le t \le T, \\ 0, & \text{elsewhere.} \end{cases}$$

The Fourier transform is

$$F(j\omega) = \int_{-\omega}^{\omega} f(t)e^{-j\omega t} \, dt$$

$$= A \int_0^T e^{-j\omega t} \, dt = A \frac{e^{-j\omega t}}{-j\omega} \bigg|_0^T$$

$$= A \left[\frac{1 - e^{-j\omega T}}{j\omega} \right], \tag{67}$$

which can be rewritten as

$$F(j\omega) = \left[A \frac{e^{-j\omega T/2}}{\omega/2} \right] \left[\frac{e^{j\omega T/2} - e^{-j\omega T/2}}{2j} \right]. \tag{68}$$

Using Eq. (41), Eq. (68) is converted to the well-known trigonometric $\sin(x)/x$. We have

$$F(j\omega) = ATe^{-j\omega T/2} \frac{\sin \omega T/2}{\omega T/2}. \tag{69}$$

The Fourier transform of the pulse is a complex function of ω having the amplitude and phase spectra shown in Fig. 16. The rectangular pulse thus can be synthesized from an infinity of sinusoids whose amplitudes and phases are depicted in Fig. 16. The set of sinusoidal components have just the correct magnitudes and phase angles for complete cancellation in the interval $(-\infty, 0)$ and (T, ∞), and add up to the value A in the interval $(0, T)$.

Observe that the $\sin(x)/x$ amplitude spectrum is concentrated over a band of frequencies around the origin, with the first zero of the major lobe occurring at a radian frequency $\omega = 2\pi/T$. In terms of frequency, the first zero is at $f = 1/T$, since $\omega = 2\pi f$. Thus, as pulse duration is increased, the first zero moves closer to the origin and the magnitude of the spectrum at $f = 0$ in-

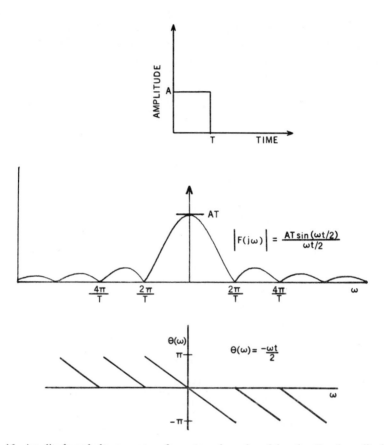

FIG. 16. Amplitude and phase spectra of a rectangular pulse of duration T and amplitude A.

creases with duration T. From inspection of Eq. (69), it is seen that the amplitude of frequency components away from the origin is independent of T. Thus, the longer the duration of the signal, the more concentrated the energy will be at the signal frequency. The inverse relationship between duration and frequency-spread characterizing the $\sin(x)/x$ spectrum is a general property of all signals.

4. Auditory Sensitivity to the $\sin(x)/x$ Spectrum

Investigations of auditory perception require that we be extremely careful about details of the frequency content of the stimulus. It is well known that the ear performs a spectral analysis of the auditory stimulus and is extremely sensitive to small differences in the spectrum. For example, Leshowitz (1971) has shown that observers can detect a 10-μsec gap between a pair of 10-μsec clicks by virtue of slight differences in the $\sin(x)/x$ amplitude spectrum in the region of 10,000 Hz.

Investigations of pure-tone masking have demonstrated that observers often base their detection of brief tones on the presence of signal energy in spectral regions remote from the signal, where signal energy is as much as 40 dB down from the on-frequency energy. In order to understand this result, it is necessary to describe the energy spectrum of a gated tonal signal.

The frequency-shifting property of the Fourier transform can be written as

$$\mathcal{F}\left[f(t)\cos\omega_0 t\right] = \tfrac{1}{2}F(\omega - \omega_0) + \tfrac{1}{2}F(\omega + \omega_0), \tag{70}$$

where $F(\omega) = \mathcal{F}\left[f(t)\right]$. Thus the amplitude spectrum of the cosine function of finite duration T is the spectrum of the pulse shown in Fig. 16 shifted along the frequency axis to $\pm\omega_0$. Although 90% of the signal's energy is located in a narrow band $2/T$ Hz wide, centered at the signal frequency, a considerable portion of the energy lies outside this frequency interval. In view of the large dynamic range of the auditory system, energy in the tails of the $\sin(x)/x$ function cannot be ignored. Indeed, Leshowitz and Wightman (1971) have argued that detection of a brief tone in the presence of a continuous tonal masker is improved when subjects monitor energy changes in regions remote from the signal. Moreover, seemingly trivial modifications of the distribution of signal energy across frequency can have profound effects on performance in both binaural and monaural masking experiments (Wightman, 1971).

5. ENERGY SPECTRUM

We have already shown that for a periodic function, the total power in a signal is the sum of the powers contained in the different discrete frequency components. The same approach can be extended to nonperiodic functions. If $f(t)$ is the voltage across a 1-Ω resistance, then the energy delivered by the source is the integral of the instantaneous power. Letting $F(j\omega)$ be the Fourier transform of $f(t)$, we have

$$E = \int_{-\infty}^{\infty} [f(t)]^2 \, dt = \int_{-\infty}^{\infty} f(t) \left[(2\pi)^{-1} \int_{-\infty}^{\infty} F(j\omega)e^{j\omega t} \right] dt. \tag{71}$$

Since the functions are uniformally continuous, we can rearrange the terms. Thus

$$E = (2\pi)^{-1} \int_{-\infty}^{\infty} F(j\omega) \left[\int_{-\infty}^{\infty} f(t)e^{j\omega t} \, dt \right] d\omega$$

$$= (2\pi)^{-1} \int_{-\infty}^{\infty} F(j\omega)F(-j\omega) \, d\omega$$

$$= (2\pi)^{-1} \int_{-\infty}^{\infty} F(j\omega)F^*(j\omega) \, d\omega$$

$$= (2\pi)^{-1} \int_{-\infty}^{\infty} |F(j\omega)|^2 \, d\omega. \tag{72}$$

Rewriting Eq. (72) in terms of frequency, we have

$$E = \int_{-\infty}^{\infty} |F(2\pi f)|^2 \, df. \tag{73}$$

Thus the total energy in the waveform is given by the quantity $|F(2\pi f)|^2$, called the *energy spectrum* or *energy spectral density*, summed across all frequencies.

6. EQUIVALENT RECTANGULAR BANDWIDTH

An especially useful description of the frequency spread of the rectangular pulse is its *equivalent rectangular* bandwidth (McGill, 1967). The *equivalent energy spectrum* is a constant and is concentrated in the region around the origin as shown in Fig. 17. The total energy of the pulse is given by the product of the equivalent energy spectral density and the equivalent bandwidth. The total energy of the pulse is equal to $(A^2 t^2)(1/T) = A^2 T$, which is as it should be.

7. MEASUREMENT OF THE CONTINUOUS SPECTRUM

In the laboratory, the continuous energy spectrum for a nonperiodic stimulus is measured as a discrete frequency spectrum. If we want to measure the frequency spectrum for the function presented in Fig. 17, we simply present the waveform as a train of identical rectangular pulses of amplitude A and duration T. The period of repetition d is generally on the order of five to ten times longer than signal duration T. It is straightforward to demonstrate that the magnitude of the Fourier series components $|C_n|$ for the periodic function is related to the magnitude of the Fourier transform of the pulse by the following relation:

$$|C_n| = 1/d \, |F_0(n\omega_0)|. \tag{74}$$

Equation (74) indicates that the Fourier components C_n are located at $\omega = n\omega_0$, where $\omega_0 = 2\pi/d$. The magnitude of each discrete component is identical to the continuous Fourier representation, except for a pro-

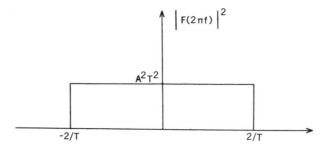

FIG. 17. Equivalent energy spectrum of a rectangular pulse. The pulse's *equivalent rectangular* bandwidth is $1/T$ Hz.

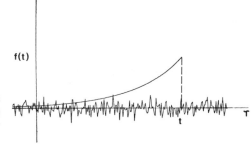

FIG. 18. Illustration of the short-time spectrum of $f(t)$. The time waveform is weighted by an exponential decay function.

portionality constant $1/d$. For example, if $d = 10$ msec and $T = 1$ msec, the envelope connecting the peaks of the components spaced 100 Hz apart traces out the $\sin(x)/x$ amplitude spectrum having its first zero at 1000 Hz. In actual laboratory measurement, the analyzing filter bandwidth of the wave analyzer should therefore be less than 100 Hz.* Calculation of the spectrum level of a transient waveform is illustrated in some detail in the appendix to a paper by Penner and Viemiester (1973).

8. SHORT-TIME SPECTRUM

From the fundamental definition of the Fourier transform in (63), it is seen that in order to determine the frequency content of a time waveform, it is necessary to perform an integration over an infinite range of time. Quite obviously, a perceiving organism does not perform an integration over an infinite range of time as required by the classical definition of *long-time* frequency spectrum. At best we carry out an integration within the limits $-\infty$ to the present time t. Moreover, a reasonable physical system does not have perfect memory for all information that has passed in time. Basic limitations imposed by memory processes must be taken into account when describing the human frequency-analyzing system.

One processing scheme that weights the most recent past history of the stimulus is the *short-time energy spectrum* (Flanagan, 1965; Kharkevich, 1960). As illustrated in Fig. 18, the spectrum is continuously computed over an integration interval given by the time constant of the exponential window. Windowing the function ensures that the most recent events are weighted most heavily. Note that the exponential weighting function is slid along the time axis, and therefore the spectrum itself is a continuous function of time. We refer to this spectrum as a *running* short-time spectrum.

* When measuring waveforms that have most of their power concentrated in a small proportion of their duration, one must be careful to avoid exceeding the *crest factor* of a true rms voltmeter. Crest factor is the ratio of the absolute value of the peak voltage to the full scale rms value and typically should not exceed 5.

The short-time spectrum is measured with real filters. Such a device is composed of a number of parallel channels. Each channel—consisting of a bandpass filter, square-law device, and a final integrator—develops the running average of the energy accumulated for some past time in a particular spectral region. The conventional speech spectrograph is an example of a short-time analyzer. It provides a record of the spectral composition of the acoustic message as a function of time. The magnitude of the energy is related to the darkness of the trace; the X and Y axes correspond to time and frequency, respectively.

In order to illustrate the time-development of the amplitude spectrum, consider a brief burst of tone gated on and off at zero crossings. Energy associated with different frequencies arrives at different times. The amplitude spectrum of the tone burst as a function of time is shown in Fig. 19, where it is seen that the spectrum is flat and of uniform amplitude near signal onset. With the passage of time a maximum develops at the frequency of the sinusoid. In the limit, as $t \rightarrow \infty$, the maximum approaches a discrete spectral line. Energy off the frequency of the signal, on the other hand, does not increase with signal duration.

The spectrum depicted in Fig. 19 is highly idealized inasmuch as it assumes a measuring instrument with perfect memory for all past time. The measurement of the spectrum by a real short-time analyzer would follow a

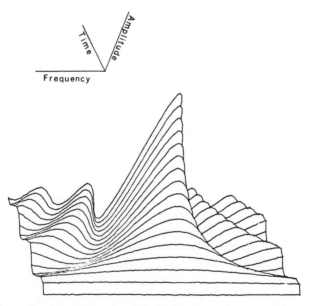

FIG. 19. The amplitude spectrum of a sinusoid plotted as a function of time. The amplitude, frequency, and time axes are shown in the inset.

somewhat different time course. To illustrate this point, consider the output of a single channel in a frequency region remote from the signal frequency. At signal onset an appreciable output is recorded as a result of energy "splatter" off the frequency of the signal. After some time has elapsed and a "steady-state" condition has been reached in which the initial burst of off-frequency energy splatter has decayed to an insignificant level, the output is considerably diminished. The short-time energy developed at the output of a filter thus reflects the arrival time of energy at different frequency regions. That the ear is extremely sensitive to the difference in arrival time has been confirmed in a number of investigations examining discrimination of auditory signals having identical long-time energy spectra (Green, 1971).

C. Addition of Sinusoidal Waveforms

One issue around which some ambiguity has developed concerns the energy spectrum of the *increment* resulting from the addition of two sinusoidal waveforms having the same frequency. Suppose a brief tone burst of duration T and amplitude S is added to a continuous sinusoid having amplitude P. The brief tone is called the *signal* and the long-duration tone, the *pedestal*. The phase difference between signal and masker is θ.

To compute the energy spectrum of the increment, we simply take the difference between the energy spectrum of the signal-plus-pedestal and the energy spectrum of the pedestal alone. Whereas the signal energy is distributed across frequency as $\sin^2(x)/x^2$, the pedestal is assumed to be a single spectral line at the pedestal frequency. Thus energy in the frequency region *off* the frequency of the signal is independent of the phase difference between signal and pedestal. As noted earlier, this off-frequency energy is also essentially independent of signal duration.

At the signal frequency, quite a different situation exists. The energy of the increment *is* sensitive to both relative phase and signal duration. Increment energy ΔE is proportional to the difference between the squared magnitudes of the two vectors corresponding to signal plus pedestal and pedestal alone. That is,

$$\Delta E = \text{SPT } \cos(\theta) + S^2 T/2. \tag{75}$$

It should also be noted that for signal and pedestal having *different* frequencies, the cross product in Eq. (75) is zero only when signal duration is greater than the reciprocal of the frequency separation.

The preceding description of the frequency content of the signal and masker in conjunction with a short-time energy detection model has been applied to several tonal masking studies. For a review of this work, see Leshowitz and Wightman (1971), Wightman (1971), and Leshowitz and Cudahy (1972).

IX. RESPONSE OF AN LTI SYSTEM TO A UNIT IMPULSE FUNCTION

Another method for measuring the system response of a device is to employ a brief pulse, called an *impulse*, as the input. The unit impulse, also known as a *delta* function, is defined by the relation

$$\delta(t) = 0 \qquad \text{if} \quad t \neq 0,$$
$$\delta(t) = \infty \qquad \text{if} \quad t = 0,$$

and

$$\int_{-\infty}^{\infty} \delta(t)\, dt = \int_{-\epsilon}^{\epsilon} \delta(t)\, dt = 1, \qquad \epsilon > 0. \tag{76}$$

The δ-function is finite only at the origin such that the integral in Eq. (76) is equal to unity. The δ-function, sometimes called the *unit* impulse, is also defined as a symbolic function by the integral

$$\int_{-\infty}^{\infty} \delta(t)f(t)\, dt = f(0). \tag{77}$$

In general we use δ-functions only in integral equations similar to Eq. (77).

A. The Convolution Integral

The response of an LTI system to a unit impulse $\delta(t)$ is denoted $h(t)$. Symbolically, this is expressed as

$$L[\delta(t)] = h(t). \tag{78}$$

If the system is time-invariant, we have

$$L[\delta(t - \tau)] = h(t - \tau). \tag{79}$$

The output $h(t)$ is the response of an LTI system to a unit impulse and is sometimes called the system's *impulse response*. From the basic property of the δ-function in Eq. (76) we can express $f_i(t)$ as

$$f_i(t) = \int_{-\infty}^{\infty} f_i(\tau)\delta(t - \tau)d\tau. \tag{80}$$

From Eqs. (39) and (78), we obtain

$$f_o(t) = L\left[\int_{-\infty}^{\infty} f_i(\tau)\delta(t - \tau)d\tau\right]$$
$$= \int_{-\infty}^{\infty} f_i(\tau)L[\delta(t - \tau)]d\tau$$
$$= \int_{-\infty}^{\infty} f_i(\tau)h(t - \tau)d\tau. \tag{81}$$

Equation (81) is a *convolution* integral, and indicates that the response of an LTI system is the convolution of the input function and the impulse response of the system. All physically *realizable* systems are *causal*. That is, $h(t) = 0$ for $t < 0$. Therefore, the integrand in Eq. (81) is zero in the interval $\tau = t$ to $\tau = \infty$. Thus, we obtain

$$f_o(t) = \int_{-\infty}^{t} f_i(\tau)h(t - \tau)\,d\tau. \tag{82}$$

The convolution integral tells us that the present output $f_o(t)$ is the sum of all past inputs weighted by the impulse response reversed in time. The short-time spectrum shown in Fig. 18 provides a visualization of convolution in which the system's impulse response is of the form $e^{-t/\lambda}$. The output $f_o(t)$ is the sum of the products of $e^{(\tau-t)/\lambda}$ and $f_i(\tau)$ for $\tau < t$.

B. Time Convolution Theorem

Convolution is expressed symbolically as

$$f_o(t) = f_i(t)*h(t). \tag{83}$$

The output is represented in the frequency domain by its Fourier transform, $F_o(j\omega) = \mathfrak{F}[f_i(t)*h(t)]$. We now make use of the time-convolution theorem which we state without proof:

$$\mathfrak{F}[f_1(t)*f_2(t)] = F_1(j\omega)F_2(j\omega). \tag{84}$$

Thus we obtain

$$F_o(j\omega) = \mathfrak{F}[f_i(t)*h(t)] = F_i(j\omega)H(j\omega), \tag{85}$$

where $H(j\omega)$ is the system function. The system function $H(j\omega)$ is thus the ratio of the response transform to the source transform, i.e.,

$$H(j\omega) = F_o(j\omega)/F_i(j\omega). \tag{86}$$

$H(j\omega)$ acts as a weighting function or filter for different frequency components in the input. This alteration of the magnitude and phase of components in the input is illustrated symbolically in Fig. 20.

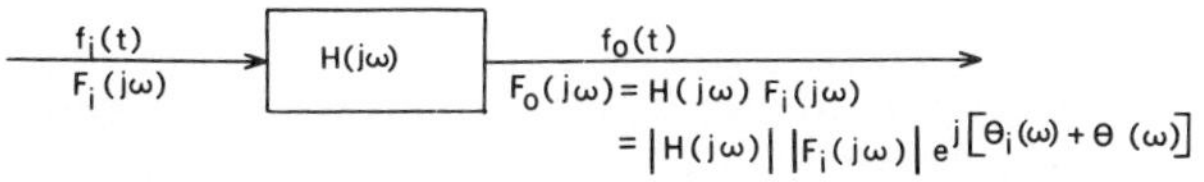

FIG. 20. Block diagram of the filtering characteristic of the linear–time-invariant system.

The energy–density spectrum of the output is computed by taking complex conjugates and we obtain

$$\begin{aligned}|F_o(j\omega)|^2 &= [H(j\omega)F_i(j\omega)][H^*(j\omega)F_i^*(j\omega)] \\ &= |H(j\omega)|^2 |F_i(j\omega)|^2. \end{aligned} \tag{87}$$

The quantity $|H(j\omega)|^2$ is called the *energy transfer function*, since it maps the input to the output energy. An example illustrating the application of energy transfer function to random signals is given in the next section.

As already mentioned, the output of an LTI system produced in response to a unit impulse at the input is the system's impulse response, $h(t)$. This result leads to a simple procedure for measuring a *real* device's system function, $H(j\omega)$. Suppose we present a brief pulse to a system whose transfer function in unknown. In general, the duration of the pulse should be less than the reciprocal of the estimated passband. The observed output waveform is the system's impulse response. The Fourier transform of $h(t)$ provides a complete description of the system. Recent advances in digital signal processing and *fast Fourier transform* techniques now enable us to compute the Fourier transform of a function extremely rapidly on small general-purpose computers. A discussion of digital signal processing techniques is beyond the scope of this chapter. For a review of digital filtering and related topics, the text by Gold and Rader (1969) is highly recommended.

X. RANDOM SIGNALS

Until now we have considered only *deterministic* signals, where a mathematical function specifies the waveform for all time. *Random* signals, on the other hand, are described in terms of their statistical properties, and therefore perfect prediction of the function at some future or past time is impossible.

A. Autocorrelation

The statistical properties of random signals are illustrated through a discussion of the *average autocorrelation functions*, denoted $\bar{R}_{11}(\tau)$ and the *average power spectra*, denoted $P(\omega)$. We begin with the autocorrelation function which is defined as

$$\bar{R}_{11}(\tau) = \lim_{T \to \infty} 1/T \int_{-T/2}^{T/2} f_1(t) f_1(t - \tau) \, dt. \tag{88}$$

As with any correlation statistic, $\bar{R}_{11}(\tau)$ provides a measure of the similarity or interdependence between two functions. For autocorrelation they are the original function $f_1(t)$ and the function delayed in time $f_1(t - \tau)$. If the autocorrelation is zero, then the original function and the function delayed by τ seconds are said to be uncorrelated.

The autocorrelation of a sine wave provides an illustrative example of the autocorrelation function and is shown in Fig. 21. For $\tau = 0$, the two functions are identical; therefore, the autocorrelation function normalized by the power of the sine wave is unity. Now suppose the sine wave is delayed by one-quarter of a period. Examination of the left panel of Fig. 21 reveals that the sum of the products of $f(t)$ and $f(t - \tau)$ over one period is zero. Therefore the autocorrelation is identically equal to zero. Now for a delay of one-half period, by inspection we can see the correlation is -1. Finally a one-period delay produces unity correlation. The average autocorrelation function of the sine wave is plotted in the right panel of Fig. 21, where it is seen that $\bar{R}_{11}(\tau)$ is a cosine wave of the same frequency as that of the sine wave. In general, $\bar{R}_{11}(\tau)$ for a periodic function is also periodic with the same period.

B. Power Spectra

The average power spectrum of $f(t)$ is defined by the quantity

$$P(\omega) = \lim_{T \to \infty} 1/T \left| \int_{-T/2}^{T/2} f(t) e^{-j\omega t} \, dt \right|^2 . \tag{89}$$

The presence of absolute value bars in Eq. (89) indicates that we cannot synthesize $f(t)$ from $P(\omega)$, since all phase information is lost in calculating the absolute value. It can be shown that the power spectrum of $f(t)$ is the Fourier transform of the average autocorrelation of $f(t)$. We define the Fourier transform pair

$$P(\omega) = \int_{-\infty}^{\infty} \bar{R}_{11}(\pi) e^{-j\omega\tau} \, d\tau, \tag{90}$$

$$\bar{R}_{11}(\tau) = (2\pi)^{-1} \int_{-\infty}^{\infty} P(\omega) e^{j\omega\tau} \, d\omega. \tag{91}$$

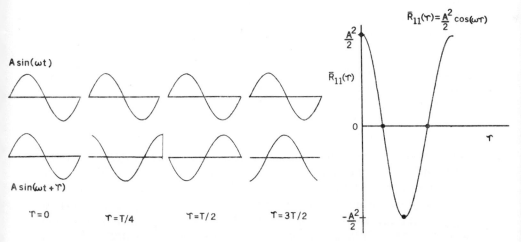

FIG. 21. Average autocorrelation of a sine wave, $A \sin \omega t$. The four values of τ yield the four values on the autocorrelation function.

From the basic definition of $\bar{R}_{11}(\tau)$ in Eq. (88), together with the definition of average power in Eq. (25), it follows that the total average power of $f(t)$ is given by

$$\bar{R}_{11}(0) = \lim_{T \to \infty} 1/T \int_{-T/2}^{T/2} [f(t)]^2 \, dt$$
$$= (2\pi)^{-1} \int_{-\infty}^{\infty} P(\omega) \, d\omega = \int_{-\infty}^{\infty} P(2\pi f) \, df. \tag{92}$$

Equation (92) is analogous to Parseval's theorem, developed for periodic signals, and states that the total average power of a random waveform is given by the integration of $P(2\pi f)$ over the entire frequency range. The quantity $P(2\pi f)$ is the average power per unit bandwidth and has the dimensions of energy.

1. WHITE NOISE

The concepts of autocorrelation and power spectrum are now applied to white noise, a random signal for which we find abundant use in psychoacoustics. White noise is defined as a random signal whose average power spectrum $P(\omega)$ is a constant, independent of frequency. In the psychoacoustic literature, white noise is usually specified in terms of the quantity $P(2\pi f)$, called *noise spectral density* and is denoted N_0. If the average power spectrum $P(\omega)$ of white noise is k, from Eq. (91) we have

$$\bar{R}_{11}(\tau) = (2\pi)^{-1} \int_{-\infty}^{\infty} P(\omega) e^{j\omega\tau} \, d\omega$$
$$= K(2\pi)^{-1} \int_{-\infty}^{\infty} e^{j\omega\tau} \, d\omega. \tag{93}$$

From the basic definition of Fourier transform in Eq. (64), the integral in Eq. (93) is recognized as the inverse transform of the constant 1. It can be shown that the Fourier transform of a constant is equal to the delta function; i.e.,

$$(2\pi)^{-1} \int_{-\infty}^{\infty} e^{j\omega\tau} \, d\omega = \delta(\tau). \tag{94}$$

Hence, we obtain

$$\bar{R}_{11}(\tau) = K\delta(\tau). \tag{95}$$

The average autocorrelation function of white noise is an impulse centered at the origin $(\tau = 0)$. For all other values of τ, $\bar{R}_{11}(\tau)$ is zero. This result is consistent with our intuitions about the random nature of a noise process.

Input–output relations characterizing linear systems discussed earlier for deterministic functions can also be developed when the input is a random signal. For random input, the output power spectrum is related to the input power spectrum through the energy transfer function as follows:

$$P_o(\omega) = |H(j\omega)|^2 P_i(\omega). \tag{96}$$

Application of power spectra to system analysis is illustrated in the following problem.

Let white noise serve as input to the r–c low-pass filter shown in Fig. 11. The system function of the rc network is given by

$$H(j\omega) = \frac{(rc)^{-1}}{j\omega + (rc)^{-1}}.$$
(50)

The power spectrum of the input white noise is

$$P_i(\omega) = K.$$

From Eq. (96) the output power spectrum is simply

$$P_o(\omega) = |H(j\omega)|^2 P_i(\omega)$$
$$= \frac{(1/rc)^2}{\omega^2 + (1/rc)^2 K}.$$
(97)

Power spectra of the input and output are shown in Fig. 22. Observe in Eq. (96) that the output power spectrum is identical to the energy transfer function $|H(j\omega)|^2$, since the power spectrum of white noise is a constant. Measurement of input–output relations for white noise is often used to specify the system's transfer function. Finally, from Eq. (99), the total power in the output can be evaluated and is

$$\lim_{T \to \infty} 1/T \int_{-T/2}^{T/2} [y(t)]^2 \, dt = (2\pi)^{-1} \int_{-\infty}^{\infty} P_o(\omega) \, d\omega$$
$$= \frac{K}{(2\pi)^{-1}(rc)^2} \int_{-\infty}^{\infty} \frac{d\omega}{\omega^2 + (1/rc)^2}$$
$$= K/2rc.$$
(98)

2. Energy Fluctuations of Noise

Additional insight into the random properties of noise is obtained through an analysis of the probability density of instantaneous noise amplitude. The

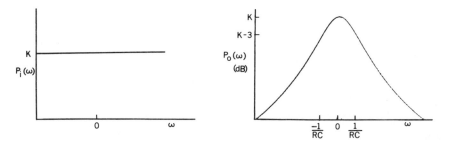

FIG. 22. The power spectrum of the output of an r–c (low-pass) filter when white noise is the input. Input power spectrum is shown on the left.

probability density function relates the probability the noise process instantaneously dwells at a given amplitude. Consider a band-limited noise waveform having bandwidth W and duration T. The probability density function is Gaussian having a mean of zero and a variance equal to the total average power [see Eq. (92)]. Therefore, approximately 68% of the instantaneous noise amplitudes will be within ± 1 *root-mean-square-power* unit.

The fluctuation of *energy* of brief noise bursts also has a familiar distribution. It is well known that a Gaussian deviate squared is distributed as χ^2 with 1 *df*. Thus the *sum* of the instantaneous noise amplitudes squared, which is the energy of a burst of noise, is distributed as χ^2 with N *df*. The product of bandwidth W and duration T determines the degrees of freedom. Now as N increases, from the central-limit theorem, we know the distribution of energy becomes Gaussian. Since the mean and variance of a χ^2 are equal to the degrees of freedom and $2 \times df$, respectively, the ratio of the mean to standard deviation is equal to $(WT/2)^{1/2}$. Hence, the reliability of noise power measurements improves with the square-root of the duration, a result which is in agreement with the $\sqrt{N}$-notion characterizing statistical reliability. The equivalence between the fluctuation statistics of noise and well-known statistical quantities is reviewed by Green and McGill (1970).

XI. NONLINEAR SYSTEMS

Thus far, we have considered the linear system in which

$$f_0(t) = Kf_i(t), \tag{99}$$

where K is a constant. Suppose that the system response is nonlinear. An example of a nonlinear response is the square law characteristic

$$f_0(t) = Kf_i^2(t). \tag{100}$$

A nonlinear system distorts the output; that is, frequency components not contained in the input are introduced into the output. The response of linear and nonlinear systems when the input is a sine wave is shown in Fig. 23.

A. Output of a Square-Law Characteristic

Let us derive the frequency content of the output of the square-law device when the input consists of two frequency components. From Eq. (100), the output is given by

$$\begin{aligned} f_0(t) &= K(A \cos \omega_1 t + B \cos \omega_2 t)^2 \\ &= K(A^2 \cos^2 \omega_1 t + B^2 \cos^2 \omega_2 t + 2AB \cos \omega_1 t \cos \omega_2 t). \end{aligned} \tag{101}$$

From the equality $\cos^2 \theta = 1/2(1 + \cos 2\theta)$, we have

$$\begin{aligned} f_0(t) = K[&(A^2/2) + (A^2/2 \cos 2\omega_1 t) + B^2/2 + (B^2/2 \cos 2\omega_2 t) \\ &+ 2AB \cos \omega_1 t \cos \omega_2 t]. \end{aligned} \tag{102}$$

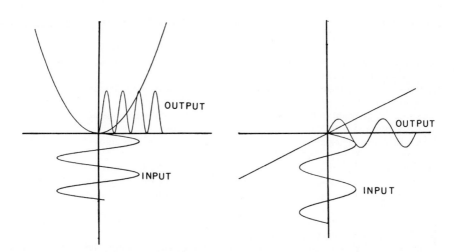

FIG. 23. Linear (right) and quadratic (left) input–output characteristics. The output points are obtained by projecting the input up to the characteristic curve. For the nonlinear case, the input sinusoid is transformed into a d–c shifted sinusoid having twice the original frequency. The linear characteristic merely attenuates the sinusoidal input.

Observe that the output consists of the following terms: A constant that produces a shift of the average value; second harmonics of the input frequencies; and a cross-product term. Rewriting the cross-product in terms of sum and difference frequencies, we have

$$2AB \cos \omega_1 t \cos \omega_2 t = AB \cos(\omega_1 + \omega_2)t + AB \cos(\omega_1 - \omega_2). \quad (103)$$

To sum up, a nonlinear system will change the average level of the input, generate higher harmonics of the input frequencies, and produce components at the sum and difference frequencies. These effects have important practical implications. In psychoacoustics, for example, it has been observed that the ear is itself nonlinear, producing distortion tones not in the original stimulus.

References

Dallos, P. Combination tone $2f_1 - f_h$ in microphonic potentials. *Journal of the Acoustical Society of America*, 1969, **46**, 1437–1444.

Denes, P. B., & Pinson, E. N. *The speech chain*. Murray Hill, New Jersey: The Bell Laboratories, 1963.

Feynman, R. P., Leighton, R. B., & Sands, M. *The Feynman lectures on physics*. Vol. 1, Reading, Massachusetts: Addison-Wesely, 1963.

Flanagan, J. L. *Speech analysis, synthesis and perception*. New York: Academic Press, 1965.

Gold, B., & Rader, C. M. *Digital processing of signals*. New York: McGraw-Hill, 1969.

Green, D. M. Temporal auditory acuity. *Psychological Review*, 1971, **78**, 540–551.

Green, D. M., & McGill, W. J. On the equivalence of detection probabilities and well-known statistical quantities. *Psychological Review*, 1970, **77**, 294–301.

Hsu, H. P. *Outline of Fourier analysis including problems with step-by-step solutions*. New York: Unitech, 1967.

Kharkevich, A. A. *Spectra and analysis*. New York: Consultants Bureau, 1960.

Leshowitz, B. Measurement of the two-click threshold. *Journal of the Acoustical Society of America*, 1971, **49**, 462–466.

Leshowitz, B., & Cudahy, E. Masking with continuous and gated sinusoids. *Journal of the Acoustical Society of America*, 1972, **51**, 1921–1929.

Leshowitz, B., & Wightman, F. L. On-frequency masking with continuous sinusoids. *Journal of the Acoustical Society of America*, 1971, **49**, 1180–1190.

McGill, W. J. Neural counting mechanisms and energy detection in audition. *Journal of Mathematical Psychology*, 1967, **4**, 351–376.

Papoulis, A. *The fourier integral and its applications*. New York: McGraw-Hill, 1962.

Penner, M. J., & Viemiester, N. F. Intensity discrimination of clicks: The effects of click bandwidth and background noise. *Jorunal of the Acoustical Society of America*, 1973, **54**, 1184–1188.

Peterson, A. P. G., & Gross, E. E., Jr. *Handbook of noise measurement*. (6th ed.) Concord, Massachusetts: General Radio Company, 1967.

Roederer, J. G. *Introduction to the physics and psychophysics of music*. New York: Springer-Verlag, 1973.

Wightman, F. L. Detection of binaural tones as a function of masker bandwidth. *Journal of the Acoustical Society of America*, 1971, **50**, 623–636.

Chapter 4

BIOPHYSICS OF THE COCHLEA*

PETER DALLOS

I. ANATOMY

The cochlea is the most highly developed and complex mechano-receptor system. Its complexity is manifested both in its functional organization and in its anatomical and structural features. Functionally, the cochlea is a multistage transducer that converts pressure changes to electrical nerve impulses with intermediate processes of mechanical deformation and electrochemical events. The salient anatomical features† of the cochlea can be followed with the aid of Figs. 1 and 2, which provide an overall view of the peripheral auditory system as well as a cross section of the actual sensory structure, the *organ of Corti*. The mammalian cochlea is a snail-shaped cavity forming a part of the bony labyrinth and communicating with the remainder of this labyrinth: the bony vestibular system. The cochlear cavity itself is divided into three longitudinal channels by a spiraling bony shelf—the osseous *spiral lamina*—that continues in the *basilar membrane* to form one of the boundaries, and by *Reissner's membrane* that consitutes the other boundary. The channel between the bony wall and Reissner's membrane is known as the *scala vestibuli*, that between the bony wall and the basilar membrane as

---

* The original work reported in this chapter was supported by grants from the National Institute of Neurological and Communicative Diseases and Stroke, NIH.

† Discussions of anatomical and morphological features are based on Iurato (1967), Spoendlin (1966), and Dallos (1973b).

the *scala tympani*. The channel between the basilar membrane and Reissner's membrane is designated as the *scala media* or *cochlear duct*. The entire structure between and including Reissner's membrane and the basilar membrane is also known as the *cochlear partition*. This partition is closed at the far end of the cochlea, proximal to the apical bony wall, and thus communication is allowed between the two outer scalae through an opening known as the helicotrema. The outer scalae are filled with perilymph, a fluid with ionic concentration quite similar to that of interstitial fluid. Perilymph is high in sodium content and low in potassium. In contrast, the fluid within the cochlear duct, endolymph, is very high in its potassium concentration and quite low in sodium. Thus, the cochlea is made up of two fluid systems, that are highly dissimilar in their ionic properties. Communication between the fluid-filled cochlea and the air-filled middle ear is via two openings in the bony wall separating these two parts of the ear. The innermost ossicle, the stapes, fills one of these openings, called the *oval window*. The footplate of the stapes is held in the window by a flexible annular ligament, and the cochlear side of this footplate is in contact with the perilymph filling the scala vestibuli. The other opening to the middle ear is the so-called *round window*,

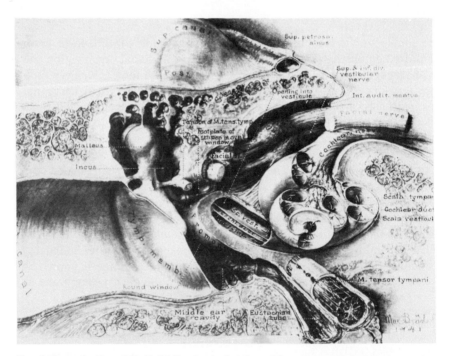

FIG. 1. Reproduction of M. Brödel's classic drawing of the cross section of the human ear. [From Brödel (1946), *Three Unpublished Drawings of the Anatomy of the Human Ear*. Copyright 1946 by W. B. Saunders.]

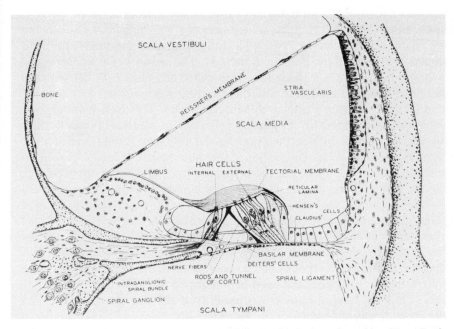

FIG. 2. Drawing of the cross section of the second turn of the guinea pig cochlea. [From Davis and associates (1953).]

which is a hole in the bony wall over the scala tympani. The opening is covered by a thin flexible layer, the *round window membrane*.

The central bony core of the cochlea is called the *modiolus*. Through it, the fibers of the cochlear branch of the 8th nerve and the blood supply enter the cochlea. The nerve fibers fan out from the modiolus in narrow channels within the *osseous spiral lamina* and approach the *organ of Corti*. The organ itself runs the length of the cochlear duct and consists of a supporting framework and the sensory cells. The supporting structures are largely cellular, they rest on the basilar membrane and form a stiff matrix that probably functions to transmit motions of the basilar membrane to the sensory cells that are embedded in the matrix. The primary stiffness of the supporting frame is provided by the two rows of pillar cells, or *rods of Corti*, that form an inverted V-shaped tunnel. Major support is also provided by *Deiters' cells*, whose bodies rest on the basilar membrane and which extend slender, stiff phalangeal processes toward the top of the organ of Corti. These processes along with extensions of the pillar cells fan out to form a rigid plate that caps the entire supporting matrix. This plate, known as the *reticular lamina*, provides the major structural support for the tops of the sensory cells that are suspended from it, as well as the primary ionic barrier between perilymph and endolymph. The various spaces within the organ of Corti are filled with a fluid that is probably not substantially different from perilymph. The organ of Corti also contains other types of supporting cells, such as the *inner phalangeal* and *border cells* toward the modiolus, and the *Hensen* and *Claudius cells* toward the outside of the coil. The sensory cells are arranged in two groups. There is a single row of so-called *inner hair cells* between the inner pillars and the modiolus, and three or four rows of *outer hair cells* are found between Hensen's cells and the outer pillars. The inner hair cells are completely surrounded by supporting cells, but in contrast, the outer hair cells are supported only at their top by the reticular lamina and at their bottom by Deiters' cells. The bodies of the outer hair cells are suspended in the fluid that fills the spaces of the organ of Corti. The nerve fibers emerge from the spongy bone of the osseous spiral lamina through openings called *habenulae perforata*, and enter the organ of Corti. The vast majority (95%) of afferent fibers approach the nearest inner hair cells and provide simple one-to-one innervation to them. About 5% of the afferents travel between the pillars and through the tunnel of Corti and innervate groups of the outer hair cells after a long and tortuous course. Each of the latter fibers can innervate about 10 outer hair cells, and each cell might be innervated from about 10 fibers. Thus the overall innervation patterns of the two groups of sensory cells are radically different.

The organ of Corti is supplied with efferent as well as afferent innervation. The efferent fibers originate in the olivary nuclei of the brainstem, about $\frac{4}{5}$ on the contralateral side, the remainder on the ipsilateral side. There are, altogether, about 500 efferent fibers aimed at each organ of Corti. These fibers provide connections with the afferent dendrites originating from the inner hair cells, and primarily with the cell bodies of the outer hair cells. The latter innervation is graded spatially, in that the richest efferent supply is in the first cochlear turn, and it gradually thins out toward the far end, the apex. There is a possibility that the efferent supply to the outer hair cells is primarily contralateral in origin.

A few more highly important cochlear structures need yet to be mentioned. Suspended above the reticular lamina from the spiral limbus (an enlargement of the epithelial lining of the bony cochlea) is the noncellular, gellike tectorial membrane. This membrane is loosely attached to the organ of Corti in the border cell region by slender processes, the *trabeculae of Hensen's stripe*, and by similar processes, the marginal net, over Hensen's cells (Lim, 1972). Some of the tallest hairs that emanate from the tops of the hair cells are in firm contact with the bottom layer of the tectorial membrane. This contact facilitates the transmission of movement from the tectorial membrane to the hair cells. We shall consider the details of the relationship between hairs and tectorial membrane later, in light of the functional significance of the physical arrangement.

The surface of the outer wall of the cochlear duct is lined with a dense layer of tissue containing a capillary network. This band of tissue is known as the *stria vascularis*. It is a site of intense metabolic activity, and its apparent primary function is the secretion of endolymph into the cochlear duct.

The morphological features of inner and outer hair cells are quite different in detail, even though some of the most significant structures show considerable similarity. As one can see from the schematic pictures of Fig. 3, the outer hair cells are regularly shaped slender cylindrical cells whose length is graded from the base to the apex of the cochlea and varies between approximately 30 and 70 μm, being longest in the apex. The diameter of the cells is fairly constant, about 6–7 μm. The inner hair cells are much more irregular in shape, they have a larger volume, and show no apparent grading in length along the longitudinal dimension of the cochlea. Both types of hair cells terminate superiorly in an irregularly shaped, very dense-appearing cuticular plate. This plate covers the entire apical pole of the cells, with the exception of a small roughly circular opening at the top border of the cell facing away from the modiolus. In this opening one can find in some species (in all species during embryonic development) a basal body that is, however, almost invariably devoid of a kinocilium. Even when the basal body is absent, the only separation between the inside of the cell and the adjacent endolymph is the cell's plasma membrane. The stereocilia, or sensory hairs, are anchored in the cuticular plate by long slender rootlets. There are 40–60 hairs on each inner hair cell, and 100–120 on each outer hair cell. The length of the latter hairs is graded from base to apex, changing between 4 and 8 μm. There is a strong spatial pattern to these hairs. Those of the outer hair cells form three or four rows, each in the shape of a "W". The open end of the "W" faces toward the modiolus. The row of hairs farthest from the modiolus is the tallest, and apparently only this tallest row of hairs contacts the bottom of the tectorial membrane. The inner hair cell hairs are also organized in an extremely shallow "W"; so shallow, that it can be considered that these hairs are aligned in relatively straight rows in the longitudinal direction.

In the vicinity of the cuticle-free region at the apical pole of the cells, there is a marked accumulation of mitochondria, lysosomes, and Golgi apparatus. A very large number of mitochondria, along with subsurface cisternae, can also be seen along the elongated free borders of the outer hair cells. These various endoplasmic organelles mark the sites of the highest metabolic activity within the cells, and suggest the location of transducer action.

In the infranuclear region of the cells (most apparently in the inner hair cells), one can distinguish numerous presynaptic structures, such as agglomerations of vesicles and synaptic bars. It is this region where adjacent nerve endings apparently form chemical synapses with the hair cell body.

The cochlea consumes a great deal of energy, and consequently it possesses an extensive network of blood vessels that supply its oxygen requirement. The cochlear artery is derived from a branch of the basilar artery, it enters the inner ear through the internal auditory meatus together with the

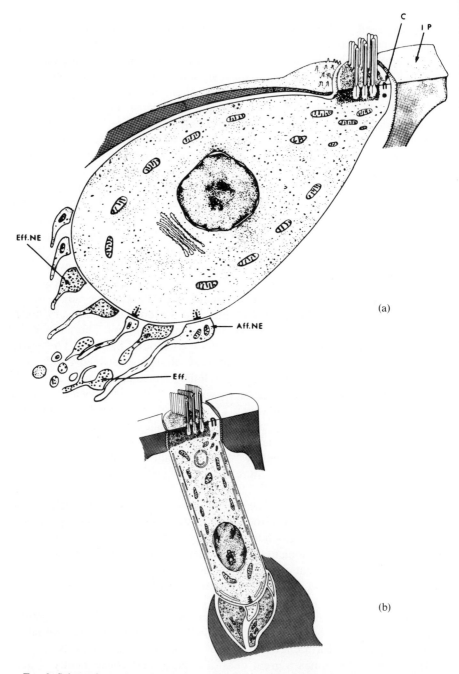

FIG. 3. Schematic cross section of inner (a) and outer (b) hair cells of the organ of Corti. Both afferent and efferent nerve terminations are shown. [From Wersäll, Flock, and Lundquist (1965), Structural basis for directional sensitivity in cochlear and vestibular sensory receptors, *Cold Spring Harbor Symposia on Quantitative Biology,* **30,** 115–145.]

cochlear nerve, and it distributes arterial blood to the cochlea via two major pathways. One of these is the stria vascularis whose extensive capillary bed is supplied by small branches of the cochlear artery. The other major source of arterial blood to the organ of Corti is obtained from the spiral vessel that runs longitudinally under the basilar membrane. The sense organ receives nutrition both from the spiral vessel and from the stria vascularis by way of the endolymph. There are no capillaries within the organ of Corti itself.

II. COCHLEAR MECHANICS

A. Gross Motion Patterns

Under most conditions, the activating signal for the cochlea is provided by the vibratory motion of the innermost ossicle, the stapes. The general scheme of events that follows the movement of *the stapes* can be described by the following simplified sequence. An inward displacement of the stapes produces a condensation (increase in density) in the perilymph adjacent to the oval window, whereas an outward motion results in rarefaction (decrease in density). Concomitant with the local density change, a pressure change also accompanies the movement of the stapes footplate. The pressure imbalance across the cochlear partition equilibrates by setting the latter in motion. The resulting mechanical energy exchange between the moving partition and the surrounding fluid is manifested by a characteristic wave pattern, which is sustained by the partition and progresses from its basal region toward the apex. This traveling wave possesses several important features, the most significant of which is the well-defined amplitude maximum that occurs at a distinct point along the partition when the stimulus is a sinusoid. The relation between the location where the amplitude achieves its maximal value and the frequency of the harmonic stimulus is such that high frequencies generate maxima toward the base, whereas low frequencies do so toward the apex. This mapping of frequencies along the spatial extent of the cochlear partition is a manifestation of the functioning of the inner ear as a mechanical frequency analyzer.

The actual motion of structures within the bone-encased, fluid-filled cochlea is made possible by the presence of the flexible round window membrane, which provides a pressure release mechanism. Since the cochlear fluids are largely incompressible, and are trapped within a rigid-walled cavity, provision of a pressure release is necessary to facilitate movements of the stapes and of the cochlear partition.

The traveling wave pattern that is sustained by the partition was first observed by Békésy (1960, pp. 429–446) in cadaver preparations. Subsequently the quantitative properties of the wave were delineated by him (Békésy, 1960, pp. 500–510; 460–469) and later by others (Johnstone & Boyle, 1967; Rhode, 1971; Wilson & Johnstone, 1972). Thus our descriptions of the various properties of the traveling wave are based on observation and measurement, rather than speculation.

A good way to become acquainted with the properties of the traveling wave is to consider the sketches of the instantaneous waveforms shown in Fig. 4a. Here the membrane positions are drawn for four successive time instants when the stimulus is a given sinusoid. The basal end of the cochlea is to the left of the picture, the amplitude of vibrations is grossly exaggerated, and the dotted lines depict an envelope, within which all vibrations are confined for a given stimulus. Figure 4b shows the first spatial derivative of the traveling wave. We shall utilize this part of the figure in later discussions. Several features are clearly shown in Fig. 4a. Among these is the gentle rise of the envelope to a peak displacement and the more rapid decay of vibrations beyond the peak. The waveforms clearly indicate the progression of the effect away from the base, these also show that the wavelength gradually decreases with distance. It has been noted, and follows from acoustic considerations as well, that along with the decrease of the wavelength, the speed of propagation also diminishes with distance. For most audio frequencies (except for the very lowest ones), the vibrations do not travel the entire length of the cochlear partition, but are extinguished before reaching the helicotrema. The decrease of amplitude, propagation velocity, and wavelength occur together distal to the location of the peak amplitude. We have already mentioned that the peak occurs at points along the membrane that are determined by the driving frequency. The relation is roughly logarithmic, in that a plot of the logarithm of the peak-frequency versus linear-peak-distance is approximately a straight line. The tuning of given cochlear locations to specific stimulus frequency is the most distinctive feature of the peripheral auditory system. An investigation of the sharpness of the tuning is one of the central concerns of auditory biophysics, a problem that is not completely resolved and is not free of controversy. The earliest measures of tuning were provided by Békésy (1960, pp. 446–460), who visually measured the relative amplitude of vibrations as a function of stimulus frequency at six positions along the cochlear partition of a cadaver. His

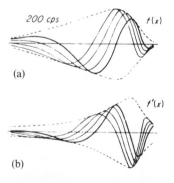

(a)

(b)

FIG. 4. Traveling waves along the basilar membrane at successive instants in time. The envelopes are indicated by the broken lines. Shown are the displacement wave (a) and its spatial derivative (b). [From *Experiments in Hearing* by G. von Békésy (1960, p. 499). Copyright 1960 by McGraw-Hill. Used with permission of the McGraw-Hill Book Company.]

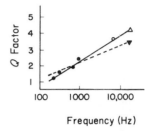

FIG. 5. Relation of Q and best frequency of cochlear tuning curves. Dashed line is after Tonndorf and Khanna (1968) who based their plot on the data of (●) Békésy (1960, pp. 460–469), and Johnstone and Boyle (1967) (▼). Solid line indicates a better fit between Békésy's data points and more recent data of Johnstone and Taylor (1970) (△), and Rhode (1971) (○). [From Dallos (1973b).]

curves are rather shallow, generally showing low-frequency slopes of the order of 6 dB/octave and high-frequency slopes of approximately − 20 dB/octave. It is also apparent from his plots that the tuning curves become more and more asymmetrical (high-frequency slope becomes sharper) as the point of measurement moves from the apex toward the base. All of Békésy's results were obtained from measurements over the apical one-half of the cochlea. Recent results gathered with the Mössbauer technique (Johnstone & Boyle, 1967; Rhode, 1971) and with capacitive probes (Wilson & Johnstone, 1972) from more basal segments of the cochlea yield sharper tuning curves. An acceptable measure of the sharpness of tuning is the so-called Q, or *quality factor*, which is computed as the ratio between the peak frequency and the 3 dB-down bandwidth. When such Q-factors are derived from Békésy's results along with some of the newer data, and plotted as a function of the peak frequency, Fig. 5 results. It is apparent that points near the base (high best frequency) appear more narrowly tuned, i.e., have higher Q's than those nearer the apex (low best frequency). The progression in Q with best frequency is quite systematic and gradual.

The contemporary measurements yield interesting details of the tuning curves that are worth discussing in some detail. To facilitate this discussion, a set of amplitude and phase responses are shown in Fig. 6. These data are from the squirrel monkey, and depict the amplitude ratio and phase difference between a point on the basilar membrane and the malleus. The data are obtained at 80 dB sound pressure level (SPL). At low frequencies the response rises at a rate of 6 dB octave^{-1}; somewhere below the best frequency the rate increases to about 24 dB octave^{-1}; above the best frequency it is of the order of − 100 dB octave^{-1}. At the peak, the basilar membrane vibrates at an amplitude that is about 10 times as great as that of the malleus. At the lowest frequencies the basilar membrane leads the malleus in phase by 90°, phase lag gradually accumulates at higher frequencies. The phase plots can be approximated by two straight lines in a linear plot. It is not shown in the figure, but both amplitude and phase responses level off to a plateau at a frequency where the amplitude drops about 30–40 dB from the peak.

The sharpness of the tuning is apparently strongly dependent upon the physiological state of the cochlea; thus the steep segment of the low-frequency slope disappears upon death, the best frequency shifts downward,

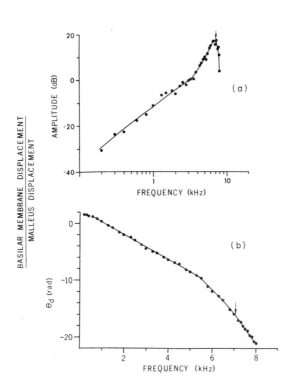

FIG. 6. Ratio of basilar-membrane and malleus displacement in decibels (a) and phase difference between the motion of the basilar membrane and the malleus (b). [From Rhode (1971).]

and the response magnitude diminishes (Rhode, 1973). One very important, and controversial finding is the presence of a pronounced nonlinearity in the basilar membrane vibration (Rhode, 1971). It appears that in the vicinity of the best frequency, the vibration amplitude shows saturation with increasing intensity. The nonlinearity is also said to disappear upon death (Rhode, 1973). Others (Békésy, 1960, pp. 446–460; Johnstone & Boyle, 1967; Wilson & Johnstone, 1972) failed to demonstrate any nonlinearity in the vibratory pattern of the basilar membrane. If the nonlinearity is indeed present (and it is doubtful that it is in most species) in the mechanical portion of the cochlea, then it would provide one plausible explanation for a variety of nonlinear phenomena observed psychoacoustically and electrophysiologically. In addition, its major significance is that it would yield much larger vibratory amplitudes at the threshold of hearing than hitherto assumed. To explain, if one linearly extrapolates from the measured (necessarily at high sound levels) basilar membrane displacement to the level of the threshold of audibility, then threshold amplitude of .001 Å results. This amplitude is contrasted with, for example, the thickness of a single cilium which is about 1000 Å. Clearly, conceptual difficulties are encountered when one attempts to envision adequate stimulation to occur when the amplitude of the movement is a millionfold smaller than the dimensions of the moving structure. If nonlinear extrapolation would be permitted, taking into account Rhode's saturating nonlinearity, then at threshold the amplitude would be of the order of 1 Å, still small but certainly more acceptable.

The very-low-frequency behavior of the amplitude and phase response of the basilar membrane verify what can be deduced on a theoretical basis, namely, that the displacement of the membrane is proportional to the velocity of the stapes. Consider that the membrane displacement is elicited by the pressure differential across it, which in turn is directly related to the pressure generated by the stapes footplate at the oval window. This pressure (p) is obtained as

$$p = Z_c v_s , \tag{1}$$

where Z_c is the acoustic input impedance of the cochlea as seen by the stapes and v_s is the volume velocity of the stapes footplate. If the input impedance is constant and resistive, then there is a direct proportionality between p and v_s. Above 100 Hz, the input impedance is resistive in most species, even though below that frequency reactive components might occur in some. In frequency plots, the derivative relationship between basilar membrane and stapes displacements is manifested by the initial 6 dB octave^{-1} slope and 90° phase lead.

It is now appropriate to consider the physical basis of the traveling wave, which is sustained by the basilar membrane. In other words, let us inquire what physical properties of the membrane determine the characteristics of its vibratory pattern. Békésy's observations again form the basis of the bulk of our knowledge of this subject. The most conspicuous feature of the basilar membrane is its shape, which is an elongated trapezoid. The membrane is narrow at the base and gradually widens toward the apex, the total change being approximately tenfold. This change in shape is accompanied by an alteration in the mass of the membrane's superstructure, which also increases from base to apex. The increase is largely due to the gradual lengthening of the hair cells and supporting cells along the cochlear spiral. The most significant physical variable that characterizes the basilar membrane is its elasticity. Békésy (1960, pp. 469–480) measured the static volume elasticity of the partition and noted that it changed drastically along the length of the cochlear canal. Figure 7 shows his numerical results. It is apparent that the cochlear partition is about one hundredfold more elastic at the apex than at the stapes, and that the change in elasticity is roughly an exponential function of the distance. This variation in stiffness is the single most important property of the basilar membrane, which determines its peculiar vibratory properties.

Aside from the variation in mass and stiffness with distance, certain other characteristics of the cochlear partition deserve attention. On the basis of some simple and ingenious experiments, Békésy (1960, pp. 469–480) determined that the basilar membrane is not under tension, and that moreover, its

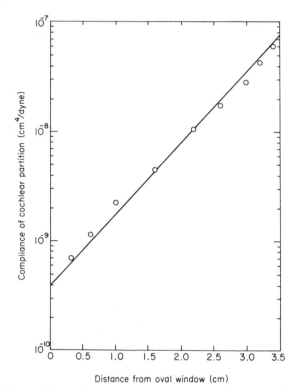

F<small>IG</small>. 7. Compliance of the cochlear partition as the function of distance from the oval window. The points are from Békésy's data, and the straight line is a mathematical approximation. [From Zwislocki (1965).]

elastic properties are the same in both longitudinal and radial directions. The importance of these contentions can be appreciated when it is considered that the cornerstone of the so-called resonance theories* of cochlear function is the assumption that the basilar membrane is stretched and that its tension is much greater in the radial than in the longitudinal direction. Lacking such features, the basilar membrane cannot be a primarily resonant system, and its frequency analyzing properties must be attributed to some other physical mechanism. As we have seen, such a mechanism is the traveling wave.

The traveling wave arises in the exchange of energy between the cochlear partition and the surrounding fluid layer. This essentially hydrodynamic process can be quantified by considering the basic equations of fluid dynamics and taking into consideration the known physical properties of the cochlear channels and the cochlear partition. Ideally, the actual mechanics of solving

---

* For a review of the various theories of cochlear frequency analysis the reader is referred to Wever (1949).

the problem of cochlear vibrations would entail solution of the three-dimensional forms of the hydrodynamic equations of continuity and force balance with the utilization of proper boundary conditions. The latter consist of the descriptions of the hydrodynamic states at the following locations: the two windows, the helicotrema, along the rigid bony walls, and along the moving partition. Even casual acquaintance with problems of this nature suggests that it is hopeless to attempt the exact analytic solution of a vibratory problem of this complexity. Fortunately, several simplifications can be made that reduce the problem to a manageable, albeit difficult, one. The two principal simplifications are the reduction of the three-dimensional problem into a one-dimensional scheme, and the elimination of the moving partition as one of the boundary conditions in the solution. The first simplification is based on the assumption that in the most significant region of basilar membrane vibrations, the wavelength of the traveling wave is greater than the transversal movements and the depth of the fluid that participates in the establishment of acoustic conditions.* If this is the case, then the so-called shallow water treatment of fluid dynamics adequately describes the situation, implying that the one-dimensional treatment is acceptable. In shallow water, the vertical velocity component is negligible, whereas the horizontal one is independent of depth. As a consequence, it is reasonable to ignore fluid movement perpendicular to the cochlear partition and to consider only longitudinal fluid flow. Such a shallow water, or long wave, solution will be appropriate to describe the properties of the traveling wave between the base and the amplitude maximum. Beyond the maximum the wavelength becomes even shorter, and thus by necessity the basic assumption of the long-wave solution is inadequate.

The second simplification involves the inclusion of the properties of the cochlear partition in the solution, not as a boundary condition, but with the aid of the concept of impedance. It is assumed that each elementary segment of the cochlear partition possesses a certain acoustic impedance (Z) that relates the pressure difference across the partition to its volume velocity:

$$p = Zv, \tag{2}$$

where all three quantities are dependent on the distance along the cochlea (x). In steady-state conditions, the partition impedance per unit length is written as

$$Z(x) = R_m(x) + j[\omega M(x) - 1/\omega C(x)], \tag{3}$$

where $R_m(x)$, $M(x)$, and $C(x)$ are the equivalent acoustic resistance, mass, and elasticity of the partition. These three functions can be determined on the basis of physical and anatomical considerations and measurements. The

* Ranke (1942, 1950) and Siebert (1974) advocate the use of the short-wave solution to the cochlear problem, while other investigators (e.g., Peterson & Bogert, 1950; Zwislocki, 1948) utilize the long-wave solution.

resulting impedance function, together with the basic hydrodynamic equations, is used to yield a solution.*

If the cochlea is considered uncoiled, with the surface area of the scala vestibuli being $S_v = S_v(x)$, that of scala tympani $S_t = S_t(x)$, and the width of the basilar membrane being $b = b(x)$, and if it is assumed that the entire cochlear partition at a given distance x vibrates in phase, then a set of hydrodynamic equations can be written for the system for a small-signal case. The first relation that can be written is based on the fact that mass is conserved in any volume element. Mathematically this yields the so-called continuity equation:

$$S_v \frac{\partial \rho_{ev}}{\partial t} + vb\rho_0 + \rho_0 \frac{\partial(u_v S_v)}{\partial x} = 0. \tag{4}$$

Here v is the partition velocity, ρ_0 the resting density of the perilymph, ρ_{ev} the excess density, and u_v the fluid particle velocity in the x-direction. This equation applies to the volume element $S_v\, dx$ in the scala vestibuli. Similar considerations yield the continuity equation for the scala tympani in the form

$$S_t \frac{\partial \rho_{et}}{\partial t} - vb\rho_0 + \frac{\partial(u_t S_t)}{\partial x} \rho_0 = 0. \tag{5}$$

Note that here the partition velocity is taken with a negative sign, for the partition moves in opposite direction when viewed from the two scalae.

The second set of relations can be obtained by considering that the forces that act on any volume element must be in equilibrium. The external force that moves element $S_v\, dx$ is due to the pressure differential that acts on the two surfaces at x and at $x + dx$. The external force is counterbalanced by inertial and frictional forces. The force balance equation for a volume element in scala vestibuli assumes the form

$$\rho_0 \frac{\partial u_v}{\partial t} + R_v u_v = -\frac{\partial p_{ve}}{\partial x}, \tag{6}$$

whereas the equation applicable to scala tympani is

$$\rho_0 \frac{\partial u_t}{\partial t} + R_t u_t = -\frac{\partial p_{te}}{\partial x}. \tag{7}$$

Here R_v and R_t are the frictional resistances in the fluids of the two scalae, and p_{ve} and p_{te} are the excess pressures. The preceding four equations can be combined to yield

---

* What follows is in essence the now classic solution provided by Zwislocki (1948). While his approach is now superseded by more contemporary techniques, Zwislocki's solution still best facilitates the understanding of cochlear hydrodynamics, and thus it is chosen for presentation. Among other approaches to the solution are those of Allaire, Raynor, and Billone (1974), Schroeder (1973), Zweig, Lipes, and Pierce (1976), and the intriguing work of Steele (1974).

$$-\frac{1}{c^2}(\ddot{p}_{ve} - \ddot{p}_{te}) - \rho_0 b\left(\frac{1}{S_v} + \frac{1}{S_t}\right)\dot{v} - \frac{1}{\rho_0 c^2}(R_v \dot{p}_{ve} - R_t \dot{p}_{te})$$

$$-b\left(\frac{R_v}{S_v} + \frac{R_t}{S_t}\right)v = -\frac{\partial^2 p_{ve}}{\partial x^2} + \frac{\partial^2 p_{te}}{\partial x^2}, \tag{8}$$

where the substitution $c^2 = p_e/\rho_e$ has been made, and where differentiation with respect to time is indicated by overdots. If we now introduce $R_v = R_t = R$, $p_{ve} - p_{te} = p$, and $1/S = (1/S_v) + (1/S_t)$, then we have the relationship

$$\frac{\ddot{p}}{c^2} + \frac{\rho_0 b}{S}\dot{v} + \frac{R}{\rho_0 c^2}\dot{p} + \frac{bR}{S}v = \frac{\partial^2 p}{\partial x^2}. \tag{9}$$

This equation contains both pressure and partition velocity, but either can be eliminated if we remember that they are related by the impedance of the partition

$$p = bvZ,$$

where bv is the volume velocity. Thus if pressure across the partition is the desired quantity, we can write

$$\frac{\ddot{p}}{c^2} + \left(\frac{\rho_0}{SZ} + \frac{R}{\rho_0 c^2}\right)\dot{p} + \frac{R}{SZ}p = \frac{\partial^2 p}{\partial x^2}. \tag{10}$$

Assuming harmonic motion, that is $p = Pe^{j\omega t}$, we obtain

$$-\left(\frac{\omega^2}{c^2} - j\omega\frac{\rho_0}{SZ}\right) + R\left(\frac{1}{SZ} + j\omega\frac{1}{\rho_0 c^2}\right) = \frac{1}{P}\frac{d^2 P}{dx^2}. \tag{11}$$

By using the relationship $p = Zbv$, we can obtain an equation in identical form that describes the velocity of the cochlear partition as a function of x and b:

$$\frac{\ddot{v}}{c^2} + \left(\frac{\rho_0}{SZ} + \frac{R}{\rho_0 c^2}\right)\dot{v} + \frac{R}{SZ}v = \frac{\partial^2 v}{\partial x^2} \tag{12}$$

and for the harmonic case, when $v = Ve^{j\omega t}$:

$$-\left(\frac{\omega^2}{c^2} - j\omega\frac{\rho_0}{SZ}\right) + R\left(\frac{1}{SZ} + j\omega\frac{1}{\rho_0 c^2}\right) = \frac{1}{V}\frac{d^2 V}{dx^2}. \tag{13}$$

The ultimately desired solution of our problem is the function $y(x)$, that is, the displacement versus distance from the stapes. This could be obtained by first solving Eq. (13) for the partition velocity v and then integrating the solution with respect to time, since

$$y = \int_0^t v\, dt, \tag{14}$$

thus $Y = V/j\omega$ in the harmonic case. Since $R = R(x)$, and $S = S(x)$ are all functions of distance, the differential equation has no general solution. One has two possible avenues of attack. Following Zwislocki (1950, 1965), it is possible to assume analytic functions for R, Z, and S and then simplify the equations so that an actual solution can be obtained, provided only steady-state conditions are considered. Another possibility is to use numerical methods to obtain a solution.

We should consider first the effects of two possible simplifications that are often invoked. First, if we neglect viscosity effects of the cochlear fluids the equation would have the following form, since neglecting these effects implies $R = 0$:

$$-\frac{\omega^2}{c^2}\left(1 - j\frac{\rho_0 c^2}{SZ_\omega}\right) = \frac{1}{P}\frac{d^2P}{dx^2} \, . \tag{15}$$

This equation is essentially that which was obtained by Peterson and Bogert (1950). Another possible simplification is to assume that the cochlear fluid is incompressible, that is $\partial\rho/\partial t = 0$. In this case, the final equation has the form

$$\frac{R + j\omega\rho_0}{SZ} = \frac{1}{P}\frac{d^2P}{dx^2} \, . \tag{16}$$

This equation is like the one that was derived by Zwislocki (1948, 1965). If we neglect both the viscosity and compressibility of the cochlear fluid, then the equation assumes the particularly simple form

$$j\omega\frac{\rho_0}{SZ} = \frac{1}{P}\frac{d^2P}{dx^2} \, . \tag{17}$$

This is essentially the equation that was solved numerically by Fletcher (1953).

Probably the most profitable way to proceed from this point is to follow the solution of one of the preceding simplified wave equations. We shall consider Zwislocki's solution because he utilized several of Békésy's physical measurements in order to affix functional and numerical values to the parameters in the equations, so as to provide the most realistic solutions. It should be noted in addition that Zwislocki did not use a curve-fitting technique in obtaining the solution to the cochlear vibration problem. Instead he used basic physical considerations and actual measurements of parameters to establish quantitative relationships, and then compared his results to experimental observations on the pattern of vibrations made by Békésy (1960, pp. 429–460). He then made small final adjustments of some parameters to achieve good harmony between the theoretical and experimental results.

The first task is to obtain the functional relationships $R = R(x)$, $S = S(x)$, and $Z = Z(x)$ in analytic form so that after substitution into the original equation, a solution can be attempted. Zwislocki (1948, 1965) derived the following expressions for the functions:

$$R(x) = R_0 \omega^{1/2} e^{ax/2},$$
$$S(x) = S_0 e^{-ax},$$
$$R_m(x) = R_{m0} e^{.175x} \approx R_{m0},$$
$$M(x) \approx 0,$$
$$C(x) = C_0 e^{hx}. \tag{18}$$

After substituting these expressions into Eq. (16) we obtain

$$\frac{1}{P}\frac{d^2P}{dx^2} = \frac{R + j\omega\rho_0}{SZ} = \frac{R_0 \omega^{1/2} e^{ax/2} + j\omega\rho_0}{S_0 e^{-ax}(R_m - je^{-hx}/\omega C_0)}. \tag{19}$$

Zwislocki had shown that an analytical solution could be obtained for Eq. (19), provided further simplifications could be made. Specifically, if it is assumed that $R_m \ll 1/\omega C$ in all regions of the cochlea where the amplitude of vibrations is substantial, and if as an approximation we assume that the following expression can be written (K is a constant):

$$K = 1 - j(\omega R_m C + R/\omega\rho_0), \tag{20}$$

then with this substitution the differential equation takes the form

$$-\frac{1}{P}\frac{d^2P}{dx^2} = \frac{KC_0\omega^2\rho_0}{S_0} e^{(h+a)x}. \tag{21}$$

This equation can be solved if the following change in variables is made

$$Z = \frac{2\omega}{h+a}\left[\frac{KC_0\rho_0}{S_0}\right]^{1/2} e^{(h+a)x/2}. \tag{22}$$

The equation then assumes the form

$$\frac{d^2P}{dz^2} + \frac{1}{z}\frac{dP}{dz} + P = 0. \tag{23}$$

Since this is the well-known Bessel differential equation, its solution can be written by inspection. One appropriate complete solution utilizes Hankel functions:

$$P = A_1 H_0^{(1)}(z) + B_1 H_0^{(2)}(z). \tag{24}$$

Let us now consider the behavior of the two functions $H_0^{(1)}$ and $H_0^{(2)}$ at very large values of the complex argument z. The function $H_0^{(1)}$ vanishes if the magnitude of the argument increases without bound, provided the imaginary part of the argument is positive. In contrast $H_0^{(2)}$ disappears at large values of z if the imaginary part of z is negative. The physical constraint provided by the helicotrema, which comprises a virtual short circuit for pressure at large values of the distance x, dictates that we cannot have solutions for the pressure that do not diminish at large arguments. This consideration necessitates that the coefficient A_1 be identically zero. Thus the solution should be written as

$$P = B_1 H_0^{(2)} \left\{ \frac{2\omega}{h + a} \frac{(KC_0\rho_0)^{1/2}}{S_0} e^{(h+a)x/2} \right\} . \tag{25}$$

When the argument of a Hankel function is large, it can be approximated by an exponential function with good accuracy. Consequently, $|P(x, \omega)|$ can be obtained as

$$|P(x, \omega)| = B_1 \frac{\exp\{-[\omega/(h + a)] (C_0\rho_0/S_0)^{1/2} - (\omega R_m C + R/\omega\rho_0)e^{(h+a)x/2}\}}{\{(\pi/2)[2\omega/(h + a)] (C_0\rho_0/S_0)^{1/2}e^{(h+a)x/2}\}^{1/2}}$$

$$= B_1'\omega^{-1/2} \exp\left[-\frac{(h + a)x}{4} - \frac{\omega}{h + a} \left(\frac{C_0\rho_0}{S_0} \right)^{1/2} \right.$$

$$\left. - \left(\omega R_m C + \frac{R}{\omega\rho_0} \right) e^{(h+a)x/2} \right] . \tag{26}$$

After the functional values for C and R are substituted, the following expression results:

$$|P(x, \omega)| = B_1'\omega^{-1/2} \exp[-(h + a)x/4 - (Q/2)\omega^2 R_m C_0 e^{(3h+a)x/2}$$
$$- (Q/2)(R_0\omega^{1/2}/\rho_0)e^{(h+2a)x/2}], \tag{27}$$

where

$$Q = 2\rho_0^{1/2} C_0^{1/2}/(h + a)S_0^{1/2} . \tag{28}$$

We note that the pressure monotonically decreases with an increase in both ω and x. At a constant frequency then, the pressure wave gradually decreases from the stapes toward the helicotrema, becoming negligible at a particular distance. The greater the frequency, the earlier the pressure magnitude diminishes to a negligible value. At a constant distance from the stapes the pressure magnitude depends on frequency: The greater the frequency, the smaller the pressure.

The phase of the pressure wave can also be determined from the exponential approximation

$$\angle P = \omega Q \, e^{(h+a)x/2} + \tfrac{1}{4}\pi. \tag{29}$$

Clearly the phase lag increases monotonically with both frequency and distance from the stapes.

The quantity of greatest interest to us is the displacement pattern of the cochlear partition. This pattern can be obtained from the pressure function with relative ease if it is considered that $p = Zbv = j\omega Zyb$. Consequently,

$$y = p/j\omega Zb.$$

The quantity $1/Z$ can be written as $j\omega C + \omega^2 R_m C^2$. Consequently, the magnitude of the impedance takes the form

$$\omega C(1 + \omega^2 R_m C^2)^{1/2} . \tag{30}$$

However, $\omega^2 R_m C^2 \ll 1$ for the values of frequency and distance of interest; consequently, we are justified to approximate $|1/Z|$ by ωC.

Let us now substitute this value of $|1/Z|$, and our equation for $|P(x, f)|$ into the formula for membrane displacement $|y|$, assuming that $b = b_0 e^{kx}$:

$$|y| = \frac{C|P|}{b} = B''_1 \omega^{-1/2} \exp\left[\frac{(3h - a)}{4} - k - \frac{Q}{2} \omega^2 R_m C_0 e^{(3h+a)x/2}\right.$$
$$\left. - \frac{Q}{2} \frac{R_0 \omega^{1/2}}{S_0} e^{(h+2a)x/2}\right]. \tag{31}$$

The phase of the partition displacement is the same as the phase of the pressure wave, provided we maintain the approximation $\omega R_m C \ll 1$. Under these circumstances the displacement function can be written as

$$y = \frac{P}{j\omega Zb} = \frac{P}{j\omega b} (j\omega C + \omega^2 R_m C^2) = \frac{pj\omega C}{j\omega b} (1 - j\omega R_m C) \approx pC/b, \tag{32}$$

consequently,

$$\angle y \approx \angle pC/b = \angle p, \qquad \text{as stated.} \tag{33}$$

The function that describes the theoretical shape of membrane displacement (to be precise, the amplitude of membrane displacement as the function of distance, which should not be confused with the instantaneous value of membrane motion) reveals that, for most frequencies, a distinct point of amplitude maximum exists. This maximum moves away from the stapes as the driving frequency decreases. At very low frequencies there is no maximum in that the magnitude of vibrations monotonically increases toward the apex. The most conspicuous property of the amplitude distribution is that points of maximal vibrations are correlated with individual frequency components. These points line up in a base-to-apex succession with decreasing input frequency. Together with changes in amplitude, the partition vibration also exhibits a gradually accumulating phase shift. It is clear that phase changes are more rapid at higher frequencies than at the lower ones, and that close to the stapes the phase changes much more slowly than in a more apical region.

One could summarize by saying that as a result of harmonic excitation, a pressure wave of monotonically decreasing magnitude and increasing phase shift travels in the cochlear fluid from base toward the apex. This pressure wave decreases to a negligible magnitude at a given point removed from its origin. The location of this point depends on the driving frequency; the lower the frequency, the greater the spatial extent of the pressure wave. This pressure wave is developed *across* the cochlear partition and is directly responsible for setting the latter in vibration. In contrast with the monotonically decreasing fluid pressure differences, the vibratory amplitude of the partition shows an extremum, that is, a point of maximal vibration. The maximum point is determined by the frequency of the stimulus. High frequencies create a peak in the basal region, and as the frequencies become lower, the peak moves closer to the apex. Very low frequencies do not elicit a clearcut maximum. As a first approximation, the phase of the fluid pressure differential across the partition and the phase of the partition displacement are the same. The theoretical results indicate that the cochlea acts as a mechanical frequency analyzer in relating a point of maximal vibration to a particular frequency. It is notable that the frequency analysis takes place without a true membrane resonance, as can be seen from the fact that in the derivation the partition mass $M(x)$ could be neglected. If some mass is included, then the computed frequency selectivity of the system improves, in other words, the tuning becomes sharper (Zwislocki, 1974).

Armed with our understanding of the properties and theoretical bases of the traveling wave, which constitutes the gross motion pattern of the cochlear partition, we can now consider how this motion is translated into the deformation of the hair cells.

B. Fine Motion Patterns

It is an almost universally accepted notion that the hair cells of the cochlea perform the essential transducer function of the hearing organ. The hair cells are ciliated cells of epithelial origin. The effective input to these cells is some sort of mechanical deformation, and it is also quite widely accepted that this deformation is mediated by the displacement of the cilia from the resting position. In different forms of mechanoreceptors the cilia are displaced by a variety of means, utilizing several physical principles (Wever, 1971). For the mammalian cochlea the scheme proposed by Ter Kuile (cf. Wever, 1971) has gained the greatest currency. We can follow this scheme with the aid of Fig. 8. The basis of Ter Kuile's argument is that the basilar membrane and the tectorial membrane rotate around different center points when displaced, the former is anchored to the osseous spiral lamina, and the latter is supported at the top of the spiral limbus. Owing to the spatial separation between the two attachments, and to the fact that the lateral margin of the tectorial membrane is not firmly supported, up and down movements of the cochlear partition result in a relative radial displacement between the tectorial membrane and the reticular lamina. The latter moves with the basilar membrane to which it is relatively firmly anchored by the pillar cells and the phalangeal processes of the Deiters cells. Since the tops of the hair cells are imbedded in the reticular lamina, the hair-bearing surfaces move with the basilar membrane. It is apparent from the illustration that there is a lateral displacement, or shear, between the top of the reticular membrane and the bottom of the tectorial membrane. If the cilia are anchored between these two surfaces, then it is inevitable that they be bent as a result of the shearing motion. A comparison of the $a-c$ and the $a'-c'$ lines in the figure vividly illustrates this idea. Not all cilia are attached to the tectorial membrane (Kimura, 1966;

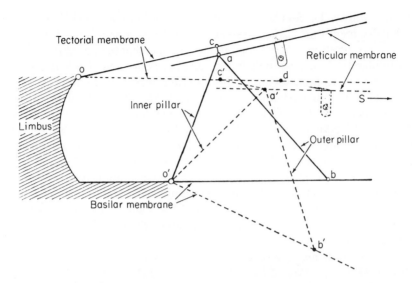

FIG. 8. The mode of hair cell stimulation according to Ter Kuile. Solid lines represent one position of the basilar membrane and associated structures, and broken lines a second position in which the basilar membrane has moved downward. [From Wever (1971), The mechanics of hair-cell stimulation, *Annals of Otology, Rhinology, and Laryngology,* **80,** 786–805.]

Lim, 1972), in fact, only the tallest row of hairs of the outer hair cells makes clear-cut contact. This means that most cilia of the outer hair cells and none of the hairs from the inner hair cells make apparent attachments with the bottom of the tectorial membrane. It is reasonable to believe that all hairs of the outer hair cells are bent when the tallest row is stimulated, since there are apparent contacts formed among the ciliary shafts by mucopolysaccharide molecules (Spoendlin, 1966). Thus Ter Kuile's scheme of hair cell stimulation applies to the outer hair cells. An alternative scheme applicable to the inner hair cells has been suggested by Billone (1972) and supported by others (Dallos, Billone, Durrant, Wang, & Raynor, 1972). According to this scheme the free-standing cilia of the inner hair cells are bent by viscous fluid drag exerted on them by endolymph streaming between the tectorial and reticular surfaces. Such viscous force is proportional to the velocity of movement, thus it follows that the two hair-cell groups receive different stimuli; the outer hair cells are stimulated in proportion to the displacement of the basilar membrane, whereas the inner hair cells are excited in proportion to the velocity of the basilar membrane. Aside from this derivative relationship between the effective input stimuli to the two hair-cell groups, a pronounced sensitivity difference between them is also evident. Because of the more efficient means of conveying energy to the outer hair cells, these units are more sensitive than the inner hair cells (Dallos & Wang, 1974).

Thus far, we have considered shear displacements between reticular and tectorial membranes and the consequent bending of the hairs in the radial direction only. The cochlea is obviously a three-dimensional structure and the basilar membrane is constrained to be at rest along both of its borders. These considerations suggest that upon displacement the membrane assumes a particular curvature not only in the radial direction but also in the longitudinal direction. In fact, owing to the differing degree of dominance between these two types of curvature, both a radial and longitudinal shear can be demonstrated, and the two types of shear have different spatial loci (Békésy, 1960, pp. 485–500; Tonndorf, 1960). Radial shear waves are directly related to the instantaneous traveling wave waveform, consequently their spatial pattern can be visualized from Fig. 4a. In contrast, the longitudinal shear is dependent on the first spatial derivative of the traveling wave and its pattern is depicted in Fig. 4b. Clearly the longitudinal shear wave is somewhat more confined to a given region of the cochlea, and it has been suggested (Tonndorf, 1970) that if it acts as the effective stimulus, then a considerable sharpening of the tuning of the mechanical system is achieved. Since the hair cells appear to be morphologically polarized in a radial direction (Engström, Ades, & Hawkins, 1962; Flock, Kimura, Lundquist, & Wersäll, 1962), it is questionable that a longitudinal shear could provide effective stimulation.

The bending of the hairs of the sensory cells initiates the transducer action within these structures. Our next concern is the scheme and details of the transducer process, including the properties of the most important ingredients of this process: the cochlear potentials.

III. TRANSDUCER PROCESSES

A. The Transducer Scheme*

Most sensory receptor organs are formed by a conglomeration of sensory receptor cells and their accessory structure. The former are specialized cells that are capable of interacting with the environment and are particularly responsive to specific factors in the environment, such as particular forms of energy. The accessory structure is a framework for the sensory cells, which has multiple functions. In general, the accessory structure strongly influences the operation of the sense organ by performing distribution and preanalysis of the stimulus. More specifically, when these structures direct and funnel the stimulus to the receptor cells, they perform filtering of the environmental stimulus, and in most cases they contribute to the dynamic response of the receptor mechanism. Much of our discussion up to this point has been devoted to the most elaborate accessory structure developed in nature: the cochlear partition. It is quite clear that the functional properties of the combined basilar-membrane–organ-of-Corti system determine to a

---

* This section is taken from Dallos (1973b).

great extent the sensitivity, the dynamic range, and the frequency range over which a particular auditory organ can function. It is also clear that via the traveling wave mechanism, the accessory structure, the basilar membrane, performs a high-level distributive and filtering function in determining which groups of sensory cells receive excitation under any stimulus condition. Clearly then, a good understanding has now been developed of the nature, purpose, and operation of the auditory accessory structure. Our task now is to examine the other major component of the sense organ, the sensory receptor cell.

All receptor cells are considered to be akin to specialized neurons, and thus they fit schemes that were developed to describe and classify the general functioning of neurons (cf. Bodian, 1962). The general scheme defines portions of a neuron according to function instead of by morphology. The typical neuron can be described as having three main functional parts. These are the receptive pole or dendritic zone, the transmission apparatus or axon, and the distribution apparatus or presynaptic zone. The receptive pole and the presynaptic region are defined functionally to be the input and output regions of the neuron. These two regions are at opposite ends of the neuronal structure, and thus both a functional and structural polarization of the neuron, both sensory and nonsensory, exist. We can develop a general classification of the sensory cells on the basis of their morphology. According to this we can distinguish primary sense cells and secondary sense cells; differentiation between the two types hinges upon the presence or absence of a transmission apparatus (axon) that is absent in the latter. Aside from the morphological differences between the two basic types, there are highly significant functional and operational differences as well.

In the vertebrate special sense organs (with the exception of the olfactory epithelium), a specialized receptor cell, of epithelial origin, receives the external stimulus, converts it into a form that is compatible with the receptive properties of adjacent cells, and activates these surrounding cells. The distinctive structural feature of the receptor cell is that it does not possess an axonal segment. With this goes hand in hand the distinguishing functional feature that this cell does not transmit pulsatile information. All-or-none signal transmission was developed in the nervous system to make "long distance" communication possible. In secondary sensory receptor systems, the sense cell is in intimate contact with the succeeding neuron; thus there is no need for pulsatile transmission. The receptive pole of the neighboring neurons is generally chemically excitable, thus the output of a sense cell is in the form of secretion of chemical transmitter substances. Between the sensory cell and the following neuron the information transfer takes place via a synaptic mechanism. Grundfest (1961) very strongly emphasizes the secretory function of the sense cell. He states that the cell is probably not electrically excitable, and it may or may not generate an electrical potential upon absorption of stimulation. If a potential does appear it might be either depolarizing, hyperpolarizing, or both, depending on stimulus parameters. In any case, if the potential does appear it might be only a secondary process, essentially an electrical sign of secretory activity of the cell. If an electrical potential does appear in the sensory cell that does not sustain pulsatile activity, this potential should not be confused with the generator potential of the simple sensory cell. Davis (1961) proposed the very useful distinction that the term *generator potential* be reserved for the graded electrical activity that is directly responsible for the initiation of all-or-none neural responses, whereas the term *receptor potential* was proposed to describe the graded electrical activity that occurs in the sensory receptor cell as a direct conse-quence of the absorption of stimulus. The microphonic and summating poten-tials of the cochlea are thought to be an aggregate external manifestation of receptor potentials originating in the hair cells (Davis, 1961, 1965).

Probably the easiest way to summarize the operation of the organ of Corti as a sensory receptor organ is with the aid of Fig. 9 which is a three-part schematic. On the left, a sketch of a hair cell is shown together with a portion of the tectorial membrane and with a few attached afferent nerve endings and fibers. In the center of the figure, the block diagram depicts the distinct structural regions of interest, whereas the block diagram on the right shows a functional classification of the different regions. The stimulus is filtered and

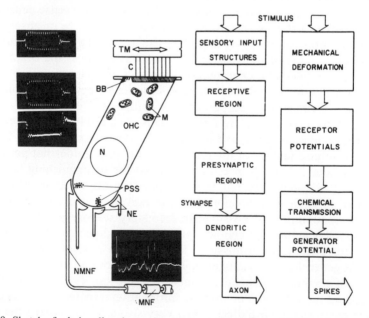

FIG. 9. Sketch of a hair cell and associated nerve endings along with structural (center) and functional (right) block diagrams of the system. The insets demonstrate the waveforms of the various quantitites that are indicated in the functional block diagram, namely, stimulus, CM, DIF SP, and neural discharges. [From Dallos (1973b).]

then distributed to the cells by the accessory structure, only a small portion of which is shown here. The accessory structure of the cochlea certainly includes the entire basilar-membrane–organ-of-Corti complex. Here only a segment of the tectorial membrane and the reticular lamina are shown. The sensory input structures in this case include the tectorial membrane, the stereocilia, and probably the reticular-membrane–cuticular-plate structure. The function of the sensory input structures is to transmit the stimulus to the receptive region of the sense cell. The most common assumption is that the stimulus is the bending of the cilia brought about by the relative sliding motion between the tectorial membrane and the reticular lamina. The receptive region is specialized to absorb the stimulus and to generate a local electric response—the receptor current, whose outward manifestation is the receptor potential. It has been assumed by most authorities that the receptive region is the uppermost portion of the cell, probably only the cuticle-free region where the basal body can be found in some species. However, it is possible that the ciliary membrane, or the central ciliary core might function as the actual sensory receptor structure which is specialized to respond to stimuli. On the far left of the figure some sample waveforms are shown for the various processes that are described in the block diagram at the right. The stimulus is assumed to be a brief sinusoidal burst. Here the actual sound pressure change is shown, but it is highly probable that the time course of the effective stimulation, that is, of the bending pattern of the cilia is quite similar. Two receptor potentials are shown—an ac and a dc component. These are presumably generated or controlled at the cell's receptive region.

The lowermost portion of the cell body is the presynaptic region. It is distinguished by the presence of characteristic structures, such as synaptic bars, accumulation of vesicles, and membrane thickening, all of which are typical at the sending end of a chemical synapse. It is presumed that the receptor potentials act on these presynaptic structures and initiate the release of packets of chemical transmitter substances.* The transmitters diffuse through the synaptic clefts clearly formed between the bottom of the cell and surrounding endings of afferent nerve fibers. The initial nonmyelinated segment of the fibers of the VIIIth nerve form the dendritic region. The chemical transmitters arriving at the nerve endings alter the local membrane permeability and thus set up a local depolarization of the membrane. This potential change is the generator potential. The generator potential is decrementally conducted in the nonmyelinated fibers to the so-called initial segment of the nerve axon, where it is instrumental in setting up all-or-none action potentials. The distinguishing feature of the initial segment is that it is electrically excitable, as opposed to the dendritic region, which probably conducts electricity in a passive manner. It is widely assumed that the initial segment of the VIIIth nerve axons is at the habenula perforata, where the

---

* The afferent transmitter substance is not yet identified.

fibers gain their myelin sheath, and where in passing through the habenulae they are severely constricted in diameter. It is a common notion that such radical structural changes as diameter shifts are the appropriate conditions for a fiber to become electrogenic, that is, for it to be electrically excitable. In the myelinated segment of the nerve fiber the information travels in the form of an impulse train. An example of such a train is given in the inset.

As our discussions indicate, the receptor potentials in a sense organ are the first electrical signs of the stimulus transduction process. In a secondary receptor system (such as the cochlea) the receptor potentials arise in the specialized sensory cell. The actual function of these potentials has never been established with certainty. Two possibilities exist. The first and more attractive possibility is that the receptor potential (or receptor current) is a direct mediator of the release of chemical transmitters at the presynaptic zone. This scheme assumes that the receptor current is set up as a direct consequence of absorption of stimulus energy by the cell and that this receptor current serves as the intermediary link between the stimulus and the cell output—the chemical transmitters. One of the most important considerations that recommend this scheme is that the receptive pole of the cell and its presynaptic region are, as a rule, on two opposite ends of the cell structure. In other words, these two regions are physically separated. The transmitter substance is stored in the synaptic vesicles that are concentrated in the presynaptic region. The excitable structure of the cell, its receptive region, is many tens of hundreds of microns away from this concentration of transmitters. Thus the excitatory process in the cell must be communicated to the presynaptic region, and the most parsimonious, indeed the most likely, assumption is that the communication between these regions takes place via the receptor potential. The scheme then functions as follows: Upon excitation, a receptor current is set up in the input region of the cell, this current generates a potential drop (receptor potential), which is passively conducted in the cell structure to the presynaptic region. There the receptor potential initiates the liberation of chemical transmitters. It should be noted that either depolarizing or hyperpolarizing receptor potentials can function as effective agents of the liberation of transmitter substances.

The second possibility is to assume that the receptor potentials are merely incidental by-products of the transducer process. In other words, whatever physical process would subserve the absorption of stimulus energy by the cell and the subsequent liberation of transmitters would have a by-product: the receptor potential. In this case the receptor potential would be a *sign* of the functioning of the cell instead of being an essential ingredient of that functioning. In this case, the receptor potential is an *epiphenomenon*. The main argument in favor of this scheme is that the function of the sense cell is secretory. Whether or not a potential accompanies this operation is incidental; even the presence of the potential is not required. This scheme is certainly more direct than the one that invokes the necessity of an intermediary process between stimulus absorption and chemical transmission. There does not seem to be, however, a clear mechanism described that would tie together the physically separated input and output processes in the cell. It is quite possible that such a mechanism is not really necessary, and that it is only our incomplete understanding of cellular and receptor function that forces us to seek such an intermediary process and feel more comfortable with it.

It should be said that experimental information concerning this problem is fragmentary and indirect. The best we can do at this juncture is to speculate on this basis and at least be aware of the problem. It is commonly assumed that the cochlear microphonic (CM) and summating potential (SP) are the receptor potentials of the cochlea. Thus, our basic problem can be stated simply in asking whether the CM and SP (or certain components of the SP) are epiphenomena or if they serve an essential intermediary role between stimulation and the release of chemical transmitters from the presynaptic region of the hair cells. An even more general question is whether or not these potentials actively (causally) participate in the initiation of neural responses in the auditory nerve. The history of this question is as old as the history of cochlear potentials themselves, and we simply do not have a convincing solution to the problem. The best that we can do at this stage of hearing research is to describe some salient properties of these receptor potentials. In the following section such a description is attempted.

B. Cochlear Potentials

A variety of electrical potentials can be recorded from within or around the cochlea. The properties of all of these potentials are strongly dependent on the exact recording site, and several are influenced by the parameters of the acoustic stimulation as well. We can classify the potentials as *resting* or *stimulus-related* depending on whether or not they are affected by the sound signal. In the former category we shall speak of an *endochlear potential* (EP) and an *organ of Corti potential* (OCP). The latter category comprises the *cochlear microphonic potential* (CM) and several types of *summating potentials* (SP).

When a microelectrode is introduced inside the scala media, it registers an unusually large positive potential (Békésy, 1960, pp. 647–654). This endocochlear potential averages about 100 mV (Peake, Sohmer, & Weiss, 1969) in healthy cochleas. Upon oxygen deprivation, the EP drops almost instantaneously, reverses polarity, and approaches about -40 mV after 2–3 min of anoxia. The EP recovers completely if the length of the anoxic period is moderate. It is now quite apparent that the recorded EP is the sum of two potentials, both of which are related to the ionic content of the endolymph. It is remembered that endolymph is high in K^+ (150 mM liter^{-1}) and low in Na^+ (1 mM liter^{-1}), whereas perilymph is reversed, that is, low in K^+ and high in

Na^+. Because of the concentration gradient across Reissner's membrane and the basilar membrane, there is a K^+ diffusion potential of 30–40 mV, which would push the endolymphatic space toward a negative potential of this magnitude. In contrast, the ionic content of the endolymph is maintained by active transport of K^+ and Na^+ by an Na^+-, K^+-ATPase activated ion pump, apparently located at the lateral margin of the border cells of the stria vascularis (see Johnstone and Sellick, 1972, for details). This pump transports K^+ into the endolymph from the bloodstream and performs the reverse action on Na^+. The pump is electrogenic, and it generates a positive potential on its endolymph side of 110–130 mV. The sum of this electrogenic potential and the K^+ diffusion potential is the commonly recorded EP. Under anoxia, or with ouabain, the pump is inhibited and the EP moves toward the negative diffusion potential. In contrast, when the K^+ gradient is reduced, by perfusing scala tympani with K^+-rich perfusates for example, the EP becomes more positive (see Johnstone and Sellick, 1972, for further details).

Electrodes penetrating the organ of Corti can record negative potentials of approximately 80 mV. Fine-tipped electrodes can "hold" this potential only for seconds, indicating that it is obtained upon penetrating cells and that it disappears when the cell becomes depolarized by injury. This organ-of-Corti potential is thus the reflection of the normal intracellular negativity of both hair cells and supporting cells. The potential is important, since it must be considered that across the cuticle-free apical portion of the hair cells, there is a resting electrical gradient of about 160–180 mV composed of the sum of the intracellular negativity and the EP. Since the ionic composition of endolymph and the interior of the hair cells is quite similar, there is no significant chemical concentration gradient across the cuticle-free pore of the cells. However, there is a significant electrical gradient, and it is likely that as a result of this gradient there is a continuous flow of K^+ ions from the endolymph into the hair cells. The excess K^+ content is drained along its chemical concentration gradient into the low K^+ fluid that fills the spaces of the organ of Corti. It is widely assumed that a modulation of the steady K^+ flow yields the receptor current of the transducer process. The modulation may be achieved by a change in the resistance or permeability of the cuticle-free pore as a direct result of mechanical deformation.

The external manifestation of the changing ionic flow through the hair cell is the receptor potential. We should be careful to distinguish between a "unit receptor potential" that could be recorded intracellularly, and the gross receptor potential that could be obtained with an electrode immersed in the cochlear fluid. The latter is the aggregate of literally thousands of unit potentials that are different in magnitude and phase for most stimulus conditions and that are seen through the complex electrical network of the fluid-filled, membraneous cochlea. Virtually all information we possess about the receptor potentials of the mammalian hearing organ is based on extracellular recordings, and thus it is proper to keep in mind that our knowledge about the properties of the unit potentials is at best indirect.

During the presence of a stimulus, the receptor current apparently consists of two components. One of these follows the instantaneous variations in the deformation of the receptive region of the hair cell, while the other is related to the envelope of these variations. Stated in other terms, both *ac* (CM) and *dc* (SP) receptor potential components are observable in the cochlea in response to sound stimulation. The asymmetry required to produce the *dc* component cannot as yet be unequivocally associated with any specific cochlear process. Any and all events in the transduction chain can be more or less asymmetrical, and they could conceivably contribute to the genesis of the *dc* receptor potential. Thus hydrodynamic, mechanical, and electrical nonlinearities could all play some role in the generation of the SP.

The *ac* receptor potential CM was discovered by Wever and Bray in 1930, and has since been the subject of innumerable studies. The site and mode of recording greatly influences the experimental findings, and it is probably prudent to utilize only microelectrode recordings from the scala media, and especially differential electrode recordings, for quantitative purposes. The latter technique involves the placement of a pair of electrodes at any given cochlear cross section, one in scala vestibuli, the other in scala tympani. The difference between the outputs of the two pickup electrodes best approximates the summed output of local generators located between the electrode tips, whereas the average of their outputs yields the sum of remotely generated responses (Dallos, 1969; Tasaki, Davis, & Legouix, 1952). The differential electrode technique provides the only available means to obtain, at least to some extent, a recording that is largely free from the contamination of remotely generated responses.

The most salient feature of the CM is that—at least at low stimulus levels where nonlinearities are not significant—at any given recording site it reflects the frequency analyzing properties of the cochlear partition. In Fig. 10 the amplitude and phase responses of three cochlear recording locations are shown. The graphs depict the magnitude of the CM when the velocity of the stapes is kept constant at all frequencies, and the phase difference between CM and stapes velocity, again while the latter is held the same over the range of frequencies. Recall that constant stapes velocity implies that the pressure at the oval window remains invariant, thus the conditions of Fig. 10 yield a situation where the input to the cochlea is held constant. It is apparent that up to a particular frequency, which is characteristic to the recording site, the CM remains constant, or in other words, its magnitude is proportional to stapes velocity. Beyond the range of flat response there is a variable size peak, beyond which the CM rapidly declines. The corresponding phase behavior shows that after the initial zero phase difference, the CM lags the stapes velocity and that phase shift accumulates rather rapidly to a

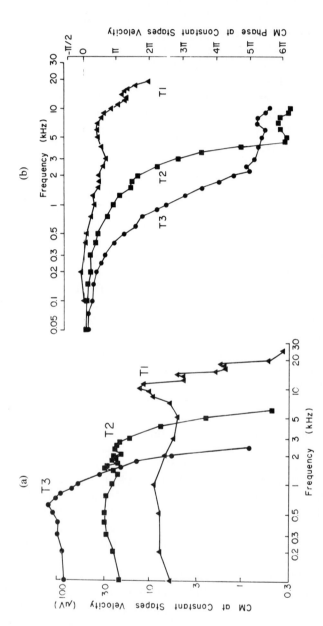

FIG. 10. (a) CM magnitude at constant stapes velocity as a function of frequency obtained from three cochlear locations. (b) CM phase referred to stapes velocity as a function of frequency from three cochlear locations. [From Dallos (1973a).]

maximum of about 5π or 6π. At the point that is 3 dB down from the CM amplitude peak, the phase difference approximates π radians.

To provide a more vivid comparison between CM and preceding mechanical events, in Fig. 11 the CM magnitude recorded at constant stapes displacement is compared with the amplitude plot of basilar-membrane displacement obtained under comparable recording conditions and from a similar cochlear site. It is apparent that the CM largely reflects the mechanical displacement pattern, particularly in the low frequency behavior and in the location of the major peak. Even the steepening of the slope below the peak is present, albeit the steep portion of the tuning curve is not as pronounced as it is for the mechanical response. The high frequency slope is considerably steeper for the mechanical plot than for the CM curve. Both plots show a flattening of the response at the highest frequencies. The discrepancies most likely result from gross electrode recording, which has the property that the response is obtained from a relatively extensive (probably about 2 mm) segment of the cochlea. Thus a flattening of the response is expected on account of the ensuing spatial averaging.

The shape of the CM tuning curves is radically influenced by the level of the stimulus. On the low-frequency slope and much above the peak frequency, the functions are only moderately altered in shape unless the signal

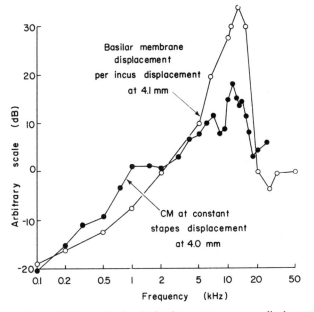

FIG. 11. Comparison of CM magnitude obtained at constant stapes displacement (1 Å) from one guinea pig with basilar-membrane displacement divided by incus displacement as measured in a guinea pig by Wilson and Johnstone (1972). In both experiments the point of measurement is approximately the same. [From Dallos *et al.* (1974).]

becomes extremely high. In other words, in these frequency regions the CM increases linearly with sound intensity up to quite high levels. In contrast, at and just above the peak, the response becomes markedly nonlinear at low stimulus levels. The result of this nonlinearity is that the higher the stimulus intensity, the flatter the CM tuning curves become. When the CM magnitude is plotted as a function of the input magnitude for a signal in this frequency range, only a very limited linear segment is seen, beyond which the CM saturates, goes through a maximum, and eventually declines. In the non-linear region, many manifestations of CM nonlinearity are seen, such as harmonic and intermodulation distortion production, interference effect, and maximal summating potential (Dallos, 1973a; Dallos, Cheatham, & Ferraro, 1974).

The CM that can be recorded from normal cochleas can be shown to be overwhelmingly generated by the outer hair cells (Davis, Deatherage, Rosenblut, Fernández, Kimura, & Smith, 1958; Dallos, 1973a). The CM output of the inner hair cell population is from 30 to 40 dB below that of the normal cochlea. Aside from the magnitude differences between inner- and outer-hair-cell-generated CM, there are highly significant dynamic differences between the two potentials. It was shown by Békésy (1960, pp. 672–684) that the CM produced in the normal ear is proportional to the displacement of the basilar membrane. We have demonstrated (Dallos et al., 1972) that the CM produced by inner hair cells alone bears a first time derivative relationship to the normal CM, thus it may be said that inner hair cells produce CM potentials in proportion to basilar membrane velocity, whereas outer hair cells generate these voltages in proportion to basilar-membrane displacement.

The summating potential was first noted by Davis, Fernández, and McAuliffe in 1950 and it has received ample attention in the years since (e.g. Davis, Deatherage, Eldredge, & Smith, 1958; Honrubia & Ward, 1969; Dallos, Schoeny, & Cheatham, 1970). This stimulus-related *dc* response of the cochlea has generally been attributed less importance than the CM, mainly because of the complex nature of the phenomenon, which made early attempts at quantification not entirely successful. It is now demonstrated that SP behavior is just as predictable as CM, the two types of potential are commensurate in magnitude, and thus there is no a priori reason to attribute less significance to the former in the transduction process.

Probably the best means of studying SP is by the differential electrode method, which allows the difference between the vestibuli and tympani electrodes and their average to be considered and investigated separately. The former potential is designated as DIF SP, and the latter as AVE SP (Dallos et al., 1970). Both components of the SP response have well-defined frequency and intensity dependence at any cochlear recording site. Figure 12 shows some sample waveforms of recordings from the first turn of the cochlea for

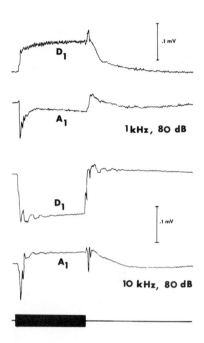

FIG. 12. DIF and AVE SP responses obtained from the basal turn in response to 1 kHz (top) and 10 kHz (bottom) tone bursts of 40 msec duration delivered at 80 dB SPL. [From Dallos (1972), Cochlear potentials: A status report, *Audiology*, **11**, 29–41.]

two frequencies delivered at the same sound pressure level. The figure demonstrates the complexity of the phenomenon when it is considered that both DIF and AVE components reverse polarity when, in this case, the stimulus changes from 1 to 10 kHz. The dependence of the SP upon frequency can best be understood with the aid of Fig. 13, where both CM and SP recordings are shown from a first turn electrode pair as a function of frequency at a constant sound pressure level. It is notable that there is a narrow frequency region, corresponding to the high-frequency slope of the CM curve, where the DIF is negative and the AVE is positive. Below this frequency band the DIF becomes positive while the AVE is negative, whereas at the highest frequencies, the DIF vanishes and the AVE is negative once again. This behavior can best be seen at low stimulus intensities. As the driving level increases, the characteristic DIF^- and AVE^+ bands extend to lower and lower frequencies. The low-intensity behavior is summarized in the schematic of Fig. 14. Here the spatial pattern of the traveling wave is indicated by the hatched envelope and the pattern and polarity of the two summating potential components are also shown. It is seen that the DIF is negative on the steep apical slope of the traveling wave envelope and that the AVE is positive in this same general region. On the basal slope of the traveling wave the DIF is positive. The AVE is negative everywhere except in the aforementioned narrow spatial extent. Both the DIF^- and AVE^+ grow linearly with stimulus intensity.

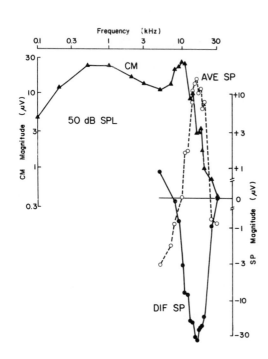
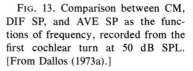

FIG. 13. Comparison between CM, DIF SP, and AVE SP as the functions of frequency, recorded from the first cochlear turn at 50 dB SPL. [From Dallos (1973a).]

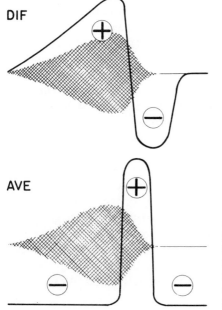

FIG. 14. Schematic spatial pattern of traveling wave envelope (shaded area) and DIF and AVE SP components at low stimulus intensity. Apex is to the right. [From Dallos (1971), Summating potentials of the cochlea. In M. B. Sachs (Ed.), *Physiology of the Auditory System.* Copyright 1971 by Natl. Educ. Cons., Baltimore.]

There is no conclusive evidence militating either for or against the proposition that CM and some components of the SP (probably DIF⁻ and AVE⁺) are important intermediary links in the cochlear transducer process. In other words, we do not know if these potentials are causally involved in the liberation of synaptic transmitters and thus the initiation of neural discharges in the fibers of the VIIIth nerve. It is more parsimonious to assume that they are, and this stance is generally taken by most authorities. However, direct experimental confirmation is yet to be obtained. The electrical phenomenon most directly associated with transmitter release is the generator potential of the VIIIth nerve dendrites. Unfortunately, experimental evidence is largely lacking that would provide information about the properties of the generator potential, and thus about the "output" of the mammalian cochlea. Voluminous data are available on the discharge characteristics of single fibers in the auditory nerve, and some information is also provided in the literature about the properties of the compound action potential (AP) of the VIIIth nerve trunk. The AP is of somewhat limited utility in quantifying cochlear output, since it arises only under specific stimulus conditions (discrete events in time, that is, transients, are required to elicit a well-synchronized volley of discharges, which is the prerequisite for a discernible AP). Unit response properties are widely used to infer cochlear processes. When this is done, however, one should consider several factors that could conceivably influence the response and thus intimate complexities that are not strictly associable with cochlear processes. One obvious item is the transformation between generator potential and discharge rate. This transformation is likely to be nonlinear and, in consequence, it may be quite complex. Another, and probably more significant factor is related to the innervation pattern of the organ of Corti. Since about 95% of the nerve fibers are innervated from inner hair cells at face value, it is thus highly probable that most information found in the literature describes the behavior of a homogeneous fiber population, namely, that which receives its primary excitation from inner hair cells. The possibility should not be ignored, however, that each fiber might receive information from multiple sources, probably from a single inner hair cell and from a group of outer hair cells. What we have seen of the dynamic differences in the operation of the two cell groups suggests that they would be likely to supply different inputs that could interact and whose dominance could shift depending on stimulus conditions. It is also conceivable that the more diffusely innervated outer hair cell population would provide only a general, facilitative, or functional input serving to set the operating point. Such mode of operation could be a counterpart to the efferent input system to the cochlea, which also possesses an extremely diffuse terminal pattern stemming from very few efferent fibers (about 500), and whose only well-defined physiological effect is a relatively moderate inhibition of the cochlear output.

IV. ADDENDUM

A number of other topics have emerged as central in the continued study of auditory biophysics. Aside from the continuing controversy about the linear versus nonlinear nature of basilar membrane motion, arguments about the necessity for two filtering processes and the physiological nature of these filters, as well as questions pertaining to the possible interaction between the two sensory cell populations have emerged. A strong argument is made (Evans & Wilson, 1973) that even the best of the contemporary mechanical measurements of the sharpness of tuning of the basilar membrane (as a frequency selective filter) cannot match the frequency selectivity exhibited by the discharge characteristics of VIIIth nerve fibers. To account for the discrepancy, it is assumed that the traveling wave mechanism constitutes a relatively crude, first filter, and that a second filter exists between basilar-membrane motion and the initial segment of the auditory nerve fibers. This second filter would provide the presumably necessary sharpening of frequency selectivity. Several suggestions have been made pertaining to the physiological identity of the second filter (e.g., Evans & Wilson, 1973; Steele, 1974; Zwislocki & Sokolich, 1974; Zwicker, 1974) but the available data do not allow one to decide among the alternatives, or indeed, to ascertain the necessity for a second filter. Similarly unresolved is the question whether or not there is an interaction between inner and outer hair cells of the cochlea. Mounting evidence suggests that some form of interaction is required, but the mechanism remains obscure.

References

Allaire, P., Raynor, S., & Billone, M. C. Cochlear partition stiffness-a composite beam model. *Journal of the Acoustical Society of America*, 1974, **55**, 1252–1258.

Békésy, G. von. *Experiments in hearing*. New York: McGraw-Hill, 1960.

Billone, M. C. Mechanical stimulation of cochlear hair cells. Unpublished Ph.D. dissertation, Northwestern Univ., Evanston, Illinois, 1972.

Bodian, D. The generalized vertebrate neuron. *Science*, 1962, **137**, 323–326.

Brödel, M. *Three unpublished drawings of the anatomy of the human ear*. Philadelphia: Saunders, 1946.

Dallos, P. Comments on the differential electrode technique. *Journal of the Acoustical Society of America*, 1969, **45**, 999–1007.

Dallos, P. Summating potentials of the cochlea. In M. B. Sachs (Ed.), *Physiology of the auditory system*. Baltimore: Natl. Educ. Cons., 1971. Pp. 57–67.

Dallos, P. Cochlear potentials: A status report. *Audiology*, 1972, **11**, 29–41.

Dallos, P. Cochlear potentials and cochlear mechanics. In A. Møller (Ed.), *Basic mechanisms of hearing*. New York: Academic Press, 1973. Pp. 335–372. (a)

Dallos, P. *The auditory periphery: Biophysics and physiology*. New York: Academic, 1973. (b)

Dallos, P., Billone, M., Durrant, J. D., Wang, C.-y., & Raynor, S. Cochlear inner and outer hair cells: Functional differences. *Science*, 1972, **177**, 356–358.

Dallos, P., Cheatham, M. A., & Ferraro, J. Cochlear mechanics, nonlinearities, and cochlear potentials. *Journal of the Acoustical Society of America*, 1974, **55**, 597–605.

Dallos, P., Schoeny, Z. G., & Cheatham, M. A. Cochlear summating potentials: Composition. *Science*, 1970, **170**, 641–644.

Dallos, P., & Wang, C.-y. Bioelectric correlates of kanamycin intoxication. *Audiology*, 1974, **13**, 277–289.

Davis, H. Some principles of sensory receptor action. *Physiological Review*, 1961, **41**, 391–416.

Davis, H. A model for transducer action in the cochlea. *Cold Spring Harbor Symposia on Quantitative Biology*, 1965, **30**, 181–190.

Davis, H., & associates. Acoustic trauma in the guinea pig. *Journal of the Acoustical Society of America*, 1953, **25**, 1180–1189.

Davis, H., Deatherage, B. H., Eldredge, D. H., & Smith, C. A. Summating potentials of the cochlea. *American Journal of Physiology*, 1958, **195**, 251–261.

Davis, H., Deatherage, B. H., Rosenblut, B., Fernández, C., Kimura, R., & Smith, C. A. Modification of cochlear potentials produced by streptomycin poisoning and by extensive venous obstruction. *Laryngoscope*, 1958, **68**, 596–627.

Davis, H., Fernández, C., & McAuliffe, D. R. The excitatory process in the cochlea. *Proceedings of the National Academy of Sciences of the United States*, 1950, **36**, 580–587.

Engström, H., Ades, H. W., & Hawkins, J. E., Jr. Structure and functions of the sensory hairs of the inner ear. *Journal of the Acoustical Society of America*, 1962, **34**, 1356–1363.

Evans, E. F., & Wilson, J. P. The frequency selectivity of the cochlea. In A. Møller (Ed.), *Basic Mechanisms of Hearing*, New York: Academic Press, 1973. Pp. 519–551.

Fletcher, H. *Speech and hearing in communication*. Princeton, New Jersey: Van Nostrand-Reinhold, 1953.

Flock, Å., Kimura, R., Lundquist, P. G., & Wersäll, J. Morphological basis of directional sensitivity of the outer hair cells in the organ of Corti. *Journal of the Acoustical Society of America*, 1962, **34**, 1351–1355.

Grundfest, H. Excitation by hyperpolarizing potentials. A general theory of receptor activities. In E. Florey (Ed.), *Nervous inhibition*. Oxford: Pergamon, 1961. Pp. 326–341.

Honrubia, V., & Ward, P. H. (1969). Properties of the summating potential of the guinea pig's cochlea. *Journal of the Acoustical Society of America*, 1969, **45**, 1443–1450.

Iurato, S. *Submicroscopic structure of the inner ear*. London: Pergamon, 1967.

Johnstone, B. M., & Boyle, A. J. T. Basilar membrane vibration examined with the Mössbauer technique. *Science*, 1967, **158**, 389–390.

Johnstone, B. M., & Sellick, P. M. The peripheral auditory apparatus. *Quarterly Review of Biophysics*, 1972, **5**, 1–57.

Johnstone, B. M., & Taylor, K. (1970). Mechanical aspects of cochlear function. In R. Plomp & G. Smoorenburg (Eds.), *Frequency analysis and periodicity detection in hearing*. Leiden: A. W. Sijthoff, 1970. Pp. 81–90.

Kimura, R. S. Hairs of the cochlear sensory cells and their attachment to the tectorial membrane. *Acta Oto-Laryngologica*, 1966, **61**, 55–72.

Lim, D. J. Fine morphology of the tectorial membrane; Its relationship to the organ of Corti. *Archives of Otolaryngology*, 1972, **96**, 199–215.

Peake, W. T., Sohmer, H. S., & Weiss, T. J. Microelectrode recordings of intracochlear potentials. In *Quarterly Progress Report*, 1969, No. **94**, 293–304. MIT Research Laboratory of Electronics, Cambridge, Massachusetts.

Peterson, L., & Bogert, B. A dynamical theory of the cochlea. *Journal of the Acoustical Society of America*, 1950, **22**, 369–381.

Ranke, O. F. Das Massenverhältnis zwischen Membran und Flüssigkeit im Innenohr. *Akustische Zeitschrift*, 1942, **7**, 1–11.

Ranke, O. F. Theory of operation of the cochlea: A contribution to the hydrodynamics of the cochlea. *Journal of the Acoustical Society of America*, 1950, **22**, 772–777.

Rhode, W. S. Observations of the vibration of the basilar membrane in squirrel monkeys using the Mössbauer technique. *Journal of the Acoustical Society of America*, 1971, **49**, 1218–1231.

Rhode, W. S. An investigation of post-mortem cochlear mechanics using the Mössbauer effect. In A. Møller (Ed.), *Basic mechanisms of hearing*. New York: Academic Press, 1973. Pp. 49–63.

Schroeder, M. R. An integrable model for the basilar membrane. *Journal of the Acoustical Society of America*, 1973, **53**, 429–434.

Siebert, W. Ranke revisited—a simple short-wave cochlear model. *Journal of the Acoustical Society of America*, 1974, **56**, 594–600.

Spoendlin, H. *The organization of the cochlear receptor*. Basel: Karger, 1966.

Steele, C. R. Behavior of the basilar membrane with pure-tone excitation. *Journal of the Acoustical Society of America*, 1974, **55**, 148–162.

Tasaki, I., Davis, H., & Legouix, J. P. The space-time pattern of the cochlear microphonics (guinea pig), as recorded by differential electrodes. *Journal of the Acoustical Society of America*, 1952, **24**, 502–518.

Tonndorf, J. Shearing motion in scala media of cochlear models. *Journal of the Acoustical Society of America*, 1960, **32**, 238–244.

Tonndorf, J. Nonlinearities in cochlear hydrodynamics. *Journal of the Acoustical Society of America*, 1970, **47**, 574–578.

Tonndorf, J., & Khanna, S. M. Displacement pattern of the basilar membrane: A comparison of experimental data. *Science*, 1968, **160**, 1139–1140.

Wersäll, J., Flock, Å., & Lundquist, P.-G. Structural basis for directional sensitivity in cochlear and vestibular sensory receptors. *Cold Spring Harbor Symposia on Quantitative Biology*, 1965, **30**, 115–145.

Wever, E. G. *Theory of hearing*. New York: Wiley, 1949.

Wever, E. G. The mechanics of hair-cell stimulation. *Annals of Otology, Rhinology, and Laryngology*, 1971, **80**, 786–805.

Wever, E. G., & Bray, C. Action currents in the auditory nerve in response to acoustic stimulation. *Proceedings of the National Academy of Sciences of the United States*, 1930, **16**, 344–350.

Wilson, J. P., & Johnstone, J. R. Capacitive probe measures of basilar membrane vibrations. In *Hearing theory*. Eindhoven: IPO, 1972. Pp. 172–181.

Zwicker, E. A "second filter" established within the scala media. In E. Zwicker & E. Terhardt (Eds.), *Facts and Models in Hearing*. Berlin: Springer-Verlag, 1974. Pp. 95–98.

Zwieg, G., Lipes, R., & Pierce, J. R. The cochlear compromise. *Journal of the Acoustical Society of America*, 1973, **59**, 975–982.

Zwislocki, J. Theorie der Schneckenmechanik. *Acta Oto-Laryngologica*, 1948, Suppl. **72**, 76.

Zwislocki, J. Theory of the acoustical action of the cochlea. *Journal of the Acoustical Society of America*, 1950, **22**, 778–784.

Zwislocki, J. Analysis of some auditory characteristics. In R. Luce, R. Bush, & E. Galanter (Eds.), *Handbook of mathematical psychology*. Vol. III. New York: Wiley, 1965. Pp. 1–97.

Zwislocki, J. Cochlear waves: Interaction between theory and experiments. *Journal of the Acoustical Society of America*, 1974, **55**, 578–583.

Zwislocki, J. J., & Sokolich, W. G. Neuro-mechanical frequency analysis in the cochlea. In E. Zwicker & E. Terhardt (Eds.), *Facts and Models in Hearing*. Berlin: Springer-Verlag, 1974. Pp. 107–117.

Chapter 5

THE NEURAL CODE

I. C. WHITFIELD

I. INTRODUCTION

The coding of information in the nervous system involves, in general, the presence of nerve impulses or "action potential spikes" in nerve fibers, although as we shall see this statement will require some modification. The amplitude of nerve impulses in a train is apparently not a significant variable so that there are three possible ways in which information could be conveyed: *(1)* the simple presence or absence of spike activity in a given nerve fiber, *(2)* the mean number of impulses in a given time, *(3)* the temporal relationship between successive impulses in a fiber or group of fibers.

Historically, all three of these mechanisms have been proposed as components of theories of hearing. The eighteenth-century resonance theories were combined by Helmholtz (1863) with Müller's theory of specific nerve energies, to form a system employing a code of type *(1)*. According to Helmholtz's original proposal, each discriminable frequency gave rise to activity in a fiber or group of fibers unique for that frequency (Fig. 1a). "Place" theories in general involve coding of type *(1)*. Implicit, if not explicit, in Helmholtz's theory was the idea that increased intensity of the stimulus would involve increased activity in the appropriate nerve fiber so that type *(2)* coding was also involved. The rival, "telephone", theories of hearing (Rutherford, 1886) employed basically a code of type *(3)*, since such theories

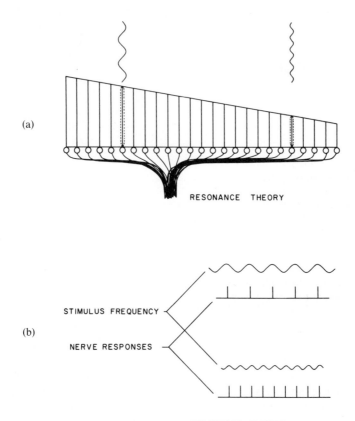

FIG. 1. Basic theories of frequency analysis. (a) Helmholtz's resonance theory; (b) Rutherford's telephone theory.

postulate a temporal relationship between the nerve impulses and the stimulating waveform (Fig. 1b).

II. THE AUDITORY NERVE

The auditory nerve forms a suitable point at which to start investigating the auditory code, since all the information from the ear must pass along it. It might be thought that all we need to do is to record the responses to a sufficient variety of stimuli and the job would be done. However, it is not as simple as that, because we have to know not only the variations that occur within the channel in response to different stimuli, but also which of those variations can be detected by the receiver (the central nervous system). Any variation which cannot be so detected, no matter that it has a one-to-one relationship with the stimulus, can provide no information. Furthermore, the existence of such epiphenomena may well confuse the outside observer attempting to break the code. Consider for example two color-blind people who use a child's paint box in order to draw designs on cards, by which they communicate with each other. They will, of course, see the patterns in various shades of gray, and the patterns will be meaningful. A person with normal color vision observing the messages passing back and forth would see something quite different which might well be meaningless. This analogy is not far-fetched; the well-known Ishihara plates used to test color vision are precisely such a set of designs which convey one message to one observer and a different message to another.

Having issued this *caveat,* let us look now at the behavior of a single auditory nerve fiber, and, since it is a dimension which has been much studied, let us look first of all at the coding of stimulus frequency. The nature of the stimulus/response pattern was first indicated in the famous experiments of Galambos and Davis (1943). Their experiments showed that each neural unit had a threshold response curve such that there was one stimulus frequency (the best, or "characteristic" frequency) for which the discharge threshold was lowest, and which served to label or characterize that fiber. As the sound intensity is raised above this best threshold, the band of frequencies to which the fiber responds gradually increases, until at an intensity 60–70 dB above the original value the fiber may respond to stimulus frequencies extending over one or two octaves. Although the results of Galambos and Davis were subsequently shown to be from cells rather than auditory nerve fibers, subsequent work by Kiang (1966) on the cat, Katsuki, Suga, and Kanno (1962) on the monkey, and Evans (1970) on the guinea pig has amply confirmed the original curves with data from undoubted single nerve fibers (Fig. 2). The

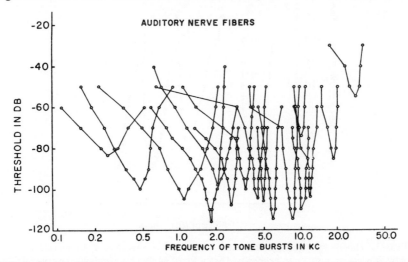

FIG. 2. Threshold/frequency response curves from single auditory nerve fibers in the cat. [From N. Y. S. Kiang, Stimulus coding in the auditory nerve. *Acta Oto-Laryngologica,* 1965, **59,** 186–200.]

"classic" curve shape is a triangle in which the rate of threshold rise is greater on the high-frequency than on the low-frequency side. However, in any study of coding, we must bear in mind that this is not universal. Some units have quite symmetrical curves and others are even mirror-imaged so that the steeper limb is on the low-frequency side. Furthermore, many units show a "break" in the low-frequency limb where the curve suddenly becomes much less steep at high intensities. This break may occur anywhere from about 60–90 dB sound pressure level (SPL).

A consistent feature of these curves is that when represented on a logarithmic (or octave) scale they become progressively narrower the higher the characteristic frequency. There is no deep significance in this; clearly if we were to choose a linear scale of frequency we would observe just the opposite—the curves would become wider with increasing frequency. The logarithmic scale is usually chosen partly on account of its musical attributes and partly because it gives an approximately straight line relationship to distance along the basilar membrane. However, if we want to generalize about nerve response areas, or compare one with another, the logarithmic scale is clearly inconvenient, and it would be better to choose one that is uniform over frequency. Ross (1968) has shown that this condition is approximated by choosing a square root frequency scale (Fig. 3). By using this transformation, it is possible to obtain figures for the mean slopes of both the high- and low-frequency limbs of the response curves together with their standard deviations. With the aid of a graph of innervation density of the cochlea (Fig. 4) it is now possible to calculate the number of fibers which would

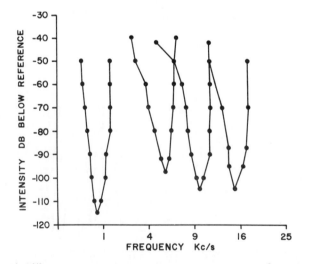

FIG. 3. Threshold/frequency response curves on a square-root frequency scale. The bandwidths are uniform over frequency. [From Ross, quoted by Whitfield, The organization of the auditory pathways, *Journal of Sound and Vibration Research,* 1968, **8**(1), 108–117.]

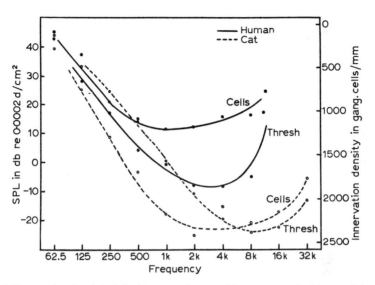

FIG. 4. Innervation density of the human and cat cochleas compared with sound threshold. [From Schuknecht (1960), Neuroanatomical correlates of auditory sensitivity and pitch discrimination in the cat. In G. L. Rasmussen & W. F. Windle (Eds.), *Neural Mechanisms of the Auditory and Vestibular Systems.* Copyright 1960 by Charles C Thomas.]

be stimulated by a given frequency at a given intensity, provided all the fibers involved had the same absolute threshold. This calculation is carried out as follows.

Suppose we choose a stimulus frequency of 4 kHz or 2 square root frequency units (sqrf). The high frequency slope is .005 sqrf/dB and the low frequency slope .01 sqrf/dB. At 40 dB above threshold the extremes of the array stimulated will lie at $2 - .2$ and $2 + .4$ sqrf, i.e., at frequencies of 3.25 kHz and 5.8 kHz. Since shift of frequency along the cochlea is about 2.8 mm per octave, this represents a distance along the cochlea of about 2.3 mm. The innervation density of the cat cochlea in the region of 4 kHz is about 2400 fibers per millimeter so that the number of fibers involved would be about 5600.

If we take a lower stimulus frequency, say 400 Hz, the number of fibers would be about 10,000, and if we take a higher one, say 16 kHz, the number would be about 2500. All these numbers will, of course, have standard deviations which are a function of the standard deviations of the response curve slopes already referred to. However, the general point to note is that any single-tone stimulus, at even a modest intensity level, involves activity in an appreciable fraction of the total available number of nerve fibers (about 40,000 in the cat).

If we raise or lower the intensity we add to or subtract from the number of active fibers at the ends of the array, and we can easily calculate this on the same basis as before. At 4 kHz, the change in the spread is about 150 fibers per decibel. This suggests that at least one possible correlate of intensity might be the extent of the active array.

III. THE CODING OF INTENSITY

So far we have assumed that every fiber within the region involved has the same absolute threshold. While fiber thresholds are fairly constant in the sense that they do not cover the whole discriminable intensity range, nevertheless there *is* some variation in threshold, amounting to perhaps 30 dB between the least and most sensitive fibers in a given region. The implication of this is that increase in stimulus intensity not only adds fibers at the ends of the array but also adds fibers within the limits of the array itself (Fig. 5).

We have then a correlation between stimulus intensity and number of active nerve fibers. Bearing in mind our early caveat (page 164), are we justified in assuming that the parameter is in fact coded in this way? We may perhaps throw some light on this by looking not at the relation of fiber number to the "input" parameter intensity, but its relation to the "output" parameter loudness. If all the nerve fibers from a restricted part of the cochlea are selectively destroyed, the result may well be loss of hearing for a particular frequency band. However, if disease destroys a proportion of the fibers in the auditory nerve without regard to their origin, a different phenomenon is seen. Surprisingly, perhaps, the hearing threshold may be quite unchanged, even though 80% of the fibers are missing. This has been shown both in humans and experimentally in the cat (Citron, Dix, Hallpike,

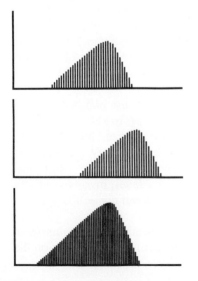

FIG. 5. Top and middle: positions of activity in the fiber array for two different frequencies at the same intensity. Bottom: activity in the fiber array for an increased intensity. Height of lines represents discharge rate in the particular channel. [From Whitfield (1967).]

& Hood, 1963; Schuknecht & Woellner, 1955). However, above threshold a deficit appears. As the intensity is raised the sound appears less loud than does a sound of similar intensity to a good ear, and the discrepancy becomes progressively greater the more intense the stimulus. The implication of this finding is that there are sufficient fibers to carry intensity information near threshold, but as the intensity is increased we no longer have sufficient fibers to mediate the increase, and so loudness is impaired.

It might be thought that because the innervation density is greater in the midfrequency region, frequencies around 1 or 2 kHz should sound relatively louder at a given intensity than those frequencies near the ends of the spectrum. To a large extent this is, of course, true, but it must be borne in mind nevertheless that at the highest intensities, when presumably all available fibers have been brought into play, the loudness of all frequencies is about the same (Fletcher & Munson, 1933) irrespective of the actual number of fibers involved. It seems that loudness is related to the proportion of fibers activated out of the total normally available rather than to the absolute number of fibers. However, it could be that a discriminable step of loudness (DL) approximates to a certain number of fibers, since at 100 Hz, a region of low innervation density, there are about 90 DL between the threshold of hearing and the threshold of pain, whereas at 1000 Hz there are over 300 DL. This relationship is not sufficiently quantitative that it should be taken too seriously however.

We may conclude, therefore, that the proposal that loudness is coded in terms of number of fibers active is not an unreasonable one. What then is the role of discharge rate? Classically, discharge rate is regarded as being linked to stimulus strength in all sensory systems, and the ear is no exception. A given primary fiber certainly shows the classical sigmoid relation between discharge rate and intensity. However, this relationship extends only over a range of about 30 dB above the threshold of the fiber, and it is thus evident that discharge rate *per se* can play only a minor role in signalling loudness over the 140-dB dynamic range of the ear. The question is rather, does it play any role at all? This is hard to answer. We cannot invoke the type of experiment where we limited the number of fibers. It is not possible artificially to hold constant the discharge rate, while changing the number of active fibers. There are two small pieces of evidence which might be invoked to suggest the relative unimportance of discharge rate. The first is the existence of "spontaneous" activity, sometimes at quite high rates, not apparently accompanied by any sensation of sound. The second is the observation that at or near threshold, the first change induced by a stimulus in a spontaneously active fiber is not an increase in the discharge rate, but an organization of the existing discharge into a more regular pattern. Neither of these points is very cogent and perhaps they raise more problems than they solve. Be that as it may, I believe we are justified in concluding, for reasons to be reinforced in what follows, that discharge rate is not a key factor in the coding of loudness.

IV. THE CODING OF PITCH

Let us consider first of all the coding of the pitch of single tones. We have seen that a single stimulus frequency at a modest intensity of 40 dB above threshold might activate perhaps 20% of all the fibers in the auditory nerve. However, we can certainly discriminate more than five different tones, so that clearly there is not a unique set of fibers activated for each tone. There must be overlap and this overlap is very very considerable. If we take a figure of 300 DL per octave around 2 kHz, then the fiber shift in the array for a single DL comes out at about *25 fibers,* i.e., 25 fibers are subtracted from one end and added to the other end of an array perhaps 5000 fibers long: in other words, 99.5% of the fibers remain the same. (It is interesting to note, in passing, that if one works out the DL for loudness in the same situation, the result is a change of 50 fibers per DL, a figure remarkably close to that for frequency, when it is remembered that an exchange of 25 fibers actually affects 50 fibers!)

We see therefore that frequency discrimination cannot involve a "specific nerve energy" type of code but is related to the position of the total active array. In signalling this position and hence enabling discrimination between two just discriminable frequencies, the 25 fibers at the edge of the array are clearly crucial. In other words all the frequency information is effectively carried by the position of the "edges"—the discontinuity between activity and inactivity.

V. THE SQUARING PROCESS

Because of the relation which exists between intensity above threshold and firing rate, the fibers near the edge of the array will fire less rapidly than those near the center. We have seen that this relationship (which exists for all receptors) plays little part in the coding of intensity. In the coding of stimulus frequency it is a positive disadvantage, because owing to the presence of "spontaneous" activity in unstimulated fibers, the slow-firing edge may be blurred or lost. It seems that the auditory system arranges to get rid of this defect at the earliest opportunity. If we look at the transfer function of the cochlear nucleus, we find in a certain proportion of the output fibers— presumably those subserving frequency discrimination if our thesis is correct—an almost step-function relationship between input and output (Fig. 6). Below a certain input rate there is no output. As the input increases, the output rises rapidly to a ceiling and then levels off; it may even fall again for very high inputs. The effect of this is to remove almost completely any remaining relation between stimulus strength and discharge rate. Fibers are now either "on" or "off". The advantage, of course, is that the edges are

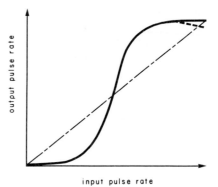

FIG. 6. Input/output relationship in the cochlear nucleus. The relationship may be non-monotonic at the highest rates.

now much more sharply defined and impervious to "noise" in the system. The result of the transformations we have been discussing then is that a given stimulus frequency produces activity in a block of fibers within the total array. The loudness appears to depend on the number of fibers activated, and the pitch on the actual position of the active fiber blocks. Because of the regular tonotopic organization of the system, at least as far up as the inferior colliculus, change of frequency causes the pattern to shift in a regular manner across the whole fiber array. It is to be noted that because of the asymmetry of the unit response curves, an increase in stimulus intensity may add fibers unevenly to the two ends of the array, thereby changing its mean position. It is understandable, therefore, that changes in intensity could potentially have a small effect on the pitch of a single tone.

It is not possible to say for certain whether the coding of pitch depends on the totality of fiber activity or whether it is purely a function of the position of the discontinuities between the active and inactive fibers. The question may well be unmeaningful. I quoted earlier the observation that destruction of 80% of the auditory nerve fibers does not affect threshold, and likewise it does not affect the pitch heard. On the other hand, reducing the "block" to one active fiber at each end of the array would clearly be insufficient, since it would be indistinguishable from two separate blocks. Presumably, therefore, we need sufficient active fibers to identify the active region as a single block and to define its limits. This suggests that at very low intensities near threshold, pitch will be poorly defined, but that the frequency DL will rapidly narrow as the intensity increases, and will then flatten off. This is, of course, precisely what is observed subjectively. It has always been an inescapable problem for proponents of the idea that pitch discrimination is in some way dependent on the width of the auditory nerve response curves (or "tuning curves" as they are sometimes unfortunately called) that however narrow they might be they inevitably result in less frequency selectivity rather than more as the intensity is raised, and this as we have just seen is at variance with observation.

A further small piece of evidence in support of the crucial role of the edges, is the proposal of Kiang, Moxon, and Levine (1970) that tinnitus arises not simply from spontaneous activity in the auditory nerve, but from a region of discontinuity between activity and inactivity brought about by selective damage.

VI. COMPLEX TONES

So far, we have been considering the coding of a single tone (that is, one comprising only a single frequency) and have discussed the relation of the coding of such a tone to the problem of its discrimination from other tones adjacent in intensity or frequency. It is to be noted that DLs for intensity and frequency are determined for successive presentations of the two stimuli. The stimuli cannot be compared in the same way when presented simultaneously, and one reason for this is inherent in the nature of the coding we have been discussing. Leaving aside problems of mechanical interaction on the basilar membrane, it is clear that two closely adjacent tones would fuse into a single active array, if singly they would have a high proportion of fibers in common.

Although we can, of course, listen to all sorts of artificially produced tone combinations, the "natural" stimulus is the so-called "complex tone" consisting of a series of harmonically related partials. Almost all sounds with a well-defined pitch are of this kind, the "pure tone" being a limiting case of rare occurrence. The "complex tone" is heard naïvely as a unitary sensation, but nevertheless it is possible to learn to distinguish separately a number of the upper partials. Estimates vary, but the number usually given is of the order of six for notes with fundamentals in the 250–1000-Hz region (Plomp, 1966). For this to be possible in terms of our single-tone coding theory, we shall need a separate block of activity for each isolable component of the sound. It is clear that the mechanics of the basilar membrane itself must eventually prove a limiting factor in the resolution of these components, but other factors may be important at the cochlear level and it may be more instructive for our purpose to look at the behavior of single auditory nerve fibers.

VII. CRITICAL BANDS

The loudness of a band of noise at constant power remains constant as the bandwidth is increased up to a certain value, the *critical bandwidth*—then the loudness starts to increase (Feldkeller & Zwicker, 1956). Similarly, the threshold of a narrow band of noise lying between two masking tones remains constant until the frequency separation between the two tones reaches the critical bandwidth, whereupon its threshold suddenly becomes lower. The critical band, then, represents some division of the auditory array within which signal power sums and within which separate signals cannot be distinguished.

[The term "critical band" was actually first used by Fletcher (1940) in investigations of the masking of a tone by a band of noise, the hypothesis being that only those components of the noise lying within a certain critical band around the tone contributed to the masking. This quantity, measured from the signal-to-noise ratio, is now more properly called the *critical ratio* (Scharf, 1970), but the two are directly related.]

Critical bands vary in width from 100 Hz at the low-frequency end of the spectrum to 2.5 kHz at 10 kHz. It has been suggested that they represent equal distances along the basilar membrane (Greenwood, 1961). This correlation tends to break down at the ends of the scale and Zwislocki (1965) has suggested that a better correlation can be obtained with innervation density so that each critical band corresponds to a certain number of auditory nerve fibers (in man about 1300).

This proposal makes it interesting to compare the critical bands with the width of the "active arrays" of nerve fibers discussed on page 167. Data for critical ratios in the cat have been determined by Watson (1963), and these may be used to estimate the critical bands. Direct measurement of critical bands in the cat has been carried out by Pickles (1975) and the results agree well with Watson's data. The bands are some 2–3 times wider than they are in man (Fig. 7).

The frequencies considered on page 167 were 400 Hz, 4 kHz, and 16 kHz and the critical bands at these frequencies in the cat are about 160 Hz, 2 kHz, and 10 kHz, respectively. Using Schuknecht's (1960) data for innervation density these figures correspond to 3000, 4800, and 5600 fibers within the respective bands. It will be remembered that for a tone around 4 kHz and 40 dB SPL the number of fibers in the active array was 5600. If we imagine two such tones situated at the two extremes of the critical band, their "peaks" will be 4800 fibers apart, and they will occupy between them 5600 fibers, i.e., there will be some overlap (Fig. 8). For the 10-kHz case, the tones will be 5600 fibers apart and occupy 2500 fibers—a considerable gap, while for the 400-Hz case, the tones are 3000 fibers apart and "occupy" 10,000 fibers, a very large overlap.

We have chosen one particular intensity of signal, and clearly by choosing different intensities we could achieve a fit at any one point, but obviously not at all points, since the trends of the sets of figures are opposite in the two cases. Furthermore, it must be remembered that critical bands, except quite near threshold, are independent of the intensity of the signals. It would

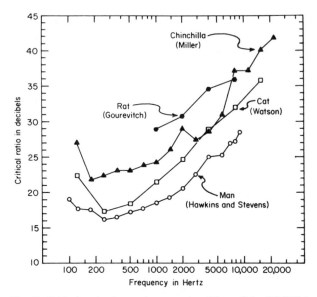

FIG. 7. Critical ratios for various species. [From Scharf (1970).]

appear therefore that the resolving power of the system for the components of a complex tone cannot be accounted for simply in terms of the way each of the components of the complex would occupy the fiber array if presented separately.

VIII. TWO-TONE INHIBITION

A defect of the "squaring hypothesis" (page 170)—the idea that the significant feature is whether fibers are "on" or "off"—is precisely that, given two overlapping responses, the positions of the separate peaks would be lost and the whole appear as one single (louder) tone situated somewhere between the two (Whitfield, 1956). However, if we try experimentally to occupy the same fiber with two different adjacent stimuli at the same time, we tend to find that the response is less than either signal alone and may be absent altogether (Fig. 8). This phenomenon of mutual inhibition (Whitfield, 1955, 1967) is an example of the very widespread phenomenon of *lateral inhibition* found throughout sensory nervous systems. The effect of the inhibitory activity is to limit the spread of the channels occupied by a particular component of a complex and to preserve its separate identity. There is some evidence that tonal interaction takes place at the auditory nerve level, resulting in suppression of activity in particular fibers, but the main site of the phenomenon we have been describing is the cochlear nucleus.

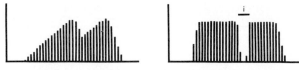

Fig. 8. Left: active array pattern due to two tones presented at the input level. Right: Inhibition (i) resulting from attempts to occupy the same channels by the two tones simultaneously. [From Whitfield (1956), Electrophysiology of the central auditory pathway, *British Medical Bulletin*, 12, 105–109.]

The filtering action of the auditory nerve fiber response curves, the "hard on/hard off" type of response imposed by the progressively restricted dynamic range of the fibers and the effects of lateral inhibition, would seem to give us a qualitative basis for the existence of something corresponding anatomically to the critical band. However, it appears that the width of these bands is not determined purely by peripheral factors but is also under central control. Pickles (1976) has shown that the magnitudes of critical bands in the cat are dependent on the activity of centrifugal fibers terminating in the cochlear nucleus, and that when this activity is blocked pharmacologically, the critical bands become abnormally wide.

IX. CENTRIFUGAL INFLUENCE

The problem of maintaining the identity of several simultaneous signals, which we have just studied, is very closely related to a number of other signal-in-noise problems.

Vietmeister (1974) has shown that, in the presence of band-stop noise, a signal located in the "gap" in the noise spectrum exhibits essentially normal loudness increments even at high signal intensities. The dilemma which, *prima facie*, presents itself is that all the fibers are saturated for firing rate, yet intensity cannot be signalled by spread along the array as we postulated on p. 168, because the needful channels are already occupied by the noise. A little thought indicates that this problem is only one special case of a more general one. Suppose we simply reduce the stop-band to zero, and have continuous wide-band white noise. If we set its intensity at a modest 60 dB, *every* fiber, the argument runs, will be saturated, and it will be impossible for any signal to be transmitted. It is a matter of experience, of course, that this is not true. It is *not* possible to mask every signal, however intense, with white noise at such a level. Obviously some modification of the discharge pattern is occurring.

This modification, like the determination of critical bandwidth, seems to be under the control of the centrifugal pathways. Pickles and Comis (1973) have shown that blocking one of the centrifugal pathways to the cochlear nucleus seriously impairs, in cats, the detection of signals against background noise, but the effect is not confined to the cochlear nucleus level. Dewson (1968) found that section of the olivo-cochlear bundle in monkeys likewise affected the discriminability of signals, but again only when presented against a noisy background. This last experiment suggests that the control begins right at the periphery—as indeed an explanation of Vietmeister's result would require.

The detailed mechanism of the centrifugal action remains to be determined. Since its operation requires a decision on which is the signal and which the noise, it is likely that it can only be seen at work in the intact behaving animal. It is possible to sketch (Fig. 9) the sort of mechanism that would be necessary. Essentially the need is to turn down the sensitivities of those fibers in the array which lie around the edges of the signal array, so that they are kept within their working range. The effect of stimulation of the olivo-cochlear bundle on the discharge of auditory nerve fibers is well known to be inhibitory (Fex, 1962), so that at least the physiological basis for this process exists, even if its precise anatomical arrangement remains to be determined.

X. THE PITCH OF COMPLEX TONES

Most complex tones have a well-defined pitch, very much more prominent than the pitches of the individual components. For example, an instrument that produces a fundamental together with, say, the third and fifth harmonics

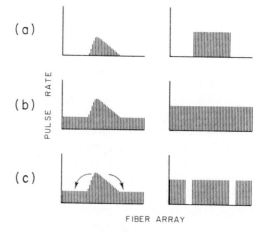

FIG. 9. A possible mechanism to explain centrifugal activity. The left-hand column shows various signal conditions; the right-hand column shows the result of saturation of the firing rate. (a) Signal alone. (b) Signal superimposed on broad band noise; the signal is lost in the transformation. (c) Activity from the signal region is fed back toward the edges of the signal array; the identity of the signal is preserved.

will, when playing A, produce frequencies of 440, 1320, and 2200 Hz. The pitch will be matched by a single tone of 440 Hz. Since 440 Hz is present in the complex, there is no conceptual difficulty about this in terms of our active fiber ("place") theory. However, if instead of omitting the second and fourth harmonics from the series of five we instead omit the first and second, we then have 1320 + 1760 + 2220 Hz. Despite the absence of the fundamental, this complex also has a pitch that can be matched by a single tone of 440 Hz. This problem of the "missing fundamental" has received a great deal of study under the heading of "periodicity pitch" in an endeavor to solve the coding process.

XI. TEMPORAL FACTORS IN CODING

In order to understand the problems involved in coding periodicity it is necessary to begin by looking at the temporal factors involved in the auditory nerve response. There is abundant evidence to show that the probability of a nerve impulse being initiated in an auditory nerve fiber is a function of the displacement, in both direction and extent, of the basilar membrane. Thus if the ear is stimulated with a single tone at a frequency of, say, 200 Hz, impulses will be preferentially initiated on one half cycle of the sine wave, although there will not necessarily, of course, be an impulse corresponding to every half cycle.

This relationship is progressively lost as the stimulus frequency is increased, because of the uncertainty in the instant of firing. This uncertainty is of the order of 200–400 μsec, so that by the time the frequency reaches about 5 kHz, the relationship is no longer apparent.

The phenomenon has been extensively studied by the Wisconsin school, who have shown that a histogram of firing probability in the auditory nerve analyzed over a period reproduces very accurately the shape of one half cycle of even a complex waveform (Fig. 10) (Rose, 1970).

Because a fiber does not fire to every cycle, a single fiber cannot contain unambiguous information about the stimulus frequency. However, a great many fibers are activated by a given tone, and since each may fire on a different cycle, they may between them provide a pulse corresponding to each cycle, and hence information about the frequency. This idea was the basis of Wever's celebrated *volley theory* (Wever, 1949) of pitch transmission for low frequencies.

A similar set of ideas has been invoked to try to explain the pitch of a complex tone from which the fundamental component is missing. Examination of Fig. 11a shows that a complex tone with components of, say, 1000, 1200, and 1400 Hz exhibits an amplitude periodicity at 200/sec. This in turn gives rise to a tendency for impulses to be released in correspondence to this periodicity.

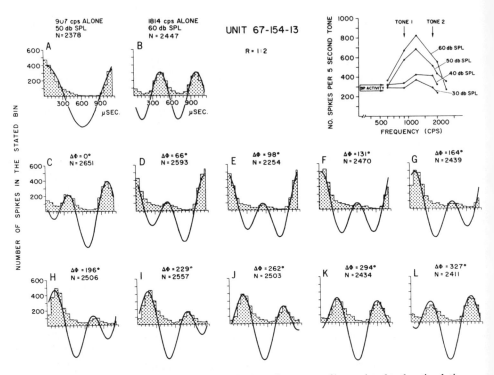

FIG. 10. Histograms of firing probability in single auditory nerve fibers related to the stimulating waveform. [From J. F. Brugge, D. J. Anderson, J. E. Hind, and J. E. Rose, Time structure of discharges in single auditory nerve fibers of the squirrel monkey in response to complex periodic sounds, *Journal of Neurophysiology,* 1969, **32,** 386–401.]

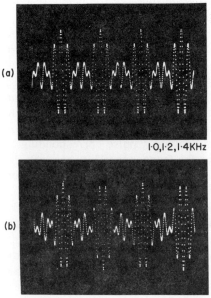

FIG. 11. (a) Waveform of complex tone composed of three harmonically related frequencies. (b) Waveform of complex composed of three anharmonically related frequencies with the same spacing as in (a). Note the "inversion" of alternate groups. [From Whitfield (1970b), Neural integration and pitch perception. In P. Andersen & J. K. S. Jansen (Eds.), *Excitatory Synaptic Mechanisms.* Copyright 1970 by Universitetsforlaget.]

Such impulses occur, of course, in our example in those fibers whose response curves cover the region 1200–1600 Hz. Nevertheless, *given some neural clock against which to measure the interpulse interval,* it is potentially possible for the nervous system to extract this periodicity information and use it in the assessment of pitch. A test of whether this information is used might be whether there is *always* a correspondence between the nerve pulse intervals and the perceived pitch. We can test this in the following way. If we follow a presentation of the harmonic series 1000, 1200, 1400 Hz by presentation of the anharmonic series 1100, 1300, 1500 Hz, then the perceived pitch in the first case corresponds as before to a simple tone of 200 Hz, but in the second case it is matched by a tone of approximately 214 Hz, i.e., about a semitone higher. Now the envelope, as shown in Fig. 11b, still retains its 200/sec periodicity (strictly speaking it is now 100/sec, since alternate groups are inverted). One might expect, therefore, that nerve impulses would continue to be generated in relation to a 50-msec period, and this would not conform with a pitch of 214 Hz, which would require an interval of about *46.7 msec.* To get over this difficulty it has been suggested that such an interval could be produced from the "fine structure" of the waveform shown in Fig. 11b. The idea here is that the distance from a single peak to the nearer of the succeeding twin peaks is less than 20 msec and so might generate the smaller interpulse interval. This prediction has been tested (Whitfield, 1970a,b) and found to be incorrect. The nerve impulses resulting from stimulation with the combination 1100, 1300, and 1500 Hz remain locked at the 50-msec interval, and no periodicity corresponding to 46.7 msec is apparent (Fig. 12). Thus in this case the perceived pitch does not correspond to the impulse periodicity.

The problem of the missing fundamental is largely a pseudoproblem and arises because of our tendency to equate pitch with frequency, forgetting in the process that frequency is a physical attribute of stimuli, while pitch is a psychological attribute of the resultant sensation. We do not make this con-

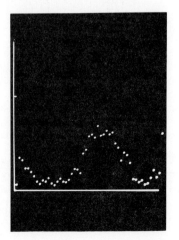

FIG. 12. Pulse periodicity histogram of a cat cochlear nucleus unit responding to a complex tone with components as in Fig. 11(b), i.e., 1.1, 1.3, and 1.5 kHz. Each bin occupies 200 μsec and successive sweeps are initiated by trigger pulses every 10 msec locked to the stimulus waveform. Peaks at zero and at 5 msec show that, although the human subjective pitch corresponds to about 214 Hz, the nerve impulse periodicity corresponds to 200 Hz. [From Whitfield (1970b), Neural integration and pitch perception. In P. Andersen & J. K. S. Jansen (Eds.), *Excitatory Synaptic Mechanisms.* Copyright 1970 by Universitetsforlaget.]

fusion in vision, and thus nobody feels the need for a temporal theory to explain why a single stimulus of $54,000 \times 10^{10}$ Hz (yellow), gives rise to the same sensation as a suitable combination of the pair of frequencies $43,000 \times 10^{10}$ and $60,000 \times 10^{10}$ Hz (red and green). We have been quite happy with a place theory (the trichromatic theory).

I have proposed an analogous explanation for the pitch of complex tones (Whitfield, 1970b). Most tones in nature are complex and, from what we have already discussed, will give rise to a series of active bands in the fiber array (Fig. 13a). It is proposed that pitch is an attribute of this total pattern. The omission of one or more of the elements of this pattern will not affect the pitch, and this is true whether the element omitted falls within or at the end of the series (Fig. 13b,c). If some of the harmonics are deliberately shifted, as in the anharmonic series experiment, the nervous system attempts, as usual, to find the "best fit" to some harmonic series, and comes up with a slightly changed pitch (Fig. 13d). Of course, if alternate harmonics are omitted (Fig. 13e), the "best fit" is an octave higher and the pitch duly rises, as experiment shows. Because pitch, on this basis, is an attribute of the whole pattern, it is not surprising that the pitch of a complex tone is more secure than that of a simple tone. Thus, for example, changes of pitch with intensity at constant frequency have been demonstrated with simple tones, but are not apparent with complex tones. Support for the pattern theory as against the periodicity theory of pitch has come from experiments of Houtsma and Goldstein (1972), who showed that the same pitch was produced irrespective of whether all the components were fed to one ear, or half the components to one ear and half to the other. Only the former would give rise to the appro-

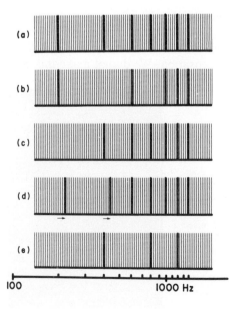

FIG. 13. (a) Neural response to a "fundamental" plus its overtones. The same pitch is assigned to such a pattern even when one or more of the components is absent (b,c). Even when the lowest components are slightly shifted so as to be anharmonic (d), the pattern may still be treated as (a). However regular omission of alternate components (e) results in a new family of patterns whose pitch is an octave higher. [From Whitfield (1970b), Neural integration and pitch perception. In P. Andersen & J. K. S. Jansen (Eds.), *Excitatory Synaptic Mechanisms.* Copyright 1970 by Universitetsforlaget.]

priate periodicity in the auditory nerve but both would, of course, give rise to the same central pattern.

At this stage, it seems reasonable to conclude that spatial patterns of activity and inactivity in the fiber array are sufficient to account for the frequency and intensity coding of both simple and complex tones. We must pass now from steady-state phenomena, to a consideration of impulsive and other time-varying stimuli.

XII. TEMPORAL CODING AND LOCALIZATION

We have seen that the temporal relationship between stimulus and response in the auditory nerve plays a very problematical role in the coding of frequency and on present evidence can be ruled out. However, it would be quite wrong to assume on that account that the temporal distribution of auditory nerve impulses plays no role in the hearing process.

In the foregoing sections we have been dealing with steady-state stimuli—stimuli, incidentally, that are rare in nature. A tone pulse has to last some 10 msec in order to be heard as having a pitch, and indeed at very low frequencies may need to last as long as 20 msec (Doughty & Garner, 1947). Below these durations, the disturbance on the basilar membrane has presumably not become stationary.

If an edge, or pressure step, is used as a stimulus, a "bulge" will travel along the basilar membrane from base to apex (Legouix, 1965) with gradually decreasing velocity, taking about 2 msec for the whole journey. Each element of the membrane performs a damped oscillation at a frequency corresponding to its position, these positions being the same as the points of maximum sensitivity to the appropriate steady-state sinusoid. Impulses are released in the auditory nerve fibers in relation to the initial deflection and, because the rate of propagation of the disturbance is very rapid near the basal end, many hundreds or even thousands of fibers will be stimulated nearly simultaneously. The first one-third of the membrane is traversed in well under 10 μsec and the first two-thirds in about 20 μsec (guinea pig, Tasaki, Davis, & Legouix, 1952). Since these figures are certainly not greater than the uncertainty of the time delay for initiating a nerve impulse, we can visualize there being a simultaneous volley in say 20,000 fibers with a time-scatter corresponding to this uncertainty.

These synchronous volleys are quite certainly treated by the cochlear nucleus in a different way from the volleys set up by tones. According to Møller (1969) a cochlear nucleus neuron (rat), which responds to a train of 1000 sound pulses per second does not necessarily respond to a 1-kHz tone. Since both stimuli are known to give rise to trains of spikes in auditory nerve fibers with similar interpulse intervals, the difference must lie in the number of such fibers available to converge on the cell. This is much greater in the case of the impulsive stimulus, as we have seen. Because of the wide distribution of activity produced by a pulse, one would expect the repetition rate not to be a critical factor for the response of the target cell, unlike the tone responding cells, where stimulus frequency must fall within a well-defined band for a response to occur.

The arrival of a volley at the pulse target cells induces not only a response, but also an inhibitory phase lasting of the order of 1 msec. This means that whereas a cell will follow a repetitive impulse train from low rates up to some critical value, above this rate the response abruptly fails. This failure point varies from cell to cell within the range of about 700–1500 pulses per second.

There is an implication in these results that, whereas the auditory nerve has to handle information in both positional and temporal forms, some division of routing is taking place at the cochlear nucleus, some cells being concerned with the place phenomena of intensity and frequency referred to in the first part of the chapter while others are concerned with the timing of impulsive and other rapidly changing stimuli. Because of the massive convergence on the latter cells it might be expected that the timing of their output pulses would be better controlled than in the case of the frequency–intensity cells.

References

Citron, L., Dix, M. R., Hallpike, C. S., & Hood, J. D. A recent clinicopathological study of cochlear nerve degeneration resulting from tumor pressure and disseminated sclerosis, with particular reference to the finding of normal threshold sensitivity for pure tones. *Acta Oto-Laryngologica*, 1963, **56**, 330–337.

Dewson, J. H. Efferent olivo-cochlear bundle: Some relationships to stimulus discrimination in noise. *Journal of Neurophysiology*, 1968, **31**, 122–130.

Doughty, J. M., & Garner, W. R. Pitch characteristics of short tones. *Journal of Experimental Psychology*, 1947, **37**, 351–365.

Evans, E. F. Narrow 'tuning' of cochlear nerve fibre responses in guinea pig. *Journal of Physiology*, 1970, **206**, 14–15P.

Feldkeller, R., & Zwicker, E. *Das Ohr als Nachrichtenempfänger*. Stuttgart: Hirzel, 1956.

Fex, J. Auditory activity in centrifugal and centripetal cochlear fibres in cat. *Acta Physiologica Scandinavica*, 1962, **55**, Suppl. 189.

Fletcher, H. Auditory patterns. *Reviews of Modern Physics*, 1940, **12**, 47–65.

Fletcher, H., & Munson, W. A. Loudness; its definition measurement and calculation. *Journal of the Acoustical Society of America*, 1933, **5**, 82–108.

Galambos, R., & Davis, H. The response of single auditory-nerve fibers to acoustic stimulation. *Journal of Neurophysiology*, 1943, **6**, 39–57.

Greenwood, D. D. Critical bandwidth and frequency coordinates of the basilar membrane. *Journal of the Acoustical Society of America*, 1961, **33**, 1344–1356.

Helmholtz, H. L. F. Die Lehre von den Tonempfindungen als physiologische Grundlage für die Theorie der Musik. Eng. In Trans. of 3rd edition by A. J. Ellis, *On the sensations of tone*. London: Longmans, Green, 1863.

Houtsma, A. S. M., & Goldstein, J. L. The central origin of the pitch of complex tones: Evidence from musical interval recognition. *Journal of the Acoustical Society of America*, 1972, **51**, 520–529.

Katsuki, Y., Suga, N., & Kanno, Y. Neural mechanism of the peripheral and central auditory system in monkeys. *Journal of the Acoustical Society of America*, 1962, **34**, 1396–1410.

Kiang, N. Y. S. *Discharge patterns of single fibers in the cat's auditory nerve*. Cambridge, Massachusetts: M.I.T. Press, 1966.

Kiang, N. Y. S., Moxon, E. C., & Levine, R. A. Auditory nerve activity in cats with normal and abnormal cochleas. In G. E. W. Wolstenholme & J. Knight (Eds.), *Ciba Symposium on sensorineural hearing loss*. London: Churchill, 1970.

Legouix, J.-P. Observations des réponses microphoniques cochleaires à des signaux de type impulsionnel. *Acustica*, 1965, **16**, 159–165.

Møller, A. R. Unit responses in the rat cochlear nucleus to repetitive, transient sounds. *Acta Physiologica Scandinavica*, 1969, **75**, 542–551.

Pickles, J. O. Normal critical bands in the cat. *Acta Oto-Laryngologica*, 1975, **80**, 245–254.

Pickles, J. O. Role of centrifugal pathways to cochlear nucleus in determination of critical bandwidth. *Journal of Neurophysiology*, 1976, **39**, 394–400.

Pickles, J. O., & Comis, S. D. Role of centrifugal pathways to cochlear nucleus in detection of signals in noise. *Journal of Neurophysiology*, 1973, **36**, 1131–1137.

Plomp, R. *Experiments on tone perception*. Soesterberg: Institute for Perception, 1966.

Rose, J. E. Peripheral nerve-fibre discharges. In R. Plomp & G. F. Smoorenburg (Eds.), *Frequency analysis and periodicity detection in hearing*. Leiden: Sijthoff, 1970. Pp. 176–192.

Ross, H. F. quoted by I. C. Whitfield. The organization of the auditory pathways. *Journal of Sound and Vibration Research*, 1968, **8**(1), 108–117.

Rutherford, W. A new theory of hearing. *Journal of Anatomy & Physiology*, 1886, **21**, 166–168.

Scharf, B. Critical bands. In J. V. Tobias (Ed.), *Foundations of modern auditory theory*. Vol. 1. New York: Academic Press, 1970.

Schuknecht, H. F. Neuroanatomical correlates of auditory sensitivity and pitch discrimination in the cat. In G. L. Rasmussen & W. F. Windle (Eds.), *Neural mechanisms of the auditory and vestibular systems*. Springfield, Illinois: Thomas, 1960. Chap. 6.

Schuknecht, H. F., & Woellner, R. C. An experimental and clinical study of deafness from lesions of the cochlear nerve. *Journal of Laryngology and Otology*, 1955, **69**, 75–97.

Tasaki, I., Davis, H., & Legouix, J.-P. The space-time pattern of the cochlear microphonics (guinea-pig) as recorded by differential electrodes. *Journal of the Acoustical Society of America*, 1952, **24**, 502–519.

Vietmeister, N. F. Intensity discrimination of noise in the presence of band-reject noise. *Journal of the Acoustical Society of America*, 1974, **56**, 1594–1600.

Watson, C. S. Masking of tones by noise for the cat. *Journal of the Acoustical Society of America*, 1963, **35**, 167–172.

Wever, E. G. *Theory of hearing*. New York: Wiley, 1949.

Whitfield, I. C. 'Two-tone' inhibition at the trapezoid body level. *Journal of Physiology*, 1955, **128**, 15–16P.

Whitfield, I. C. Electrophysiology of the central auditory pathway. *British Medical Bulletin*, 1956, **12**, 105–109.

Whitfield, I. C. *The auditory pathway*. London: Arnold, 1967.

Whitfield, I. C. Central nervous processing in relation to spatio-temporal discrimination of auditory patterns. In R. Plomp & G. F. Smoorenburg (Eds.), *Frequency analysis and periodicity detection in hearing*. Leiden: Sijthoff, 1970. Pp. 136–152. (a)

Whitfield, I. C. Neural integration and pitch perception. In P. Andersen & J. K. S. Jansen (Eds.), *Excitatory synaptic mechanisms*. Oslo: Universitetsforlaget, 1970. (b)

Zwislocki, J. Analysis of some auditory characteristics. In R. D. Luce, R. R. Bush, & E. Galanter (Eds.), *Handbook of mathematical psychology*. New York: Wiley, 1965.

Part III

Analyzing Mechanisms of Frequency, Intensity, Time, and Period

Chapter 6

LOUDNESS*

BERTRAM SCHARF

I. INTRODUCTION

Loudness is the subjective intensity of a sound. *Subjective* means a listener must consciously respond to the sound. *Intensity* means the response indi-

* Preparation of this chapter was supported in part by a grant, R01 NS07270, from the National Institute of Neurological Diseases and Stroke, U.S. Public Health Service. The author is pleased to acknowledge suggestions by William Coan, David Fishken, Rhona Hellman, and Igor Nabelek that led to the elimination of some errors and ambiguities in the final draft.

cates how strong the sound seems to the listener. This definition is vague, but in experiments on loudness it usually suffices to elicit consistent responses. The responses then become the basis for describing the relation between loudness and the experimentally manipulated physical and observer variables. Functional relationships replace definitions. Although this chapter can be understood without a better definition of loudness, the problem is not trivial, and Section IX takes it up again.

Loudness depends upon both the sound and the listener. The stimulus variables can be divided among four categories: intensity, spectral content, time, and background. Sound intensity is most important in determining loudness, but spectral variables like signal frequency and bandwidth must also be considered. Duration and intermittency are among the significant temporal determinants. Finally, the loudness of a sound may be strongly affected by other, background sounds.

The stimulus variables interact with subject variables. Loudness resides in the listener, not in the stimulus. Whether the subject listens with one ear or two ears, with a fresh ear or one just exposed to noise, with a healthy or impaired ear, and whether he listens (pays attention) to the sound or merely hears it—all play a role in determining how loud a sound seems.

After discussions of the four stimulus categories and the listener, come discussions of physiological correlates and of models of loudness. The last section is about the meaning of loudness and about alternative response measures, such as reaction time, evoked potentials, and muscular changes.

II. INTENSITY

A. Loudness Function

1. STANDARD LOUDNESS FUNCTION

Loudness is a monotonic function of stimulus intensity. Figure 1 gives the loudness in *sones* of a 1000-Hz tone as a function of loudness level in *phons*. Table I lists the sone values as a function of sound pressure level. Since *loudness level* is the sound pressure level (SPL) of an equally loud 1000-Hz tone, the loudness level in phons of a 1000-Hz tone is the same as its sound pressure level in decibels.* The straight line in Fig. 1 is based on the standard loudness function (ISO R131-1959). At 40 phons, a 1000-Hz tone has by definition a loudness of 1 sone. A sound twice as loud has a loudness of 2 sones; a sound half as loud has a loudness of .5 sone, and so on. The loudness function is based on direct psychophysical procedures such as halving and

---

* We owe the origin of the concept of loudness level and its unit, the phon, to the German acoustician Barkhausen (1926).

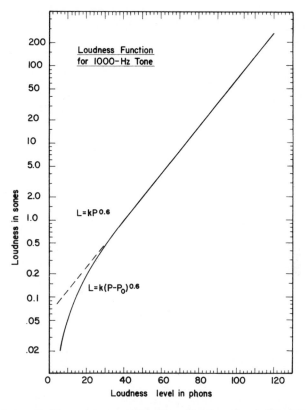

Fig. 1. Loudness of a binaural tone as a function of loudness level. The dashed line shows how the loudness function would look were the simple power function valid down to threshold, which is around 6 phons. The solid line corresponds more closely to loudness as measured; this empirical curve is roughly approximated by the equation with a small constant P_0 subtracted from the signal's sound pressure.

doubling and magnitude estimation (see Stevens in Volume 2 of the *Handbook* and Stevens, 1955, 1957; for a listing of relevant papers, see Marks, 1974a). The equation for the standard loudness function is a simple power law.

$$L = kP^{.6} . \tag{1}$$

In Eq. (1) L is loudness, P is sound pressure, and k is the intercept. For loudness measured in sones and P in micropascals (or micronewtons per square centimeter), the value of k is .01. For P measured in dynes per square centimeter, the value of k is 10.45. Plotted on the log–log coordinates of Fig. 1, a power function is a straight line.

The physical magnitude of a sound may be characterized in several different ways (see Leshowitz, Chapter 3 of this volume). Sound pressure is most

TABLE I
Sone Values for 1000-Hz Tone and for White Noise

SPL dB	Tone	Noise	SPL dB	Tone	Noise	SPL dB	Tone	Noise
10	.052	—	50	2.00	3.85	90	32.0	46.0
12	.072	—	52	2.30	4.45	92	36.8	50.5
14	.095	—	54	2.64	5.20	94	42.2	57.5
15	.110	—	55	2.83	5.60	95	45.3	61.0
16	.125	—	56	3.03	6.00	96	48.5	65.0
18	.155	—	58	3.48	7.00	98	55.7	72.0
20	.190	—	60	4.00	7.85	100	64.0	80
22	.230	—	62	4.59	8.9	102	73.5	91
24	.280	—	64	5.28	10.2	104	84.4	102
25	.305	—	65	5.66	10.9	105	90.5	108
26	.330	—	66	6.06	11.5	106	97.0	114
28	.395	.450	68	6.96	13.0	108	111	128
30	.460	.580	70	8.00	14.7	110	128	—
32	.550	.720	72	9.19	16.4	112	147	—
34	.640	.900	74	10.6	18.5	114	169	—
35	.700	1.00	75	11.3	19.5	115	181	—
36	.750	1.10	76	12.1	20.6	116	194	—
38	.860	1.36	78	13.9	23.2	118	223	—
40	1.00	1.65	80	16.0	26.0	120	256	—
42	1.15	2.00	82	18.4	29.0			
44	1.32	2.40	84	21.1	32.5			
45	1.41	2.60	85	22.6	34.8			
46	1.52	2.80	86	24.3	36.5			
48	1.74	3.28	88	27.9	41.0			

commonly measured, but reference is often made to intensity or energy. Given that pressure is proportional to the square root of intensity, we can substitute $I^{.5}$ for P in Eq. (1) to obtain

$$L = k'I^{.3} .\qquad(2)$$

The exponent and intercept change, but not the form of the equation.

The loudness of sounds other than 1000 Hz can be determined by matching procedures (see Section III,B) or by one of several calculation schemes (see Section VIII). Approximate sone values for a few common sounds are 1 sone for the average level in a quiet residential neighborhood at night; 4 sones for normal conversation; 16 sones for a nearby vacuum cleaner; 250 sones for a clap of thunder.

In general, the power function means that equal stimulus ratios produce equal sensation ratios. Stevens (Volume 2 of the *Handbook,* and 1975) shows this to be the prevailing psychophysical relationship for most sensory attributes. In particular, Eq. (1) means that when the SPL increases 10 dB (a ratio of over 3 : 1), the loudness doubles. Loudness doubles regardless of the SPL to which the 10 dB are added; going from 40 to 50 dB doubles the loudness of a 1000-Hz tone, just as going from 100 to 110 dB does. An increase of 20 dB (a ratio of 10 : 1) makes the 1000-Hz tone four times louder. The relative simplicity of the psychophysical function relating sensation magnitude and stimulus magnitude reflects the fundamental operating mode of all the sensory systems, a mode based on the equivalency of ratios.

The function in Fig. 1 is defined for a 1000-Hz pure tone presented in a free field, where the sound reaches the listener directly from the sound source without being reflected from any nearby surfaces. Presenting the tone through a pair of earphones does not alter the loudness function. Furthermore, the free-field and earphone functions are not altered by changing the abscissa from loudness level in phons to *sensation level* (SL), which is the number of decibels above threshold. The threshold for a 1000-Hz tone appears to be about the same, 6 dB SPL, whether presented through earphones or in a free field (Anderson & Whittle, 1971). So, subtracting 6 dB from the loudness levels in Fig. 1 gives the sensation levels. (The near identity of a 1000-Hz loudness function under earphone and free-field listening justifies the use of loudness level, without corrections, for sounds presented through earphones. Technically, the loudness level of any sound is defined as the SPL of an equally loud 1000-Hz tone presented as a plane progressive wave in the listener's frontal plane.)

2. VARIATIONS IN THE STANDARD FUNCTION

The loudness function is defined specifically for a 1000-Hz pure tone. If the frequency is changed or if a complex sound such as a band of noise replaces the pure tone, the function may change. The effect of such spectral changes is treated in Section III. A tonal stimulus implies a stimulus duration longer than about .5 sec. At shorter durations, it is more often called a *tone burst* or *pulse*. The standard loudness function is based primarily on tones lasting about 1 sec. Changing the duration of the tone seems to have little effect on the shape of the function, although shortening the duration below about 200 msec reduces the loudness at a given SPL, thus moving down the whole function in Fig. 1. Loudness and duration are discussed in Section IV. It is also assumed that the 1000-Hz tone is presented in the quiet. A noise background usually steepens the function near threshold as shown in Section V.

The loudness function is meant to represent the responses of listeners with normal hearing who listen with both ears. If the threshold is elevated because the listener has impaired hearing or has just been exposed to noise, the function often changes, as described in Section VI.

The loudness or sone function is largely based on the efforts of S. S. Stevens (e.g., Stevens, 1955), who in 1972, suggested that a critical band of noise centered at 3150 Hz would be a better standard than a 1000-Hz tone. The loudness function for a 1000-Hz tone appears to wobble a bit, deviating from the simple power function at middle and high levels (Hellman & Zwislocki, 1961; Robinson, 1957). According to Stevens, the function for a critical band of noise at 3150 Hz follows the power function more closely. Stevens has also suggested that the exponent at 3150 Hz (and also at 1000 Hz) is greater than .60, being more like .67. Since experimental evidence for these proposals is hard to come by (Hellman, 1976), and since the function in Fig. 1 is the international standard and is commonly used, it will serve as the reference standard in the rest of this chapter.

3. LOUDNESS NEAR THRESHOLD

The curved section in Fig. 1 is based on Hellman and Zwislocki's (1961) summary of their own data and those collected by a number of other investigators (Robinson, 1957; Scharf & Stevens, 1961; Zwicker, 1958). Unlike the full straight line, it shows the true course of loudness near threshold. Loudness grows more rapidly from threshold to about 30 phons than at higher levels. The solid curve in Fig. 1 can be adequately approximated by a modification of the power law:

$$L = k (P - P_0)^{.6} , \tag{3}$$

where P_0 is a value that approximates the effective threshold.* Since sound

---

* A value of 45 μPa for P_0 yields a fair approximation of the modified power function in Fig. 2. The equation then reads

$$L = .01(P - 45)^{.6} ,$$

where L is loudness in sones and P is sound pressure measured in micropascals. The chosen value for P_0 corresponds to a loudness level of 8 phons, 2 phons above our assumed detection threshold. If P is measured in dynes per square centimeter, the modified equation reads

$$L = 10.45(P - 4.5 \times 10^{-4})^{.6} .$$

pressure first begins to have a sensory effect at threshold, the appropriate measure of the stimulus may be its distance above subjective zero, that is, threshold, rather than above physical zero.

Other modifications of the power law can also eliminate the curvature near threshold. Zwislocki (1965), for example, has proposed that loudness is a linear function of stimulus intensity near threshold. Lochner and Burger (1961) have proposed the following modification:

$$L = k (P^{.6} - P_0^{.6}) \ .$$

Since curvature near threshold is true of most sensory continua, not only of loudness, these different proposals are fraught with theoretical significance (see Marks, 1974b, pp. 21–24; Zwislocki, 1974), but there is scant empirical justification for choosing among them (Marks & J. C. Stevens, 1968). Equation (3) has the advantage of being the simplest and most straightforward of the proposed modifications.

B. Difference Limen

The loudness function tells how loud a 1000-Hz tone is at a given level. A classical question has been: What is the minimum intensity difference between two sounds, otherwise identical, that allows a listener to report reliably that one sound is louder than the other? In 1928, Riesz provided the answer to this question (see also Knudsen, 1923). Riesz asked 12 listeners to detect beating between two tones set 3 Hz apart in frequency. For example, the intensity of a 1003-Hz tone was increased in the presence of a fixed 1000-Hz tone until loudness just began to fluctuate. This minimum intensity change is the just noticeable difference (jnd) or ΔI.

At 1000 Hz, ΔI decreases from about 3 dB at 10 dB SL to less than .5 dB at 70 dB SL. (Expressed in decibels, which are the logarithms of ratios, ΔI is a relative value equivalent to $\Delta I/I$. Hence, a constant decibel change means that the relative increase in intensity is constant, not the absolute increase.) The ΔI decreases as the tone becomes more intense at all frequencies, but at different rates. Figure 2 gives ΔI in decibels as a function of the SL at five frequencies. Differential sensitivity is best at higher sensation levels and at frequencies between about 1000 and 4000 Hz. Investigators since Riesz have generally confirmed his results although precise values differ somewhat (e.g, Harris, 1963; Miller, 1947; Tonndorf, Brogan, & Washburn, 1955; Zwicker & Feldtkeller, 1967). Modern psychophysical procedures and analyses, however, reveal a small but consistent departure from Weber's law which increases with level above 25 dB SL (McGill & Goldberg, 1968; Viemeister, 1972). In their summary of 15 modern studies of intensity discrimination of 1000-Hz tone pulses, Rabinowitz, Lim, Braida, and Durlach (1976) noted that discrimination improves from threshold to 10 dB SL, is then constant between 10 and 40 dB SL, and again improves at levels above 40 dB SL.

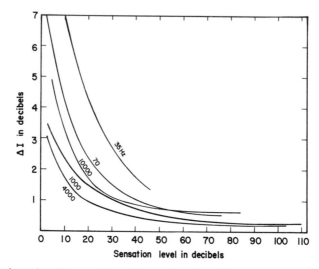

FIG. 2. The intensity difference limen, ΔI, as a function of the sensation level. Each curve is for a pure tone at the indicated frequency. [Adapted from Stevens and Davis (1938, p. 138).]

The comprehensive study of intensity discrimination by Jesteadt, Wier, and Green (1977) reveals a somewhat simpler picture than did Riesz's. Using an adaptive, two-interval, forced-choice procedure with three well-trained observers, Jesteadt *et al.* found that $\Delta I/I$ was independent of frequency over the whole range they tested from 200 to 8000 Hz. Like Riesz, they found that $\Delta I/I$ decreases with increasing sensation level, but near threshold their observers discriminated better than Riesz's and above about 30 dB SL they discriminated more poorly. These differences in the results probably arise from differences in the stimuli (500-msec tone bursts as opposed to two continuous sinusoids separated by 3 Hz) and procedures (e.g., forced choice as opposed to a method of limits).

What is the relation between the size of ΔI and loudness? Since the detection of an intensity difference between two sounds requires that the sounds have different effects on the listener, it is reasonable to expect that those effects can be expressed in terms of loudness. Detection of a difference ought to depend on how much two sounds differ in loudness, not in intensity. It follows that the more rapidly loudness changes with intensity, the smaller the relative ΔI a listener should need in order to detect a difference between two sounds. A comparison of Fig. 1 with Fig. 2 shows just the opposite. For a 1000-Hz tone, ΔI is largest near threshold where loudness changes most rapidly. According to Riesz's data, a listener requires an intensity change as large as 3 dB near threshold in order to detect that a change has occurred, but requires a change of only .5 dB or less at levels above about 60 dB where the loudness function is flatter. Likewise, according to Jesteadt *et al.*, a listener requires a ΔI of approximately 1.6 dB near threshold and .5 dB at 80 dB. Clearly, the slope of the loudness function does not predict the size of the jnd.*

Translating ΔI, as measured by Riesz, into equivalent loudness values reveals that neither the relative loudness change nor the absolute loudness change corresponding to ΔI is constant. The absolute loudness change increases with level over the whole intensity range. The relative loudness change decreases as level increases up to about 60 dB; at higher levels it is fairly stable, varying between only 1.5 and 3%.

III. SPECTRUM

The loudness of a pure tone depends on its frequency as well as its intensity. The loudness of a complex sound—a sound with energy at two or more frequencies—depends on overall intensity, on the frequency of its components, and also on the distance between the component with the lowest frequency and that with the highest frequency.

A. Equal-Loudness Contours

In a number of studies, loudness matches have been made between a 1000-Hz tone and tones at other frequencies. Three large-scale studies are those of Fletcher and Munson (1933), Churcher and King (1937), and Robinson and Dadson (1956). Fletcher and Munson had their subjects match a binaural tone of variable frequency to a binaural 1000-Hz tone presented through earphones. Their data, the most widely cited, are presented as equal-loudness contours in Fig. 3. On the ordinate is the SPL at which a tone, the frequency of which is given on the abscissa, sounds as loud as a 1000-Hz tone. The parameter on the curves is loudness level. All the combinations of SPL and frequency on a given contour describe pure tones equal in loudness. For example, a tone at 500 Hz set to 50 dB is equal in loudness to a tone at 10,000 Hz set to 71 dB; both have a loudness level of 48 phons,

---

* Why is a steeper loudness function not accompanied by smaller ΔIs? (The same question applies to brightness and other continua.) One possible reason is that a steeper function means that any variation in the stimulus or its transmission through the ear (and possibly in transduction) are magnified within the auditory nervous system. Consequently, the variance of the distribution of events elicited in the sensory domain by a signal at a given level is increased where the loudness function is steeper. Since discrimination requires distinguishing between two distributions of the sensory events produced by two stimuli, any increase in the variance of those distributions must lead to reduced discrimination. However, the whole relation between discrimination and sensory-magnitude functions is unclear, but is coming under closer scrutiny (see e.g., Durlach & Braida, 1969; Teghtsoonian, 1971).

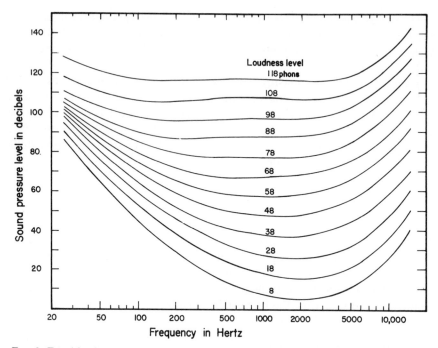

Fᴵɢ. 3. Equal-loudness contours for pure tones presented through earphones. The ordinate gives the sound pressure level required for a tone, at the frequency specified on the abscissa, to reach the loudness level indicated as the parameter on each curve. [Adapted from Stevens and Davis (1938, p. 124).]

which means they are as loud as a 1000-Hz tone at 48 dB SPL.* By showing how SPL must be varied in order to keep loudness constant as frequency varies, equal-loudness contours tell us, indirectly, how loudness depends on frequency.

The bottom contour at 8 phons is the threshold curve computed by Fletcher and Munson (1933) for earphone listening. The next curve at 18 phons is nearly parallel to the threshold curve. This similarity is important because the 8-phon curve is based on threshold measurements, whereas the 18-phon curve is based on judgments of equal loudness. Despite the gross difference in the listener's task, both sets of results reveal the same basic relation between loudness (or sensitivity) and frequency. With increasing level, however, the equal-loudness contours change shape. The large differ-

---

* These statements assume that transitivity holds for loudness matches, i.e., that if sounds A and B are equal in loudness to sound C, say a 1000-Hz tone, at a given level, then sound A is equal in loudness to sound B. Robinson and Dadson (1956) and Ross (1967) have shown experimentally that transitivity holds within the limits of variability of loudness matches between tones of different frequency.

ences in SPL between equally loud low and medium frequencies lessen at higher levels. At 18 phons, a 100-Hz tone must be 37 dB more intense than an equally loud 1000-Hz tone, but at 78 phons the difference is less than 10 dB, and at 118 phons there may be no difference.

Since the equal-loudness contours change shape with level and are not parallel to one another, loudness cannot grow as a function of sound pressure in the same way at all frequencies. The standard loudness function for the 1000-Hz tone is not valid for every frequency. In particular, the loudness functions for the lower frequencies, where the contours bunch together, must differ from the standard function. Before examining those differences, let us look at the equal-loudness contours measured in a free field. Robinson and Dadson (1956) published a large set of data, which are summarized in Fig. 4.

The free-field contours differ strikingly from those measured for earphone listening at frequencies above 1000 Hz. At the higher frequencies, the presence of the listener's head significantly affects the sound pressure at the eardrum. The SPL shown on the ordinate is measured in an anechoic room where the specially constructed walls, floor, and ceiling reflect almost no sound. Introducing the listener alters the sound field so that the sound pressure in the ear canal is greater around 4000 Hz and smaller around 8000 Hz.

At low frequencies, the free-field and earphone contours differ less obviously, but the earphone contours do rise more steeply as frequency decreases below 1000 Hz. Anderson and Whittle (1971) ascribe this difference to low-frequency noise under the ear cushions. The noise raises the threshold for low-frequency tones, the more so the lower the frequency (see Chapter 8 by Zwislocki on masking). The noise also reduces the loudness of suprathreshold, low-frequency tones. The loudness reduction becomes less as the level of the tone increases (see Section V). At high levels the noise has little effect, and the differences between the earphone and free-field contours at low frequencies diminish. The differences do not disappear, however, possibly because Robinson and Dadson did not use the same measuring techniques and psychophysical procedures to obtain their free-field contours as Fletcher and Munson used to obtain their earphone contours.

Unlike the contours at low frequencies, the earphone and free-field contours at high frequencies are equally dissimilar at all levels, because they reflect differences in the sound pressure at the eardrum. These differences in the sound pressure generated by the earphone and in the free field are invariant with level. Were we to substitute sound pressure in the ear canal for sound pressure in the field on the ordinate of Fig. 4, the new contours would become very similar to those in Fig. 3 at frequencies above 1000 Hz. Such a change in the ordinate is unwarranted because sound pressure in the ear canal, being difficult to measure, is seldom known precisely in the free field.

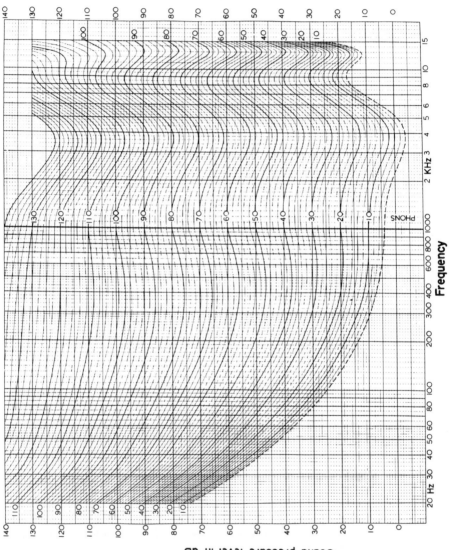

Frequency

Sound pressure level in dB

B. Loudness Functions at Frequencies Other than 1000 Hz

Loudness functions at other frequencies can be calculated from the equal-loudness contours and the standard loudness function. For a tone at a chosen frequency, each equal-loudness contour provides the loudness level of the tone and its corresponding SPL. For example, the 18-phon contour in Fig. 3 shows that the 100-Hz tone at 52.5 dB SPL has a loudness level of 18 phons, the 28-phon contour shows that the 100-Hz tone at 60 dB has a loudness level of 28 phons, the 58-phon contour that the tone at 75 dB has a level of 58 phons, and so forth. The loudness levels are then converted to loudness in sones from the standard function in Fig. 1 or from Table I. The derived set of SPLs and associated loudnesses in sones contains all the information needed to plot the loudness function for the tone at the chosen frequency.

In this manner, loudness functions were derived for tones at 100, 250, 500, 4000, and 8000 Hz. Figure 5 presents these functions along with the standard function at 1000 Hz. Loudness in sones is plotted as a function of SPL in decibels. Functions derived for 2000 and 3000 Hz lie between the 1000-Hz and 4000-Hz curves; to avoid confusion, they are omitted. The derived loudness functions are nearly congruent or parallel at frequencies above 1000 Hz, where the equal-loudness contours are parallel.

The bunching of the equal-loudness contours at frequencies below 1000 Hz produces loudness functions at 100, 250, and 500 Hz that are steeper near their respective thresholds than is the standard 1000-Hz function near its threshold. Near their elevated thresholds, the tones at lower frequencies are softer than an equally intense 1000-Hz tone, but their loudness grows so rapidly with sound pressure as to catch up with the 1000-Hz tone at the higher SPLs. Similarly steep functions for tones at 100 and 250 Hz were obtained by Hellman and Zwislocki (1968), who used the direct psychophysical procedures of magnitude estimation and magnitude production. Using magnitude estimation only, Schneider, Wright, Edelheit, Hock, and Humphrey (1972) also measured steeper functions at low frequencies. In general, steep loudness functions are associated with elevated thresholds, and, as already suggested by the low-frequency functions in Fig. 5, the higher the threshold, the steeper the function.

FIG. 4. Equal-loudness contours for pure tones presented in a free field. Ordinate, abscissa, and loudness level as in Fig. 3. [Adapted from ISO/R 131-1959E with permission of the original authors, D. W. Robinson and R. S. Dadson, 1956, Crown copyright C.S. 10986 held by National Physical Laboratory, Teddington, England, and with permission from International Organization for Standardization Recommendation R226, Normal Equal-Loudness Contours for Pure Tones and Normal Threshold of Hearing Under Free Field Listening Conditions, December 1961, copyrighted by the American National Standards Institute, 1430 Broadway, New York, N.Y. 10018.]

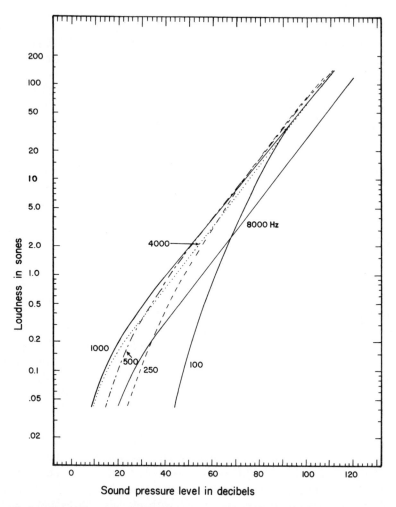

FIG. 5. Loudness of tones at different frequencies as a function of sound pressure level. Functions are derived from the equal-loudness contours of Fig. 3 and 1000-Hz loudness function of Fig. 1.

C. Bandwidth Effects

The greater the frequency range covered by a sound (which is not close to threshold), the louder it is. For a complex sound made up of discrete components (line spectra), the frequency range is the separation in hertz between the components with the lowest and highest frequencies. For a complex sound with a continuous spectrum, i.e., with energy at all frequencies, the frequency range or bandwidth is the distance between the lowest and highest frequencies with significant amounts of energy. (The bandwidth is usually measured between the half-power points.) Since the same rules apply to

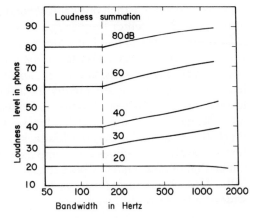

FIG. 6. Loudness level of a band of filtered white noise as a function of its width. Parameter on the curves is the overall sound pressure level of the noise bands. The dashed line indicates the location of the critical band for these noises centered on 1000 Hz. [Adapted from Feldtkeller and Zwicker (1956, p. 82), *Das Ohr als Nachrichtenempfänger*. Copyright 1956 by S. Hirzel Verlag.]

line spectra and continuous spectra, both overall frequency separation and bandwidth will be represented by the same symbol, ΔF. This section deals first with the relation between loudness and ΔF, and then specifically with the loudness function for white noise.

1. LOUDNESS AND ΔF

The loudness of a complex sound increases with ΔF, although the overall intensity of the sound is held constant. This effect is often referred to as *loudness summation*. Loudness does not begin to increase, however, until ΔF exceeds a minimum value called the *critical band* or *Frequenzgruppe* (Zwicker & Feldtkeller, 1955; Zwicker, Flottorp, & Stevens, 1957; and see Zwislocki, Chapter 8 of this volume). The width of the critical band varies with the center frequency of the complex sound as shown in Table I of Zwislocki's chapter (p. 290).

Figure 6 shows how the loudness level of a band of noise centered on 1000-Hz changes as a function of bandwidth. Results are similar for a complex sound comprising only two tones (Scharf, 1970a). The curves in Fig. 6 were obtained by having subjects adjust the level of a 1000-Hz tone until it sounded as loud as the band of noise, the overall SPL of which remained at the value shown on each curve. Up to 160 Hz, which is the critical bandwidth at the center frequency of the noise, loudness is independent of bandwidth. Within the critical band, loudness depends only on SPL and center frequency in a manner predictable from the equal-loudness contours (see Fig. 3 or 4). This rule, however, does not apply at bandwidths narrower than about 30 Hz, where loudness fluctuations of the noise become audible; there, loudness measurements are highly variable and depend on whether the subject judges maximum loudness, average loudness, minimum loudness, or makes some compromise judgment (Bauch, 1956). Bauch's subjects, listening to three-tone complexes, mostly judged average loudness. Outside the range of audible fluctuations or beating, a complex sound whose ΔF is the same as or narrower than one critical band is equal in loudness to a pure tone at the geometric center frequency of the complex and at the same SPL.*

Beyond the critical band, the loudness level of a complex sound increases with ΔF except at sensation levels below 10 or 15 dB (Scharf, 1959a). At successively higher sensation levels up to between 40 and 60 dB, loudness increases more and more rapidly as a function of ΔF. But at still higher levels, above 60 dB SPL, loudness increases progressively less rapidly with ΔF. The general rule is that loudness summation is greatest at moderate levels (Pollack, 1952). Because loudness summation is a nonmonotonic function of level, the loudness of complex sounds wider than a critical band, unlike that of midfrequency pure tones, cannot be a simple power function of SPL. This observation leads us to consider the loudness function for the widest possible sound, white noise.

2. Loudness Function for White Noise

After the 1000-Hz tone, the artificial sound most often studied has been white noise. Because the threshold for white noise is about 10 dB higher than for a 1000-Hz tone (e.g., Gässler, 1954; Hellman, 1976), to achieve equal loudness near threshold, the overall SPL of the noise must be greater than that of the tone. At moderate levels, however, the tone must be considerably more intense than the noise. At high levels, the tone must still be more intense in order to be as loud as the noise, but the intensity difference is smaller than at moderate levels. These basic relations have been revealed by loudness matches between tone and white noise (Brittain, 1939; Hellman, 1976; Miller, 1947; Pollack, 1951; Robinson, 1953; Stevens, 1955; Zwicker, 1958) and agree with an extrapolation from matches between pure tones and bands of noise (see Fig. 6).

Data based on loudness matches also agree reasonably well with direct estimates of the loudness of white noise as summarized in Fig. 7 and Table I (Scharf & Fishken, 1970). Figure 7 also reproduces the tone function of Fig. 1. The white-noise function was obtained by magnitude estimation and magnitude production. Subjects judged white noise and a 1000-Hz tone, which were presented in a mixed order—within the same series—at eight different levels. On any given trial, the subject heard either the noise or the tone. In this way, the resulting functions for tone and noise could be directly compared. Although the measured loudness function for the tone was flatter than the standard 1000-Hz function, it was clearly a power function. The same factors that caused a flatter tone function presumably also flattened the noise function. To compensate for this distortion, the noise function presented in

---

* An apparent exception to this rule has been reported for bands of noise at 8500 Hz where loudness begins to increase with bandwidth well before the critical band is reached (Fastl, 1975). Fastl, however, seems not to have taken into account the steep slope of the equal-loudness contours around 8500 Hz (see Fig. 3 of this chapter). The bands of white noise contained energy at frequencies that may have contributed disproportionately to overall loudness.

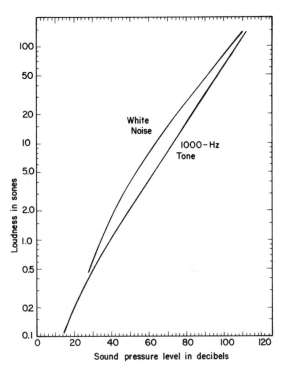

FIG. 7. Loudness of white noise and a 1000-Hz tone as a function of sound pressure level. The tone function is taken from Fig. 1.

Fig. 7 has been steepened by the same amount necessary to bring the measured tone function into accord with the standard sone function (see Fig. 1).

As predicted from matching data, the white-noise function is concave downward in log–log coordinates, with a distinct midlevel bulge. Starting from its higher threshold, the noise first grows more rapidly in loudness than the tone. But the noise loses steam, and above 60 dB SPL or so, its loudness grows less rapidly. Owing to their different shapes and threshold, the tone and noise functions must cross, probably near 25 dB SPL. At the cross point a white noise and a 1000-Hz tone are equally loud when both are at the same SPL (cf. Hellman, 1976). This equality implies that the loudness of a band of noise is independent of its width when the overall SPL is held constant near 25 dB. Such a finding is suggested in Fig. 6 and was apparent in the multitone data of Scharf (1959a).

Although there is general agreement that the white-noise loudness function is curved relative to the 1000-Hz function (see Stevens, 1972), the precise size of the difference in loudness between noise and tone is more difficult to determine. Loudness matches between a pure tone and white noise are highly variable, probably because matching the loudness of two such different sounds is a difficult and uncertain task. Not only is there much variability between subjects, but when subjects adjust the tone to match the noise, their judgments may differ as much as 10 dB, on the average, from their judgments when they adjust the noise (e.g., Zwicker, 1958). Also, the perceived volume or size of the white noise is much greater than that of a pure tone, which could lead to overestimation of its loudness. Both these problems may have been partly solved in the direct estimation procedure used by Scharf and Fishken (1970).

3. SECONDARY SPECTRAL FACTORS

For multitone complexes, loudness level is highest when the component tones are evenly spaced with respect to critical bands (Zwicker et al., 1957). For example, as many as four phons are gained by spacing four tones an equal number of critical bands apart instead of bunching three of them together. Similarly, loudness is greatest when the components are all about equally loud (Scharf, 1962). If the loudness of some components is reduced relative to others (without reducing the overall intensity or changing ΔF), the loudness of a supercritical sound goes down. However, despite the effects of component loudness and internal spacing, overall loudness does not seem to change as the number of components within given frequency limits (ΔF) is increased from two to the infinite number contained within a band of white noise (Scharf, 1959b). Loudness summation is also the same whether the sound comes from a single earphone to one ear, from a pair of phones to both ears, from a single loudspeaker, or even if the lower frequencies come from one loudspeaker and the higher frequencies from another speaker (Niese, 1960, 1961; Scharf, 1974).

IV. TIME

Up to about half a second, temporal variables such as signal duration and repetition rate affect loudness. Precise values for these effects are, however, often undefined, owing to conflicting experimental results. This section reviews the data on duration, double pulses, and repetition rate. [The effect of rise–fall time is usually negligible (Gjaevenes & Rimstad, 1972).]

A. Duration

The study of the relation between loudness and signal duration divides into two distinct domains. In the study of brief sounds, the aim is to discover how rapidly loudness reaches maximum value as duration is lengthened from a few milliseconds to hundreds of milliseconds. In the study of loudness adaptation or perstimulatory fatigue, the aim has been to discover how rapidly loudness decreases, if at all, as duration lengthens well beyond 1 sec.

1. BRIEF SOUNDS

First, a word about thresholds. As the duration of a tone increases up to about 200 msec, threshold intensity decreases in direct proportion to time; the total sound energy, which is the product of time and intensity, thereby

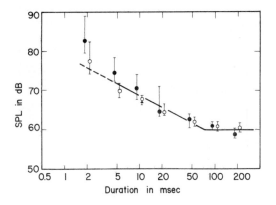

Fig. 8. Sound pressure level at
which narrow-band noise at various
durations is judged equal in loudness
to a long-duration band at 60 dB SPL.
[Adapted from Port (1963a), Ueber
die Lautstärke einzelner kurzer
Schallimpulse, *Acustica*, 1963, **13**,
212–223.]

remains constant. This finding implies that the ear integrates energy over time up to about 200 msec. However, knowledge of the auditory system suggests very strongly that the ear integrates neural energy, not acoustical or mechanical energy (Zwislocki, 1969).

The auditory system integrates neural energy also at suprathreshold levels, where loudness replaces threshold or detection as the response variable. In the typical experiment, listeners make loudness matches between short-duration and long-duration stimuli. Results are treated by plotting the intensity of the brief sound, at which it is judged equal in loudness to the standard sound, as a function of its duration. Figure 8 is one such plot (Port, 1963a). The sounds were third-octave bands of filtered white noise, and the standard was at 60 dB SPL. Since all the loudness matches were made to the same long-duration stimulus, the data map out an equal-loudness contour, which is approximated by the solid line.

We can pose three questions about such data. At what duration does intensity become constant and independent of duration? Before becoming constant, how does intensity change as a function of time, i.e., what is the trading relation between intensity and time? Does the shape of the contour depend on stimulus variables such as frequency, level, and bandwidth? Answers to these questions have been many and varied. Table II summarizes them, first for white noise and then for pure tones, mostly at 1000 Hz.

The column labeled trading relation indicates whether *(a)* intensity changed in direct inverse proportion to time, thus maintaining constant sound energy (as at threshold); *(b)* intensity changed more rapidly than time, so that energy decreased as time increased; or *(c)* intensity changed less rapidly, so that energy increased with time. The next column gives the duration at which intensity became constant. Usually, the equal-loudness contour showed a rather gradual transition from a decreasing to a constant intensity, so that the values for the critical duration are not precisely defined. The next column gives the value of the time constant τ calculated by the experimenter for his data from an exponential function of the form, $I(t) =$

TABLE II

SUMMARY OF STUDIES OF HOW LOUDNESS VARIES AS A FUNCTION OF DURATION

Author(s) & year	Number of subjects	Stimulus	Rise-fall time (in msec)	Trading relation[a]	Critical duration[b] (in msec)	Time constant (in msec)	Effect of level
Miller, 1948	3	white noise	abrupt	energy increases	60–140	—	CD decreases as level increases
Pollack, 1958	7–10	white noise	abrupt	energy constant	100	—	—
Small, Brandt, & Cox, 1962	12	white noise	—	energy decreases	15–50	—	CD decreases as level increases
Stevens & Hall, 1966	12	white noise	—	energy decreases	150	—	none
Zwicker, 1966	83	white noise	abrupt	energy constant	200–400	100	—
	74	1000 Hz	1–2	energy constant	200–400	100	—
Békésy, 1929	—	800 Hz	abrupt	energy increases	120–180	—	CD shorter at higher level
Boone, 1973	14–20	500, 1000, 4000 Hz	5	energy constant	150	120	—
Ekman et al., 1966	10	1000 Hz	10	energy increases	over 500	—	steeper trading relation at high levels
Garner, 1949	6	1000 Hz	abrupt	energy increases	500	—	steeper trading relation at higher level
Munson, 1947	—	125, 1000, 5650 Hz	3	energy decreases	200	—	steeper trading relation at higher level
Niese, 1956	12	500, 1000, 3000 Hz	abrupt	energy constant	65	23	steeper trading relation at higher level
Niese, 1959	10	1000 Hz	1–2	energy increases	100	23	none
Pedersen, Lyregaard, & Poulsen, 1977	381	1000 Hz	1–2	energy constant or decreases	160–320	80	steeper trading relation at lower levels
Reichardt & Niese, 1970	50	1000 Hz	3	energy constant	100	30	—
Stephens, 1974	10	250 Hz	abrupt	energy constant	100	—	—
		1000			90		
		4000			10		
Port, 1963a	8	narrow-band noise at 350, 2000, 10,000 Hz	1–2	energy constant	70	70	none

[a] Trading relation refers to the relation between intensity and time. As stimulus duration increases up to the critical duration, total sound energy ($I \times t$) has been found to remain constant, decrease, or increase.

[b] For constant loudness, intensity must be reduced as duration is increased up to the critical duration.

NOTE: A dash means the information either was not relevant to the study or was not provided.

$I_\infty/(1 - e^{-t/\tau})$, where I_∞ is the asymptotic intensity at long durations t of the sound. The exponential function does not exhibit a sharp discontinuity, and would fit the data in Fig. 8 somewhat better than the solid lines do. However, the pictured discontinuity may be real.

Variability among subjects in their critical duration or trading relation would smear the discontinuity and produce a slow transition. Accordingly, the calculated time constant and measured critical duration can both be treated as estimates of the same discontinuity in an intensity-by-time contour having two expressions, each equal to a constant.

For $t <$ CD: $I \times t = k$.   (This first expression becomes more complicated if the equal-energy rule does not hold.)

For $t \geq$ CD: $t = k'$.

Table II reveals no striking differences between the trading relations and critical durations or time constants measured for white noise and those measured for pure tones. This finding is consistent with the observation that loudness increases as a function of bandwidth or ΔF in the same way whether a sound lasts a few milliseconds or hundreds of milliseconds (Port, 1963a; Scharf, 1970b; Zwicker, 1965). Nevertheless, the large variability among the measurements in Table II may obscure real differences. For both tone and noise, the measured trading relation has revealed all three possibilities: increasing, decreasing, and constant energy. The critical duration or time constant also varies over a wide range of values, but has almost always been 150 msec or less. The effect of sound level is unclear. Some studies show no effect on either the critical duration or trading relation. Other studies show a decrease in the critical duration with increasing level. A few studies suggest that the higher the level, the more rapidly intensity decreases as duration increases. Frequency seems to have little, if any, effect. Signal frequency was varied in five ştudies (Boone, 1973; Munson, 1947; Niese, 1956; Port, 1963a; Stephens, 1974); the first three authors reported no frequency effect, Port noted a lengthening of the critical duration at 10,000 Hz, and Stephens noted a shortening at 4000 Hz, his highest frequency.

Owing to the disagreement in the data and to the importance of a time constant in the calculation of loudness and assessment of sound annoyance, an international experimental program—a so-called "round robin"—has been undertaken in over 20 laboratories to measure the relation between loudness and duration. Part of the final report (Pedersen, Lyregaard, & Poulsen, 1977) is summarized in Table II. Despite nearly uniform experimental conditions and procedures, results from different laboratories showed considerable scatter. Nevertheless, the carefully averaged data at 95 phons are best summarized by a constant-energy function with a time constant of 80 msec. At 55 and 75 phons the same time constant was adopted by the authors, although the trading relation is steeper than at 95 phons; in order to keep the loudness level constant at 55 or 75 phons, the overall energy must be reduced as duration increases from 5 msec to approximately 20 msec.

Investigators come up with many different conclusions about the relation between loudness and duration mainly because matching the loudness of a brief sound to a long sound is difficult. The outcome is readily affected by variations in experimental parameters, such as the interstimulus time, repetition rate, and difference in the duration of the variable and standard sounds (Reichardt, 1965), and by instructions and method (Stephens, 1974). (Even when many of these pitfalls are avoided, as in the international round robin, different laboratories come up with different results.) Possibly the auditory system handles temporal factors differently from person to person. More likely, normal listeners vary because they use different criteria in their loudness matches, rather than because their auditory systems differ significantly. Some listeners may have trouble abstracting the loudness of a sound from its subjective duration, others may be confused by what Reichardt (1965) calls a roughness component.

Criterion differences are especially important when the stimuli are tone bursts. As its duration is shortened, a tone steadily loses its pitch and tonal quality, partly because the auditory system does not have time enough to build a full pitch percept and partly because an increasing portion of the sound energy falls at frequencies other than that of the original long-duration tone. The effective bandwidth of a tone, which is turned on and off abruptly, increases in nearly direct inverse proportion to duration. Turning a tone on and off gradually instead of abruptly keeps the bandwidth narrow but limits the shortest possible duration. Spectral changes contribute to the variability of the loudness judgments by making the sounds more dissimilar and thereby harder to match in loudness. (The increase in bandwidth is usually too small to influence loudness directly, in the manner described in Section III,C; unless the duration is shortened to less than 1 to 10 msec, depending on frequency, almost all the sound energy remains confined to a single critical band.)

Two of the studies in Table II did not require subjects to match short and long sounds for equal loudness. Ekman, Berglund, and Berglund (1966) and J. C. Stevens and Hall (1966) had their subjects make magnitude estimations of the loudness of signals presented at various durations and levels. These results provided a direct measure of how loudness increases with duration. Ekman *et al.* found that the loudness of a pure tone increases as the logarithm of duration, with the rate of increase faster at higher than at lower levels. Stevens and Hall found that the loudness of white noise increases at all levels as the .35 power of duration.

The data vary so much that it is difficult to say how the loudness function looks at short durations. Stevens and Hall (1966) have, however, directly measured loudness functions for sounds (white noise) of different durations. They found that signal duration had no effect on the exponents of the power functions they fitted to their data. (Actually, the data would be better fitted by a bowed function similar to the one shown in Fig. 7.) The results of the round robin (Pedersen *et al.*, 1977) agree essentially with those of Stevens and Hall. Limited to three levels over a range of 40 phons, the round-robin data suggest only small changes, if any, in the exponent of the loudness function for a 1000-Hz tone at short durations.

The discord in the literature precludes definitive answers to all three questions posed at the beginning of this section about the loudness of brief sounds. However, by giving special weight to the outcome of the international round robin, involving as it did so many subjects, laboratories, and careful measurements, we can arrive at some reasonable generalizations. Best agreement has been reached with respect to the question of the duration at which loudness reaches its full value. (In terms of the equal-loudness contour of Fig. 8, the question is when must one stop decreasing intensity in order to keep loudness constant as duration gets longer.) A time constant of 80 msec summarizes the round-robin data very well and is close to most of the values for the time constant previously proposed. Beyond 80 msec, loudness continues to increase with duration but more gradually. Loudness may be considered, within the error of measurement, to reach full value between 150 and 300 msec. Evidence is meager for the sharp discontinuity implied by a critical duration.

The second question concerned the trading relation between intensity and time that yields constant loudness at brief durations. The data are highly discordant, even those from the round robin. A simple, descriptive summary of the data in the literature is a trading relation with sound energy constant up to approximately 80 msec.

The third question concerned the effects of stimulus variables such as level, frequency, and bandwidth on the time constant and trading relation. On the whole, none of these variables has been shown to have a consistent effect on either the time constant or trading relation. Thus, the best current summary of the literature on the loudness of brief sounds goes as follows: The dependence of the loudness of a brief sound on duration can be described by an exponential function with a time constant of 80 msec. (Accordingly, loudness level comes within 1 phon of its asymptotic value when duration reaches 180 msec.) Put another way, loudness increases with duration up to approximately 180 msec; it increases more gradually between 80 and 180 msec than at shorter durations.

2. LONG-DURATION STIMULI

Loudness first reaches full value a fraction of a second after the onset of stimulation. Does loudness then remain steady or decrease? Is there loudness adaptation? A number of studies have revealed little or no decline in the loudness of sounds lasting as long as 30 min (Bray, Dirks, & Morgan, 1973; Fraser, Petty, & Elliott, 1970; Grube & Braune, 1974; Mirabella, Taug, & Teichner, 1967; Petty, Fraser, & Elliott, 1970; Stokinger, Cooper, Meissner, & Jones, 1972; Wiley, Small, & Lilly, 1973). So far, loudness adaptation has been found only at high frequencies near thresholds elevated by cochlear impairment or masking noises (Dirks, Morgan, & Bray, 1974; Margolis & Wiley, 1976; Wiley, Small, & Lilly, 1976) and, in one study (Mirabella *et al.*, 1967), at 1000 Hz near normal thresholds.* Consequently, except perhaps near threshold, the loudness function in Fig. 1 is valid for any binaural 1000-Hz tone whose duration exceeds about 200 msec.

A kind of loudness adaptation does occur when one ear receives a continuous sound while the other ear receives an intermittent or occasional sound. Many earlier studies showed that the loudness level of the continuous sound dropped as much as 30 to 50 phons within a few minutes (e.g., Egan, 1955; Hood, 1950; Palva & Kärjä, 1969). Since this remarkable loudness reduction can be measured only when both ears are stimulated, it must result from binaural interaction, possibly involving the same mechanisms that underlie lateralization (Ward, 1973, pp. 334–337).

B. Double Pulses

The overall loudness of two tone bursts, each lasting less than 10 msec, depends on the time interval separating them. At brief intervals of 1 or 2 msec, the loudness level of two equally loud bursts is 3 phons higher than the level of either one alone. As the interval lengthens, this advantage decreases, disappearing altogether, according to some data, when the interval reaches 25 msec (Niese, 1956) or 50 msec (Schwarze, 1963). Other data suggest that there is some loudness summation up to intervals as long as 200 msec (Irwin & Zwislocki, 1971; Scharf, 1970b). Even when presented dichotically and separated by 150 msec, two clicks are louder than a single monaural click (Botte, 1974). The 200-msec estimate is based also on data for two tones very different in frequency, which have as much as a 10-phon advantage in loudness level at brief temporal separations. Such a large difference in loudness level made it possible to trace the decay of loudness over time more precisely than the 3-phon difference measured with identical stimuli. Apparently, then, loudness summates over a longer time period for two tone bursts separated by a silent interval than for a single burst. The inserted silent interval may permit recovery from inhibitory off-effects (Zwislocki, 1969). (The near absence of such poststimulus inhibitory effects at threshold may be why the critical duration at threshold is longer than above threshold.)

Besides the overall loudness of two pulses, one can measure the loudness of each member of the pair. The first pulse may strongly affect the loudness of the second, but the second pulse seems hardly to affect the first (Elmasian & Galambos, 1975; Irwin & Zwislocki, 1971). For example, Elmasian and

---

* Loudness is a principal component of sound aversiveness (see Berglund, Berglund, & Lindvall, 1976). It would then be strange, indeed, if intense sounds, which can damage the ear after prolonged exposure, became softer and hence less aversive over time. Loudness adaptation at high levels would be comforting but costly.

Galambos have shown that the loudness level of the second pulse may be enhanced as much as 30 phons owing to a preceding, more intense pulse. Although loudness enhancement is strongest when both pulses go to the same ear (or ears), a pulse to one ear can enhance the loudness of a later pulse that goes to the other ear (Galambos, Bauer, Picton, Squires, & Squires, 1972). Since loudness enhancement is absent when the two pulses are equally intense, it is probably irrelevant to the overall loudness of two equally intense or equally loud pulses. Indeed, Zwislocki (Zwislocki, Ketkar, Cannon, & Nodar, 1974; Zwislocki & Sokolich, 1974) presents evidence that loudness enhancement and loudness summation (overall loudness) are fundamentally different processes.

C. Pulse Trains

A pulse repeated over and over has a repetition rate or pulse frequency expressed in pulses per second (pps). Several investigators have measured the loudness of a pulse train as a function of its rate (Garner, 1948; Niese, 1961; Pollack, 1958; Port, 1963b). Their subjects matched a continuous tone or noise to the interrupted sound. When the pulse frequency equals $1/T$, where T, in seconds, is the duration of each single pulse, then the interrupted sound is indistinguishable from a continuous sound. [For example, a 10-msec (.01 sec) burst repeated 100 times per second is identical to a continuous sound.] At $1/T$, the "interrupted" sound is set to the same level as the continuous sound for equal loudness. At slower rates, the interrupted sound must have a higher level for loudness to be equal.

At repetition rates so slow that only one or two brief pulses are presented each second, the duration of the pulse determines how much higher the level of the interrupted sound must be. The shorter the pulse, the larger the difference between the levels of the interrupted and continuous sounds. For a given duration, however, the level difference reaches its maximum between 2 and 5 pps; slowing the rate below 2 pps has no effect on the loudness of the interrupted sound. Further reduction of the repetition rate is ineffective because at 2 pps, the individual pulses are already almost 500 msec apart, beyond the range of loudness summation as already noted in studies of double pulses.

As repetition rate slows from its maximum value, $1/T$, to its lower effective limit, near 2 pps, the level of the interrupted sound required to maintain constant loudness increases too slowly to maintain constant sound energy. The interrupted sound requires less energy than an equally loud steady sound. (Energy is computed over the whole presentation period, including the silent intervals.) Hence, for a given amount of sound energy, greater loudness is attained by distributing the energy over time with interspersed silent intervals than by making it a continuous sound. Perhaps the advantage comes from a reduction of poststimulus inhibitory effects during the silent intervals.

V. BACKGROUND

In the quiet, a 1-sec, 1000-Hz tone at 80 dB SPL has a loudness of 16 sones and is loud. Heard against a 90-dB white noise, the same 80-dB tone is soft. The reduction of loudness by a background noise is called *partial masking,* to distinguish it from complete masking, in which the noise makes the signal inaudible. A masking sound, then, raises the threshold for the signal and reduces its loudness. At the same time, the masker makes the loudness function for the signal steeper, and the more intense the masker, the steeper the loudness function (Chocholle & Greenbaum, 1966; Hellman & Zwislocki, 1964; Lochner & Burger, 1961; Scharf, 1964; Stevens & Guirao, 1967). Partial masking depends not only on the intensity of the masker, but also on its bandwidth and its frequency location relative to the frequency of the signal.* Each of these factors is treated in turn.

A. Intensity of Masker

Figure 9 presents some of the data collected by Stevens and Guirao (1967). The listeners adjusted a 1000-Hz tone in the quiet to match the loudness of another 1000-Hz tone presented against a white noise. The noise was set at the level given as the parameter on the curves. If the noise had no effect on the loudness of the tone, the data would fall on the dashed line, where the levels of the unmasked and masked tones are equal. Stevens and Guirao drew the solid lines through the data on the basis of a model that included the following three assumptions.

(1) A tone in noise must be more intense than an equally loud tone in the quiet, but the intensity difference decreases as the level of the partially masked tone increases. In other words, the loudness of the tone in noise grows more rapidly than the loudness of the tone in quiet.

(2) Loudness grows more rapidly in noise up to a level 30 dB above the effective masked threshold for the tone. Above 30 dB, the loudness of the tone in noise grows at the same rate as the loudness of the tone in quiet; the solid line is then parallel to the dashed line.

(3) The more intense the noise, the steeper the function.

Although not predicted by the model, it turned out that the tone in noise must be more intense than the equally loud tone in quiet even at high signal levels where the noise no longer steepens the function. Zwicker (1963) noted a similar failure of a tone in wide-band noise to attain normal loudness.

By means of the standard sone values in Table I, the data of Stevens and

---

* Signal duration appears also to be a factor in partial masking. Chocholle (1975) reports that the loudness functions for partially masked tone bursts become even steeper when signal duration is reduced to 50 or 100 msec.

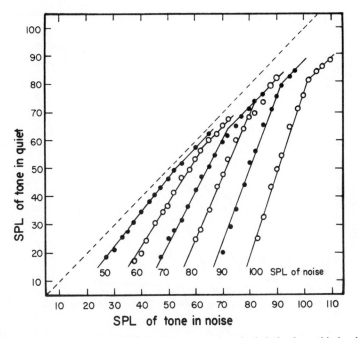

FIG. 9. Sound pressure level at which a 1000-Hz tone in quiet is judged equal in loudness to a tone partially masked by white noise. Parameter on the curves is the level of the masking noise in decibels. Symbols are filled and unfilled for clarity. [Adapted from Stevens and Guirao (1967), Loudness functions under inhibition, *Perception and Psychophysics*, **2**, 459–465.]

Guirao were converted to sones. Figure 10 presents the loudness of the 1000-Hz tone in noise as a function of the sound pressure level of the tone. These curves are based on the data in Fig. 9 and on other data, which Stevens and Guirao obtained by having listeners adjust the tone in noise to match the tone in quiet. The slope of the loudness functions in Fig. 10 increases monotonically with the level of the masking noise. Put another way, the higher the masked threshold for the tone, the steeper its loudness function up to about 30 dB above threshold.

No attempt was made to draw the loudness functions in Fig. 10 with a sharp change of slope at a level 30 dB above threshold. Stevens and Guirao suggested such a discontinuity, but most available data do not show it, perhaps because averaged data tend to obscure discontinuities. Nevertheless, it is clear that within about 30 dB of the masked threshold, the loudness function is steeper; at higher levels it has the usual slope of about .6. The question remains whether the transition zone is smooth or sharp.

The corrected power law $L = k(P - P_0)^{.6}$ does not appear to provide a good fit to these masked functions. In general, a simple modification of the power

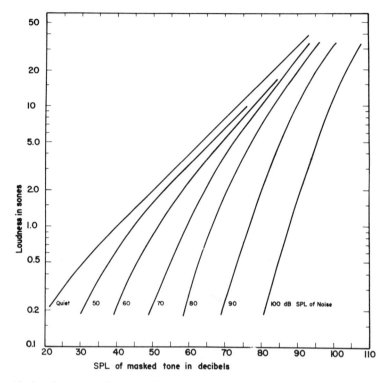

FIG. 10. Loudness as a function of the sound pressure level of a 1000-Hz tone partially masked by white noise. Curves are derived from the loudness matching data of Stevens and Guirao (1967) and the standard loudness function in Fig. 1.

function is insufficient. Stevens (1966) has suggested that in masking, as in other cases of elevated thresholds, such as in deafness, and for low-frequency tones, the relation between loudness and intensity undergoes a *power transformation,* in which the slope of the function decreases abruptly at some level above threshold. Zwicker (1963) and Zwislocki (1965) have suggested other modifications.

That noise steepens the loudness function was first quantitatively demonstrated by Steinberg and Gardner (1937) in a paper that pointed out the similarity with loudness recruitment in certain types of deafness. Loudness recruitment refers to the abnormally steep growth of loudness so clearly shown in Fig. 10. Recruitment in hard-of-hearing listeners is discussed in Section VI,C.

B. Bandwidth

The slope of the loudness function under masking increases when the bandwidth of the masking noise is narrowed while its overall level is kept constant (Hellman, 1970; Zwicker, 1963). This rule holds provided the frequency of the masked tone remains within the frequency limits of the masking band. Heard against a masker no more than one critical band wide, the loudness of a tone grows so rapidly that it reaches its normal value at a level 10 to 15 dB above the masked threshold. Heard against a noise wider than a critical band, the tone may never reach normal loudness. Nevertheless, the *slope* of the loudness function does become normal at some point, in white noise at about 30 dB above threshold.

Bandwidth is also a relevant variable when the noise is the signal and a pure tone is the masker. The tone masks a narrow-band noise somewhat better than it masks a wide-band noise. In both cases, however, the tone is a much less effective complete and partial masker, by about 20 dB at high intensities, than an equally loud narrow-band noise (Hellman, 1972).

C. Frequency Relations between Masker and Signal

How much one sound masks another depends very much on their frequency relations. Figure 11 shows how a narrow band of white noise reduces the loudness of a pure tone whose frequency is given on the abscissa. The noise, set at 70 dB SPL, was one critical band wide and centered on 1000 Hz. The parameter on the curves is the loudness level to which the masked tone was set, so that all points on a given contour were equally loud. The top contour is the threshold curve. The ordinate shows masking in decibels, defined as the amount by which the sound pressure level of the masked tone had to be increased, owing to the presence of the noise, in order for the tone to reach the given loudness level.

The spread of masking is the same at threshold as at 15 phons. But as the loudness level increases, the pattern becomes less skewed toward the higher frequencies until at 75 phons, it is slightly skewed toward the lower frequencies. This change means that at low loudness levels, a given noise is more effective in completely or partially masking higher-frequency tones, whereas at high levels it is more effective in masking lower-frequency tones. Put another way, the loudness functions for tones lying above the frequency limits of the noise are steeper than the functions for tones lying the same distance in frequency below the noise. Once again, steeper loudness functions are associated with higher thresholds. These relations hold as well for a masking noise at 90 dB SPL and for a subcritical band of noise (Scharf, 1971). Similar results have been obtained for a pure tone partially masking another pure tone (Chocholle & Greenbaum, 1966).

VI. LISTENER

People hear in much the same way, permitting a large number of generalizations about loudness with hardly a reference to the listener. Neverthe-

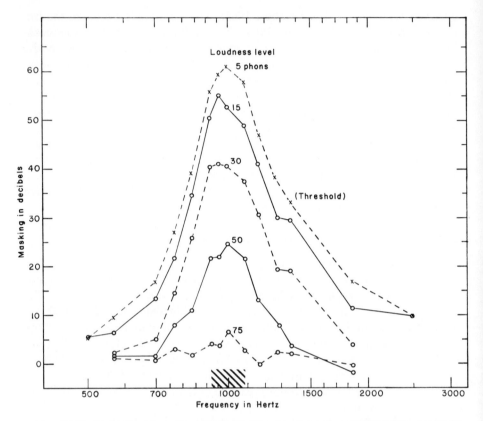

FIG. 11. Masking of pure tones by a narrow-band noise centered on 1000 Hz and set at 70 dB SPL. Masking is the difference between the sound pressure level of the masked tone and that of an unmasked tone when judged equally loud. The loudness level of the masked tone, measured by matching it to the unmasked tone of the same frequency, is the parameter. Hatched area gives the ideal spectral limits of the masking noise. Data are based on four subjects. [Adapted from Scharf (1971), Fundamentals of auditory masking, *Audiology*, **10**, 30–40.]

less, listeners do differ from one another; and the same person's judgment may change from one time to another. It makes a difference whether the subject listens with one ear or two ears, and whether or not he or she has recently been exposed to loud sounds. Both these factors can be controlled by the experimenter. Factors outside of experimental control include pathology of the auditory system and normal individual differences. Normal differences may include small physiological variations in the auditory system and complex variations in those aspects of decision making and personality that could affect the judgment of sound. This section deals with each of these factors in turn—binaural loudness, fatigue, deafness, and individual differences.

A. Binaural Loudness

A sound is louder in two ears than in one. The question that has intrigued investigators for many years is how much louder. The most recent answer is that a pure tone or narrow-band noise is about 1.7 times louder in two ears than in one (Scharf & Fishken, 1970). A wide-band noise, such as white noise, is also about 1.7 times louder in two ears, on the average, but the ratio of binaural-to-monaural loudness increases with SPL until at high levels it may be 2 : 1.

An invariant binaural-to-monaural ratio means that the binaural and monaural loudness functions for pure tones have the same exponent; only the constant of proportionality differs. The ratio of the constants k in the power function $L = kP^n$ is equal to the ratio of binaural to monaural loudness. Accordingly, the loudness function of Fig. 1 holds for both binaural and monaural tones, except that the monaural curve should lie about 8 phons to the right of the binaural curve at loudness levels higher than 40 phons and less than 8 phons to the right at lower loudness levels. The white-noise function in Fig. 7 is for binaural loudness. The monaural function for noise has a similar bowed shape, but lies to the right of the binaural function; the decibel difference between the two functions increases with SPL.

The data of Scharf and Fishken are based on magnitude estimation and production. The tonal data agree with those of Hellman and Zwislocki (1963), who used similar procedures to measure the binaural and monaural loudness of a 1000-Hz tone. The data on white noise differ somewhat from those of Reynolds and Stevens (1960) who used a moderately wide band of noise; they measured a larger binaural-to-monaural ratio, which increased more rapidly with level.

The conclusions of Scharf and Fishken also agree with most of the matching data in the literature (Caussé & Chavasse, 1942; Porsolt & Irwin, 1967; Scharf, 1968). Only the matching data of Fletcher and Munson (1933) suggested a larger binaural-to-monaural ratio for a pure tone. Their overestimation was constant across frequency, which shows that binaural loudness summation is independent of frequency. Scharf (1969) went further to show that loudness summation is the same even when the tone in one ear differs greatly in frequency from the tone in the other ear. This *dichotic summation of loudness* is the same in different parts of the frequency spectrum. Some loudness summation also seems to occur between a tone in one ear and a noise in the other, since the tone is often judged louder with a contralateral noise than without one (Rowley & Studebaker, 1971; Vigran, 1965).

While independent of frequency differences between the two ears, binaural loudness summation is not independent of intensity differences. Irwin (1965) showed that binaural summation is greatest when the sound power is about equal in the two ears.

Given a constant binaural-to-monaural loudness ratio, the monaural loudness function for a pure tone or narrow-band noise can be derived from the standard binaural function by changing the value of k so that $L_m = 10.45/1.7$ $(P - 1.4P_0)^{.6}$, where L_m is monaural loudness in sones, P is the sound pressure in dynes per square centimeter of a 1000-Hz tone, and P_0 is the correction factor used in the binaural formula. (Because the monaural threshold is 3 dB higher than the binaural threshold, the value of P_0 is increased by the corresponding ratio.)

B. Auditory Fatigue

A loud sound fatigues the ear. Auditory fatigue has been demonstrated many times as a temporary increase in the normal threshold, known as the *temporary threshold shift* (TTS) (see Zwislocki, Chapter 8 of this volume). Near an elevated threshold, loudness must be depressed; there is also a temporary loudness shift (TLS).

Short exposure to very intense sounds or long exposure (measured in years) to weaker sounds may result in a permanent threshold shift and a permanent loudness shift, a condition dealt with in the section on auditory pathology.

The reduction in loudness caused by a fatiguing sound is analogous to partial masking, except that in the former the masking sound is turned off at least several seconds before the signal is turned on. The temporal separation of masker and maskee reduces the threshold shifts and changes their pattern. Instead of maximum loudness reduction and threshold elevation at the same frequency as the fatiguing sound, the maximum TLS and TTS are at a frequency a half octave higher (Davis, Morgan, Hawkins, Galambos, & Smith, 1950).

Riach, Elliott, and Reed (1962) measured the loudness function for a 2800-Hz tone 4 min after one ear had been fatigued by a 2000-Hz tone. Presented between 100 and 110 dB SL, the fatiguing tone was left on long enough to raise threshold 10, 20, or 30 dB. Magnitude estimation of the 2800-Hz tone presented separately to the fatigued and rested ears showed that the loudness function was steeper in the fatigued ear up to about 60 dB above the normal threshold. Above 60 dB SL, the loudness functions were approximately the same in both ears. Here is clear evidence of loudness recruitment like that shown in Fig. 10. And the greater the TTS, the steeper the function; the slope of the lower part of the loudness function increased from .62 to 1.06 as TTS increased from 10 to 30 dB. Once again, higher thresholds mean steeper loudness functions. Davis *et al.* (1950) and Hickling (1967) have reported similar evidence for loudness recruitment after exposure to noise.

The strong effects of fatigue on loudness may seem at variance with the lack of loudness adaptation. If a sound can be turned off and still reduce the loudness of another sound presented 4 min later, then the fatiguing sound ought to reduce its own loudness during continuous stimulation. However, the fatiguing sound reduces the loudness only of sounds at intensity levels much lower than its own. The published curves of Riach *et al.* show that for loudness to be reduced, the judged tone has to be at least 40 to 50 dB weaker than the fatiguing tone. Furthermore, the fact that the loudness function under fatigue is steeper than the normal function means that the reduction of loudness is greatest near threshold. Perstimulatory loudness adaptation apparently does not occur because the level of the "test" sound (later segment of a sound) is too high relative to the level of the "fatiguing" sound (early segment).

C. Auditory Pathology

Changes in the loudness function have long been important in the clinical diagnosis of auditory pathology. Loudness recruitment (a term first used by Fowler, 1928) often occurs in cochlear pathology but seldom in either conductive or retrocochlear neural pathology (Hallpike, 1967). Patients with high thresholds caused by Ménière's disease (Hallpike & Hood, 1959) or noise exposure (Ward, Fleer, & Glorig, 1961), both of which lead to damage of the hair cells, often report they are disturbed by loud sounds. Thus a person with a midfrequency threshold at 60 dB SPL, 50 dB higher than normal, may call sounds at 90 dB SPL very loud, even annoyingly loud.

Quantitative measurements are usually obtained by loudness matches either between a good ear and a bad ear in cases of unilateral pathology (alternate binaural loudness balance) or between a tone at a frequency with an abnormal threshold and a tone in the same ear at a frequency with a normal threshold. Such tests are routine in many audiological clinics. Miskolczy-Fodor (1960) pooled 300 loudness matches by patients who showed loudness recruitment. In all the cases, recruitment was complete, meaning that loudness eventually reached a normal level after starting from an elevated threshold. The data indicate that the greater the hearing loss, the steeper the loudness function. Stevens and Guirao (1967) have suggested that the data fit their power-transformation model. The data are too scattered to distinguish between a double power function and a smooth curve, but they do fit the model's prediction that the slope of the loudness function increases with threshold. The data also are similar to those collected from normal listeners for a partially masked tone (Hellman & Zwislocki, 1964).

Although loudness adaptation is generally absent in normal ears, might it occur in impaired ears? In certain types of deafness, usually involving lesion of the auditory nerve or more central parts of the auditory system, a tone not far above threshold soon becomes inaudible if left on continuously (Ward, 1973). Harbart, Weiss, and Wilpizeski (1968) could not find a corresponding decay of loudness at suprathreshold levels. Of course, a tone near threshold must decrease in loudness before it disappears, but at higher levels even severely impaired auditory systems do not show significant amounts of loudness adaptation. On the other hand, in ears with a noise-induced hearing loss, which do not adapt abnormally at threshold, some suprathreshold loudness adaptation has been measured at low sensation levels (Margolis & Wiley, 1976; Wiley et al., 1976; see also Section IV,A,2).

While recruitment is the most striking loudness anomaly in cochlear impairment, another more subtle change has been noted. Listeners with severe cochlear impairment show no loudness summation over bandwidth. For such listeners, the loudness of four equally loud tones does not increase with ΔF or bandwidth even when the tones cover a frequency range much wider than the normal critical bandwidth (Martin, 1974; Scharf & Hellman, 1966). For normal listeners who heard the four tones against an intense masking noise, loudness summation was less than in the quiet but still measurable and as much as predicted by a model of loudness summation developed for normal ears (Zwicker & Scharf, 1965). These results suggested the possibility that the critical band is abnormally large in ears with a cochlear impairment. Also, despite the similarity of loudness recruitment in cochlear deafness and under masking, the underlying processes may be quite different in the two conditions.

Listeners with a conductive hearing loss show normal loudness summation. They also have normal loudness functions—no recruitment—an exception to the rule that loudness grows more rapidly from elevated thresholds than from normal, midfrequency thresholds. This exception suggests that loudness recruitment occurs only when threshold is raised by changes beyond the middle ear, such as occur in masking, fatigue, and cochlear impairment.

D. Individual Differences

Not all listeners with normal hearing exhibit loudness functions like the standard function (Fig. 1). Some listeners do not give a good power function; more important, listeners give functions with different slopes. Stevens and Guirao (1964) measured functions for 11 listeners under a combined estimation–production procedure in which the subject both set the level of the stimulus and assigned a number proportional to its loudness. The exponents in the first session ranged from .4 to 1.1. Other investigators (de Barbenza, Bryan, & Tempest, 1970; McGill, 1960; Reason, 1968) have also found large individual differences in the slopes of loudness functions. (A steep loudness function from a normal listener may be distinguished from a steep function from a listener with impaired hearing not only because threshold is normal, but because the normal listener's function does not become flat at 30 or 40 dB SL.) Loudness functions probably differ among normal listeners for many and complex reasons, some of a stable nature and some less stable. Stable variations could include variations in the auditory system or less specifiable variations in personality. Nonstable variation could be random, or accidental influences that affect judgments from one stimulus presentation to another and from one session to another. To a limited extent, each of these possibilities has been treated experimentally.

Ross (1968a) showed that much of the variability among the equal-loudness contours measured on three subjects could be ascribed to differences in the impedance of the middle ear. However, since the impedance was independent of intensity below about 100 dB SPL, impedance differences could not account for possible differences in the slope of the loudness function. Slope differences are more likely to be based on variations in the cochlea. But Ross's analysis does point up the possibility of accounting for at least some of the variability in loudness judgments on the basis of specifiable and presumably stable physiological differences.

Stephens (1970) has reported some tentative conclusions based on magnitude estimations that link personality differences, as measured by a standard test of anxiety, with differences in the slope of the loudness function. High-anxiety scorers gave steeper loudness functions than did low-anxiety scorers. Similarly, de Barbenza *et al.* (1970) reported that excitable subjects tended to give steep loudness functions. While highly tentative, these data suggest, quite reasonably, that different kinds of people use different strategies in estimating loudness, or any other subjective continuum. Reason (1972) provides further support for this hypothesis. He measured significant correlations between the slope of the loudness function and other, nonauditory measures such as persistence of a visual illusion, susceptibility to motion sickness, and the slope of the function for perceived weight. Reason ascribed the correlations, which varied from .30 to .75, to individual differences in the way the central nervous system handles stimulus intensity.

At least two studies have looked at how loudness estimations change from one session to another. Stevens and Guirao (1964) noted that their subjects gave a different exponent in a second session, one to six months after the first session. The correlation between the exponents from the first and second sessions was .53. For a fixed interval of 11 weeks between sessions, Logue (1976) reported a correlation of .59. Since these correlations account for only about one-third of the variance of the individual exponents, much of the difference among subjects in their judgment of loudness is not constant and stable but is unstable, perhaps random. Consequently, differences among the loudness functions from normal listeners are apparently not, for the most part, directly related to the way the auditory system works. Therefore, pooling loudness judgments from a group of normal subjects is a suitable procedure for arriving at the best estimate of the slope of the loudness function. Personality and other such individual differences may account for little of the variance in loudness functions. To the extent that "central" nonsensory factors randomly affect loudness, it is wise to attempt to cancel them out by averaging across subjects.

VII. PHYSIOLOGICAL CORRELATES OF LOUDNESS

Auditory physiologists seldom look directly for physiological correlates of loudness; rather, they try to discover how the auditory system codes sound pressure. Physiological events that are monotonic functions of sound pressure are likely correlates of loudness. Changes in sound pressure give rise to a sequence of mechanical events in the middle ear and cochlea that culminate in the bending of the "cilia" of the hair cells. Just how the deformation of the cilia, which apparently triggers neural activity, varies with sound pressure is not known. It is known, however, that the maximum amplitude of displacement of the basilar membrane, on which the hair cells sit, is a linear or nearly linear function of sound pressure (just how linear is uncertain; see Johnstone and Yates, 1974; and Rhode and Robles, 1974). Consequently, up to the point of transduction, the major physiological correlate of loudness is amplitude of displacement.

Beyond transduction, the great unknown of all sensory physiology, what is the *neural* correlate of loudness? The classical answer has been the quantity of neural activity as measured by the number of nerve impulses per second (Davis, 1959). The more active the auditory nervous system, the greater the loudness. More activity is achieved by a higher *rate* of firing in single neurons and by a larger *number* of active units.

In all sensory modalities, neurons respond more rapidly to stronger stimuli. The auditory system, in addition, has more units active at higher stimulus intensities. A sound wave displaces the basilar membrane not at a single point but along much of its length—how much depends on sound pressure. Thus, with increasing pressure, both the depth and breadth of displacement increase; so too does the number of active fibers because the hair cells and their nerve fibers are distributed along the whole bsilar membrane. The depth or amplitude of displacement determines how fast the neurons fire, and the breadth or extent of the displacement determines how many of them fire.

Widening the bandwidth of a sound, even without increasing overall intensity, broadens the area of displacement on the basilar membrane. Presumably that is why loudness increases with stimulus bandwidth. It is not known, however, why loudness does not begin to increase until bandwidth exceeds the critical band; perhaps displacement only then begins to broaden.

Loudness depends on stimulus frequency as well as on bandwidth and sound pressure. Threshold, measured as the SPL of a barely detectable stimulus, also depends on frequency. However, measured as the relative amplitude of displacement on the basilar membrane, threshold hardly varies with frequency (Zwislocki, 1965). Differences in sensitivity arise largely from the frequency-dependent transmission of sound pressure through the peripheral auditory system to the hair cells. For the same reason, the equal-loudness contours are not flat over frequency. But below 1000 Hz, they are also not parallel to each other or to the threshold curve. They become flatter at higher levels, which means that loudness increases more rapidly with level at low frequencies than at middle or high frequencies. No doubt, they become flatter at higher intensities partly because the low-frequency internal noise, which raises the threshold for low-frequency tones, masks strong tones less effectively than it masks weak tones. Another factor may be the rapid increase in the area of displacement on the basilar membrane as a low-frequency tone is intensified. With increasing level, the displacement pattern spreads mainly from the place of maximum displacement toward the stapes. Since a low-frequency sound produces a displacement pattern on the basilar membrane with a maximum toward the apical end, the pattern has plenty of room to spread out. [Partly to avoid this influence, Stevens (1972) advocated using a reference sound located near 3000 Hz instead of a 1000-Hz tone.]

Much of the variance in loudness seems related to the displacement pattern on the basilar membrane. However, loudness also depends on time. Up to 200 msec or so, loudness increases with duration. Zwislocki (1969) suggests that this temporal summation occurs in some central part of the auditory nervous system. He ascribes the observed shortening of the time constant at suprathreshold levels to temporal decay of the neural firing rate at the input to an hypothesized integrator. An essential and almost unavoidable assumption is that the auditory system does not integrate acoustic energy, but neural energy. For a change, the mechanical events in the cochlear are secondary.

The approach that equates loudness with the amount of neural activity usually ascribes the effects of masking, fatigue, and cochlear pathology to a reduction in the number of units available for responding to the test signal. But why is there a rapid increase in loudness once threshold is exceeded? One answer has been that *inner* hair cells first become active at high intensities, perhaps at 50 dB and higher; unaffected by the masking or fatiguing sound, they are able to respond as the signal increases above the masked or fatigue threshold (e.g., Simmons & Dixon, 1966). Becoming active, these cells signal high loudness levels. Data by Kiang (1968), however, fail to give evidence for high-threshold units in the peripheral auditory system.

Although intuitively appealing and supported by many data, the notion that loudness is a simple correlate of total neural activity may be wrong or, at best, incomplete. Kiang (1968) undermines the notion with data from the cat's auditory nerve. He notes that single units increase their firing rate in response to increased sound pressure over a maximum stimulus range of only 40 dB. Furthermore, those units maximally sensitive to the same stimulus frequency all begin to respond at about the same level of stimulation; the threshold range is little more than 20 or 30 dB. Kiang finds no evidence for a population of high-threshold units that could be served exclusively by the inner hair cells. How then can loudness increase from threshold to well over

120 dB SPL? The dynamic range of a single unit is at most 40 dB and the maximum difference in threshold between units is 30 dB; these together account for a range of only 70 dB. Can the spread of excitation to larger numbers of fibers account for the missing 60 or more decibels? Perhaps, but how then does a low-frequency tone manage to increase in loudness in the presence of a high-frequency, band-pass noise (Hellman, 1974)? And what about white noise whose loudness also continues to grow over at least 120 dB? A white noise already stimulates the whole basilar membrane, since it contains all the audible frequencies. As intensity increases, additional units can come in at low and high frequencies where thresholds are high. But by about 100 dB the equal-loudness contours are nearly flat over much of the audible region; yet the loudness of white noise continues to increase above 100 dB. Loudness coding may involve more than simply the quantity of neural activity. [See Goldstein (1974) for an analysis of some of these discrepancies between current physiological models and psychophysical data.]

Despite these difficulties, some direct physiological measurements have shown that neural activity does continue to increase up to high SPLs. Teas, Eldredge, and Davis (1962) found that the amplitude of the action potential, produced by the guinea pig's auditory nerve, grew with sound pressure from a level of 50 dB to over 100 dB. Moreover, the amplitude increased as a reasonably good power function of sound pressure (Stevens, 1970). Boudreau (1965) also measured power functions for the amplitude of the integrated neural response in the superior olivary complex, but the range over which the neural response increased seldom was as large as 60 dB. Evidence from other modalities suggests that the power function may be determined right at the sensory receptor where stimulus energy is transduced to neural energy (Stevens, 1970); just how the auditory system manages it is an intriguing question.

Other approaches to the problem of loudness coding are possible. For example, Luce and Green (1972) have presented a model of sensory magnitude based primarily upon the interval between "neural" pulses. The model accommodates a variety of data on discrimination, recognition, magnitude estimation, and reaction time with heavy emphasis on hearing. It works so nicely for a variety of psychophysical tasks that hopefully the model can be applied more generally to loudness and such critical variables as bandwidth, masking, and fatigue.

VIII. MODELS OF LOUDNESS

Investigators have long sought to calculate loudness from the physical characteristics of a sound. A system for calculating the loudness of a sound from its spectrum often entails a model that transforms acoustical parameters into quasi-physiological analogues. One of the earliest models was based on masking (Fletcher & Munson, 1937). The model had two basic principles:

(1) The spread and amplitude of the excitation evoked by a sound in the auditory system can be approximated from the sound's masking pattern, i.e., the degree to which the sound completely masks pure tones over a wide range of frequencies.

(2) Loudness is directly related to this excitation.

These principles reappear in the models of Harris (1959), Howes (1950), and Munson and Gardner (1950) and also serve in Zwicker's comprehensive model (Zwicker, 1958, 1963; Zwicker & Scharf, 1965). Other schemes for calculating loudness (Reichardt, Notbohm, & Jursch, 1969; Stevens, 1972) or its close relative, noisiness (Kryter, 1970), are designed primarily to yield the correct loudness estimate rather than to model the auditory system.

The top curve of Fig. 11 is an example of the kind of masking pattern used in Zwicker's model, a pattern obtained from the complete masking of pure tones by a narrow-band noise. Zwicker's model converts masking in decibels first to excitation and then to *specific loudness*, the loudness per critical band. Frequency on the abscissa is converted to *tonalness*, a scale based on critical bands and approximately proportional to distance along the basilar membrane. Specific loudness plotted against tonalness yields a loudness pattern, whose integral is the loudness of the narrow-band noise that was the original masker. The same loudness pattern serves for any subcritical sound, including a pure tone, with the same intensity and center frequency as the original noise. The same loudness pattern can be used for a whole set of subcritical bandwidths because equally intense sounds narrower than a given critical band are all equally loud (see Section III,C).

Sounds wider than a critical band require broader excitation and loudness patterns. Each component critical band is then represented by its own excitation pattern. All the patterns are geometrically combined. Where patterns from different critical bands overlap, they are adjusted to take into account mutual inhibition, which reduces the contribution from each component to the overall loudness. Despite this reduction, a broader pattern means greater loudness for supercritical sounds.

Zwicker's model also permits the calculation of loudness against a masking noise. Figure 12 shows how the model is applied to a tone masked by a narrow-band noise. (Data for such a combination are given in Fig. 11.) The ideal spectra for the tone and noise are at the top of the figure. Below them are the theoretical excitation patterns, based on masking, which the tone and various levels of noise produce in the auditory system. To simplify the example in Fig. 12, let us assume that whichever pattern has a higher excitation level completely suppresses the other at a given tonalness. Accordingly, the shaded portions of the tone's pattern contribute nothing to the loudness of the tone, which is calculated by converting excitation level to specific loudness and integrating.

Not only does the model provide a measure of loudness, but more important for present purposes, it illustrates probable interactions within the audi-

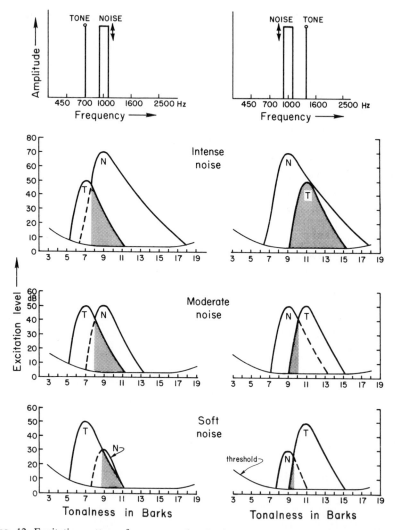

FIG. 12. Excitation patterns for a narrow-band noise and two pure tones. Ideal spectra are shown at the top. [Adapted from Scharf (1964), Partial masking, *Acustica,* **14,** 16–23.]

tory system. For example, Fig. 12 shows why one sound completely masks another sound at a higher frequency more easily than a sound at a lower frequency. The pattern produced by the intense noise is skewed toward the higher frequencies, and completely envelopes the pattern produced by the higher-frequency tone, making it inaudible. The same noise pattern only partially covers the pattern of the lower-frequency tone, and so that tone is faint but easily heard. When the noise intensity is reduced, however, much of its pattern now lies under that of the higher-frequency tone, and so most of the tone's pattern is free to contribute to loudness. In contrast, a good part of the lower-frequency tone continues to be suppressed even by the soft noise. Thus, on the basis of the skewed masking patterns and the assumption that loudness is the integral of the whole excitation pattern, the model explains why the loudness of the higher-frequency tone grows very rapidly as the noise is softened (or if the tone is intensified and the noise held constant), while the loudness of the lower-frequency tone grows more slowly.

Other calculation schemes also take into account the mutual inhibition among the components of a wide-band sound, but they do not provide the geometrical picture that Zwicker does and that Fletcher and Munson did. If one's prime purpose is to compute loudness level, then Stevens's (1972) procedure is simpler to use, but if the prime purpose is to analyze possible interactions within the auditory system or to predict loudness under masking and for narrow-band signals, then Zwicker's system is better.

Except for a calculation system developed by Niese (1965; Reichardt, *et al.*, 1969), none of the systems takes temporal summation into account. They are meant to apply to sounds that last longer than about 200 msec and that have no significant short-duration components. Uncertainty about the appropriate time constant is one reason for this omission.

At present Stevens's system is the United States standard for the calculation of the loudness of sounds (USA Standard, 1968), and both his method and Zwicker's are recommended by the International Standards Organization (ISO, 1966). Stevens (1972) has suggested some modifications of his procedure. In addition, Kryter's (1970) procedure is frequently used in the calculation of noisiness, an attribute often indistinguishable from loudness. The increasing concern with noise pollution may compel adoption of a single calculation scheme. Nonetheless, the various procedures provide results similar enough to permit reasonable decisions on the basis of any one of them.

IX. MEANING OF LOUDNESS

A. Loudness as Subjective Intensity

Loudness is the subjective intensity of a sound. Subjective means a sentient listener, human or animal, must respond to the sound. Intensity is normally a physical term, but the modifier "subjective" puts intensity in the observer and brings along all the other senses where subjective intensity seems to be part and parcel of every sensation. The many experiments in which subjects have successfully equated the intensity of one sensation to that of another—of loudness to brightness, force of handgrip to vibratory strength, loudness to roughness, etc. (Stevens, 1966)—show that subjective intensity is common to all the sensory modalities. Sound, in the definition, assigns loudness to hearing.

Any sound, even one as simple as a pure tone, is more than just louder or softer. People can respond to its pitch, size, density, duration, vocality, and annoyingness. A complex sound such as a band of noise, a bird's song, a pile driver has still more attributes: meaning, timbre, roughness, intermittency, and color. Telling a subject to judge loudness and ignore all other attributes of a sound leaves the experimenter who attempts to measure an equal-loudness contour or a loudness function at the mercy of the subject's interpretation of loudness (or intensity or strength).

Striving for a rigorous definition, Stevens (1934) proposed that a sensory attribute must have *independent invariance*. It must be possible to hold the given attribute constant while all other attributes vary. For example, Stevens told his subjects to make two tones of different frequency equal in loudness by adjusting the sound pressure of one of them. Presenting tones at different frequencies, Stevens mapped out an equal-loudness contour. He then told the subjects to make two tones of different frequency equal in density, or volume (size), or pitch—again by adjusting the intensity of one of the two tones. Figure 13 shows the four different equal-sensation contours these matches produced. Instructions to match for "brightness" or other possible attributes did not yield a fifth equal-sensation contour. Apparently, a pure tone manipulated as in these experiments has only four attributes, one of which is loudness. Note that varying two physical parameters of a sound, frequency and intensity, yields four sensory attributes. The equal-loudness contour is so labeled to correspond to the instructions given in the experiment.

Once established as an independent attribute, its functional relation to the relevant stimulus properties can be mapped out. That is what much of this chapter has been about. Loudness, as subjective intensity, is sometimes incorrectly identified with physical intensity, primarily because loudness is so closely associated with physical intensity, being a relatively simple, monotonic function of sound pressure. One could perhaps define loudness as

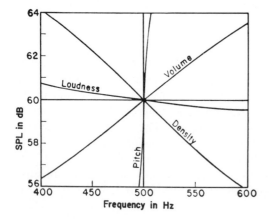

FIG. 13. Equal-sensation contours for pure tones. The sound pressure level is shown to which a pure tone must be set in order to remain constant in loudness, volume, density, or pitch as its frequency is varied. [Adapted from Stevens (1934), The attributes of tones, *Proceedings of the National Academy of Sciences*, **20**, 457–459.]

the attribute of a sound that changes most readily when sound intensity is varied.

No matter how hard we try, we seem unable to measure loudness without using language. Somehow, the subject must be told to judge loudness by one means or another. The experimenter has no way of determining that a judgment is right or wrong; only the listener can say what the loudness ratio is between two sounds. The experimenter hopes that the subject chooses the right criteria. (The experimenter also hopes that the subject listens, not only to the instructions but to the stimuli. A subject may report a sound as much softer—even nonexistent—when he pays no heed to it than when he listens carefully. In the laboratory, getting subjects to pay attention to the stimuli is seldom a problem, but in the real world of intrusive noise, attention and habituation are often critical variables.)

Stevens could label one of the equal-sensation contours of Fig. 13 an equal-loudness contour, because loudness or some similar term was used in the instructions. Had the subject been an animal, trained to respond to equality, the problem would have been to get the animal to respond only on the basis of loudness. How do you train for loudness without knowing what makes different sounds equally loud? You might assume the animal's loudness contours are like human contours; but that is an unfounded assumption, which, in any case, returns you once again to verbally based judgments. Training and language can be avoided with both human and animal subjects by measuring response latency or physiological changes that follow auditory stimulation. These nonverbal measures can be only indirectly related to loudness, and not always successfully, as we see in the next section.

B. Nonverbal Measures of Loudness

A sound evokes many kinds of responses—some voluntary, most involuntary. Only voluntary responses, often verbal and always under the control of verbal instructions, have provided data about loudness. Other kinds of responses, entirely nonverbal, must be used to study loudness in animals, very young children, and severe retardates. The problem is to find nonverbal responses that are highly correlated with loudness. The search has concentrated on evoked potentials, a normally involuntary physiological change, and reaction time, one aspect of a normally voluntary behavioral response. These responses, like certain other electrical, muscular, and vascular changes, can be measured without disturbing the auditory system. Those physiological measures that require surgical intervention within the auditory nervous system are discussed in Section VII.

The nonverbal procedures, like the standard psychophysical procedures, are used to find out how the response depends on stimulus variables such as frequency, bandwidth, background noise; and observer variables such as pathology and noise exposure. First, we look at measurements of reaction time in humans and animals, and then measurements of involuntary, physiological changes.

1. REACTION TIME

Chocholle (1940) pioneered in showing how the time it takes to react to a sound depends on intensity and frequency. The subject's task was to press a telegraph key as soon as he heard the sound. The data established two important facts. Reaction times to equally loud sounds are equal; and the louder the sound, the shorter the reaction time.* Thus, tones at very different frequencies and sensation levels but at the same *loudness* levels yielded the same reaction times. Chocholle (1954) could represent a subject's reaction times to frequencies ranging from 50 Hz to 10,000 Hz by a single curve, which is reproduced in Fig. 14. Reaction time stopped decreasing at loudness levels above 80 or 90 phons, no doubt owing to a lower limit of the order of 100 msec for human motor responses. These same data could be used to estimate equal loudness among different frequencies. The derived equal-loudness contours resemble those Fletcher and Munson (1933) obtained by loudness matching (see Fig. 3).

If nonsensory factors place a lower limit on auditory reaction time, then subtracting 100 msec from the measured values ought to provide a better estimate of the sensory component and its functional relation to sound intensity. Thus "corrected," reaction time is a good power function of loudness level between 20 and 90 phons. Below 20 phons the function steepens. The slope of the power function, however, is only about .2, much lower than the .6 of the standard loudness function. Such a low exponent means not only that reaction time changes with level much more slowly than does loudness, but also that it would be difficult to determine whether a power function, a logarithmic function, or some other function best fits the data. Despite the many nonauditory factors that enter into the auditory reaction time and those that affect loudness estimations, Reason (1972) obtained a significant correlation of .45 between the slopes of the loudness function and the function relating reaction time to sound intensity.

Whatever their precise relation, so long as reaction time is a simple monotonic function of level, loudness and reaction time can be simply related. For example, if reaction time is a power function of sound pressure with an exponent of .2 then reaction time is a power function of loudness with an exponent of .33. A crucial question is whether a similar transform works when the slope of the loudness function is altered by background noise, cochlear pathology, noise exposure, etc. Reaction time, like loudness, does change faster with signal level in the presence of a partially masking

---

* Kohfeld (1971) also found that reaction time decreased as loudness level increased, from 30 to 60 phons, but his subjects' reactions were about 100 msec slower than Chocholle's. On the other hand, Angel (1973) noted that sound intensity was related less lawfully to reaction time than to the muscular tension in the responding finger. Muscular tension increased as a power function (exponent = .2) of intensity.

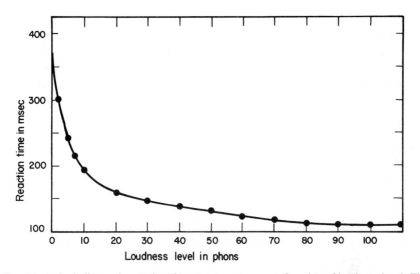

FIG. 14. A single listener's reaction time to a pure tone as a function of loudness level. The same curve represents tones varying in frequency from 50 to 10,000 Hz. [Adapted from Chocholle (1954), Les temps de réaction: Leur utilization possible en audiologie, *Annales d'Oto-Laryngologie*, **71**, 379–389. Copyright 1954 by Masson et Cie, Paris.]

sound than in the quiet (Chocholle & Da Costa, 1971; Chocholle & Greenbaum, 1966). Likewise, it changes faster for an impaired ear with recruitment than for a normal ear (Pfingst, Hienz, Kimm, & Miller, 1975). But the precise relation between reaction-time functions and loudness functions under masking or in the impaired ear seems not to have been determined. It would also be interesting to compare the binaural-to-monaural loudness ratio to the binaural-to-monaural reaction-time ratio, measured in the same experiment. Binaural reaction times are faster (Chocholle, 1946). [It is rather puzzling that whereas reaction time to sound fails to match loudness functions, reaction time to light appears to duplicate human brightness functions very well (Mansfield, 1973).]

The reaction times of animals to sound also depend in a lawful manner on stimulus parameters. Stebbins (1966; Stebbins & Lanson, 1961) trained monkeys to depress a bar upon onset of a warning signal and then release it as soon as the auditory signal comes on. The monkey's reaction time or response latency is over twice as long as a well-trained human's, but it changes with intensity in similar fashion, decreasing rapidly at near-threshold levels and much more slowly at higher levels. Variability in the monkey is not much greater than the average standard deviation of 10% for man reported by Chocholle (1954). Moody (1970, 1973) and Pfingst *et al*. (1975) have uncovered another similarity. After exposure to a loud tone, monkeys have longer latencies to tones near the elevated threshold, but with increasing intensity, the latency quickly becomes normal. This rapid drop in latency is similar to that in humans with loudness recruitment.

Response latency to tones of different frequency has been used to construct the monkey's equal-latency contours. The contours are not the same as equal-loudness contours for man (see Figs. 3 and 4)—partly because the monkey can hear much higher frequencies, up to 45 kHz—but they are similar enough to support the assumption that equal response latency means equal loudness.

2. INVOLUNTARY, PHYSIOLOGICAL RESPONSES

Among the many involuntary responses elicited by a sound are the electrical changes in the nervous system observable most readily as evoked potentials on the scalp. Much attention has also been given to the acoustic reflex, the contraction of the stapedial muscle in response to intense sounds.

The brain produces so much electrical activity, that a change evoked by a sound can be recognized only by averaging over the time-locked responses to many repetitions of the same sound. The averaged waveform bares recognizable features that correlate with various stimulus parameters. The amplitude of the evoked potential is commonly measured, although latency also often provides relevant information. Distinct amplitude peaks that occur within about 12 msec of stimulus onset are called early components; those within 12–60 msec are the middle components, and still later ones are the late components.

Keidel and Spreng (1965) found that the amplitude of a late component of the evoked potential increases as a power function of sound pressure. The exponent was smaller than the standard .6 but how much smaller was not reported (the authors gave only the exponent multiplied by an unstated factor). Davis and Zerlin (1966) also measured a power function with a small exponent, .24. Davis, Bowers, and Hirsh (1968) measured a still smaller exponent for a 1000-Hz tone, .11. Madell and Goldstein (1972) reported similarly low exponents for early and middle components. Since the data both between and within subjects were highly variable, power functions with such small exponents are not easily distinguished from linear, logarithmic, or other functions. However, Davis et al. (1968) did find that the cortical potential grows much more rapidly from a masked threshold in the presence of a band of noise than in the quiet. The steep rise resembles loudness recruitment. Despite this resemblance, late cortical potentials and loudness are poorly correlated, even when measured simultaneously (Botte, Bujas, & Chocholle, 1975; Davis, 1974).

Although poorly correlated with the loudness function, evoked potentials do seem to have roughly the same amplitude when stimuli are equally loud. Tones different in frequency and level but equal in loudness evoke similar cortical potentials (Davis et al., 1968; Davis & Zerlin, 1966; Keidel & Spreng, 1965). Equally loud binaural and monaural signals also evoke equal potentials, but if equally intense, then the louder binaural signal evokes a larger potential (Allen, 1968; Davis & Zerlin, 1966). Sounds made louder by increasing their bandwidth, without increasing their intensity, also evoke bigger potentials (Davis *et al.*, 1968; Spreng, 1967). However, while loudness increases with duration up to about 180 msec, neither the early nor the late components do (Davis & Zerlin, 1966; Hecox, Squires, & Galambos, 1976). Furthermore, enhancing the loudness of one pulse by a preceding stronger pulse is not reflected in the evoked potential (Bauer, Elmasian, & Galambos, 1975).

With respect to loudness, evoked potentials and reaction times bare some striking similarities. Both change more slowly than loudness as a function of sound pressure, both may be power functions of sound pressure, and each is roughly invariant for equally loud sounds. It remains to compare evoked potentials, especially their latencies, and reaction times to each other in the same experiment with the same listeners.

The evoked potential reflects gross activity in unspecifiable parts of the brain. Potentials from the human auditory nerve have also been measured by inserting an electrode through the back wall of the ear canal to bring it close to the ear drum (Salomon & Elberling, 1971) or inserting it right through the ear drum (Aran, Portmann, Portmann, & Pelerin, 1972; Yoshie & Ohashi, 1969). As the intensity of a click stimulus increases, the amplitude of selected components of the auditory potential goes up and their latency goes down. These techniques, being developed primarily in the clinic, have revealed recruitment of the nerve response in some patients who have cochlear impairment with evidence of loudness recruitment. Perhaps, data will become available to indicate the extent to which the shape and slope of the loudness function are determined at the transducer.

A different approach to the measurement of auditory responses involves the acoustic reflex. An intense sound causes the stapedial muscle to contract, resulting in a change in the impedance of the middle ear. The amount of change has been measured as a function of sound pressure, frequency, and bandwidth (Hung & Dallos, 1972). Measurements have been restricted to levels above 70 dB SPL; at lower levels, the reflex is too weak to measure, if present at all. Nevertheless, the acoustic reflex has been shown to reflect the relation between loudness and frequency (Ross, 1968b), between loudness and intensity or bandwidth in cochlear pathology (Ewertsen, Filling, Terkildsen, & Thomsen, 1958; Jerger, Burney, Mauldin, & Crump, 1974), and between binaural loudness and monaural loudness (Simmons, 1965). Loudness and the acoustical reflex differ, however, in the way they vary with stimulus bandwidth and the number of components in a multitone complex (Djupesland & Zwislocki, 1973; Flottorp, Djupesland, & Winther, 1971; Margolis & Popelka, 1975; Sesterhenn & Breuninger, 1976). These differences suggest that the acoustical reflex is not a direct or simple corollary of loudness (Scharf, 1976).*

---

* There is also much uncertainty about how the acoustic reflex affects loudness (Reichardt & Müller, 1969; Ward, 1974). Despite the changes in middle-ear impedance, the acoustic reflex seemingly affects the loudness of only low-frequency pure tones above 100 dB (Morgan & Dirks, 1975).

Few reports on physiological responses to sound seem to concern responses outside the auditory system. Hovland and Riesen (1940) found that the galvanic skin response (measured as the Tarcharoff potential) increased as a power function of sound pressure, with an exponent of about .1. Epstein and Eldot (1972) and Sokolov (1968) also measured changes in skin resistance, which became larger as sound intensity increased; moreover, Epstein and Eldot observed, using a classical conditioning procedure, more rapid changes with level under masking than in the quiet. Sokolov and Vinogradova (1968) measured changes in the volume blood flow in the vessels of the head and hand as a function of sensation level. Muscular action potentials in the forearm also depend on sound intensity, but Davis (1948) could find a correlation between response amplitude and intensity only at levels above 90 dB.

All the various nonverbal responses to sound are clearly and meaningfully related to many of the same stimulus and observer variables that determine loudness. Some measures, notably the cortical evoked potential and reaction time, seem to be invariant when loudness is constant. None seems to correlate very well with loudness ratios, and so leaves unfulfilled the hope of finding "objective" validation for the loudness function.

References

Allen, D. Spatial summation in the evoked cortical response to auditory stimuli. *Perception & Psychophysics,* 1968, **4**, 355–356.

Anderson, C. M. B., & Whittle, L. S. Physiological noise and the missing 6dB. *Acustica,* 1971, **24**, 261–272.

Angel, A. Input–output relations in simple reaction time experiments. *Quarterly Journal of Experimental Psychology,* 1973, **25**, 193–200.

Aran, J.-M., Portmann, M., Portmann, Cl., & Pelerin, J. Electro-cochléogramme chez l'adulte et chez l'enfant. *Audiology,* 1972, **11**, 77–89.

de Barbenza, C. M., Bryan, M. E., & Tempest, W. Individual loudness functions. *Journal of Sound and Vibration,* 1970, **11**, 399–410.

Barkhausen, H. Ein neuer Schallmesser für die Praxis. *Zeitschrift für Technische Physik,* 1926, **7**, 599–601.

Bauch, H. Die Bedeutung der Frequenzgruppe für die Lautheit von Klängen. *Acustica,* 1956, **6**, 40–45.

Bauer, J. W., Elmasian, R. O., & Galambos, R. Loudness enhancement in man. I. Brainstem-evoked response correlates. *Journal of the Acoustical Society of America,* 1975, **57**, 165–171.

Békésy, G. von. Zur Theorie des Hörens; Über die Bestimmung des einem reinen Tonempfinden entsprechenden Erregungsgebietes der Basilarmembran vermittelst Ermüdungserscheinungen. *Physikalische Zeitschrift,* 1929, **30**, 115–125.

Berglund, B., Berglund, U., & Lindvall, T. Scaling loudness, noisiness, & annoyance of community noises. *Journal of the Acoustical Society of America,* 1976, **60**, 1119–1125.

Boone, M. M. Loudness measurements on pure tone and broad band impulsive sounds. *Acustica,* 1973, **29**, 198–204.

Botte, M. C. Effet du délai interaural pour des clics binauraux sur la sonie et sur les réponses évoquées. *Acustica,* 1974, **31**, 256–265.

Botte, M. C., Bujas, Z., & Chocholle, R. Comparison between the growth of the averaged electroencephalic response and direct loudness estimations. *Journal of the Acoustical Society of America*, 1975, **58**, 208–213.

Boudreau, J. C. Stimulus correlates of wave activity in the superior-olivary complex of the cat. *Journal of the Acoustical Society of America*, 1965, **37**, 779–785.

Bray, D. A., Dirks, D D., & Morgan, D. E. Perstimulatory loudness adaptation. *Journal of the Acoustical Society of America*, 1973, **53**, 1544–1548.

Brittain, F. H. The loudness of continuous spectrum noise and its application to loudness measurements. *Journal of the Acoustical Society of America*, 1939, **11**, 113–116.

Caussé, R., & Chavasse, P. Différence entre l'écoute binauriculaire et monauriculaire pour la perception des intensités supraliminaire. *Comptes rendus des séances de la Société de Biologie*, 1942, **136**, 405–406.

Chocholle, R. Variation des temps de réaction auditifs en fonction de l'intensité à diverses fréquences. *Année Psychologique*, 1940, **41**, 65–124.

Chocholle, R. Les temps de réaction absolus binauraux. *Comptes rendus des séances de la Société de Biologie*, 1946, **140**, 496–497.

Chocholle, R. Les temps de réaction: Leur utilization possible en audiologie. *Annales d'Oto-Laryngologie*, 1954, **71**, 379–389.

Chocholle, R. Les effets de masque, tant totaux que partiels, sur des sons de durée courte ou brève, de sons homolatéraux de longue durée. *Journal de Psychologie*, 1975, **72**, 5–22.

Chocholle, R., & Da Costa, L. Les temps de réaction à un son pur partiellement masqué contralatéralement par deux autres sons purs simultanés choisis de part et d'autre du premier. *Comptes rendus des séances de la Société de Biologie*, 1971, **165**, 36–41.

Chocholle, R., & Greenbaum, H. B. La sonie de sons purs partiellement masqués. *Journal de Psychologie*, 1966, **4**, 385–414.

Churcher, B. G., & King, A. J. The performance of noise meters in terms of the primary standard. *Journal of the Institute of Electrical Engineering*, 1937, **81**, 57–90.

Davis, H. Excitation of auditory receptors. In J. Field, H. W. Magoun, & V. E. Hall (Eds.), *Handbook of Physiology*. Section 1, Vol. 1. Neurophysiology. Baltimore: Waverly Press, 1959.

Davis, H. Relations of peripheral action potentials and cortical evoked potentials to the magnitude of sensation. In H. R. Moskowitz, B. Scharf, & J. C. Stevens (Eds.), *Sensation and measurement—Papers in honor of S. S. Stevens*, Dordrecht: Reidel Press, 1974.

Davis, H., Bowers, C., & Hirsh, S. K. Relations of the human vertex potential to acoustic input: Loudness and masking. *Journal of the Acoustical Society of America*, 1968, **43**, 431–438.

Davis, H., Morgan, C. T., Hawkins, J. E., Galambos, R., & Smith, F. W. Temporary deafness following exposure to loud tones and noise. *Acta Otolaryngolica Supplement*, 1950, **88**, 1–87.

Davis, H., & Zerlin, S. Acoustic relations of the human vertex potential. *Journal of the Acoustical Society of America*, 1966, **39**, 109–116.

Davis, R. C. Motor effects of strong auditory stimuli. *Journal of Experimental Psychology*, 1948, **38**, 257–275.

Dirks, D. D., Morgan, D. E., & Bray, D. A. Perstimulatory loudness adaptation in selected cochlear impaired and masked normal listeners. *Journal of the Acoustical Society of America*, 1974, **56**, 554–561.

Djupesland, G., & Zwislocki, J. J. On the critical band in the acoustic stapedius reflex. *Journal of the Acoustical Society of America*, 1973, **54**, 1157–1159.

Durlach, N. I., & Braida, L. D. Intensity perception. I. Preliminary theory of intensity resolution. *Journal of the Acoustical Society of America*, 1969, **46**, 372–383.

Egan, J. P. Perstimulatory fatigue as measured by heterophonic loudness balances. *Journal of the Acoustical Society of America*, 1955, **27**, 111–120.

Ekman, G., Berglund, B., & Berglund, U. Loudness as a function of the duration of auditory stimulation. *Scandanavian Journal of Psychology*, 1966, **7**, 201–208.

Elmasian, R., & Galambos, R. Loudness enhancement: monaural, binaural, and dichotic. *Journal of the Acoustical Society of America*, 1975, **58**, 229–234.

Epstein, A., & Eldot, H. An approach to an objective measure of loudness. *Audiology*, 1972, **11**, (supplement) 124–125.

Ewertsen, H., Filling, S., Terkildsen, K., & Thomsen, K. A. Comparative recruitment testing. *Acta Oto-Laryngolica* (Stockholm), 1958, Supplement **140**, 116–122.

Fastl, H. Loudness and masking patterns of narrow noise bands. *Acustica*, 1975, **33**, 266–271.

Feldtkeller, R., & Zwicker, E. *Das Ohr als Nachrichtenempfänger*. Stuttgart: S. Hirzel Verlag, 1956.

Fletcher, H. F., & Munson, W. A. Loudness, its definition, measurement and calculation. *Journal of the Acoustical Society of America*, 1933, **5**, 82–108.

Fletcher, H. F., & Munson, W. A. Relation between loudness and masking. *Journal of the Acoustical Society of America*, 1937, **9**, 1–10.

Flottorp, G., Djupesland, G., & Winther, F. The acoustic stapedius reflex in relation to critical bandwidth. *Journal of the Acoustical Society of America*, 1971, **49**, 457–461.

Fowler, E. P. Marked deafened areas in normal ears. *Archives of Otolaryngology*, 1928, **8**, 151–155.

Fraser, W. D., Petty, J. W., & Elliott, D. N. Adaptation: Central or peripheral? *Journal of the Acoustical Society of America*, 1970, **47**, 1016–1021.

Galambos, R., Bauer, J., Picton, T., Squires, K., & Squires, N. Loudness enhancement following contralateral stimulation. *Journal of the Acoustical Society of America*, 1972, **52**, 1127–1130.

Garner, W. R. The loudness of repeated short tones. *Journal of the Acoustical Society of America*, 1948, **20**, 513–527.

Garner, W. R. The loudness and loudness matching of short tones. *Journal of the Acoustical Society of America*, 1949, **21**, 398–401.

Gässler, G. Ueber die Hörschwelle für Schallereignisse mit verschieden breitem Frequenzspektrum. *Acustica*, 1954, **4**, 408–414.

Gjaevenes, K., & Rimstad, E. R. The influence of rise time on loudness. *Journal of the Acoustical Society of America*, 1972, **51**, 1233–1239.

Goldstein, J. L. Is the power law simply related to the driven spike response rate from the whole auditory nerve? In H. R. Moskowitz, B. Scharf, & J. C. Stevens (Eds.), *Sensation and measurement—Papers in honor of S. S. Stevens*. Dordrecht: Reidel Press, 1974.

Gruber, J., & Braune, H. Auditory adaptation measured by cross-modality matching. *Eighth international congress on acoustics*. Trowbridge, England: Goldcrest Press, 1974, p. 130.

Hallpike, C. S. The loudness recruitment phenomenon: A clinical contribution to the neurology of hearing. In A. B. Graham (Ed.), *Sensorineural hearing processes and disorders*. Boston: Little, Brown, 1967. Pp. 489–499.

Hallpike, C. S., & Hood, J. P. Observations upon the neurological mechanism of the loudness recruitment phenomenon. *Acta Oto-laryngolica*, 1959, **50**, 472–486.

Harbart, F., Weiss, B. G., & Wilpizeski, C. R. Suprathreshold auditory adaptation in normal and pathologic ears. *Journal of Speech and Hearing Research*, 1968, **11**, 268–278.

Harris, C. M. Residual masking at low frequencies. *Journal of the Acoustical Society of America*, 1959, **31**, 1110–1115.

Harris, J. D. Loudness discrimination. *Journal of Speech and Hearing Disorders*, 1963, Monograph Supplement II, 1–63.

Hecox, K., Squires, N., & Galambos, R. Brainstem auditory evoked responses in man. I. Effect of stimulus rise-fall time and duration. *Journal of the Acoustical Society of America*, 1976, **60**, 1187–1192.

Hellman, R. P. Effect of noise bandwidth on the loudness of a 1000 Hz tone. *Journal of the Acoustical Society of America*, 1970, **48**, 500–504.

Hellman, R. P. Asymmetry of masking between noise and tone. *Perception & Psychophysics*, 1972, **11**, 241–246.

Hellman, R. P. Effect of spread of excitation on the loudness function at 250 Hz. In Moskowitz, H. R., Scharf, B., & Stevens, J. C. (Eds.), *Sensation and measurement—Papers in honor of S. S. Stevens*. Dordrecht: Reidel Press, 1974, pp. 241–249.

Hellman, R. P. Growth of loudness at 1000 and 3000 Hz. *Journal of the Acoustical Society of America*, 1976, **60**, 672–679.

Hellman, R. P., & Zwislocki, J. J. Some factors affecting the estimation of loudness. *Journal of the Acoustical Society of America*, 1961, **33**, 687–694.

Hellman, R. P., & Zwislocki, J. J. Monaural loudness function at 1000 cps and interaural summation. *Journal of the Acoustical Society of America*, 1963, **35**, 856–865.

Hellman, R. P., & Zwislocki, J. J. Loudness function of a 1000 cps tone in the presence of a masking noise. *Journal of the Acoustical Society of America*, 1964, **36**, 1618–1627.

Hellman, R. P., & Zwislocki, J. J. Loudness determination at low sound frequencies. *Journal of the Acoustical Society of America*, 1968, **43**, 60–64.

Hickling, S. Hearing test patterns in noise induced temporary hearing loss. *Journal of Auditory Research*, 1967, **7**, 63–76.

Hood, J. D. Studies in auditory fatigue and adaptation. *Acta Oto-Laryngologica* 1950, Suppl. **92**, 1–57.

Hovland, C. I., & Riesen, A. H. The magnitude of galvanic and vasomotor responses as a function of stimulus intensity. *Journal of General Psychology*, 1940, **23**, 103–121.

Howes, D. H. The loudness of multicomponent tones. *American Journal of Psychology*, 1950, **63**, 1–30.

Hung, I. J., & Dallos, P. Study of the acoustic reflex in human beings. I. Dynamic characteristics. *Journal of the Acoustical Society of America*, 1972, **52**, 1168–1180.

International Organization for Standardization. *Expression of the physical and subjective magnitudes of sound*. ISO/R 131–1959 (E).

International Organization for Standardization. *Method for calculating loudness level*. ISO/R 532–1966 (E).

Irwin, R. J. Binaural summation of thermal noises of equal and unequal power in each ear. *American Journal of Psychology*, 1965, **78**, 57–65.

Irwin, R. J., & Zwislocki, J. J. Loudness effects in pairs of tone bursts. *Perception and Psychophysics*, 1971, **10**, 189–192.

Jerger, J., Burney, P., Mauldin, L., & Crump, B. Predicting hearing loss from the acoustic reflex. *Journal of Speech and Hearing Disorders*, 1974, **39**, 11–22.

Jesteadt, W., Wier, C. G., & Green, D. M. Intensity discrimination as a function of frequency and sensation level. *Journal of the Acoustical Society of America*, 1977, **61**, 169–177.

Johnstone, B. M., & Yates, G. K. Basilar membrane tuning. *Journal of the Acoustical Society of America*, 1974, **55**, 584–587.

Keidel, W. D., & Spreng, M. Neurophysiological evidence for the Stevens power function in man. *Journal of the Acoustical Society of America*, 1965, **38**, 191–195.

Kiang, N. Y. A survey of recent developments in the study of auditory physiology. *Annals of Otology, Rhinology, and Laryngology*, 1968, **77**, 656–675.

Knudsen, V. O. The sensibility of the ear to small differences of intensity and frequency. *Physics Review*, 1923, **21**, 84–102.

Kohfeld, D. Simple reaction time as a function of stimulus intensity in decibels of light and sound. *Journal of Experimental Psychology*, 1971, **88**, 251–257.

Kryter, K. D. *The effects of noise on man*. New York: Academic Press, 1970.

Lochner, J. P. A., & Burger, J. F. Form of the loudness function in the presence of masking noise. *Journal of the Acoustical Society of America*, 1961, **33**, 1705–1707.

Logue, A. W. Individual differences in magnitude estimation of loudness. *Perception & Psychophysics*, 1976, **19**, 279–280.

Luce, R. D., & Green, D. M. A neural timing theory for response times and the psychophysics of intensity. *Psychological Review*, 1972, **79**, 14–57.

Madell, J. R., & Goldstein, R. Relation between loudness and the amplitude of the early components of the averaged electroencephalic response. *Journal of Speech and Hearing Research*, 1972, **15**, 134–141.

Mansfield, R. J. W. Latency functions in human vision. *Vision Research*, 1973, **13**, 2219–2234.

Margolis, R. H., & Popelka, G. R. Loudness and the acoustic reflex. *Journal of the Acoustical Society of America*, 1975, **58**, 1330–1332.

Margolis, R. H., & Wiley, T. L. Monaural loudness adaptation at low sensation levels in normal and impaired ears. *Journal of the Acoustical Society of America*, 1976, **59**, 222–224.

Marks, L. E. On scales of sensation: Prolegomena to any future psychophysics that will be able to come forth as science. *Perception & Psychophysics*, 1974, **16**, 358–376. (a)

Marks, L. E. *Sensory processes*. New York: Academic Press, 1974. (b)

Marks, L. E., & Stevens, J. C. The form of the psychophysical function near threshold. *Perception and Psychophysics*, 1968, **4**, 315–318.

Martin, M. C. Critical bands in sensori-neural hearing loss. *Scandinavian Audiology*, 1974, **3**, 133–140.

McGill, W. J. The slope of the loudness function; a puzzle. In Gulliksen, H. and Messick, S. (Eds.), *Psychological scaling, theory and applications*. New York: Wiley & Sons, 1960. pp. 67–81. Also in Moskowitz, H. R. *et al.* (Eds.), *Sensation and measurement*. Dordrecht: Reidel, 1974. pp. 295–307.

McGill, W. J., & Goldberg, J. P. Pure-tone intensity discrimination and energy detection. *Journal of the Acoustical Society of America*, 1968, **44**, 576–581.

Miller, G. A. Sensitivity to changes in the intensity of white noise and its relation to masking and loudness. *Journal of the Acoustical Society of America*, 1947, **19**, 609–619.

Miller, G. A. The perception of short bursts of noise. *Journal of the Acoustical Society of America*, 1948, **20**, 160–170.

Mirabella, A., Taug, H., & Teichner, W. H. Adaptation of loudness to monaural stimulation. *Journal of General Psychology*, 1967, **76**, 251–273.

Miskolczy-Fodor, F. Relation between loudness and duration of tonal pulses. III. Response in cases of abnormal loudness function. *Journal of the Acoustical Society of America*, 1960, **32**, 486–492.

Moody, D. B. Reaction time as an index of sensory function. In W. C. Stebbins (Ed.), *Animal psychophysics*. New York: Appleton, 1970. Pp. 277–303.

Moody, D. B. Behavioral studies of noise-induced hearing loss in primates: Loudness recruitment. *Advances in Otorhinolaryngology*, 1973, **20**, 82–101.

Morgan, D. E., & Dirks, D. D. Influence of middle-ear muscle contraction on pure-tone suprathreshold loudness judgments. *Journal of the Acoustical Society of America*, 1975, **57**, 411–420.

Munson, W. A. The growth of auditory sensation. *Journal of the Acoustical Society of America*, 1947, **19**, 584–591.

Munson, W. A., & Gardner, M. B. Loudness patterns—A new approach. *Journal of the Acoustical Society of America*, 1950, **22**, 177–190.

Niese, H. Vorschlag für die Definition und Messung der Deutlichkeit nach subjektiven Grundlagen. *Hochfrequenztechnik und Elektroakustik*, 1956, **65**, 4–15.

Niese, H. Die Trägheit der Lautstärkebildung in Abhängigkeit vom Schallpegel. *Hochfrequenztechnik und Elektroakustik*, 1959, **68**, 143–152.

Niese, H. Subjektive Messung der Lautstärke von Bandpassrauschen. *Hochfrequenztechnik und Elektroakustik*, 1960, **68**, 202–217.

Niese, H. Die Lautstärkebildung bei binauralem Hören komplexer Geräusche. *Hochfrequenztechnik und Elektroakustik*, 1961, **70**, 132–141.

Niese, H. Eine Methode zur Bestimmung der Lautstärke beliebiger Geräusche. *Acustica*, 1965, **15**, 117.

Niese, H. Die Lautstärke impulsiver Dauergeräusche. *Acustica*, 1966, **17**, 335–344.

Palva, T., & Kärjä, J. Suprathreshold auditory adaptation. *Journal of the Acoustical Society of America*, 1969, **45**, 1018–1021.

Pedersen, O. J., Lyregaard, P. E., & Poulsen, T. E. The round robin test on evaluation of loudness level of impulsive noise. Acoustics Laboratory, Technical University of Denmark. Report No. 22, September 1977.

Petty, J. W., Fraser, W. D., & Elliot, D. N. Adaptation and loudness decrement: A reconsideration. *Journal of the Acoustical Society of America*, 1970, **47**, 1074–1081.

Pfingst, B., Hienz, R., Kimm, J., & Miller, J. Reaction-time procedure for measurement of hearing. I. Suprathreshold functions. *Journal of the Acoustical Society of America*, 1975, **57**, 421–430.

Pollack, I. On the measurement of the loudness of white noise. *Journal of the Acoustical Society of America*, 1951, **23**, 654–657.

Pollack, I. The loudness of bands of noise. *Journal of the Acoustical Society of America*, 1952, **24**, 533–538.

Pollack, I. Loudness of periodically interrupted white noise. *Journal of the Acoustical Society of America*, 1958, **30**, 181–185.

Porsolt, R. D., & Irwin, R. J. Binaural summation in loudness of two tones as a function of their bandwidth. *American Journal of Psychology*, 1967, **80**, 384–390.

Port, E. Ueber die Lautstärke einzelner kurzer Schallimpulse. *Acustica*, 1963, **13**, 212–223. (a)

Port, E. Zur Lautstärkempfindung und Lautstärkemessung von pulsierenden Geräuschen. *Acustica*, 1963, **13**, 224–233. (b)

Rabinowitz, W. M., Lim, J. S., Braida, L. D., & Durlach, N. I. Intensity perception. VI. Summary of recent data on deviations from Weber's law for 1000-Hz tone pulses. *Journal of the Acoustical Society of America*, 1976, **59**, 1506–1509.

Reason, J. T. Individual differences in auditory reaction time and loudness estimation. *Perceptual and Motor Skills*, 1968, **26**, 1089–1090.

Reason, J. T. Some correlates of the loudness function. *Journal of Sound and Vibration*, 1972, **20**, 305–309.

Reichardt, W. Zur Trägheit der Lautstärkebildung. *Acustica*, 1965, **15**, 345–354.

Reichardt, W., & Müller, S. Die Abhängigkeit der Lautstärke vom akustischen Reflex. *Hochfrequenztechnik und Elektroakustik*, 1969, **78**, 92–102.

Reichardt, W., & Niese, H. Choice of sound duration and silent intervals for test and comparison signals in the subjective measurement of loudness level. *Journal of the Acoustical Society of America*, 1970, **47**, 1083–1090.

Reichardt, W., Notbohm, K., & Jursch, H. Verbesserung des Lautstärkeberechnungverfahrens nach Niese. *Acustica*, 1969, **21**, 134–143.

Reynolds, G. S., & Stevens, S. S. Binaural summation of loudness. *Journal of the Acoustical Society of America*, 1960, **32**, 1337–1344.

Rhode, W. S., & Robles, L. Evidence for nonlinear vibrations in the cochlea from Mössbauer experiments. *Journal of the Acoustical Society of America*, 1974, **55**, 588–596.

Riach, W., Elliott, D. N., & Reed, J. C. Growth of loudness and its relationship to intensity discrimination under various levels of auditory fatigue. *Journal of the Acoustical Society of America*, 1962, **34**, 1764–1767.

Riesz, R. R. Differential intensity sensitivity of the ear for pure tones. *Physics Review*, 1928, **31**, 867–875.

Robinson, D. W. The relation between the sone and phon scales of loudness. *Acustica*, 1953, **3**, 344–358.

Robinson, D. W. The subjective loudness scale. *Acustica*, 1957, **7**, 217–233.

Robinson, D. W., & Dadson, R. S. A re-determination of the equal-loudness relations for pure tones. *British Journal of Applied Physics*, 1956, **7**, 166–181.

Ross, S. Matching functions and equal sensation contours for loudness. *Journal of the Acoustical Society of America*, 1967, **42**, 778–793.

Ross, S. Impedance at the eardrum, middle-ear transmission, and equal loudness. *Journal of the Acoustical Society of America*, 1968, **43**, 491–505. (a)

Ross, S. On the relation between the acoustic reflex and loudness. *Journal of the Acoustical Society of America*, 1968, **43**, 768–779. (b)

Rowley, R. R., & Studebaker, G. A. Loudness–intensity relations under various levels of contralateral noise. *Journal of the Acoustical Society of America*, 1971, **49**, 499–504.

Salomon, G., & Elberling, C. Cochlear nerve potentials recorded from the ear canal in man. *Acta Oto-laryngolica*, 1971, **71**, 319–325.

Scharf, B. Critical bands and the loudness of complex sounds near threshold. *Journal of the Acoustical Society of America*, 1959, **31**, 365–370. (a)

Scharf, B. Loudness of complex sounds as a function of the number of components. *Journal of the Acoustical Society of America*, 1959, **31**, 783–785. (b)

Scharf, B. Loudness summation and spectrum shape. *Journal of the Acoustical Society of America*, 1962, **34**, 228–233.

Scharf, B. Partial masking. *Acustica*, 1964, **14**, 16–23.

Scharf, B. Binaural loudness summation as a function of bandwidth. *Reports of the Sixth International Congress on Acoustics*, 1968, 25–28, (Paper A-35).

Scharf, B. Dichotic summation of loudness. *Journal of the Acoustical Society of America*, 1969, **45**, 1193–1205.

Scharf, B. Critical bands. In J. V. Tobias (Ed.), *Foundations of modern auditory theory*. Vol. I. New York: Academic Press, 1970. Pp. 157–202. (a)

Scharf, B. Loudness and frequency selectivity at short durations. In R. Plomp & G. F. Smoorenburg (Eds.), *Frequency analysis and periodicity detection in hearing*. Leiden, Netherlands: A. W. Sijthoff, 1970. Pp. 455–461. (b)

Scharf, B. Fundamentals of auditory masking. *Audiology*, 1971, **10**, 30–40.

Scharf, B. Loudness summation between tones from two loudspeakers. *Journal of the Acoustical Society of America*, 1974, **56**, 589–593.

Scharf, B. Acoustic reflex, loudness summation, and the critical band. *Journal of the Acoustical Society of America*, 1976, **60**, 753–755.

Scharf, B., & Fishken, D. Binaural summation of loudness: Reconsidered. *Journal of Experimental Psychology*, 1970, **86**, 374–379.

Scharf, B., & Hellman, R. P. A model of loudness summation applied to impaired ears. *Journal of the Acoustical Society of America*, 1966, **40**, 71–78.

Scharf, B., & Stevens, J. C. The form of the loudness function near threshold. *Proceedings of the Third International Congress of Acoustics*, Vol. 1. Amsterdam: Elsevier, 1961.

Schneider, B., Wright, A. A., Edelheit, W., Hock, P., & Humphrey, C. Equal loudness contours derived from sensory magnitude judgments. *Journal of the Acoustical Society of America*, 1972, **51**, 1951–1959.

Schwarze, D. Die Lautstärke von Gausstönen. Unpublished Ph.D. dissertation, Technische Universität Berlin, 1963.

Sesterhenn, G., & Breuninger, H. Lautheitsfunktion und Frequenzgruppeneffekt beim akustischen Stapediusreflex. *Acustica*, 1976, **35**, 37–46.

Simmons, F. B. Binaural summation of the acoustic reflex. *Journal of the Acoustical Society of America*, 1965, **37**, 834–836.

Simmons, F. B., & Dixon, R. F. Clinical implications of loudness balancing. *Archives of Otolaryngology*, 1966, **83**, 449–454.

Small, A. M., Jr., Brandt, J. F., & Cox, P. G. Loudness as a function of signal duration. *Journal of the Acoustical Society of America*, 1962, **34**, 513–514.

Sokolov, E. N. The use of cutaneous-galvanic reactions for the objective study of loudness perception. In R. W. West (Ed.), *Russian translations on speech and hearing*. Washington, D. C.: American Speech and Hearing Association Report No. 3, 1968. Pp. 34–44.

Sokolov, E. N., & Vinogradova, O. S. The correlation of oriented and defensive reflexes during the action of sound stimuli. In R. W. West (Ed.), *Russian translations on speech and hearing*. Washington, D.C.: American Speech and Hearing Association Report No. 3, 1968. Pp. 57–69.

Spreng, M. Ueber die Messung der Frequenzgruppe und der Integrationszeit des menschlichen Gehörs durch vom Schall abhängige Hirnspannungen längs der Kopfhaut. Unpublished Ph.D. dissertation, Technische Hochschule Stuttgart, 1967.

Stebbins, W. C. Auditory reaction time and the derivation of equal loudness contours for the monkey. *Journal of the Experimental Analysis of Behavior*, 1966, **9**, 135–142.

Stebbins, W. C., & Lanson, R. N. A technique for measuring the latency of a discriminative operant. *Journal of the Experimental Analysis of Behavior*, 1961, **4**, 149–155.

Steinberg, J. C., & Gardner, M. B. The dependence of hearing impairment on sound intensity. *Journal of the Acoustical Society of America*, 1937, **9**, 11–23.

Stephens, S. D. G. Personality and the slope of loudness function. *Quarterly Journal of Experimental Psychology*, 1970, **22**, 9–13.

Stephens, S. D. G. Methodological factors influencing loudness of short duration sounds. *Journal of Sound and Vibration*, 1974, **37**, 235–246.

Stevens, J. C., & Guirao, M. Individual loudness functions. *Journal of the Acoustical Society of America*, 1964, **36**, 2210–2213.

Stevens, J. C., & Hall, J. W. Brightness and loudness as functions of stimulus duration. *Perception and Psychophysics*, 1966, **1**, 319–327.

Stevens, S. S. The attributes of tones. *Proceedings of the National Academy of Sciences*, 1934, **20**, 457–459.

Stevens, S. S. The measurement of loudness. *Journal of the Acoustical Society of America*, 1955, **27**, 815–829.

Stevens, S. S. Concerning the form of the loudness function. *Journal of the Acoustical Society of America*, 1957, **29**, 603–606.

Stevens, S. S. Matching functions between loudness and ten other continua. *Perception and Psychophysics*, 1966, **1**, 5–8.

Stevens, S. S. Neural events and the psychophysical law. *Science*, 1970, **170**, 1043–1050.

Stevens, S. S. Perceived level of noise by mark VII and decibels (E). *Journal of the Acoustical Society of America*, 1972, **51**, 575–601.

Stevens, S. S. *Psychophysics*. New York: John Wiley, 1975.

Stevens, S. S., & Davis, H. *Hearing—Its psychology and physiology*. New York: Wiley, 1938.

Stevens, S. S., & Guirao, M. Loudness functions under inhibition. *Perception and Psychophysics*, 1967, **2**, 459–465.

Stokinger, T. E., Cooper, W. A., Jr., Meissner, W. A., & Jones, K. O. Intensity, frequency, and duration effects in the measurement of monaural perstimulatory loudness adaptation. *Journal of the Acoustical Society of America*, 1972, **51**, 608–616.

Teas, D. C., Eldredge, D. H., & Davis. H. Cochlear responses to acoustic transients: An interpretation of whole-nerve action potentials. *Journal of the Acoustical Society of America*, 1962, **34**, 1438–1459.

Teghtsoonian, R. On the exponents in Stevens' law and the constant in Ekman's law. *Psychological Review*, 1971, **78**, 71–80.

Tonndorf, J., Brogan, F. A., & Washburn, D. D. Auditory DL of intensity in normal hearing subjects. *Archives of Oto-Laryngology*, 1955, **62**, 292–305.

U.S.A. Standard Procedure for the Computation of Loudness of Noise. 1968, USAS S3.4.

Viemeister, N. F. Intensity discrimination of pulsed sinusoids: The effects of filtered noise. *Journal of the Acoustical Society of America*, 1972, **51**, 1265–1269.

Vigran, E. Loudness change of pure tones with contralateral noise stimulation. *Journal of the Acoustical Society of America*, 1965, **37**, 1134–1138.

Ward, W. D. Adaptation and fatigue. In J. Jerger (Ed.), *Modern developments in audiology*. New York: Academic Press, 1973. Ch. 9.

Ward, W. D. Psychophysical correlates of middle-ear-muscle action. In Moskowitz, H. R. *et al.* (Eds.), *Sensation and measurement—Papers in honor of S. S. Stevens*. Dordrecht: Reidel, 1974. Pp. 315–324.

Ward, W. D., Fleer, R. E., & Glorig, A. Characteristics of hearing losses produced by gunfire and by steady noise. *Journal of Auditory Research,* 1961, **1**, 325–356.

Wiley, T. L., Small, A. M., Jr., & Lilly, D. J. Monaural loudness adaptation. *Journal of the Acoustical Society of America,* 1973, **53**, 1051–1055.

Wiley, T. L., Small, A. M., & Lilly, D. J. Loudness adaptation in listeners with noise-induced hearing loss. *Journal of the Acoustical Society of America,* 1976, **59**, 225–227.

Yoshie, N., & Ohashi, T. Clinical use of cochlear nerve action potential responses in man for differential diagnosis of hearing losses. *Acta Oto-Laryngolica,* (Stockholm), 1969, Supplement **252**, 71–87.

Zwicker, E. Ueber psychologische und methodische Grundlagen der Lautheit. *Acustica,* 1958, **8**(Beiheft 1), 237–258.

Zwicker, E. Ueber die Lautheit von ungedrosselten und gedrosselten Schallen. *Acustica,* 1963, **13**(Beiheft 1), 194–211.

Zwicker, E. Temporal effects in simultaneous masking and loudness. *Journal of the Acoustical Society of America,* 1965, **38**, 132–141.

Zwicker, E. Ein Beitrag zur Lautstärkemessung impulshaltiger Schalle. *Acustica,* 1966, **17**, 11–22.

Zwicker, E., & Feldtkeller, R. Ueber die Lautstärke von gleichformigen Geräuschen. *Acustica,* 1955, **5**, 303–316.

Zwicker, E., & Feldtkeller, R. *Das Ohr als Nachrichtenempfänger.* Stuttgart: S. Hirzel Verlag, 1967.

Zwicker, E., Flottorp, G., & Stevens, S. S. Critical bandwidth in loudness summation. *Journal of the Acoustical Society of America,* 1957, **29**, 548–557.

Zwicker, E., & Scharf, B. A model of loudness summation. *Psychological Review,* 1965, **72**, 3–26.

Zwislocki, J. Analysis of some auditory characteristics. In R. D. Luce, R. R. Bush, & E. H. Galanter (Eds.), *Handbook of mathematical psychology.* Vol. III. New York: Wiley, 1965.

Zwislocki, J. J. Temporal summation of loudness: An analysis. *Journal of the Acoustical Society of America,* 1969, **46**, 431–441.

Zwislocki, J. J. A power function for sensory receptors. In H. R. Moskowitz, B. Scharf, & J. C. Stevens (Eds.), *Sensation and measurement—Papers in honor of S. S. Stevens.* Dordrecht: Reidel Press, 1974.

Zwislocki, J. J., Ketkar, I., Cannon, M. W., & Nodar, R. H. Loudness enhancement and summation in pairs or short sound bursts. *Perception & Psychophysics,* 1974, **16**, 91–95.

Zwislocki, J. J., & Sokolich, W. G. On loudness enhancement of a tone burst by a preceding tone burst. *Perception & Psychophysics,* 1974, **16**, 87–90.

Chapter 7

FREQUENCY AND PERIODICITY ANALYSIS

JAN O. NORDMARK

I. NATURE OF THE AUDITORY STIMULUS

A. Historical Introduction

If the pressure variations caused by a steady sound are displayed as a function of time, we obtain an irregular wave that repeats itself over and over again. The time in which the wave repeats itself is known as its *period*. Such a wave can be represented by sinusoidal waves in such a manner that sinusoids of appropriate amplitude and starting time will add together to make up a particular complex wave. For a sound wave we generally use the term *frequency*, the reciprocal of the period, and call the multiples of the fundamental frequency *harmonics*.

HANDBOOK OF PERCEPTION, VOL. IV

By means of suitably tuned resonators a listener's attention can be focused on the harmonics. This was Helmholtz's method to assist the ear in hearing pitches other than that of the fundamental when listening to a complex sound. The ear thus works somewhat like a frequency analyzer. At the same time it is obvious that aural analysis is difficult and only partially successful. It is also true that on hearing a steady complex sound we hear a tone of one definite pitch and timbre rather than a set of separate tones.

The question as to what extent the ear is a frequency analyzer has given rise to much research in hearing since the middle of the nineteenth century. In fact, the last few years have seen a renewal of activity in this field accompanied by arguments vaguely reminiscent of the much earlier debate started by Seebeck, Ohm, and Helmholtz.

The debate concerned the interpretation of some of the results Seebeck (1841) had obtained in his experiments with a siren, where the holes could be arranged to give various spacings between the impulses resulting from air blown through the holes. The pitch assigned to the waveform in Fig. 1(b) is, not unexpectedly, the octave of that in (a). When alternate holes were slightly displaced, the lower tone could be heard along with the higher, despite the small magnitude of the lower component. The higher harmonics, however, could not be heard separately, Seebeck noticed. Instead he assumed that, because they have a period equal to that of the fundamental, they somehow enhance the loudness of the fundamental tone. He therefore rejected Ohm's (1843) hypothesis, which said that only sinusoidal components can give rise to an impression of pitch.

Ohm (1843) objected that Seebeck's effect must be due to an auditory illusion. Helmholtz (1863) also disagreed with Seebeck's interpretation, arguing that Seebeck was not a listener good enough to be able to hear the higher harmonics separately.

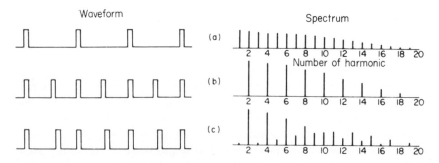

FIG. 1. The pitch of waveform (b) (400) is an octave above that of waveform (a) (200). In waveform (c), a component of pitch 200 is distinctly audible in spite of the fact that very little energy exists at the fundamental frequency as shown in the spectrum at the right. [After Schouten (1940a), The residue and the mechanism of hearing, *Proceedings of the Koninklijke Nederlandsche Akademie van Wetenschappen*, 1940, **43**, 991–999.]

Helmholtz's further development of his conception of the ear as a frequency analyzer rests on four ideas.

1. Fourier's purely mathematical theorem, according to which every periodic function can be represented by sinusoidal functions.

2. Ohm's purely physical definition of a simple tone as a sinusoidal oscillation of the air and of every periodic sound wave as a sum of simple sine waves. [This formulation is due to Stumpf (1926, p. 358), who pointed out, correctly, in my opinion, that the view of the ear as an analyzer of a complex sound into constituent partials is perhaps implied, but never explicitly stated by Ohm.]

3. Helmholtz's purely physiological hypothesis that there existed resonators in the cochlea capable of accomplishing sound analysis.

4. Helmholtz's psychological conception, according to which two levels of perceptual processes must be distinguished. The higher level is the analytical awareness of a sensation as a part of the sum of sensations, for instance, the identification of an upper partial in a complex tone. These are always somehow sensed, even if it may take some effort to perceive them analytically. The lower level is that the influence of the sensation makes itself felt only in the conception we form of external things and processes, and assists in determining them. We ascribe certain characteristics to the sound of a violin because we are used to connecting the perceived partials with a particular external object.

Helmholtz here clearly follows the British empiricist tradition. His emphasis on learning and on association of sensations in perceptual processes has probably been more important for auditory research than is commonly realized. For a long time the sheer weight of his authority prevented the phenomenological and nativist viewpoints from having significant influence. Helmholtz's belief that an elucidation of the elementary analytical processes will also lead to an understanding of complex phenomena is even today widely—if subconsciously—shared by workers in the auditory field.

Although Wolfgang Köhler (1923), one of the founders of the Gestalt psychology movement, considered the "summative" theory of Helmholtz inadequate for explaining the facts of vowel perception, Gestalt psychologists in general made few purely auditory experiments, concentrating instead on the study of visual form and motion. Furthermore, at the time when the movement appeared, its phenomenological and nativist ideas ran counter to the prevailing mood in, above all, American psychology. In addition the empiricist bias was strongly reinforced by the sudden influx into the field of electronic engineers thoroughly trained in Fourier analysis and predisposed to ascribe phenomena like the perceived fundamental in Seebeck's experiment to the effects of nonlinear distortion.

When Helmholtz's theory finally had to be modified because Békésy (1943) had demonstrated the impossibility of sharply tuned resonators in the cochlea, the empiricist, analytical part of the resonance concept remained virtually intact. Not even Schouten's (1940b) vindication of Seebeck's results, showing that the pitch Seebeck heard should indeed be attributed to the periodicity of the higher harmonics made any direct allusion to Gestalt ideas. Conversely, recent arguments that instead we hear a periodicity pitch because we are used to associating the harmonics with an actual fundamental have been put forth without any reference to the implied empiricist assumptions.

The absence of a serious discussion of basic philosophical attitudes in audition does not mean that they are unimportant. To a large extent they determine what type of problems should be tackled. Basically Helmholtz's approach to perceptual problems is static, not dynamic. This is true of his research in vision (Johansson, in preparation), as well as in audition. The scarcity of investigations on how sounds with changing characteristics are perceived and identified is probably due to the predominantly analytical attitude among auditory experimenters.

B. Description of Auditory Stimuli

In audition, both the success and the limitations of the analytical approach is, to a large extent, bound up with its utilization of Fourier mathematics. Fourier analysis is of unique value if the time-varying quantity is a periodic function. If it is nonperiodic, it can sometimes be represented by the Fourier series extension called a *Fourier integral*. But this kind of mathematics is ill suited to describing the constantly changing sounds typical of our everyday experience. Also, as we shall see, the identification of the mathematical variables with physical quantities like time and frequency is not as straightforward as is customarily assumed.

As an illustration let us consider a pure tone that we change in either amplitude of frequency. If we turn the dials controlling amplitude or frequency back and forth, we hear a tone whose loudness or pitch varies. This amplitude modulation (am) or frequency modulation (fm) can be achieved mechanically or electronically, so that the quantity we want modified varies sinusoidally at any desired rate. We could take oscillographic records of the resulting waveforms and analyze them into their Fourier components. We would then find that the strongest component is that of the tone we modulated, the carrier. There are also sidebands of smaller amplitude distributed symmetrically around the carrier frequency at a distance equal, in hertz, to the rate of modulation. When the amplitude of a tone is modulated sinusoidally there are only two sidebands, whereas for sinusoidal fm the number of sidebands depends on the strength of the modulating wave.

Stevens and Davis (1938), after a similar description of the modulating process, offered the following commentary.

Since any type of modulated wave can be analyzed into a spectrum containing several steady components, the ear would, if its tuning were sufficiently sharp, hear all the components independently, just as it hears at once the flute and the cello in an orchestra. Then, when the tuning dial of an oscillator is turned back and forth, instead of hearing a pitch which rises and falls, we should hear only a group of steady tones spaced a certain distance apart. Even though the tuning dial were moved continuously, so that, to all appearances, the change in frequency is likewise continuous, there would be certain frequencies which we should hear and intermediate frequencies which we should not hear! Such is the nature of fm—a continuous change in frequency produces a discontinuous spectrum. Nothing, perhaps, is more contrary to intuition than that we should be able to change the frequency of an oscillator continuously between two limits without producing all intermediate frequencies, but that is precisely what we do when we generate a sinusoidal fm. And if the ear were a better analyzer it would tell us so [p. 226].

For all its lucidity of exposition the argument contains one debatable point. Interestingly, it concerns the failure to apply strictly operational criteria to the definition of a physical concept, and Stevens, the probable author of the passage, had tried harder and more consistently than anyone to make his fellow psychologists adopt the operational viewpoint.

It is commonly forgotten that the analytic functions of Fourier cannot properly be identified with concepts like time and frequency. The concept of frequency as used in the preceding argument is meaningful only so long as it refers to some physical measuring procedure. A sinewave of long duration can be ascribed a frequency of a precision sufficient for our purposes if we lead it through a sharply tuned variable filter. The setting that gives maximum output defines the frequency of the sinewave. If the duration is short, however, there is a range of settings that give practically equal output and, strictly speaking, we can no longer say that the stimulus we present is a pure frequency. Auditory scientists are, of course, well aware of the inverse relationship between precision in time and frequency. Yet occasionally a concept like frequency is used as if it had a meaning independent of any measuring apparatus.

In order to make it easier to avoid such mistakes, Nordmark (1968) adopted Kneser's (1948) distinction between group frequency, which is identical to the one we have been discussing so far, and phase frequency, which is simply the reciprocal of the time interval between two events of equal phase. The theories that consider the neural identification of the maximally stimulated portion of the similar membrane to be the basis for frequency discrimination—the place theories—use frequency in the first sense. In the formulation of existing nonplace theories, the second definition may or may not have been implied. Nordmark considers the distinction fundamental in frequency discrimination theory.

Considerations very similar to those of Nordmark led Korn (1968) to examine the definition of fm in sound analysis. One of his conclusions is that given an optimal analyzing procedure, the information uncertainty of variable-frequency signals may well exceed that of the analyzing mechanism. Although Korn does not consider the case of periodic fm, it appears clear that the description by Stevens and Davis of how the ear would react to fm tones if it were a perfect analyzer could be true only for very special stimuli. Nor are Feth, Wolf, and Bilger (1969) quite correct in stating that the auditory system would exhibit infinite resolving power if its integration time were not limited to 200 msec.

The complex task of describing a sound stimulus is thus intimately bound up with the analyzing procedure. A possible consequence of this would be to make use of data on the analytical ability of the ear in our descriptions of auditory stimuli. In cases where an unnecessarily detailed specification should be avoided, this might be of some advantage, and has, as will be discussed later, been tried, but more often the usual type of specification will do, so long as its limitations are kept in mind.

A more interesting possibility would be to include the motion of the basilar membrane of the cochlea in the *description* of the stimulus. Adopting a distinction common in vision (see Zener & Gaffron, 1962) we could call the stimulus directly affecting the receptors the *proximal* stimulus and the sound as it leaves the source the *distal* stimulus. Although the mechanism for transducing basilar membrane motion into neural impulses is unknown, a consideration of the proximal stimulus will often give information that is new and at times even contrary to our intuitive conceptions.

A similar distinction was made by Békésy (1972) in what may have been his last paper. He states that the brain does not process the external stimulus, but it processes the stimulations at the nervous end organ produced by an internal stimulus, which can be different from the external stimulus. In his opinion the results of Seebeck's experiment may be differently interpreted when we look at the internal (proximal) stimulus. We saw that for short clicks like those used by Seebeck, the fundamental will be weak or absent when we displace alternate clicks up to about 10%. Békésy found that if we make the clicks longer by using condenser discharges with a decay time longer than a period, a spectral analysis will show the presence of a fairly strong fundamental. However, as the oscillogram shows, the time pattern will still have a periodicity of twice the fundamental. Since a click produces a traveling wave that takes quite a long time to travel from the stapes to the helicotrema in the cochlea, we have, according to Békésy, exactly the same type of lengthening of the stimulus in the ear.

Duifhuis (1970) has also pointed out that describing a stimulus in terms of a frequency spectrum does not necessarily present the best correspondance with subjective sensation. One of Duifhuis's findings was that separately eliminating a high harmonic in the spectrum of a periodic pulse train paradoxically made the listener hear a clear tone whose pitch corresponded to that of the suppressed harmonic. We can understand why this might happen only by considering the basilar membrane motion. As we have

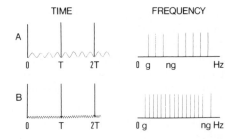

FIG. 2. Time patterns and frequency amplitude spectra of periodic pulses of which the *n*th harmonics *(ng)* have been suppressed. [After Duifhuis (1970).]

known since Békésy measured the cochlear response to pure tones, a sinusoid will give rise to a much broader displacement than Helmholtz had assumed. The membrane will respond to an input of harmonics that are closely spaced and approximately in phase, somewhat like a filter to a sudden impulse: The initially large response amplitude will gradually decay to zero and, provided the pulse rate is low enough, the membrane will not be set in motion until the next pulse arrives. But if the stimulus has the appearance shown in Fig. 2, in the formerly silent interval between consecutive pulses then, the basilar membrane will reflect the wavy form of the stimulus, and a listener will hear a tone of corresponding pitch. The phenomenon is a consequence of the limited resolving power of the mechanical analyzer of the ear. If instead one of the lower harmonics, say the fourth or the fifth (Fig. 2A), were to be eliminated, a trained observer would indeed be expected to notice that a tone that had been a part of the complex-tone sensation had disappeared.

The usefulness of a closer consideration of what constitutes the proximal stimulus is by no means limited to occasional phenomena where spectral analysis happens to be insufficient. A more direct approach to picturing the proximal stimulus has been made by Flanagan (1962) in an attempt to relate psychoacoustic phenomena to a computational model for the mechanical operation of the ear.

At present, our attempts to describe the proximal stimulus are hampered by difficulties in visualizing the detailed response of the basilar membrane to complex stimuli. Also, its precise significance for perception is not clear, as we do not know exactly how the membrane motion is represented in the auditory nerve. A further refinement in our conception of cochlear mechanics will eventually permit a much fuller description by means of computer display or similar kinds of representation.

II. THE SELECTIVITY OF THE EAR

A. Mechanical Selectivity

We have seen that the frequency selectivity of the ear is not as complete as Helmholtz thought. Studies of the basilar membrane motion, of the response in the auditory nervous system, and of the ability of a subject to separate closely spaced tones from one another have all been used to estimate the limits of the resolving power of the ear. We should not expect a wholly unambiguous picture to emerge from these studies. At each level, the estimates vary according to the criteria employed. It is, furthermore, far from obvious how the activity at the different levels should be related.

When Békésy (1943) first managed to measure the response of the basilar membrane to low-frequency tones of very high intensity, he could show that a pure tone stimulates a portion of the membrane that is fairly broad, but that the point of maximal excursion of the membrane is unique for each frequency. The idea of a one-to-one correspondance between pitch and position on the membrane could therefore, in principle, be maintained. To explain, however, why less than maximally stimulated parts do not give rise to a sensation of pitch, Békésy invoked the concept of neural inhibition. The idea of an aural effect similar to the Mach bands in vision was central to Békésy's thinking. In fact, it may have preceded his working out of the model of the traveling wave in the cochlea. By means of a cochlear model applied to the skin, he tried to show that phenomena analogous to inhibition in the ear exist for the tactual sense. For many years the presence of neural inhibition in the ear was widely accepted.

A number of studies using the Mössbauer technique have considerably increased our knowledge of the basilar membrane movement. Experiments on the guinea pig (Johnstone & Boyle, 1967; Johnstone, Taylor, & Boyle, 1970) and on the squirrel monkey (Rhode, 1971) show that the movement caused by a pure tone is more narrowly confined to an area close to the point of maximum stimulation than Békésy's measurements led us to believe. Another way of expressing these findings is to say that the basilar membrane motion is less heavily damped than was formerly thought.

Recordings from cochlear fibers give results that point in the same direction. With certain kinds of stimuli, neurophysiologists can make inferences about the behavior of the basilar membrane. The conclusions to be drawn from the studies by de Boer (1967), Møller (1970), and Evans and Wilson (1973) appear to be that the filtering performed by the membrane is linear and that there is no evidence of lateral inhibition. Whether there is any discrepancy between the data on mechanical and neural tuning—in other words, whether the mechanical selectivity of the membrane can account for the spectral resolution of the stimulus—is at present a matter for debate. Recordings from single auditory fibers, however, appear to show somewhat sharper filter characteristics than could be expected from a purely mechanical analysis. An interesting scheme to account for the discrepancy has recently been suggested by Zwislocki (1974). On the basis of single-nerve recordings of normal and kanamycin-treated gerbils, Zwislocki concluded that the inner and outer hair cells of the cochlea interact, and that their inputs to the auditory nerve fibers are in phase opposition. This arrangement is held to provide the required sharpening of the mechanical filter action of the basilar membrane.

B. Psychophysical Studies

1. FILTER CONCEPTS

Attempts have also been made to estimate the mechanical selectivity of the cochlea on the basis of results of psychophysical experiments. Obviously the appropriateness of such procedures is critically dependent on the particular assumptions made to relate the presumed mechanical behavior to the perceptual effect under investigation. It is perhaps not entirely unfair to say that experiments of this kind are at least as much a test of the correctness of the basic assumptions as of any mechanical characteristics of the cochlea. Wilson and Evans (1971), who made a number of ingenious experiments to relate mechanical, physiological, and psychological behavior, were forced to the conclusion that their assumptions about the mechanism resulting in the perceptual effect may have been only partially correct. Duifhuis (1972) also stresses that his estimate of the Q, or filter sharpness, of the high-frequency part of the basilar membrane arrived at through psychological experiments is tentative. His reasoning, however, may have been sound, as his estimated Q, merely described as being larger than seven, is of the same order as that which could be deduced from the physiological studies just mentioned. Furthermore, it is in line with some estimates for high frequencies of the so-called critical bandwidth (Zwicker, Flottorp, & Stevens, 1957).

This concept grew out of various studies showing abrupt changes in subjective responses when a certain bandwidth is exceeded. The loudness of a band of noise, for instance, remains constant as the bandwidth increases up to the critical bandwidth, after which it begins to increase. Similarly, the threshold of a narrow band of noise surrounded by two masking tones remains constant with increasing frequency separation up to the critical bandwidth. Beyond this point, the threshold drops sharply. These and related studies form the empirical core of the concept.

In other experiments, especially those concerned with wide-band noise, the estimates of bandwidths depend on specific assumptions and measurement criteria (Reed & Bilger, 1973). As we proceed in our examination of auditory analysis we shall meet further examples of such dependency. In one area of auditory analysis, the concept must be considered irrelevant: The frequent assertion that the difference limen (DL) for pitch is related to the critical bandwidth is completely lacking in empirical support (Nordmark, 1968).

If the critical-band concept at present does not have the degree of generality many experimenters assume, the function generated by its more well-established measures is nevertheless useful as a frame of reference for a variety of studies.

2. The Separability of Pure Tones

A number of procedures can be used to investigate the frequency analyzing ability of the ear. The most direct would be to have a subject identify the constituents of a set of regularly spaced pure tones. His success would determine the limit of the analyzing ability. As few of us have a sense of pitch accurate enough to be able to assign a label or a number to a tone, identification would have to mean equating the pitch of a generator under the subject's control with each constituent tone in turn.

One disadvantage with this method lies in the difficulty in identifying tones in a complex stimulus without using an auxiliary tone to assist the listener. Despite its attraction the direct method has therefore not been employed in recent investigations.

Methods using auxiliary tones, however, have been common in such studies. The subjects in the experiments by Plomp (1964) and Plomp and Mimpen (1968) had a three-position switch at their disposal. In the middle position a subject heard a complex tone. In the other positions pure tones were presented, one with a frequency equal to the frequency of one of the harmonics, and the other one with a frequency midway between this harmonic and the adjacent higher or lower one. The listener's task was to decide which auxiliary tone was also present in the complex tone. The method may not be ideal (Moore, 1972), but there is little doubt that it is adequate. Plomp's results are also indirectly supported by the poststimulus masking curve generated by the complex tone. The experiments show that not more than seven and generally only five harmonics of a complex tone can be heard separately. Plomp's conclusion is that the ear is able to distinguish partials of a tone only if there frequency separation exceeds the critical bandwidth. Using Plomp's method, a direct test of this hypothesis was made by Soderquist (1970) for inharmonic tones. The deviation found was not considered by the author to justify a rejection of this hypothesis, and Plomp's results were thus replicated.

Plomp (1964) used a very similar method to examine the separability of two pure tones. As can be seen from Fig. 3, which also shows the critical-band and the complex-tone curve, the high-frequency portion of the curve is reasonably close to the critical-band function, but as the frequencies become lower, separation becomes increasingly difficult. Plomp does not comment on this change in the curve.

A different procedure for determining two-tone separability was employed by Terhardt (1968a). His subjects had to decide whether one pitch or two pitches should be assigned to the beating two-tone complex. Intuitively this seems an easier task than that given in Plomp's experiment. For frequencies above 200 Hz his results do indeed show a somewhat smaller frequency difference necessary for separability. The considerable decrease in separability below 200 Hz is also absent (Fig. 3).

FIG. 3. Three experiments to determine separability for pure tones. One curve (Plomp & Mimpen, 1968) shows the frequency difference between the harmonics of a complex tone required to hear them separately as a function of frequency. In the second curve (Plomp, 1964), separability, similarly determined, for only two tones is plotted. In Terhardt's experiment the stimulus was also a tone pair, the criterion the perception of more than one pitch. ——, critical bandwidth; - - -, Plomp and Mimpen (1968); · · ·, Plomp (1964); · - · -, Terhardt (1968a).

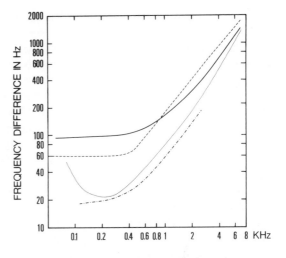

I found this low-frequency divergence sufficiently intriguing to justify a small-scale study where the subject had to adjust a generator to agree with his impression of one or more pitches when presented with a two-tone stimulus of varying frequency-separation. An adjustment that came within 2% of either of the physical frequencies was taken as constituting identification.

For frequencies above about 200 Hz the results agreed quite well with those of Terhardt. Below 200 Hz, however, the subjects' task was experienced as considerably more difficult. Adjustments within 5–10% had to be accepted to obtain a meaningful curve. With this altered criterion, the deterioration was similar to but slightly more pronounced than that found by Plomp.

The distribution curve for the settings made by the subjects, however, had a third maximum situated in between the frequencies of the two tones. This is clearly the intertone referred to in some earlier writings on beats (Wever, 1929) and empirically established by Ekdahl and Boring (1934). An intermediate pitch was also noticed by Plomp. For frequency separations up to about 30 Hz, the settings were almost exclusively limited to frequencies corresponding to the intertone. It is audible at even larger separations. Terhardt's criterion is therefore insufficiently precise. The poor resolution of the ear in this range is most remarkable. Pure tones of 100 and 160 Hz still cannot be accurately identified. What is most intriguing is that in music this is an important frequency range, where simultaneous complex tones without any doubt are separately perceived. This matter will be taken further in a later section. It is also obvious that the separability curve for complex tones is the only one to show a reasonable agreement with the critical-band curve.

Further evidence for a spectral resolution sharper than would be expected if the critical bandwidth determines the limit has been provided by Duifhuis (1972). According to Duifhuis his method is similar to that used by some other authors (Cardozo & Neelen, 1967; Gibson, 1971). The essence of the method lies in having the subject distinguish between periodic pulses where a certain harmonic is attenuated or completely suppressed. Cardozo and Neelen determined the threshold for a harmonic by asking his subjects to raise its level from zero until it became audible. The procedure was also used in Duifhuis's experiment. If the point where the harmonic has a level no higher than the other constituents of the complex tone is taken as the limit, values for the highest audible harmonic of between 12 and 20 were found in these studies. In an experiment by Gibson (1971) a complex tone could be deprived of any partial by means of interruption by an electronic switch, and the observers were asked to duplicate the frequency of the interrupted partial. In the middle-frequency range partials as high as the eleventh and the twelfth could be separately perceived with some consistency.

It occurred to me that another way of determining the limits of audibility for harmonics could make use of the phenomenon of binaural beats. These beats are heard, for example, when a tone of 600 Hz is fed to one ear and a tone of 601 Hz is fed to the other ear. The sound will then appear to move across the head once per second. I found that the phenomenon can be heard when two harmonics of different complex tones are close in frequency. When, for instance, a complex tone of 70 Hz is heard in one ear, and one of 80.1 Hz is heard in the other, the eighth and seventh harmonics, respectively, neither of which is perceptible in the monaural condition, will stand out with great clarity as a tone moving across the head about once every second. Harmonics up to at least the tenth and the eleventh can be heard in this way.

The limits of audibility of harmonics clearly depend on the experimental method employed. It is still true, however, that when listening to one complex tone the unaided ear can only hear a few harmonics.

C. Hypotheses on Auditory Resolution

We are now in a position to look more closely at suggested mechanisms of auditory selectivity. To make the problem somewhat easier to visualize, in Fig. 4 I have drawn idealized patterns of excitation on the basilar membrane in response to (a) a two-tone and (b) a multitone signal. The steep part of the curves had a slope of 100 dB per octave, and the flat part of the curves has a slope of 24 dB per octave, which appears to be representative of recent measurements. I have assumed that the selectivity is the same in all frequency ranges, which may not be true at all. What is important here is that the slope on the high-frequency side is extremely unlikely to be appreciably steeper. Unless there is further filtering, mechanical or neural, the curves can be expected to give an idea of what sort of frequency resolution occurs in the cochlea.

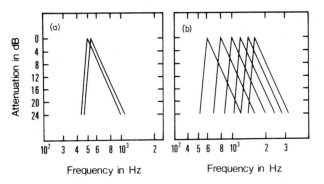

FIG. 4. Idealized excitation patterns on the basilar membrane in response to (a) a tone pair, and (b) a complex tone consisting of harmonics 5–9.

The curves on the left represent two just separable tones. Those on the right show the fifth to ninth harmonics of a complex tone with a fundamental frequency of 200 Hz. The lower four harmonics are spaced so that their maxima will not fall within the same critical band. We can see that even for these harmonics a good deal of mechanical interaction will take place.

We shall now consider how the results on auditory analysis could be explained in terms of either the place theory or a temporal theory.

The primary condition that must be fulfilled if two tones are to give rise to separate pitches according to place theory is clearly that the peaks and valleys of the mechanical response are of sufficiently different amplitude to be distinguished by the neural fibers (Wilson & Evans, 1971). In order to keep its identity, each tone must further exert an influence on the pitch-determining elements similar to that of the isolated tone.

There appear to be two ways in which a place principle could work. First, only the maximally stimulated nerves determine the sensory impression. Since it is known (Geisler, Rhode, & Kennedy, 1973; Kiang & Moxon, 1973; Rose, Hind, Anderson, & Brugge, 1971) that auditory nerve fibers respond to stimulation from an extensive area of the basilar membrane, we would have to assume that when, for instance, the signal is a loud, low-frequency tone, all except a few nerves are inhibited. A few years ago a neural sharpening in successive parts of the auditory pathway was held in many quarters to be the answer to the problem of place pitch. It is now known (Møller, 1972; Whitfield, 1967) that instead of becoming progressively sharper, the neural response areas will, if anything, be wider as one goes beyond the auditory nerve and the cochlear nucleus. Psychophysical attempts to show perceptual sharpening have led to inconclusive results (Carterette, Friedman, & Lovell, 1969; Rainbolt & Small, 1972). Most psychophysicists who accept neural place as the main basis of pitch no longer appear to feel the need for invoking neural sharpening (Zwicker, 1965).

The second possibility for a place principle is to assume instead that for every pure tone, a whole block of nerves—the size of which varies with intensity—is stimulated, and that pitch is determined by the "location" of the block (Allanson & Whitfield, 1956; Whitfield, 1967).

Whitfield's proposed scheme to account for decomposition of complex tones involves two effects: a clearer definition of the edges of the neural activity, and mutual inhibition between two stimulated areas. The effects, which take place at neural stations later than the auditory nerve, are shown in Fig. 5 of Chapter 5 of this book. The inhibition of some fibers that are activated by either tone separately is necessary, as two tones could be expected to give rise to a distribution of active neural fibers indistinguishable from a single much broader tone.

Terhardt (1972) has pointed to a possibility for additional peripheral analysis that does not involve inhibition. When two pure tones are close, there will be a point where both tones have the same amplitude. At this point, the resulting amplitude will fluctuate between zero and a maximum value at the beat frequency, that is, at the rate corresponding to the difference in frequency between the pure tones. On either side of the point, however, the maxima may be considered to be more stationary. If the ear could take account of the other maxima, the discrepancy between the critical bandwidth and the much smaller bandwidth sufficient for frequency separation could, in Terhardt's view, be explained.

This scheme appears to dispose of the problem Whitfield considered by accepting the existance of the intertone, although Terhardt does not refer to this phenomenon explicitly. To some extent, the assumption is based on facts. An intertone is, as we have seen, heard in certain frequency combinations. But it is prominent only in the low-frequency range. What the proximal stimulus looks like during a beat period is also difficult to visualize. Basing himself on Ranke's basilar membrane model, Albert (1951) made a number of drawings showing the excitation pattern for two tones at 1000 and 1066.7 Hz, which happens to be almost exactly the frequency difference required by Terhardt's subjects to hear separate tones in this range. Albert's picture of the beating complex bear out Terhardt's suggested pattern only partially. Regardless of the actual form of the proximal stimulus, the proposal is valuable as it points to the possibility that local maxima may be transitory and still give rise to a pitch impression.

The place principle embodies the idea that pitch is determined by activity in a particular group of nerves. By definition, not more than one kind of pitch information can be effectively transmitted by a group of nerves of pitch-determining size. With a temporal mechanism it is, on the contrary, conceivable that effective pitch information could be mixed in the same neural channel. Psychophysicists with leanings toward a temporal mechanism appear nevertheless to have been as prone as the adherents of the rival principle to imply separate channels for pitch. The idea was formalized with the acceptance of the critical-band concept. But it is a weakness of temporal theories of pitch, which few, if any, of either their critics or proponents seem to have spotted, that mixing of temporal information is bound to occur when simultaneous tones are close in frequency. The limited mechanical resolution of the basilar membrane is thus as much a problem for a temporal as it is for a place theory. It is somewhat a less acute problem now than a few years ago, as the mechanical filtering has been found to be sharper than Békésy's measurements indicated. If the assumptions on which Fig. 4 is based are accepted, the figure shows that the fourth harmonic, which is clearly audible, has about half the amplitude of the next harmonic at the point of that harmonic's maximum. The sixth, which is separated by just about a critical bandwidth from its neighbors, has slightly less than twice the amplitude of the fifth. The sixth harmonic is audible to some but not to most of the observers, according to Plomp and Mimpen. The condition that must be fulfilled if a temporal mechanism is to be considered acceptable is that a combination of two harmonics at points where they are in a 2:1 amplitude ratio will show peaks sufficiently well defined to account for the perceived harmonic. This condition is reminiscent of the one we discussed for place theory. The difference, of course, is that in one case the word peak has a temporal meaning and in the other case, a spatial. Either theory, however, is easier to defend if mechanical filtering is sharp and correspondingly embarrassed by a lower degree of high-frequency attenuation. It is uncertain whether the mechanical resolution suggested by recent studies is quite sufficient to explain discriminability in terms of either principle.

A further requirement which must be met is that the temporal pattern of the basilar membrane movements will be represented in the firing patterns of the auditory nerve. Brugge, Andersson, Hind, and Rose (1969) have studied the time structure of discharges in single auditory nerve fibers in response to two tones locked to each other in a ratio of small integers. The authors found that there was a close correspondence between the various waveforms and the shapes of the respective period histograms, provided it is assumed that the auditory nerve is stimulated by excursions of the cochlear partition in one direction only. Some of the ratios investigated were 5:6, 6:7, and 7:8. It appears that even in these cases, it was usually quite simple to construct a waveform from the compound sinusoids that matched the period histograms reasonably well.

The crucial question for a temporal theory of auditory analysis is therefore perhaps rather if the periodicities corresponding to separable harmonics are represented in a sufficiently distinct way in the excitation pattern of the basilar membrane. At present we cannot answer this question.

III. INTERACTION PHENOMENA

A. Beats and Modulated Signals

The last section dealt with some of the phenomena of auditory analysis. The complementary aspect of complex-tone hearing, phenomena resulting from an absence of tonal analysis, will form the content of the next section.

As is well known, the interaction of two tones close in frequency is perceived as *beats*. Helmholtz devoted much attention to beats, particularly to the variation in the strength of beats with increasing frequency difference between the tones. According to Wever (1929) three stages can be distinguished in this development:

(1) The loudness appears to surge up and down continuously.
(2) The beats are heard as a series of intermittent impulses.
(3) There is roughness without intermittence.

The second stage begins at about six or seven beats per second, and the transition to roughness takes place around a frequency difference of 25 (Terhardt, 1968b). Roughness was considered by Helmholtz to be largest for frequency differences of 30–40 Hz. This maximum became important in his writings on dissonance, a concept he came, to a large extent, to equate with roughness.

Very similar changes are noticed when the rate of amplitude modulation is gradually increased. In frequency modulation the ear can follow the pitch changes at rates up to 7 Hz sec^{-1}. We would therefore expect that low rates would give smaller DLs for pitch than rates about 10 Hz. Feth *et al.* (1969), however, have shown that the earlier studies that confirmed this expectation were based on incorrectly computed spectra, and that the DL does not increase with modulation rates from 1 to 16. This interesting and surprising finding shows how difficult, but also potentially rewarding, the study of human frequency modulation discrimination can be. When the rate of frequency modulation is 20 Hz—beyond the range where pitch changes can be heard—the impression is one of a complex warbling or fluttering sound rather than roughness (McClelland & Brandt, 1969). With further increases in the modulation rate the warbling changes to a roughness and then disappears.

A somewhat different approach was adopted by Zwicker (1952). He discovered that amplitude modulation (am) is more readily detected than frequency modulation (fm) for low modulation rates. The sensitivity to the two forms of modulation becomes identical at frequencies that depend on the carrier frequency. They turn out to correspond to half the critical band value at the carrier frequency. In other words, when the sidebands are no longer within one critical band, phase relations are not perceived. Goldstein (1967) confirmed Zwicker's main findings, but found that in contrast to other critical-band measures the modulation limit was dependent on the intensity of the stimulus.

The difference between am and fm can be understood by looking more closely at the shape of the signals involved. The envelope of an approximately frequency-modulated tone is relatively smooth, whereas a 100% amplitude-modulated tone has a sharply peaked waveform. Mathes and Miller (1947) could show that roughness is connected with these differences in waveform. In the modulation range between 25 and 75 Hz, the switch from the am to the fm case was marked by the disappearance of the roughness. For higher rates the differences between the modulation conditions gradually diminished, but some difference could be detected when the modulation rate was as high as 40% of the carrier. Vogel (1975) has been able to show in greater detail how roughness correlates with the difference between minimum and maximum values of the amplitude of the sound pressure.

B. Limits for Beats, Roughness, and Dissonance

The smallest frequency difference at which two tones at a loudness level of 60 phon do not interfere is shown as Curve 2 in Fig. 5. The curve is taken from a study by Plomp and Steeneken (1968). Under similar conditions but using a different procedure, Terhardt (1968b) obtained results for beats and am tones that followed the critical-band curve at low frequencies, but deviated even more sharply than Curve 2 at higher frequencies. In both studies, the deviation was attributed to the inability of the ear to perceive very fast amplitude fluctuations.

To measure the maximum frequency difference giving an impression of

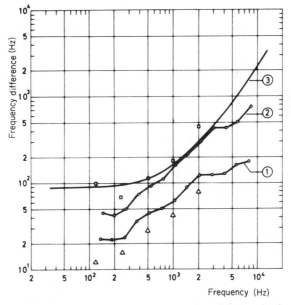

FIG. 5. Frequency difference between two pure tones adjusted for maximal roughness (Curve 1) and for absence of interference (Curve 2), plotted as a function of the mean frequency of the two tones. Curve 3 represents the critical bandwidth. The other data points correspond to the frequency difference for maximal dissonance (□) and the difference at which the consonance plateau is reached (△). [Data adopted from Plomp and Levelt (1965) and Plomp and Steeneken (1968); figure from Plomp (1971).]

roughness as a function of frequency, Terhardt (1968b) employed am tones, but in view of the close connection believed to exist between roughness and dissonance—which is a concept most easily defined for two tones—it has been more natural to study interference for pure-tone intervals only. Plomp and Steeneken had their subjects determine (1) the frequency combination giving maximal roughness and (2) the lowest value for which the tones did not interfere. The results can be seen in the figure. Also shown are data from an earlier study by Plomp and Levelt (1965) on the frequency difference for tone pairs giving maximal dissonance and the difference beyond which intervals were no longer judged increasingly consonant.

Using a different scaling technique, Kameoka and Kuriyagawa (1969) estimated the consonance and dissonance values for tonal combinations where the lower frequency varied from about 60 to 7000 Hz. The authors also found that after the point of maximum dissonance, consonance increases with the frequency separation between the primary tones, and in addition it continues to increase even beyond the octave. In this respect their results differ from those shown in Fig. 5. The somewhat less consonant character of tones in a simple frequency ratio in the low-frequency area mentioned in the older literature was confirmed by Kameoka and Kuriyagawa. In fact, a single pure low-frequency tone also gets less consonant. A tone of 56 Hz obtained a rating of 4.5 on a 10-point scale and should be considered a dissonance!

The separation that gives maximum dissonance also increases with frequency, but the authors point out that it is not simply proportional to the critical bandwidth. Furthermore, it increases with intensity, whereas the critical bandwidth is generally supposed to be independent of intensity. As the frequency increased, the point of maximum dissonance was found at a progressively smaller musical interval. Dissonance for tones at a sound-pressure level (SPL) of 57 dB could be quite accurately represented by a power function with an exponent near .5. The data of Plomp and Steeneken for maximum roughness would seem to fit this curve quite well, and the data on maximum dissonance reasonably well. The critical bandwidths, of course, cannot be described by a power function.

C. Beats of Mistuned Consonances

Beats, however, will also occur between tones that are nearly but not quite in a harmonic relationship. Such beats of mistuned consonances were attributed by Helmholtz to various forms of distortion. As beats also occur between tones in a relationship such as 5 : 9, very complex distortion products are required to account for the phenomena, and a number of scientists objected to this explanation (for an historical review, see Plomp, 1967). Using masking noise Plomp (1967) could show that combination tones could not be responsible for these beats. To prove that the same is true of aural harmonics, Plomp asked his subjects to adjust the intensity of the higher tone of various tone combinations in numerically simple ratios until the beats were maximally prominent. For a constant high-intensity lower tone of 125 Hz, the points for best beats as a function of frequency could be connected by a smooth curve. This shows that frequency difference, not frequency ratio, is the important variable, and that aural harmonics could not be responsible for the effect. Similar curves could be drawn for a number of basic frequencies of various intensities. On the assumption that best beats are heard when the tones have equal amplitude, these curves could be expected to give information on the attenuation slope toward higher frequencies from the point of maximum excursion on the basilar membrane, which we discussed earlier. The results in this study indicate a somewhat less sharp slope than that pictured in Fig. 4. Plomp, however, gives some reasons why the assumption may not be entirely correct. Also, there is the puzzling fact that, whereas the subjects could hear beats up to a ratio of 1:13 for a lower tone of 125 Hz, ratios beyond 1:2 were ineffective at 2000 Hz. What is clear beyond any doubt is that low-frequency tones exert an influence on tones over a range of several octaves.

There is another effect connected with beats of mistuned consonances, especially those in which the tones are in a 1:2, 1:3, or 1:5 relationship. This phenomenon, however, is not connected with loudness variations, but with recurrent pitch changes occurring over a range of about a musical fourth. The effect was very briefly described by Nordmark (1960), who related it to the time-separation pitch phenomenon discovered by Thurlow and Small (1955). The first quantitative study was made by Plomp (1967), who called the phenomenon the sweep-tone effect. His subjects were required to adjust the pitch of a comparison tone to match the sweep tone as the phase of a 600-Hz tone, locked to a 200-Hz tone, was varied in steps. Over the phase range covering all possible waveform variations, the pitch was found to change from one close to the 600-Hz tone to one a major third higher. Similar results have been obtained for two-tone octave complexes (Lamoré, 1975).

Again it appears difficult to understand how nonlinear distortion by the hearing mechanism could explain these results. Plomp (1967) and Nordmark (1970) have both argued that the phenomenon is also difficult to understand in terms of place pitch, and have suggested instead that the pitch is related to the temporal pattern of impulses in the auditory nerve generated by the stimulus waveforms. Variations in the stimulus waveform resulting from superimposed sinusoids are, according to Plomp, likely to be responsible for both pitch and loudness variations connected with beats of mistuned consonances.

D. Conclusions about the Resolution of the Ear

In the view of most observers the primary requirement for the phenomena of beats and modulation is that in one area on the basilar membrane tones must, to some extent, overlap. The limits of the various phenomena can therefore be expected to be related to the limits of the ear's resolving power. The relationship, however, is far from simple.

Terhardt (1968b) relates roughness to the critical-band function in the following way: Increasing the modulation rate for a given carrier increases roughness until the sidebands reach the critical bandwidth. Beyond this point roughness begins to decrease. It disappears completely when the components are all separated by a critical band, as under these conditions there will be hardly any overlap at all. Maximum roughness for two tones, however, does not reach a maximum when the frequency difference amounts to a critical-band. Other attempts to establish a similar relationship cannot be said to have been quite successful either. According to Plomp and Levelt maximum tonal dissonance is produced by intervals subtending 25% of the critical bandwidth. Apart from the difficulty in understanding why a maximum would be reached at this particular bandwidth, the data, as pointed out earlier, fit a rather different function at least as well.

Minimum values for tones up to 1 kHz, on the other hand, are much better correlated with the critical-band function. This must not be interpreted to mean, however, that no interaction occurs for tones separated by more than one critical bandwidth. The beats of mistuned consonances show that such interaction does occur and are another manifestation of the relatively low degree of selectivity in the ear, which other data lead us to infer. They also show that phase relations for tones outside one critical band may be important. Quite small changes in phase for three-component tones are in fact noticeable both when the frequency difference between the outer components is smaller than one critical band and when it is considerably larger (Fleischer, 1976). The attempt to explain this discrimination as due to interactions of the excitation patterns of the partial tones or to aural distortion products cannot conceal the fact that the results imply a weakening of the critical-band concept.

IV. PERIODICITY PITCH

A. Spectral Origin of Periodicity Pitch

The best known of all phenomena that have been attributed to the collective behavior of a group of pure tones has come to be labeled *periodicity pitch*. The effects discovered by Seebeck discussed in an early part of this chapter are examples of periodicity pitch.

The modern development in the area starts with Schouten's (1938, 1940a,b) studies. He showed that cancelling the fundamental of a low-intensity complex tone with an externally supplied sinusoid left what he termed a *residue* with an impure sharp timbre but with the same pitch as the fundamental. Distortion at moderate intensities was found to be negligible.

Cancellation of the fundamental could also be expected to remove at the same time any difference frequency generated in the ear. The pitch could therefore not be due to distortion. Instead Schouten attributed it to the collective behavior of the higher harmonics, none of which was supposed to be individually perceptible.

Later experiments have confirmed that periodicity pitch must arise in channels other than those which carry low-frequency information. A powerful method to demonstrate this employs selective masking. A tone in any part of the spectrum may be masked by a sufficiently intense band of noise affecting the same part of the basilar membrane as the pure tone. If periodicity pitches were due to nonlinear distortion, we would expect that a band of low-frequency noise capable of masking a pure tone equal in energy to the complex tone would also mask the difference tone. Licklider (1954), however, could show that under such circumstances the pitch corresponding to the fundamental could still be heard. The same conclusion was arrived at independently by Thurlow and Small (1955).

Small and Campbell (1961) extended these studies by examining the masking pattern for (a) bursts of a 2200-Hz sinusoid repeated about 150 times per second, and for comparison, (b) pure tones of 2200 and 150 Hz. Both high- and low-pass noise was used as maskers. The pulsed tones yielded a masking pattern very similar to that of a 2200-Hz pure tone and quite unlike that of a 150-Hz tone. The results of this study have been confirmed by Patterson (1969). The hypothesis that periodicity pitch is mediated by the high-frequency channels is further supported by a study involving selective fatigue (Small & Yelen, 1962), as well as by neurophysiological evidence (Glattke, 1969).

In the first section, we saw that Békésy tried to explain Seebeck's effect by assuming that considerable low-frequency energy could be present on the basilar membrane without being part of the distal stimulus. But, as pointed out by Broadbent (1971, p. 121), it is hard or even impossible to see how the masking experiments described here could be explained in terms of a low-frequency stimulus. Nor, to the best of my knowledge, has this explanation been invoked by place theorists. The particular kind of mechanism by which Békésy accounted for periodicity phenomena in terms of place theory has not gained widespread acceptance, and few place theorists today assume that the periodicity pitch originates at the same position on the membrane as the pure tone giving an identical pitch. This does not mean that a nonplace mechanism is generally accepted. But the classical hypothesis of reintroduced low-frequency energy now appears to have been abandoned.

B. The Pitch Shift for Inharmonic Stimuli

Further evidence against the distortion hypothesis was found by Schouten (1940b). If all components of a harmonic complex, 1800, 2000, 2200, etc., are shifted 30 Hz in frequency, the resulting complex 1230, 2030, 2230, etc., is no longer harmonic. Schouten discovered that under these conditions the periodicity pitch will correspond to that of a pure tone of about 203 Hz. The pitch continues to move upward as the frequency shift of the harmonics increases. The am tones in Fig. 6 represent one kind of such complex stimuli.

If the periodicity pitch were due to a difference tone, it would remain unchanged as the carrier frequency moved from 2000 to 2030 Hz. This would be true also if the pitch corresponded to the envelope (the dashed curve). There are, at present, two principal explanations for the pitch shift and periodicity pitch in general. The first hypothesis is based on the observation by de Boer (1956) that the pitch shift, to a first approximation, corresponds to the decrease of 1.5% in time intervals 1–1', 2–2', and 3–3' in the lower graph. The pitch shift thus appears to be linearly dependent on the change in frequency of the carrier, which is also 1.5%. Furthermore, the fact that additional pitches, less prominent than the main pitch, can often be heard is well explained by other periodicities in the temporal fine structure, such as 1–2' and 2–3', or 2–1', and 3–2' (Schouten et al., 1962). However, the hypothesis has not been able to account for the fact that the pitch shift has been found to be slightly, but consistently, larger than predicted from a linear relationship when the center frequency is changed.

Other hypotheses discard the idea of a temporal fine-structure analysis. They are similar to the first hypothesis in that they assume that the basis for

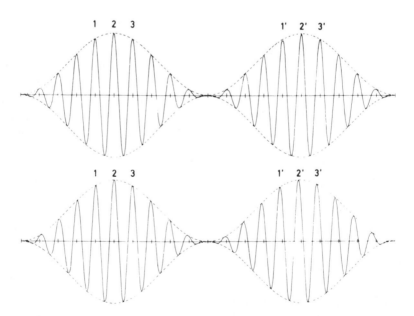

FIG. 6. Carrier frequencies of 2000 and 2030 Hz (upper and lower graph, respectively) am with 200 Hz. [From Plomp (1968), Pitch, timbre, and hearing theory, *International Audiology*, 7, 322–344.]

the pitch of complex tones is derived from higher harmonics, but different in that they require that at least one harmonic should be resolved. Some of the models are vague about the possible mechanisms for the pitch shift. Others, such as the complex model of Walliser (1969), are highly specific in the sense that they try to derive mathematically the observed pitch shifts, and the deviations from the linear relationship, from the pitch of a particular harmonic. Even in Walliser's model, however, the predicted pitch does not agree completely with experimental values (Smoorenburg, 1970).

No entirely satisfactory account of the pitch shift for inharmonic signals has been given. Van den Brink (1970), in fact, believes that we cannot expect simple, purely mathematical models to describe the phenomena in detail. In what follows I shall limit the discussion to other aspects of periodicity pitch.

C. Parameters Influencing the Perception of Periodicity Pitch

1. NUMBER OF COMPONENTS

In early studies of the residue phenomenon, it was observed that periodicity pitch was most prominent when the number of harmonics was large. De Boer even considered residues with less than five harmonics atonal. It was later shown that three or even two (Smoorenburg, 1970) could be sufficient. We must expect, however, that the impression of pitch becomes less clear as the number of components is reduced. Unfortunately no attempts have been made to measure the degree of this variation. Nor do I know of any data that would permit an indirect estimate.

The main reason for the lack of data on this point is to be found in the absence of a standard procedure for measuring pitch discrimination that would allow a comparison between various stimuli giving rise to periodicity pitch. Many investigators have commented on the difficulty of matching such stimuli with a pure tone and have therefore preferred to use another complex tone with a similar timbre as the matching signal. Yet a general use of a pure-tone matching signal, as in the studies by Small (1955) and Walliser (1969), would probably have led to a wider realization of the vast differences in clarity between various periodicity pitch stimuli and helped in avoiding some of the confusion in the theoretical area.

The absence of any reference to a common pitch discrimination standard in certain studies using indirect methods of investigating periodicity pitch is one reason why it is very hard to evaluate the results. In one such study, Houtsma and Goldstein (1971, 1972) examined what they called musical pitch by having the listener identify the melodic steps resulting from the consecutive presentation of pairs of successive partials. They presumed that in each pair, the listener heard the pitch corresponding to the fundamental. This presumption, however, was never put to a test. Their reasons for omitting such a test in a study on periodicity pitch are not presented very clearly or convincingly. In view of the results, the omission is even more surprising. According to the authors, the perceptibility of the musical pitch remains about the same when both partials are heard in one ear as when one partial is fed to one ear and the next higher partial is fed to the other. Houtsma (1971) has stated that the fundamental is heard somewhere near the center of the head, so there should have been no difficulty for a trained observer to match it with a tone from an external source. The authors have apparently overlooked Maronn's (1964) study, where a number of subjects had to report all the pitches they could hear when presented various binaural intervals. All subjects were connected with music in a professional capacity, yet none of the additional pitches reported corresponded to the fundamental. But the authors should have been aware of the fact that many other investigators have listened without success for binaural periodicity pitches and should have been particularly careful in demonstrating their findings.

Regardless of what interpretation we put on the two-tone phenomena, there can be little doubt that a three-tone combination leads to a stronger periodicity pitch. With good reason, we could expect a similar strengthening with a further addition of one or two components. Somewhat surprisingly, however, three-tone combinations have come to be regarded as representative for complex, residue-producing signals in general. Again the absence of a common measuring procedure for perceptual clarity has resulted in a failure to resolve the discrepancy between earlier and present assumptions.

The adoption of three-tone combinations in the form of am pure tones as standard periodicity pitch signals can be traced to two studies by Ritsma (1962, 1963). In the first series of experiments, Ritsma explored the conditions under which a periodicity pitch for am tones of different modulation depths could be heard. His subjects were instructed to decide whether or not the residue was tonal, which was taken to mean that the stimulus had the same pitch as a harmonic reference tone. From Fig. 7, showing the so-called existence region of the tonal residue, it can be seen that for some carrier frequencies and modulation rates, very low modulation depth, that is sidebands of small amplitude, will give rise to a periodicity pitch. For other conditions not even a 100% modulation depth is sufficient. Ritsma concludes that a tonal residue can be perceived only if its frequency value lies between 40 and 800 Hz. Moore (1972) has confirmed these results, except for the slightly higher modulation range found in his study. Ritsma (1963) extended his investigation on the existence region to tones with wide frequency spectra. His main finding was that periodicity pitch exists only when at least three signal components below a frequency of about 3 kHz are present.

This is a modification of Schouten's original conception, which was that a residue could be heard only when component frequencies above about 2 kHz were present. At this time, it was still commonly held that an unanalyzed complex was responsible for the pitch phenomenon. Ritsma (1962) pointed out that one critical bandwidth is not exceeded for most stimulus configura-

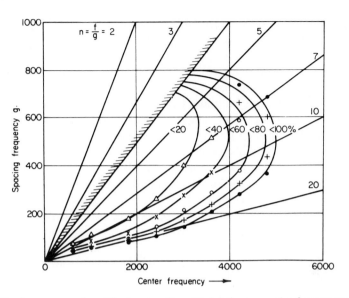

FIG. 7. The frequency region of the tonal residue. Modulating or spacing frequency g is shown on the ordinate, and carrier or center frequency f appears on the abscissa. The solid lines radiating from the origin represent constant values of the ratio f/g, M is the modulation index. [From Ritsma (1962).]

tions in the existence area shown in the figure. However, the opposite hypothesis has since gained widespread acceptance: Periodicity pitch is heard only when at least a few components can be separately perceived. To understand this complete reversal of position, we must examine the concept of spectral dominance.

2. POSITION OF HARMONICS

The concept of spectral dominance was defined in a paper by Ritsma (1967), where he claimed that a rather limited spectral region is utilized by the ear in producing a well-defined periodicity pitch. The dominant spectral region corresponds to about four times the fundamental pitch value, although individual variations are said to be considerable. Much of the evidence for spectral dominance is unconvincing. In some studies where one of two pitches has been found to dominate the perceptual impression, it seems as if attention rather than pitch is being investigated. When one pitch is truly masking another pitch, as in Nordmark's (1963) study on filtered pulse trains, the spectral dominance hypothesis could, in retrospect, be said to have been supported by the results, but no conclusion can really be drawn, as only one pitch condition was studied.

There are, however, two studies that indicate that there may be some substance to the concept. Patterson (1973) found that while a signal with components at 1260, 1460, and 1660 Hz produces a pitch of 209 Hz, and one with components at 1860, 2060, and 2260 Hz, produces a pitch of 206 Hz (Schouten *et al.*, 1962), all six tones together give rise to a pitch of 209 Hz, showing that the components close to a low multiple of the periodicity pitch are dominant in its production.

A study from Ritsma's laboratory also indicates that spectral dominance may imply more than a fixed region of maximum effectiveness in bringing about a fundamental pitch impression. Hoekstra (1973) measured pitch discrimination for ⅓-octave filtered periodic pulses. Least discriminable change in fundamental frequency as a function of filter frequency was constant so long as the signal passed by the filter included harmonics up to the eighth. The DL increased for harmonics 8–20. For still higher harmonics, the relative DL was constant at about 2%, irrespective of fundamental frequency. The same value for relative DL was also obtained for white noise periodically interrupted at rates below 100 kHz. Hoekstra's conclusion was that spectral resolution—not to be confused with the ability to identify spectral components—is necessary for periodicity pitch.

3. Phase of Components

It is commonly supposed that the waveform of a narrow-band signal that enters the ear is more or less identical to the pattern of displacement on the basilar membrane. This belief rests on two assumptions. First, the phase-shift introduced by the middle ear is not large enough to affect the waveform. Second, the waveform remains unchanged as it travels down the basilar membrane. While the second assumption is probably valid (Nordmark, Glattke, & Schubert, 1969), the first is supported by just a few scattered observations, mainly from the well-known study by Mathes and Miller (1947). The different character of am and fm tones noticed by these authors was the first instance of a clear influence of phase on complex stimuli. What must be borne in mind, however, is that most of the observations concerned modulation rates in the 25- to 75-Hz range. It is obviously less probable that any variations in the rate of change of phase will be noticeable when the spectral components are closely spaced. The modulation characteristics are in fact prominent also for signals with a faster modulation rate: When the distal stimulus is an am tone, the sound complex is raucous and the periodicity pitch is reasonably clear; when the stimulus is an fm tone, the sound is smooth and a periodicity pitch is absent or very weak. But for modulation rates between 250 and 500 Hz, it is only seldom that these relations apply. In fact, there are cases where the am signal presented by the earphone has the character of an fm tone, and *vice versa!*

We have to make the charitable assumption that most experimenters have been aware of the possibility of waveform changes during the passage through the inner ear, but have regarded these changes as insignificant for the signals they have been using. Only once, however, have I seen this assumption explicitly stated (Ritsma, 1967).

The fact that the phase shift of the middle ear cannot be neglected has implications for many aspects of periodicity pitch, particularly for the question whether pitch is different for three-component am and fm tones, as reported by Ritsma and Engel (1964). In an exploratory study I had six subjects adjust the phase of a 2000-Hz carrier in a three-component signal until the complex sounded maximally smooth. The settings differed from the approximate fm condition by 27–35 degrees. For the condition where the proximal stimulus can be assumed to have corresponded to an fm signal, no low-frequency pitch could be detected. A change in phase of 5–10 degrees would bring back a weak periodicity pitch. It is hard to say how these findings affect the interpretation Ritsma and Engel put on the pitch changes they observed. In any case, it is obvious that the possible effect of phase on periodicity pitch must be carefully considered in future studies in this area.

D. Hypotheses on Periodicity Pitch

Spectrally resolved components have been suggested by a number of workers as a prerequisite for periodicity pitch. Houtsma and Goldstein (1971, 1972), based on their own results and on Ritsma's hypothesis that the third, fourth, and fifth harmonics are the dominant pitch conveyors, suggest that fundamentals of complex tones are retrieved by means of a central mechanism that operates on resolved tones in the cochlea. The authors note that this conclusion is a radical departure from the original residue concept, which was defined as "joint perception of those higher Fourier components which the ear fails to resolve" (Schouten *et al.*, 1962).

Other experimenters have argued that periodicity pitch is a learned response derived from our life-long experience of harmonic sounds (Terhardt, 1972; Thurlow, 1963; Whitfield, 1967). Terhardt has described a model to account for what he calls the virtual pitch, which involves our stored memories of the first eight harmonics of complex tones. The memory hypothesis appears to come perilously close to the extreme empiricist doctrine of subconscious inference, which was an important part of Helmholtz's theory of perception. I doubt that it will ever prove more widely persuasive than did Helmholtz's conception. It is, nonetheless, an interesting example of how the nativist–empiricist controversy survives even in present-day auditory theory.

Do the new findings on perceptibility of harmonics mean that Schouten's residue concept must be abandoned? Before we embrace the new doctrine let us consider some facts that appear to have been overlooked. A closer examination of Fig. 7 will show that perceptibility of harmonics is neither a necessary nor a sufficient basis for periodicity pitch. We can see that the minimal modulation depth required to produce a tonal residue of 100 Hz for three components centered at 1000 Hz is about 20%. As the existence region hardly undergoes any change when the loudness level is raised from 20 dB above threshold (Ritsma, 1962), any masking curve with the stationary frequency at 1000 Hz will show that the very weak sidebands in this case cannot possibly be separately perceived. We may also notice that in parts of the existence area all three components are within one critical band. But it is also true that the three components may be separated by more than one critical band and be clearly audible, yet produce no periodicity pitch. No low-frequency pitch is heard in a complex consisting of harmonics 4, 5, and 6 of fundamentals above 800 Hz, although the components are all in the spectral dominance region.

Nor is it quite clear in what sense the harmonics 8–20 in Hoekstra's pitch discrimination experiment can be said to be separately perceived. Furthermore, while it is true that the DL increases as harmonic numbers get higher, even periodicity tones from harmonics above 20 are discriminated with an accuracy of 2%. The fact that pulsed noise is discriminated with a similar accuracy is highly suggestive, but only serves to confirm the observations of Miller and Taylor (1948), Small (1955), and Pollack (1969) that even noise without any spectral cues can give low-frequency information.

There are some earlier experiments that also show that harmonics that cannot possibly be resolved may give rise to a periodicity pitch. On the record accompanying Plomp's (1966) thesis, one example illustrating timbre shows that periodicity pitch can be heard when all frequencies below 8000 Hz are filtered out and fundamental frequencies are in the region of 400 Hz. An even earlier record illustrating a paper by Meyer-Eppler, Sendhoff, and Rupprath (1959) reproduced a melody consisting of filtered tones with fundamental frequencies between 65 and 98 Hz. The high-pass filter settings were increased in steps from 180 Hz to 8000 Hz. When the first 21 harmonics are removed, the melody is still easily recognizable, and even without the first 80–122 harmonics the melody is faintly recognizable.

Considering the evidence presented in this section, we are permitted to draw the interesting conclusion that periodicity effects somehow are additive. Three tones spaced at a distance of 100 Hz will produce no periodicity pitch above 2500 Hz. But an alternative way of describing the results of Meyer-Eppler et al. would be that an undetermined number of adjacent groups, any one of which is ineffective alone, will together give rise to a pitch of 100 Hz. The result is inexplicable from the point of view of the spectral resolution doctrine. The harmonics will, if anything, be more difficult to resolve when their number is increased.

At present, place theory offers no acceptable hypothesis that could explain periodicity pitch. The resolution doctrine, which recently has constituted a second line of defense, is untenable. But temporal theories, while basically more probable, can give no satisfactory answer to a number of questions. How are the pitch shifts to be explained? If the fine structure and not the envelope of the stimulus is responsible for periodicity pitch, why is this pitch absent for fm tones where the fine structure is no less well defined? Why does periodicity pitch disappear if the number of harmonics is decreased to three in some frequency areas? What is the reason for the better pitch discrimination for low-numbered harmonics found by Hoekstra? If the answer to the last question is, let us say, a better temporal resolution with low-numbered harmonics, why will harmonics 4, 5, and 6 of a 900-Hz tone not produce the periodicity pitch that a stimulus which includes some higher harmonics apparently produces? We can only speculate about the answer to these questions.

V. PERCEPTION OF A COMPLEX SOUND AS A WHOLE

A. Timbre

Since the early 1970s we have witnessed a renewal of interest in the field of timbre or sound quality. A problem that has concerned investigators since Helmholtz is to what extent phase influences timbre. To Helmholtz, any such influence was incompatible with the resonance theory, but later workers have shown, as we have seen, that at least under certain conditions, phase plays a role in tone perception. As often before, Plomp has instituted or taken part in the application of new methods to this old problem. Plomp and Steeneken (1969) used the method of triadic comparisons in judging the timbre differences for tones of various phase patterns. They found that the maximal possible effects were obtained for a tone consisting exclusively of sine or cosine terms, and one consisting of alternating sine and cosine terms. The effect was more pronounced for complex tones of low fundamental frequencies. To understand the observed effects Schroeder (1970) assumed that the ear can detect differences in the degree of amplitude modulation of all triplets of adjacent frequency components falling in the same critical band. The findings on the influence of these particular phase configurations on timbre may be correct, but the larger effects for low-frequency tones would be expected if the phase changes occurring before the components reach the basilar membrane were taken into consideration. The probability that anyone has ever heard a proximal stimulus consisting of, for example, only cosine terms is vanishingly small. Until a network capable of correcting the phase shift of the middle ear can be made, the maximum effects for phase differences cannot be determined with certainty.

What is established beyond doubt is that for the timbre of ordinary signals the amplitude spectrum is much more important than the phase spectrum. It has been known for a long time that, to a large extent, timbre is determined by spectral peaks or formants. These peaks are the results of the interaction of the acoustic energy from an energy source with some sort of passive acoustic system. It is the resonances in the passive system that give the peaks in the spectrum envelope. Broadbent (1971) has presented another way of looking at the same facts: The resonances of a passive system correspond to carriers, which are modulated by pulses produced by the source. In speech, for instance, the separate cavities activated by the pulses from the vocal chords will have different frequencies but the same modulation frequency. To a large extent, these factors are independent. Timbre for vowels and many instruments is little affected by changes in source or modulation frequency with fixed formants, and greatly affected by changes in formant frequency (Slawson, 1968).

In order to describe the frequency characteristics of a stimulus, however, the best method may not necessarily be to present the relative SPLs of the individual harmonics. Plomp (1970) and Pols (1970) have argued that it would be more logical to take the limits of the ear's frequency-analyzing power into account and present spectra in the form of levels for frequency ranges roughly corresponding to critical bands only. Using m bandfilters, we can consider the SPLs in these bands as coordinates of a point in an m-dimensional Euclidian space. Experiments have therefore been made to determine if distances in the multidimensional physical space correspond to distances in a timbre space. A multidimensional scaling technique was applied to complex tones of equal loudness and pitch. The stimuli were single periods of vowels (Pols, Kamp, & Plomp, 1969) and various instruments (Plomp, 1970). The comparison between perceptual and physical space permitted the conclusion that differences in sound spectrum, measured in one-third octave bands, was a good first-order approximation of the physical correlate of timbre dissimilarity. For the further development of these concepts the reader is referred to a paper by Pols, Tromp, and Plomp (1973).

Another method for studying the dimensionality of timbre has been called the semantic differential. In this technique sounds are rated by the subjects on a number of bipolar scales, where the endpoints are characterized by opposite verbal attributes, such as sharp–dull, or rough–smooth. In one study von Bismarck (1974a,b) asked his subjects to rate 35 synthetic sounds along 30 scales. Factor analysis showed that four factors could almost completely account for the differences in timbre. On the other hand, only the dull–sharp scale, which accounted for the largest part of the variance, appeared to be suitable for the description of timbre in general. In its dependence on frequency composition, the attribute of sharpness showed a remarkable similarity to that of density (Guirao & Stevens, 1964), but sharpness, in contrast to density, appeared to be independent of loudness.

Strictly speaking, the preceding conclusions are valid only for the particular kind of stimuli employed, that is, complex tones of unvarying characteristics. For instrumental timbres the changes in spectral composition during the sounding of a note are very important (see Risset, Chapter 12, Section III,B). The two-dimensional Euclidian representation for the timbre of nine orchestral instruments obtained by Wessel (1973) suggests, according to the author, that one direction corresponds to a perceptual attribute determined by the rapidity with which low- and high-order harmonics reach full amplitude. The vertical direction might be interpreted as a perceptual attribute associated with the distribution of energy in the steady-state region of the spectrum. The use of natural instrumental tones in this study may explain why the similarities found by Wessel agree with our intuitive ideas far better than those in Plomp's experiment.

B. Fusion

Considering the number of studies devoted to the analysis of complex tones, it is highly surprising that so little attention has been directed to the question what makes certain combination of pure tones cohere, or fuse. A group of pure tones spaced at equal frequency distances that has a reasonably smooth spectral envelope will be perceived as a unit with a pitch corresponding to the spacing frequency and a timbre determined by the spectral envelope. With an irregular spacing, the unitary impression is lost. Changing the configuration from a regular to an irregular one, at which point does the complex begin to lose its unity? Slaymaker (1970) has reported some interesting observations on tones with partials having frequencies proportional to N^s, where N is the partial number and s is the stretch exponent. As s increases, the tone quality becomes notably different from true harmonic tones. By the time $s = 1.08$, the tone sounds somewhat bell- or chimelike, and for $s = 1.26$, the chime effect is quite pronounced. The same effect is obtained when the partials are compressed. The observations do not permit us to draw any firm conclusions as to the degree of unitariness of the percept, but it is obvious from listening to a tape recording of chords of stretched partial tones that for larger stretch exponents, all sense of unity for the individual "tone" is lost.

Another way of causing a unitary perception to disintegrate was described in an important study on fusion by Broadbent and Ladefoged (1957). The authors produced synthetic speech sounds by exciting resonant circuits with repetitive pulses. So long as the two formants had the same fundamental frequency, the subjects heard one voice only, but a different fundamental, or modulation, frequency made them all report two voices, or voicelike sounds. Fusion could even be achieved if formants with identical modulation frequency were fed to separate ears. Apparently, central mechanisms group together information from receptors sharing a single modulation frequency. Broadbent (1971) has argued that place mechanism will transmit information about the carrier frequencies that are present, that is the formants, whereas the frequency mechanism will convey information about the modulation frequency.

It is not certain, however, if we are allowed to regard the mechanisms for periodicity pitch and that of fusion as identical. Leakey, Sayers, and Cherry (1958) showed that am tones at 200 Hz would give a fused image if the carrier frequency in one ear was 4000 Hz and 4100 Hz in the other. We must expect, however, that the pitch in the latter, inharmonic, case was slightly higher than the harmonic periodicity pitch. We may compare these psychophysical results with the pulse-interval histogram obtained by Whitfield (1970) in recordings from the cochlear nucleus. His stimuli were carrier frequencies of 1200 and 1300 Hz amplitude modulated at 200 Hz. An envelope periodicity of 200 Hz was found also in the inharmonic case, where the pitch would be expected to be about 214 Hz. Whitfield's conclusion is that periodicity pitch does not depend on neural periodicity. Another possibility would be that envelope periodicity is related to the phenomenon of fusion and periodicity pitch—at most investigators in the field appear to believe at present—is related to the temporal fine structure.

C. Mixed Complex Sounds

The problem of how we can identify a sound in a mixture of sounds is central to auditory theory. Yet there is an almost complete absence of systematic studies or even speculation related to possible mechanisms of separate identification. On the other hand, the history of music can be said to constitute one vast experiment in auditory perception, from which at least one firm conclusion emerges: Music would be a meaningless activity if, in general, the constituent tones of chords are not in some sense separately perceived. This is not to say that ordinary listeners could be expected to be able to identify the notes in a complex chord, or that interaction phenomena among the tones are unimportant. But listeners who have an exceptionally acute sense of absolute pitch and thus can label their sensory impressions will correctly identify pitch and timbre of instruments in sustained orchestral chords. How can we explain this remarkable ability?

The timbre of a sound, as we have seen, largely depends on the distribution pattern of energy for its harmonics. Mixing of sounds will, consequently, result in a mixing of these distribution patterns. We nevertheless hear separate timbres instead of a new composite timbre, except for the case where the fundamentals are identical. In this case the timbres do lose their identity, as Broadbent and Ladefoged (1957) could show. The suggestion by the authors that the fusion of formants with a common fundamental is responsible for separate identification again appears to be the most likely one.

Helmholtz, who clearly realized that the separation of simultaneous sound sources constituted a serious problem for his theory, attributed identification of timbre to different starting times of the various instruments, melodic context, and similar extraneous factors. Nordmark (1970), however, pointed out that such factors cannot explain why the different sound qualities of am tones, square waves, or filtered pulse trains retain enough of their quality in a mixture to allow identification, even when all dynamic factors in the presentation of the tones are excluded. Stern (1972), working with synthetic instrumental timbres, has shown that it is possible to perceive two different timbres presented simultaneously, without external cues, such as melodic context, provided that the sounded notes are separate in frequency. Slaymaker's (1970) experiment, although primarily intended to show the influence of stretched partials on beats and dissonance perception, also makes it clear that identification of different instruments in a chord can be accomplished so long as the degree of stretching is small. With larger degrees of stretching it is no longer possible to identify timbre or pitch, or even, it appears to me, to say how many instruments are taking part.

Identification of the timbre of a sound in the presence of other sounds is thus apparently related to a periodicity common to a group of harmonics in a complex sound. Is the same true of perception of pitches in a complex-tone mixture? Strange as it may appear, it seems that no study has been made on how the pitch of a complex tone is influenced by the presence of one or more other complex tones. Again, of course, the literature of music indicates that discrimination is better than we could expect from experiments on pure tones. To take one musical example: Tschaikovsky's well-known *Pathétique* symphony opens with a passage for three instrumental parts moving within an approximate compass of 45 Hz in the 100-Hz area. We may recall that spearability for two simultaneous pure tones in this region is extremely poor. Yet this passage, while appropriately lugubrious, is always wholly intelligible.

In order to quantify the difference in discriminability, I had the two subjects taking part in the pure-tone experiment described earlier match the pitches of two simultaneous trains of short pulses with a pure tone. The task turned out to be so easy even for closely spaced tones that a criterion of better than 1% frequency deviation was adopted. When the complex tones had fundamental frequencies of 100 and 106 Hz, respectively, they could be matched with the required degree of accuracy. For this frequency region, discrimination for two complex tones is consequently at least 15 times better than that for pure tones. Obviously the dramatic improvement must be related to the presence of harmonics. But the maximum difference in frequency between any two harmonics of the complex tones in no case amounts to more than a fraction of the critical band or the frequency difference necessary for resolution of harmonics (see Fig. 3).

These findings suggested some further experiments. Would two simultaneous complex tones led through a filter passing frequencies within one critical band give rise to two separable periodicity pitches, and if so, how accurately would they be discriminated? The stimuli were filtered pulse trains whose fundamental frequencies were at a distance of a minor second and a major third, respectively. The critical-band filter was centered near 2000 Hz in order to permit a comparison with the results plotted for the discrimination of $\frac{1}{3}$-octave filtered pulses in Hoekstra's experiment. Although matching with a pure tone was used instead of a constant-stimulus method, the results for one subject when each tone was tested separately agreed on the whole with Hoekstra's curve, confirming his finding that discrimination deteriorates sharply as the harmonic constituents of the filtered pulse become increasingly high-numbered. When the pulse trains formed an interval of a minor second with the lower tone at 196 Hz (G_3), the spectrum obtained was that plotted in Fig. 8. In this case the relative DL for the higher tone was about .9%, and that for the lower tone about .8%. When the pulse trains formed a major third, the DL for the higher tone was .6%, whereas that for the lower was .4%. These values should be compared with the values of .5–1% reported by Ritsma (1963) for ordinary residue tones.

We can draw a number of conclusions from this experiment. As we have seen, a number of authors have suggested that the resolution of harmonics is a necessary condition for periodicity pitch. The hypothesis has been championed by adherents of a place theory of pitch as well as by workers leaning toward some form of a temporal mechanism. In no conceivable sense of the word, however, can the harmonics in Fig. 8 be said to be resolvable.

Furthermore, the critical band is commonly thought of as a nonreducible analytic unit, and it has been stated that spectral analysis with a bandwidth smaller than the critical bands of the ear makes no sense. Clearly, however, some sort of analysis can take place within one critical band.

These considerations have wider implications. As an explanation of periodicity pitch in terms of place theory no longer appears possible, the alternative temporal hypothesis, in particular in its fine-structure form, becomes increasingly likely. The DL for periodicity pitch should therefore be represented as least discriminable difference in time interval instead of in frequency. We then find that the temporal resolution required of the nervous system is in the microsecond range. Neural-fiber recordings of responses to

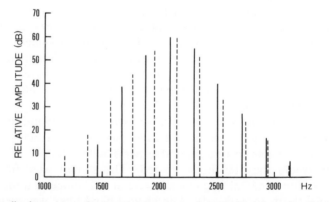

FIG. 8. Amplitude spectrum for two simultaneous pulse trains led through a filter of approximately one critical bandwidth. The dashed lines represent harmonics of a 196-Hz pulse train, and the solid line harmonics of a 209-Hz pulse train.

periodic stimuli do not show any such high degree of spike-interval precision. Both Whitfield (1967) and Nordmark (1968) have argued that there lies the real problem for a temporal theory of pitch. The alleged inability of the nervous system to follow higher frequencies is only a consequence of this imprecision.

The two authors have, however, drawn opposite conclusions from these facts: Whitfield (1967, 1970) that a temporal analysis for periodicity pitch, or pitch in general, is improbable; Nordmark (1968, 1970) that a temporal pitch mechanism for all frequencies is probable and that consequently, neurophysiological data in some way must be misleading. This could be the case, for instance, if the neural information from a group of identically stimulated neurons could be assumed to give a more accurate representation of the temporal structure of a stimulus than one single neuron. From what we know of neuronal mechanisms, it appears inherently unlikely that a single neuron could fire with the accuracy of a few microseconds, which the neuron system as a whole is capable of for the localization of a sound source. It seems more likely that the individual neurons of the different sensory modalities can achieve only limited accuracy, and that precision is brought about through the interaction of a larger number of neurons. It is perhaps significant that the interval and cycle histograms from responses to a stimulus of about 200 Hz show similar temporal variability when recorded from a fiber innervating the subcutaneous tissue of the monkey hand (Talbot, Darian-Smith, Kornhuber, & Mountcastle, 1968) or a single unit in the monkey cochlear nucleus (Rose, Brugge, Anderson, & Hind, 1967). Nevertheless, at this frequency the DL for pitch (Nordmark, 1968) and vibration frequency (Franzén & Nordmark, 1975) differ by a factor 20. Conceivably the larger number or the organization of the neurons involved in auditory discrimination could explain the greater precision.

There is a further implication of the experiment with filtered pulses. We saw in the section on the selectivity of the ear (Section II,C) that place and frequency theorists have always presupposed, or implied separate representation of pitch in the nerve or group of nerves that carry pitch information. In my view, the elevation of this assumption to unchallenged dogma has been the single most important mistake of auditory theory. We may assume, however, that the successful mixing of temporal information with critical-band-filtered pulses is typical for the behavior of the auditory system in the situations where sounds are presented simultaneously. It is interesting to note that two or more filtered pulse trains exhibit the phenomena of beats and consonances. There is a very strong feeling of consonance when a major triad is put through a narrow-band filter, and a corresponding sense of dissonance for dissonant chords. As these differences exist even for sounds where the energy is limited to one critical band, the hypothesis of Plomp and Levelt (1965) on the nature of consonance and dissonance must at least be modified.

References

Albert, K. Die Schwebung 15:16 im Innenohr nach Ort und Zeit. *Zeitschrift für Biologie,* 1951, **104,** 321–336.

Allanson, J. T., & Whitfield, I. C. The cochlear nucleus and its relation to theories of hearing. In C. Cherry (Ed.), *Third London Symposium on information theory.* London: Butterworth, 1956. Pp. 269–286.

Békésy, G. von. Über die Resonanzkurve und die Abklingzeit der verschiedenen Stellen der Schneckentrennwand. *Akustische Zeitschrift,* 1943, **8,** 66–76.

Békésy, G. von. The missing fundamental and periodicity detection in hearing. *Journal of the Acoustical Society of America,* 1972, **51,** 631–637.

Bismarck, G. von. Timbre of steady sounds: A factorial investigation of its verbal attributes. *Acustica,* 1974, **30,** 146–159. (a)

Bismarck, G. von. Sharpness as an attribute of the timbre of steady sounds. *Acustica,* 1974, **30,** 159–172. (b)

Broadbent, D. E. *Decision and stress.* New York: Academic Press, 1971.

Broadbent, D. E., & Ladefoged, P. On the fusion of sounds reaching different sense organs. *Journal of the Acoustical Society of America,* 1957, **29,** 708–710.

Brugge, J. F., Anderson, D. J., Hind, J. E., & Rose, J. E. Time structure of discharges in single auditory nerve fibers of the squirrel monkey in response to complex periodic sounds. *Journal of Neurophysiology,* 1969, **32,** 386–401.

Cardozo, B. L., & Neelen, J. J. M. Frequentie-analyse en maskering. I.P.O. Report No. 104, 1967.

Carterette, E., Friedman, M. P., & Lovell, J. D. Mach bands in hearing. *Journal of the Acoustical Society of America,* 1969, **45,** 986–998.

de Boer, E. One the residue in hearing. Unpublished Ph.D. dissertation, Univ. Amsterdam, 1956.

de Boer, E. Correlation studies applied to the frequency resolution of the cochlea. *Journal of Auditory Research,* 1967, **7,** 209–217.

Duifhuis, H. Audibility of high harmonics in a periodic pulse. *Journal of the Acoustical Society of America,* 1970, **48,** 888–893.

Duifhuis, H. Perceptual analysis of sound. Unpublished Ph.D. dissertation, Eindhoven Techn. Highschool, 1972.

Ekdahl, A. G., & Boring, E. G. The pitch of tonal masses. *American Journal of Psychology,* 1934, **46,** 452–455.

Evans, E. F., & Wilson, J. P. The frequency selectivity of the cochlea. In A. R. Møller (Ed.), *Basic mechanisms in hearing.* New York: Academic Press, 1973. Pp. 519–554.

Feth, L. L., Wolf, R. V., & Bilger, R. C. Frequency modulation and the difference limen for frequency. *Journal of the Acoustical Society of America,* 1969, **45,** 1430–1437.

Flanagan, J. L. Models for approximating basilar membrane displacement—Part II. *Bell System Technical Journal,* 1962, **41,** 959–1009.

Fleischer, H. Über die Wahrnehmbarkeit von Phasenänderungen. *Acustica,* 1976, **35,** 202–209.

Franzén, O., & Nordmark, J. O. Vibrotactile frequency discrimination. *Perception & Psychophysics,* 1975, **17,** 480–484.

Geisler, C. D., Rhode, W. S., & Kennedy, D. T. Responses of squirrel monkey auditory-nerve fibers to tones. *Journal of the Acoustical Society of America,* 1973, **54,** 282(A).

Gibson, L. The ear as an analyzer of musical tones. *Journal of the Acoustical Society of America,* 1971, **49,** 127(A).

Glattke, T. J. Unit responses of the cat cochlear nucleus to amplitude-modulated stimuli. *Journal of the Acoustical Society of America,* 1969, **45,** 419–425.

Goldstein, J. L. Auditory spectral filtering and monaural phase perception. *Journal of the Acoustical Society of America*, 1967, **41**, 458–479.

Guirao, M., and Stevens, S. S. Measurement of auditory density. *Journal of the Acoustical Society of America*, 1964, **36**, 1176.

Helmholtz, H. von *Die Lehre von den Tonempfindungen*. Braunschweig: F. Vieweg u. Sohn, 1863.

Hoekstra, A. Het frekwentie analyserend vermogen van het gehoor en het tonale residu. Audiological Institute, Groningen, Report, April, 1973.

Houtsma, A. J. M. What determines musical pitch? *Journal of Music Theory*, 1971, **15**, 138–157.

Houtsma, A. J. M., & Goldstein, J. L. Perception of musical intervals: evidence for the central origin of the pitch of complex tones. *M.I.T. Quarterly Progress Report*, No. 484, 1971.

Houtsma, A. J. M., & Goldstein, J. L. The central origin of the pitch of complex tones from musical interval recognition. *Journal of the Acoustical Society of America*, 1972, **51**, 520–529.

Johansson, G. Visual event perception. In *Handbook of sensory physiology*. (In preparation).

Johnstone, B. M., & Boyle, A. F. J. Basilar membrane vibration examined with the Mössbauer technique. *Science*, 1967, **158**, 389–390.

Johnstone, B. M., Taylor, K. J., & Boyle, A. F. J. Mechanics of the guinea pig cochlea. *Journal of the Acoustical Society of America*, 1970, **47**, 504–509.

Kameoka, A., & Kuriyagawa, M. Consonance theory, part 1: Consonance of dyads. *Journal of the Acoustical Society of America*, 1969, **45**, 1451–1459.

Kiang, N. Y. S., & Moxon, E. C. Tails of tuning curves of auditory-nerve fibers. *Journal of the Acoustical Society of America*, 1973, **54**, 274–275(A).

Kneser, H. O. Bemerkungen über Definition und Messung der Frequenz. *Archiv der Elektrischen Übertragung*, 1948, **2**, 167–169.

Köhler, W. Tonpsychologie. In G. Alexander & O. Marburg (Eds.), *Handbuch der Neurologie des Ohres*. Vol. 1. Berlin: Urban und Schwarzenberg, 1923.

Korn, T. S. La notion de la fréquence du son. *Acustica*, 1968, **20**, 55–61.

Lamoré, P. J. J. Perception of two-tone octave complexes. *Acustica*, 1975, **34**, 1–14.

Leakey, D. M., Sayers, B. Mca., & Cherry, C. Binaural fusion of low- and high-frequency sound. *Journal of the Acoustical Society of America*, 1958, **30**, 222.

Licklider, J. C. R. 'Periodicity' pitch and 'place' pitch. *Journal of the Acoustical Society of America*, 1954, **26**, 945(A).

Maronn, E. Untersuchungen zur Wahrnemung sekundärer Tonqualitäten bei ganzzahligen Schwingungsverhältnissen. *Kölner Beiträge zur Musikforschung*, 1964, **30**, 1–102.

Mathes, R. C., & Miller, R. L. Phase effects in monaural phase perception. *Journal of the Acoustical Society of America*, 1947, **19**, 780–797.

McClelland, K. D., & Brandt, J. F. Pitch of frequency-modulated sinusoids. *Journal of the Acoustical Society of America*, 1969, **45**, 1489–1498.

Meyer-Eppler, W., Sendhoff, H., & Rupprath, R. Residual tone and formant tone. *Gravesaner Blätter*, 1959, **4**, 70–91.

Miller, G. A., & Taylor, W. G. The perception of repeated bursts of noise. *Journal of the Acoustical Society of America*, 1948, **20**, 171–182.

Møller, A. R. Studies of the damped oscillatory response of the auditory frequency analyzer. *Acta Physiologica Scandinavica*, 1970, **78**, 299–314.

Møller, A. R. Coding of sounds in lower levels of the auditory system. *Quarterly Review of Biophysics*, 1972, **5**, 59–155.

Moore, B. C. J. Audibility of partials in a complex tone in relation to the pitch of the complex as a whole. In *Symposium on hearing theory*. Eindhoven: Institute for Perception Research, 1972. Pp. 96–104.

Nordmark, J. Perception of distance in animal echo-location. *Nature,* 1960, **188,** 1009–1010.
Nordmark, J. O. Some analogies between pitch and lateralization phenomena. *Journal of the Acoustical Society of America,* 1963, **35,** 1544–1547.
Nordmark, J. O. Mechanisms of frequency discrimination. *Journal of the Acoustical Society of America,* 1968, **44,** 1533–1540.
Nordmark, J. O. Time and frequency analysis. In J. Tobias (Ed.), *Foundations of modern auditory theory.* New York: Academic Press. 1970. Pp. 55–83.
Nordmark, J. O., Glattke, T. J., & Schubert, E. D. Waveform preservation in the cochlea. *Journal of the Acoustical Society of America,* 1969, **46,** 1587–1588.
Ohm, G. S., Über die Definition des Tones. *Annalen der Physik und Chemie,* 1843, **59,** 513–565.
Patterson, R. D. Noise masking of a change in residue pitch. *Journal of the Acoustical Society of America,* 1969, **45,** 1520–1524.
Patterson, R. D. The effects of relative phase and the number of components on residue pitch. *Journal of the Acoustical Society of America,* 1973, **53,** 1565–1572.
Plomp, R. The ear as a frequency analyzer. *Journal of the Acoustical Society of America,* 1964, **36,** 1628–1636.
Plomp, R. Experiments on tone perception. Unpublished Ph.D. dissertation, Univ. of Utrecht, 1966.
Plomp, R. Beats of mistuned consonances. *Journal of the Acoustical Society of America,* 1967, **42,** 462–474.
Plomp, R. Pitch, timbre, and hearing theory. *International Audiology,* 1968, **7,** 322–344.
Plomp, R. Timbre as a multidimensional attribute of complex tones. In R. Plomp & G. F. Smorrenburg (Eds.), *Frequency analysis and periodicity detection in hearing.* Leiden: A. W. Sijthoff. 1970. Pp. 397–411.
Plomp, R. Old and new data on tone perception. In W. D. Neff (Ed.), *Contributions to sensory physiology.* New York: Academic Press. 1971. Pp. 179–220.
Plomp, R., & Levelt, W. J. M. Tonal consonance and critical bandwidth. *Journal of the Acoustical Society of America,* 1965, **38,** 548–560.
Plomp, R., & Mimpen, A. M. The ear as a frequency analyzer. II. *Journal of the Acoustical Society of America,* 1968, **43,** 764–767.
Plomp, R., & Steeneken, H. J. M. Interference between two simple tones. *Journal of the Acoustical Society of America,* 1968, **43,** 883–884.
Plomp, R., & Steeneken, H. J. M. Effect of phase on the timbre of complex tones. *Journal of the Acoustical Society of America,* 1969, **46,** 409–421.
Pollack, I. Periodicity pitch for interrupted white noise—fact or artifact? *Journal of the Acoustical Society of America,* 1969, **45,** 237–238.
Pols, L. C. W. Perceptual space of vowel-like sounds and its correlation with frequency spectrum. In R. Plomp & G. F. Smorrenburg (Eds.), *Frequency analysis and periodicity detection in hearing.* Leiden: A. W. Sijthoff. 1970. Pp. 463–473.
Pols, L. C. W., Kamp, L. J. T. van der, & Plomp, R. Perceptual and physical space of vowel sounds. *Journal of the Acoustical Society of America,* 1969, **46,** 458–467.
Pols, L. C. W., Tromp, H. R. C., & Plomp, R. Frequency analysis of Dutch vowels from 50 male speakers. *Journal of the Acoustical Society of America,* 1973, **53,** 1093–1101.
Rainbolt, H., & Small, A. M. Mach bands in auditory masking: An attempted replication. *Journal of the Acoustical Society of America,* 1972, **51,** 567–574.
Reed, C. M., & Bilger R. C. A comparative study of S/N and E/No. *Journal of the Acoustical Society of America,* 1973, 1039–1044.
Rhode, W. S. Observations of the vibration of the basilar membrane in squirrel monkeys using the Mössbauer technique. *Journal of the Acoustical Society of America,* 1971, **49,** 1218–1231.
Ritsma, R. J. Existence region of the tonal residue I. *Journal of the Acoustical Society of America,* 1962, **34,** 1224–1229.

Ritsma, R. J. Existence region of the tonal residue II. *Journal of the Acoustical Society of America*, 1963, **35**, 1241–1245.

Ritsma, R. J. Frequencies dominant in the perception of the pitch of complex sounds. *Journal of the Acoustical Society of America*, 1967, **42**, 191–198.

Ritsma, R. J., & Engel, F. L. Pitch of frequency-modulated singals. *Journal of the Acoustical Society of America*, 1964, **36**, 1637–1644.

Rose, J. E., Brugge, J. F., Anderson, D. J., & Hind, J. E. Phase-locked responses to low-frequency tones in single auditory nerve fibers of the squirrel monkey. *Journal of Neurophysiology*, 1967, **30**, 679–793.

Rose, J. E., Hind, J. E., Anderson, D. J., & Brugge, J. F. Some effects of stimulus intensity on response of auditory nerve fibers in the squirrel monkey. *Journal of Neurophysiology*, 1971, **34**, 685–699.

Schouten, J. F. The perception of subjective tones. *Proceedings of the Koninklijke Nederlandse Akademie van Wetenschappen*, 1938, **41**, 1086–1093.

Schouten, J. F. The residue and the mechanism of hearing. *Proceedings of the Koninklijke Nederlandsche Akademie van Wetenschappen*, 1940, **43**, 991–999.(a)

Schouten, J. F. The perception of pitch. *Philips Technical Review*, 1940, **5**, 286–294.(b)

Schouten, J. F., Ritsma, R. J., & Cardozo, B. L. Pitch of the residue. *Journal of the Acoustical Society of America*, 1962, **34**, 1418–1424.

Schroeder, M. R. Model for phase perception of complex tones. *Journal of the Acoustical Society of America*, 1970, **48**, 70(A).

Seebeck, A. Beobachtungen über einige Bedingungen der Entstehung von Tönen. *Annalen der Physik und Chemie*, 1841, **53**, 417–436.

Slawson, A. W. Vowel quality and musical timbre as functions of spectrum envelope and fundamental frequency. *Journal of the Acoustical Society of America*, 1968, **43**, 87–101.

Slaymaker, F. H. Chords from tones having stretched partials. *Journal of the Acoustical Society of America*, 1970, **47**, 1569–1571.

Small, A. M. Some parameters influencing the pitch of amplitude modulated signals. *Journal of the Acoustical Society of America*, 1955, **27**, 751–760.

Small, A. M. Periodicity pitch. In J. V. Tobias (Ed.), *Foundations of modern auditory theory*. Vol. 1. New York: Academic Press. 1970. Pp. 3–54.

Small, A. M., & Campbell, R. A. Masking of pulsed tones by bands of noise. *Journal of the Acoustical Society of America*, 1961, **33**, 1570–1576.

Small, A. M., & Yelen, R. D. Fatigue as an indicator of pitch channels. *Journal of the Acoustical Society of America*, 1962, **34**, 1987(A).

Smoorenburg, G. F. Pitch perception of two-frequency stimuli. *Journal of the Acoustical Society of America*, 1970, **48**, 924–942.

Soderquist, D. R. Frequency analysis and the critical band. *Psychonomic Science*, 1970, **21**, 117–119.

Stern, R. M. Perception of simultaneously presented musical timbres. *M.I.T. Quarterly Progress Report*, No. 106, 1972.

Stevens, S. S., & Davis, H. *Hearing, its psychology and physiology*. New York: Wiley, 1938.

Stumpf, C. *Die Sprachlaute*. Berlin: J. Springer. 1926.

Talbot, W. H., Darian-Smith, I., Kornhuber, H. H., & Mountcastle, V. B. The sense of flutter-vibration: Comparison of the capacity with the response patterns of mechano-receptive afferents from the monkey hand. *Journal of Neurophysiology*, 1968, **31**, 301–334.

Terhardt, E. Über die durch amplitudenmodulierte Sinustöne hervorgerufen Hörempfindung. *Acustica*, 1968, **20**, 210–214.(a)

Terhardt, E. Über akustische Rauhigkeit und Schwankungsstärke. *Acustica*, 1968, **20**, 215–224.(b)

Terhardt, E. Zur Tonhöhenwahrnehmung von Klängen II. Ein Funktionsschema. *Acustica*, 1972, **26**, 187–199.

Thurlow, W. R. Perception of low auditory pitch: A multicue mediation theory. *Psychological Review*, 1963, **70**, 461–470.

Thurlow, W. R., & Small, A. M. Pitch perception for certain periodic auditory stimuli. *Journal of the Acoustical Society of America*, 1955, **27**, 132–137.

Van den Brink, G. Two experiments on pitch perception: Diplacusis of harmonic AM signals and pitch of inharmonic AM signals. *Journal of the Acoustical Society of America*, 1970, **48**, 1355–1365.

Vogel, A. "Über den Zusammenhang zwischen Rauhigkeit und Modulationsgrad", *Acustica*, 1975, **32**, 300–306.

Walliser, K. Zusammanhänge zwischen dem Schallreiz und der Periodentonhöhe. *Acustica*, 1969, **21**, 319–329.

Wessel, D. L. Psychoacoustics and music. *Bulletin of Computer Arts Society*, 1973.

Wever, E. G. Beats and related phenomena resulting from the simultaneous sounding of two tones. *Psychological Review*, 1929, **36**, 402–523.

Whitfield, I. C. *The auditory pathway*. London: Arnold, 1967.

Whitfield, I. C. Central nervous processing in relation to spatio-temporal discrimination of auditory patterns. In R. Plomp & G. F. Smorrenburg (Eds.), *Frequency analysis and periodicity detection in hearing*. Leiden: A. W. Sijthoff. 1970. Pp. 136–152.

Wilson, J. P., & Evans, E. F. Grating acuity of the ear: psychophysical and neurophysiological measures of frequency resolving power. *Proceedings of 7th International Congress of Acoustics*, Vol. 3. Akademiai Kiado, Budapest 1971. Pp. 393–400.

Zener, K., & Gaffron, M. Perceptual experience: An analysis of its relation to the external world through internal processing. In S. Koch (Ed.), *Psychology: A study of a science*. Vol. 4. New York: McGraw-Hill, 1962. Pp. 515–618.

Zwicker, E. Die Grenzen der Hörbarkeit der Amplitudenmodulation und der Frequenzmodulation eines Tones. *Acustica*, 1952, **2**, (Beiheft 3), 125–133.

Zwicker, E. Temporal effects in simultaneous masking and loudness. *Journal of the Acoustical Society of America*, J. acoust. 1965, **38**, 132–141.

Zwicker, E., Flottorp, G., & Stevens, S. S. Critical band width in loudness summation. *Journal of the Acoustical Society of America*, 1957, **29**, 548–557.

Zwislocki, J. J. A possible neuro-mechanical sound analysis in the cochlea. *Acustica*, 1974, **31**, 354–359.

Chapter 8

MASKING: EXPERIMENTAL AND THEORETICAL ASPECTS OF SIMULTANEOUS, FORWARD, BACKWARD, AND CENTRAL MASKING

J. J. ZWISLOCKI

I. INTRODUCTION

Auditory masking may be defined as decreased audibility of one sound due to the presence of another. The term *partial masking* is used for situations where the masked sound is clearly audible, but its loudness is decreased. This chapter addresses itself to total masking, the magnitude of which is determined by means of detection measurements. Usually, the intensity of a test stimulus is varied so as to produce a criterion probability of detection. This is done once in the presence of and again in the absence of the masking sound, or *masker*. The difference between the two intensity levels so obtained, often called *threshold shift,* is taken as a measure of the masking effect.

Originally, the concept of masking was applied to situations in which the masking and masked sounds occurred simultaneously. But numerous experiments showed that sounds decreased the audibility of other, weaker sounds that just followed or just preceded them. The term *masking* was extended to these effects, and currently, the term *forward masking* is applied to stimuli following the masking sound, and the term *backward masking,* to stimuli preceding it.

The definition of masking is strictly operational, and should not imply any

HANDBOOK OF PERCEPTION, VOL. IV

specific physiological process. In fact, it will be pointed out later that forward masking probably results from at least two processes and that the same seems to be true of backward masking. Even simultaneous masking appears to be a complex phenomenon.

Although we seem to be far removed from a general theory of masking processes, it appears reasonable to accept the view of the psychophysical theory of signal detection (Green & Swets, 1966) that masking results from the inherent difficulty in detecting a signal in the presence of a randomly varying amplitude of the masker. Under many conditions, the variance of this amplitude is directly proportional to the average power of the masker, and the detectability of a test sound, or signal, remains constant for a constant ratio between the powers of the test and masking sounds, often called *constant signal-to-noise ratio*. Although the detection-theory concept of masking is most easily understood when the masker consists of a random noise, it appears to remain basically valid even for deterministic maskers. This is so because of the probabilistic response of the nervous system to deterministic stimuli. Experiments show that even when the masker consists of a sinusoid, the signal-to-masker ratio remains approximately constant for constant detection under certain experimental conditions. A more specific use of this concept is made in further sections of this chapter.

Perhaps more auditory experiments have been performed on masking than on any other auditory phenomenon. Masking experiments are reasonably straightforward, and their popularity seems to be supported by the belief that masking characteristics reflect in a reasonably simple way various internal characteristics of the auditory system. This has been particularly true for simultaneous, monaural masking experiments in which the masking and test sounds are delivered to the same ear, and for binaural masking experiments in which the masking and test sounds are delivered to both ears under various phase and intensity combinations. The variety of masking experiments makes it impossible to include all aspects of masking phenomena in one chapter. This chapter is limited to some fundamental characteristics of monaural masking—simultaneous, forward, and backward; furthermore to some aspects of central masking that occurs when the masker is introduced to one ear, the test sound to the other, and acoustic leakage between the two ears is prevented. Central masking does not seem to have been included in any previous handbook on a systematic basis. Although its effect is quite small, it is of interest, since it results from a strictly neural interaction between the two stimuli.

In a final section of the chapter, a few theoretical considerations of simultaneous monaural and simultaneous central masking are discussed. According to these considerations, certain characteristics of monaural masking are consistent with the sensory power transformation proposed by S. S. Stevens (1962), but monaural masking does not give any unequivocal information about internal characteristics of the auditory system. On the other hand, it appears that central-masking characteristics are related in a simple way to certain processes in the peripheral and low central auditory system.

II. EXPERIMENTAL RESULTS

A. Monaural Simultaneous Masking

1. MASKING BY WIDE-BAND NOISE

Simultaneous monaural masking depends on many stimulus parameters. Their number is minimized when broad-band random noise is masked by a noise with an identical frequency spectrum. In a classical experiment, Miller (1947) investigated the detectability of such a noise with an approximately uniform frequency spectrum, when it was added to a background noise from the same noise generator. In fact, Miller modulated the amplitude of the noise according to a rectangular time pattern. Since the signal to be detected and the background stimulus were identical and coherent, his procedure resembled that of experiments on just noticeable differences (jnd's) rather than on masking. Accordingly, the original data were plotted in the jnd form. They are shown in Fig. 1.

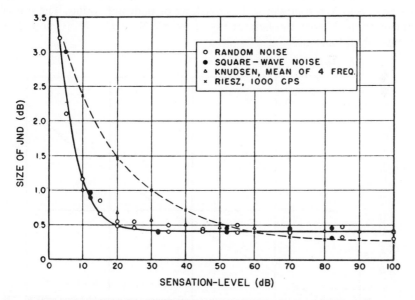

FIG. 1. Intensity increments of wide-band random noise detected 50% of the time, as a function of the noise SL. For comparison, analogous results obtained with different sound stimuli are shown. Note that jnd's obtained with a nearly sinusoidally modulated 1000-Hz tone (Riesz) differ from jnd's obtained with stimuli having broad frequency spectra. [From Miller (1947). By permission of the Acoustical Society of America.]

In order to make Miller's results comparable with other masking experiments, a recalculation of his data is necessary. When a signal is added to a coherent pedestal, the ratio between the total power and the background power amounts to

$$D_1 = (P + \Delta_1 P)^2/P^2, \tag{1}$$

where P denotes the pedestal sound pressure, and ΔP the just noticeable incremental sound pressure. This ratio is plotted in Fig. 1. When the signal and the masking noise are not coherent, the ratio becomes

$$D_2 = (P^2 + \Delta_2^2 P)/P^2, \tag{2}$$

with $\Delta_2 P$ meaning the just noticeable increment under the modified conditions. For equal ratios, $D_2 = D_1$, so that

$$(P^2 + \Delta_2^2 P)/P^2 = (P^2 + \Delta_1^2 P + 2P\Delta_1 P)/P^2, \tag{3}$$

and

$$\Delta_2^2 P/P^2 = (\Delta_1^2 P + 2P\Delta_1 P)/P^2. \tag{4}$$

This relationship may be expressed in decibels as follows

$$10 \log(S_M/N) = 10 \log[S_D/N + 2(S_D/N)^{1/2}], \tag{5}$$

where S_M is the power of the noncoherent signal, S_D the power of the coherent signal, and N the power of the masking or pedestal sound. The conversion can be made with the help of Fig. 2, where $10 \log(S_M/N)$ is plotted as a function of $10 \log(S_D/N)$.

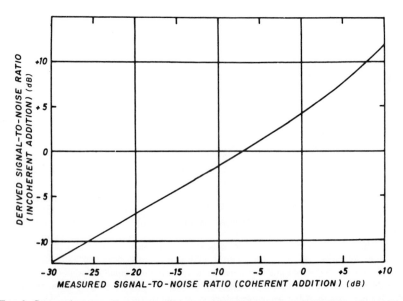

FIG. 2. Conversion curve between coherent and noncoherent sound additions. [From Bos and de Boer (1966). By permission of the Acoustical Society of America.]

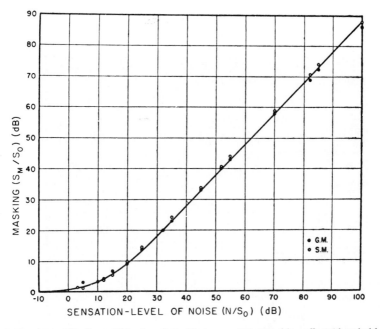

FIG. 3. Random-noise data of Fig. 1 replotted in terms of the masking effect (threshold shift). The curve is derived from the data of Hawkins and Stevens (1950). [From Miller (1947). By permission of the Acoustical Society of America.]

At pedestal sensation levels (SL) greater than about 20 dB, Miller obtained an approximately constant signal-to-noise ratio on the order of -25 dB. This is equivalent to about -12 dB for noncoherent summation. Miller's results converted to noncoherent summation are shown in Fig. 3. They are expressed in terms of $10 \log(S_M/S_0)$ as a function of $10 \log(N/S_0)$, where S_0 means the threshold signal power in the absence of the masker. At SLs exceeding 20 dB, the masked threshold is directly proportional to the masker power, so that

$$10 \log(S_M/S_0) = 10 \log(N/S_0) + 10 \log M , \qquad (6)$$

with $M = S_M/N$.

When the masker consists of broad-band noise but the test signal is limited to a narrow band or even one spectral line, two additional degrees of freedom are introduced—the center frequency and the bandwidth of the test signal. The classical experiments for such stimulus conditions were performed by Hawkins and Stevens (1950), who masked pure tones by a broad-band random noise of approximately uniform spectral power. As in masking of broad-band noise by broad-band noise, the signal-to-noise ratio remained independent of noise SL for constant detection, except at very low levels. However, the numerical value of the ratio varied with the test fre-

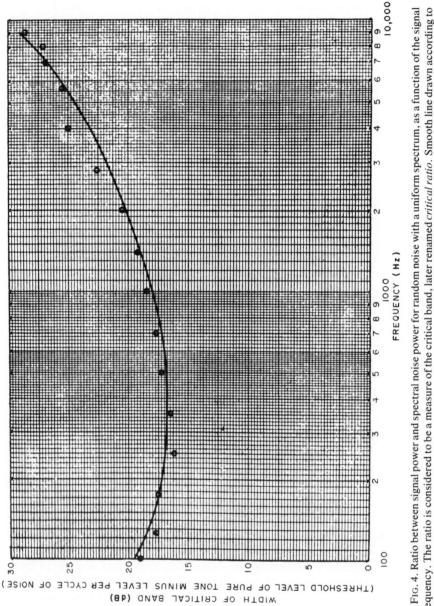

FIG. 4. Ratio between signal power and spectral noise power for random noise with a uniform spectrum, as a function of the signal frequency. The ratio is considered to be a measure of the critical band, later renamed *critical ratio*. Smooth line drawn according to measurements at the Bell Telephone Laboratories. [From Hawkins and Stevens (1950). By permission of the Acoustical Society of America.]

quency, as shown in Fig. 4. The signal-to-noise ratio is expressed here in terms of spectral power, i.e.,

$$M_S(f) = S_M(f)/N_S, \tag{7}$$

where $S_M(f)$ means the signal power as a function of sound frequency, and N_S, the noise power per cycle.

Hawkins and Stevens interpreted their results according to Fletcher's (1940) hypothesis that the auditory system functions as a bank of parallel bandpass filters. The bandwidth of these filters was assumed to be such that, at the masked threshold, the ratio between the signal power and the noise power in each filter remained constant. Fletcher also postulated that this ratio was equal to one. Accordingly, the masking ratio $M_S(f)$ became a measure of the filter bandwidth. In Fig. 4, the bandwidth is plotted in terms of decibels:

$$10 \log M_S(f) = 10 \log S_M(f)/S_0 - 10 \log N_S/S_0, \tag{8}$$

where S_0 means a reference level. The minimum bandwidth is shown to be located around 400 Hz and to amount to 50 Hz. At 9000 Hz, it increases to 950 Hz. In general, the bandwidth remains reasonably constant up to 500 Hz and becomes nearly proportional to the center frequency above 1000 Hz.

Hawkins and Stevens' results are in good agreement with results obtained by Fletcher's group, as indicated in Fig. 4. They have since been confirmed repeatedly. However, the numerical values included in Fletcher's assumption of auditory filters had to be modified. Feldtkeller and Zwicker (1956) and their co-workers found by means of a large number of experiments dealing not only with masking but also with other auditory phenomena that the auditory filter bandwidth was about 2.5 times greater. Nevertheless, the dependence of the bandwidth on center frequency remained almost the same. These results have been confirmed and extended in experiments performed at Harvard by Zwicker, Flottorp, and Stevens (1957), and by Scharf (1959). They changed the name of the filter bandwidth derived by Fletcher from *critical band* to *critical ratio* and transferred the critical-band designation to the modified bandwidth.

The critical band as a function of center frequency is tabulated in Table I and plotted in Fig. 5. For comparison, the critical ratio and the frequency jnd are also shown in the figure. The jnd curve is almost exactly parallel to the critical-band curve. The same is approximately true for the critical ratio curve, except at low frequencies. As has been discussed elsewhere (Zwislocki, 1965), the critical band and the jnd curves are approximately parallel to the pitch function. They all appear to follow the location of the vibration maximum in the cochlea. The agreement is particularly close when distances along the cochlear spiral are weighted by the density of corresponding innervation. According to Wever (1949), the density of the ganglion-cell population in the spiral ganglion, as projected longitudinally on the basilar mem-

TABLE I

CRITICAL BANDWIDTHS AT THE INDICATED CENTER FREQUENCIES[a]

ΔF	Center and cutoff frequencies		ΔF
	20		
90		65	
	110		90
90		155	
	200		95
95		250	
	295		95
100		345	
	395		105
108		450	
	503		110
120		560	
	625		130
130		690	
	755		140
145		830	
	900		150
160		980	
	1,060		175
190		1,155	
	1,250		200
210		1,355	
	1,460		225
240		1,580	
	1,700		255
270		1,835	
	1,970		295
320		2,130	
	2,290		350
380		2,480	
	2,670		420
450		2,900	
	3,120		500
560		3,400	
	3,680		620
680		4,020	
	4,360		760
840		4,780	
	5,200		920
1,000		5,700	
	6,200		1,150
1,300		6,850	
	7,500		1,550
1,800		8,400	
	9,300		2,100
2,400		10,500	
	11,700		2,800
3,300		13,300	
	15,000		4,000
	17,300		

[a] From Zwicker et al. (1957).

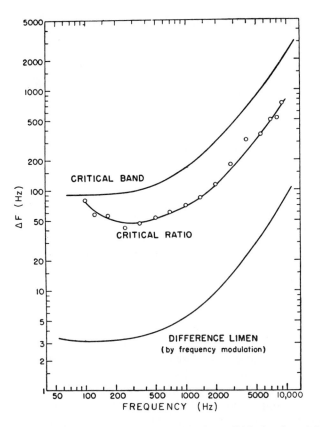

FIG. 5. Critical bandwidth as a function of center frequency. Critical-ratio and frequency-jnd data are shown for comparison. [From Zwicker *et al.* (1957). By permission of the Acoustical Society of America.]

brane, is greatest in the midsections of the cochlea and smallest near the apex. The neural scale compresses the cochlear distances somewhat in the sections responding maximally to low frequencies.

The critical band and related auditory functions can be described rather accurately by the following empirical equation (Zwislocki, 1965):

$$W_C(f) = Af^{1.5} + W_1. \tag{9}$$

For the critical-band function, $A = 2 \cdot 10^{-3}$ (sec$^{-.5}$) and $W_1 = 10^2$ (sec^{-1}). The masking ratio can now be defined in terms of

$$M_C(f) = S_M(f)/N_C(f), \tag{10}$$

with $N_C(f) = N_S W_C(f)$ denoting the noise power per critical band. If the critical band were directly proportional to the critical ratio, the masking ratio $M_C(f)$ would have to be constant. However, according to Zwicker and

Feldtkeller (1967), and others, it decreases slightly as the bandwidth increases. It may be approximated by

$$M_C(f) = BW_C^\alpha(f), \tag{11}$$

where $B \simeq 1/2.5$ and $\alpha \simeq -.3$. By rewriting Eq. (10) with reference to the threshold in the absence of masking noise, we obtain

$$S_M(f)/S_0(f) = M_C(f)N_C(f)/S_0(f) \tag{12}$$

or, introducing the appropriate expressions for $N_C(f)$ and $M_C(f)$, and also $W_C(f)$,

$$S_M(f)/S_0(f) = [B(Af^{1.5} + W_1)^{1+\alpha}N_S]/S_0(f). \tag{13}$$

Accordingly, the threshold shift produced by broad-band noise with a uniform spectrum should grow as

$$10 \log[S_M(f)/S_0(f)] = (1 + \alpha)\ 10 \log(Af^{1.5} + W_1)$$
$$+ 10 \log[BN_S/S_0(f)] \tag{14}$$

and should depend on frequency somewhat less than does the critical band, since $\alpha < 1$. In practice, experimental variability tends to obscure the difference. The signal-to-noise ratio changes by only about 4 dB, from $M_C(f) \simeq -2$ dB at low frequencies to $M_C(f) \simeq -6$ dB at high frequencies (Zwicker & Feldtkeller, 1967), the exact values depending on experimental conditions.

The numerical relationships discussed thus far concern masker SLs at which the signal-to-noise ratio remains approximately constant. As is evident in Figs. 1 and 3, this does not hold at low levels. The departure was already observed by Fechner (cit. Miller, 1947) and was emphasized by Miller (1947). It may be accounted for by assuming an intrinsic masking noise whose effective power is added arithmetically to the power of the extrinsic noise. With this correction, the masking equations (7) and (10) become

$$M_S(f) = S_M(f)/[N_S(f) + N_{IS}(f)] \tag{15}$$

and

$$M_C(f) = S_M(f)/[N_C(f) + N_{IC}(f)], \tag{16}$$

respectively, with N_{IS} indicating the intrinsic noise per cycle, and N_{IC}, per critical band. The correction implies that the threshold in the absence of extrinsic noise is itself a masked threshold. For $N_C(f) = 0$,

$$S_0(f) = M_C(f)N_{IC}(f). \tag{17}$$

If $M_C(f)$ is assumed to be independent of SL, the effective intrinsic noise may be calculated from threshold measurements (Zwislocki, 1965):

$$N_{IC}(f) = S_0(f)/M_C(f). \tag{18}$$

At medium audible frequencies, where $M_C \simeq .4$, it appears to exceed the threshold of audibility by 4 dB.

The signal-to-noise ratio of -12 dB obtained by Miller for a broad-band noise masked by a broad-band noise disagrees with the ratio obtained by Hawkins and Stevens and by others for pure tones masked by broad-band noise. Taken per critical band, this ratio amounts to about -4 dB. The discrepancy of 8 dB seems to be related to the difference in spectral width between the two signals. This follows from experiments on masking by noise of variable spectral width, to be discussed next.

2. MASKING BY NARROW-BAND NOISE

Many experiments were conducted on masking various signals by random noise of varying bandwidth. Fletcher (1940) sought to strengthen his critical-band hypothesis by determining the masking of pure tones by narrow-band noise. His affirmative results were confirmed by Schafer, Gales, Shewmaker, and Thompson (1950). However, later results obtained by Feldtkeller and Zwicker and their co-workers (1956), by Hamilton (1957), and by others showed that the masking effect of narrow-band noise was more complex than was realized in the interpretation of earlier data. As already mentioned, these and other results led to a correction of Fletcher's critical bands by a factor of about 2.5.

The partial misinterpretation of the earlier results seems to have resulted from the assumption that the masking effect is independent of the noise bandwidth as long as this bandwidth is smaller than the critical band. In fact, the masking effect increases slightly as the bandwidth decreases and the total noise power remains constant. The phenomenon is ascribed to audible fluctuations of noise amplitude, which make the signal detection more difficult.

The effects inherent in narrow-band masking and their transition to the conditions of broad-band masking are evident in the results obtained by Bos and de Boer (1966). They are shown in Fig. 6 for one of the two listeners participating in their experiments. The various symbols indicate the sound frequency of the test signal, which was the same as the center frequency of masking noise bands and was varied parametrically. The filled symbols refer to the masking of pure tones, the open ones to that of bands of noise. In the second instance, the test sound and the masker had identical frequency spectra and were added coherently, as in Miller's (1947) experiments. The data were converted to equivalent noncoherent addition with the help of the curve in Fig. 2 and were expressed in terms of the jnd and of the signal-to-noise ratio based on the total noise power. Both dependent variables are plotted as a function of the noise bandwidth. The dash–dot curve follows the trend of the data obtained with the noise signal. The slanted lines, which coincide with the part of pure-tone data, follow constant noise power per cycle; the horizontal lines, constant total power. If, for instance, we follow

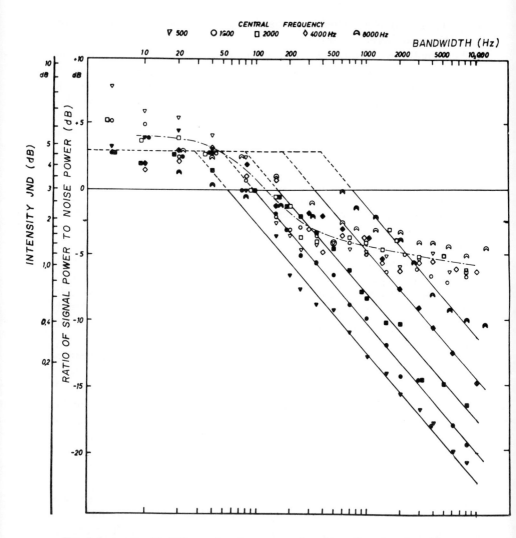

FIG. 6. Just noticeable difference in noise power and masking effect of random noise on pure
tones, as a function of noise bandwidth for several test frequencies. Filled symbols refer to the
masking experiment; open symbols, to the differential–sensitivity experiment. Dash–dot line
follows the main trend of the jnd data. Slanted, solid lines indicate constant noise powers per
cycle; horizontal, intermittent line, constant total power. [From Bos and de Boer (1966). By
permission of the Acoustical Society of America.]

the locus of the unfilled circles, which correspond to a center frequency of
1000 Hz, we can see that, at very narrow bandwidths, the signal-to-noise
ratio approaches the high value of 5 dB. Between the bandwidths of 50 and
200 Hz, the signal-to-noise ratio decreases rapidly. It continues to do so at

greater bandwidths, but at a lesser rate, and it tends toward an asymptote of about −6 dB.

The filled circles refer to the detection of the 1000-Hz tone. They indicate that, for bandwidth of the masking noise smaller than 50 Hz, the detection of the masked tone is somewhat better than of the masked noise. This is not surprising, since the variance of the noise signal is greater than that of the tone signal. However, at greater bandwidth, the detection advantage disappears and even reverses.

The slanted line that follows the filled circles indicates that the signal-to-noise ratio for the 1000-Hz sinusoid amounts to −2.5 dB when the computation is based on the noise power within the critical band centered at 1000 Hz. The computation is performed by taking the signal-to-noise ratio for the bandwidth of 10 kHz, for instance, multiplying it by the ratio between 10 kHz and 170 Hz, the critical bandwidth of 1000 Hz, and converting the result to decibels.

By comparing the data of Miller and of Hawkins and Stevens, we saw that wide-band noise masked a pure tone more than it did a wide-band noise. Bos and de Boer's experiment confirms this difference, although their absolute decibel values are somewhat smaller.

Why a wide-band noise should affect the detectability of a sinusoid more than it affects the detectability of a wide-band noise is not clear. It is likely that the noise is processed on many more parallel channels than is the sinusoid. Such parallel processing would tend to reduce the variability inherent in the signal as well as the variability resulting from responses of single neurons.

It should be evident that masking relationships are complex and that extrapolations from one masking situation to another should be made with great caution. In particular, masking produced by narrow-band noise is not directly predictable from masking experiments with wide-band noise, and vice versa.

A further complication in the masking phenomenon was found by Greenwood (1961), who varied both the bandwidth and the intensity level of the masker. When random noise of subcritical bandwidth masked a tone located at the center of its spectrum, a discontinuity appeared at a masker SL of about 50 dB. Below and above the discontinuity, the signal-to-noise ratio was independent of the masker intensity but, around 50 dB, the numerical value of the ratio dropped suddenly by approximately 3.5 dB. The discontinuity was absent when the noise bandwidth exceeded the critical band. The phenomenon is illustrated in Fig. 7, which contains four sets of individual results. The threshold shift is plotted as a function of the masker SL for two different frequency regions. The open circles and intermittent curves follow the data obtained with supracritical bands; the filled circles and solid lines, those obtained with subcritical bands. The discontinuity is clearly visible, especially in the higher frequency range.

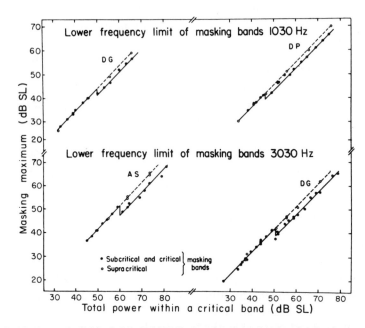

FIG. 7. Maximum individual threshold shifts produced by bands of noise in two different frequency regions, as a function of noise power. [From Greenwood (1961). By permission of the Acoustical Society of America.]

By varying the frequency of the signal, Greenwood discovered that the discontinuity in the intensity domain was accompanied by a discontinuity in the frequency domain. For critical or narrower bands of noise, the frequency distribution of masking was approximately triangular at sufficiently low SPLs. Near an SL of 50 dB, the pattern suddenly became trapezoidal. For wider bands, the trapezoidal pattern occurred at all SPLs, but the width of the plateau increased with the level. These results are shown in Fig. 8 for one listener. Other listeners produced similar results.

Individual masking data determined by Greenwood (1971) over a wide frequency range for two different noise bandwidths are shown in Fig. 9. Several additional features become evident. The frequency distribution of the threshold shift produced by the narrower, subcritical band is asymmetric. It exhibits a steep monotonic decay toward the low frequencies, and a more gradual nonmonotonic decay toward the high ones. The masking curve is almost flat-topped; however, the edges of the flat portion are somewhat elevated, especially the lower frequency one. The pronounced dip around 2500 Hz is attributed to audible combination tones produced by the interaction of the test tone with distortion products of the masking noise. The phenomenon will be discussed in the next section.

The masking pattern produced by the noise with the wider spectrum is

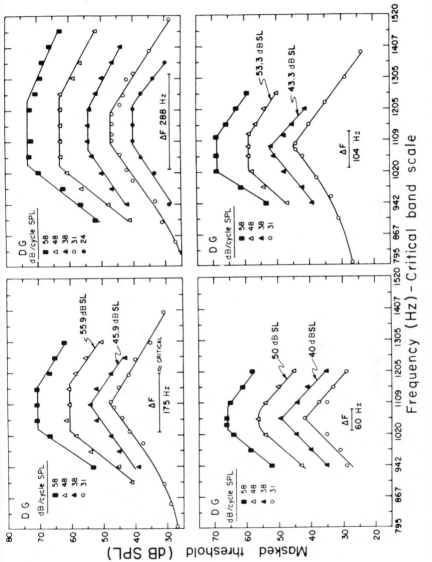

FIG. 8. Individual frequency distributions of masked thresholds produced by noise bands of various widths and SPLs. The frequency scale follows critical bandwidths. The two lower graphs correspond to subcritical bandwidths; the upper left graph, to the critical bandwidth; the upper right graph to a supracritical bandwidth. [From Greenwood (1961). By permission of the Acoustical Society of America.]

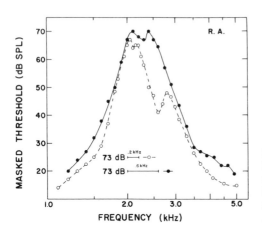

FIG. 9. Individual frequency distributions of masked thresholds produced by two different bands of noise with steep skirts. Both bands were at 73 dB SPL. [From Greenwood (1971). By permission of the Acoustical Society of America.]

almost symmetrical. In particular, it does not contain a pronounced dip at the high-frequency roll off. The flattened top of the pattern is wider than with the narrower noise and the elevation of its edges is more pronounced. Although such an elevation is not always present, as evident from the preceding figure, its significance should not be underestimated. It may be analogous to the well-known Mach-band phenomenon in vision (Ratliff, 1965). Mach bands may be observed at the borders of visual fields with unequal reflectance. The edge of the darker field appears darker and the edge of the brighter field brighter than the rest of the corresponding field surfaces. Mach bands are a special case of contrast phenomena produced by lateral neural inhibition, as has been demonstrated by Hartline and his co-workers on the eye of the horseshoe crab (Ratliff, 1965).

Demonstration of spatial contrast phenomena in audition is much more difficult than in vision where sharp intensity transitions can be effected at the receptor surface. Especially, in the compound eye of the horseshoe crab it is possible to illuminate one of several separate receptors while leaving the rest in darkness. In the mammalian ear spatial stimulus distribution on the receptor surface is controlled by the frequency spectrum of sound, as has been demonstrated in many physiological experiments. Because of mechanical coupling in the cochlea, sharp transitions are not possible, and even a single spectral component stimulates a substantial portion of the receptive surface. This is illustrated in Fig. 10, which shows amplitude distributions along the cochlear partition, as observed by Békésy (1943, 1960a). Similar distributions produced by single sinusoids can be calculated theoretically (Zwislocki, 1948, 1965) and demonstrated on mechanical and electrical models (Békésy, 1928, 1960a; Tonndorf, 1960; Zwislocki, 1948). With the help of such models, it is possible to show that a noise stimulus with a band-limited flat-topped spectrum, like the one of Fig. 11, produces not a flat topped but, rather, a rounded amplituded distribution in the cochlea. According to Bé-

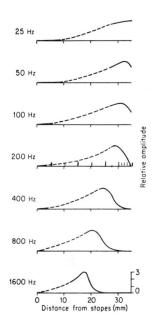

FIG. 10. Optically observed spatial distributions of vibration amplitude of human cochlear partition for several sound frequencies. [From *Experiments in Hearing* by G. von Békésy. Copyright 1960 by McGraw-Hill. Used with permission of McGraw-Hill Book Company.]

késy's (1960b) model of lateral inhibition, a rounded stimulus distribution would be unlikely to produce Mach bands. However, it would produce neural excitation whose distribution would be more flat topped than the stimulus distribution. Some of Greenwood's masking audiograms, shown in Fig. 8, seem to reflect flat-topped excitation distributions. The noise spectrum of Fig. 11 produced individual masking results shown in Fig. 12 (Carterette, Friedman, & Lovell, 1970). Some of the curves suggest the possibility of Mach bands, but most do not. Nevertheless, they are consis-

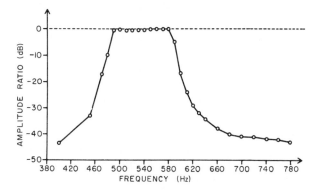

FIG. 11. Frequency spectrum of a flat-topped, narrow band of noise with steep skirts. [From Carterette *et al.* (1970). By permission from A. W. Sijthoff.]

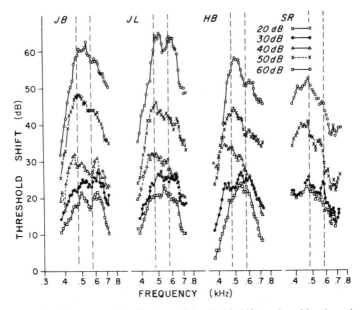

FIG. 12. Individual frequency distributions of threshold shift produced by the noise band of Fig. 11, at several SLs. [From Carterette *et al.* (1970). By permission from A. W. Sijthoff.]

tent with the hypothesis of a mechanism enhancing the differences in mechanical amplitude distribution along the cochlea.

3. Masking by Pure Tones

When a pure tone is masked by a pure tone, the interpretation of detection results is complicated by the occurrence of beats between the two stimuli. In order to avoid the beats, a narrow-band noise is sometimes used as a test stimulus. Experiments combining pure tones as maskers with narrow-band noise as test sound were used by Zwicker (1954) and Greenwood (1961) for the determination of auditory critical bands. Both series led to mutually consistent results. In Greenwood's experiments two simultaneously masking sinusoids were used, one at a fixed lower frequency and another at a higher frequency varied in steps. A 60-Hz band of random noise with variable center frequency served as the signal to be detected. The sinusoids were kept at a reasonably low SPL to avoid complicating effects of auditory distortion products. When their frequency difference was small, a unimodal distribution of masking effect resulted. At greater separations, the distribution became bimodal, as is evident in Fig. 13. Greenwood found that the frequency separation at which the transition occurred agreed with the critical bandwidth measured by different methods (Zwicker *et al.*, 1957).

Greenwood's (1961) results, when combined with computations of mechanical amplitude distribution along the cochlear partition, can serve as an

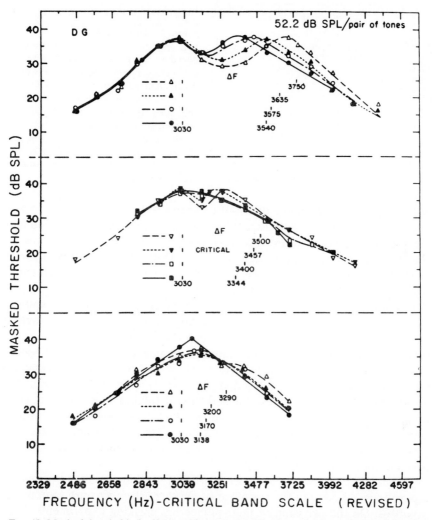

FIG. 13. Masked threshold of a 60-Hz-wide band of noise with variable center frequency in the presence of a pair of sinusoidal maskers spaced by a variable frequency interval. In the lowest graph, the frequency interval is subcritical; in the middle graph, approximately critical; in the highest graph, supracritical. [From Greenwood (1961). By permission of the Acoustical Society of America.]

indication of auditory Mach bands (Zwislocki, 1965). The computations indicate that, for a frequency separation of one critical band, the amplitude distribution is not bimodal but has a flat top. The same is true even for a separation of two critical bands, as illustrated in Fig. 14. Since the masking curves are bimodal at these separations, a neural enhancement of the edges

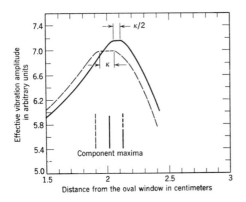

FIG. 14. Theoretical distributions of vibration amplitude of cochlear partition produced by two pairs of sinusoids with different intercomponent frequency intervals. The distribution indicated by the solid line corresponds to frequency components marked by solid lines; the distribution indicated by the intermittent line corresponds to the components marked by intermittent lines. The critical bandwidth is indicated by κ. [From Zwislocki (1965). By permission from John Wiley and Sons, Inc.]

of the flat-topped amplitude distribution seems to be taking place. It may be of corollary interest to note that these edges are more closely spaced along the cochlear spiral than are the maxima of vibration produced by the two sinusoidal components presented separately (Fig. 14). Correspondingly, the masking maxima of Fig. 13 are more closely spaced along the frequency scale than are the two masking sinusoids.

That some sort of mutual inhibition takes place among sound components has been demonstrated repeatedly by means of microelectrode studies (for instance, Sachs & Kiang, 1968), although the nature of this inhibition has remained unknown. The still-continuing arguments on the subject seem to arise from the lack of anatomical evidence of inhibitory connections and from the circumstance that the inhibition, if present, appears to act practically instantaneously. The well-established lateral inhibition in the eye of the horseshoe crab, by contrast, develops gradually with stimulus duration. It should be noted, however, that all neural processes in this animal are much slower than in warm blooded animals. Also, different mechanisms of inhibition are known to exist.

As already mentioned, the interpretation of masking results obtained with a pure tone sounded in the presence of another, stronger pure tone is quite involved. On the occasion of their pioneering masking experiments, Wegel and Lane (1924) noted that the test tone could signal its presence by means of beats with the masking tone or with its higher harmonics, and by formation of combination tones. More recently, Greenwood (1971) has presented extensive evidence that the most important combination tone affecting the masking results is the cubic combination tone arising as a difference between the second harmonic of the masker and the test tone ($2f_M - f_T$). When the frequency of the test tone (f_T) is gradually increased, the frequency of the cubic combination tone decreases and reaches a region of rapidly diminishing effectiveness of the masker. As a consequence, the combination tone becomes more audible than the test tone itself. This effect is counteracted by the rapidly decreasing amplitude of the combination tone (Goldstein, 1967).

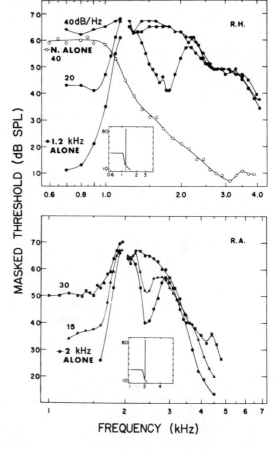

FIG. 15. Individual frequency distributions of masked threshold produced by a 2-kHz tone in the absence and in the presence of a low-frequency noise with a cutoff at 1050 Hz. The pure-tone masker was at 85 dB SPL; the noise had spectral SPLs indicated at corresponding curves. The masking effect produced by the strongest noise alone is shown by means of unfilled circles in the upper graph. [From Greenwood (1971). By permission of the Acoustical Society of America.]

The interaction leads to a frequency region of maximum audibility of the combination tone, which is reflected as a notch in the masking curves. Such a notch can be seen at about 2.5 kHz in Fig. 9 and near 1.7 and 2.4 kHz in Fig. 15. The notch at 1.7 kHz corresponds to a cubic combination tone of .7 kHz located near the low-frequency foot of the pure-tone masking curve. This kind of coincidence was found by Greenwood independent of the frequency of the masker. To prove that the notch was actually produced by a low-frequency distortion product, Greenwood masked the low frequencies by means of a low-pass-filtered random noise. With even moderate noise intensities that did not directly affect the notch region, the notch disappeared. Such a change in the masking pattern can be seen in Fig. 15. The upper graph of this figure shows the masking effect of the strongest noise used when presented alone. It is about 15 dB below the lowest point in the notch.

In addition to beats and combination tones, side bands produced by switching transients may affect the measured amount of masking. Although the problem of audible transients has been known for a long time, more recent experiments by Leshowitz and Wightman (1971) brought it particularly clearly into focus. They have been able to prove that listeners actually detect the side bands before they detect the carrier. They did this with the help of two well-known psychophysical phenomena. When a sinusoidal signal is added to a sinusoidal pedestal of the same frequency, the power increment depends on their mutual phase relationship.

$$\Delta S_{\mathrm{T}} = P_{\mathrm{S}}P_{\mathrm{P}} \cos(\Theta_{\mathrm{S}} - \Theta_{\mathrm{P}}) + P_{\mathrm{S}}^2/2 \ , \tag{19}$$

where ΔS_{T} means the increment in total power; P_{S} and P_{P} are the sound pressures of the signal and pedestal, respectively; and $\Theta_{\mathrm{S}} - \Theta_{\mathrm{P}}$ is their phase difference. A maximum increment results when the phase difference is zero; at a phase difference of 90°, the power increment is reduced to $P_{\mathrm{S}}^2/2$. In the first situation, the increment should be more easily detectable than in the second. The second phenomenon they used concerns temporal auditory summation. A longer signal is more easily detected than a short one. Leshowitz and Wightman added rectangular increments of various durations to a 1300-Hz continuous pedestal, both in phase and in quadrature and determined the signal SPL for 75% correct detections. Some of their results obtained on three listeners are shown in Fig. 16. The left side of the figure shows what happened when the signal was unfiltered. The filled squares indicate the expected results for quadrate signal addition, using the empirical results for in-phase addition as reference. As is evident, the prediction was not confirmed, and detection was practically independent of the phase relationship. In addition, it did not depend on signal duration. Very different relationships prevail in the right side of the figure, which shows results obtained with a signal filtered through a bandpass filter to minimize the side bands. Here, detection strongly depends on both phase difference and signal

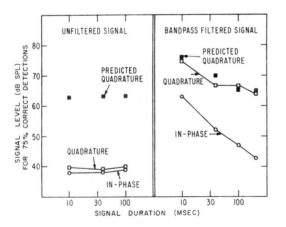

FIG. 16. Detectability of amplitude increments of a 1300-Hz tone added in phase or in quadrature to a 1300-Hz pedestal. SPL of increments for constant detectability is plotted as a function of increment duration. [From Leshowitz and Wightman (1971). By permission of the Acoustical Society of America.]

duration. The results of the left side of the figure are consistent with the hypothesis that the listeners detected the side bands before they detected the carrier, since the energy of the side bands does not depend on either the phase relationship between the signal and the pedestal or the signal duration. The results of the right side indicate that the filtering was effective and that the listeners detected the carrier before the side bands.

The energy ratio between the carrier and the side bands depends on signal duration and amplitude envelope. It increases with both the signal duration, the rise time and the decay time. However, the latter effect is not straightforward, since the detailed shape of the envelope is also important. For instance, a Gaussian envelope produces smaller side bands than an exponential one. The magnitude of the side bands resulting from trapezoidal modulation of a 2000-Hz carrier with various rise times is shown in Fig. 17 (Wightman, 1971). Note that, at a frequency 1000 Hz higher than the carrier frequency, the energy is reduced by less than 20 dB when the rise time is 1 msec, and only 30 dB for a rise time of 10 msec.

The results of Leshowitz and Wightman confirm the suspicion that some experiments on auditory masking performed in the past are invalid because of side-band effects.

4. TEMPORAL EFFECTS

The detectability of a sound burst in the presence or in the absence of a masking noise increases with burst duration within a time interval of about 200 msec. Apparently, neural excitation is cumulated over this time period. If the masking effect depended on accumulated excitation produced by the masker, we would expect it to increase with the masker duration preceding the test stimulus. In other words, the detectability of a short sound burst would decrease as its delay from the masker onset increased. Empirical evidence indicates that this does not happen. A possible explanation can be found in the psychophysical theory of signal detection (Green & Swets, 1966) according to which detectability is not determined by the average magnitude of the masker but by the variability of its instantaneous magnitude. Whereas the average excitation may increase with duration through a process of temporal summation, the variability may remain constant.

Numerous experiments have shown that monaural masking either remains time invariant or decreases slightly with the delay from the masker onset. Several articles have been devoted to the question of under what conditions a decrement takes place and how large it is. Some investigations showed a very dramatic effect (Elliot, 1965, 1967; Green, 1969), others, hardly any effect at all (Osman & Raab, 1963). The most substantial effects occurred when the masker consisted of bursts cut out of sound with a narrow-band spectrum, the frequency of the test tones was outside this spectrum, and the masker was turned on abruptly or nearly so. Green (1969) suggested that energy splatter produced by the sharp masker onset could be responsible. It

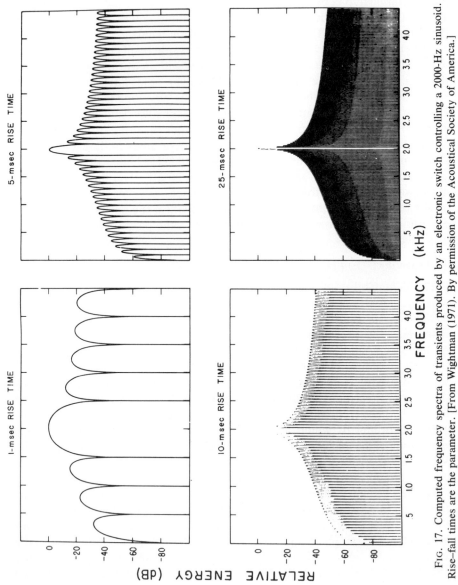

FIG. 17. Computed frequency spectra of transients produced by an electronic switch controlling a 2000-Hz sinusoid. Rise-fall times are the parameter. [From Wightman (1971). By permission of the Acoustical Society of America.]

does temporarily broaden the effective masker spectrum and could produce increased transient masking at off-masker frequencies. Green's suggestion is supported by Zwicker's (1965a,b) experiments in which transient energy splatter was either held within reasonable limits or made ineffective by the use of broad-band maskers. Zwicker showed that the dependence of masking on the time delay from the masker onset increases with the difference in spectral bandwidth between the masking and test stimuli. The relationships appear particularly clear when the bandwidth is expressed in terms of auditory critical bands. Figure 18 shows some of Zwicker's results. The SPL of a 5-kHz, 2-msec tone burst required for criterion detection is plotted as a function of time delay Δt from the masker onset. The spectral width of the masker was varied parametrically from 1 to 24 critical bands. One critical band at 5 kHz amounts to about 800 Hz. For maskers one or two critical bands wide, the masking is practically independent of the time delay. Wider bands produce a gradually increasing masking effect, *overshoot*, near the masker onset. In another experiment, Zwicker could demonstrate that the overshoot is absent even when the test sound is outside the masker frequency band, provided both have the same bandwidth in critical-band units.

What physiological mechanisms underly the masking relationships found by Zwicker is not clear, but it is reasonable to assume, as Green (1969) did, that neural short-term adaptation is involved. Many experiments on VIIIth nerve fibers (e.g., Kiang, 1965) have shown that the firing rate is greatest at the stimulus onset and decays asymptotically to a steady-state level with a time constant of about 50 msec (Zwislocki, 1970). Experiments on single units of the cochlear nucleus with characteristics similar to those of VIIIth nerve units produced the unexpected result that, within certain intensity ranges, incremental responses are independent of adaptation (Smith & Zwislocki, 1971). When a short intensity increment is added to a longer pedestal, the response to the increment remains constant or even increases with the time delay from the pedestal onset, while the response to the pedestal itself decreases. As a consequence, the ratio of signal-to-noise increases.

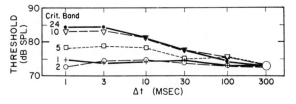

FIG. 18. Masked threshold of 2-msec bursts of a 5-kHz tone in the presence of bands of noise of various bandwidths. The noise bandwidth is indicated in numbers of critical bands. The threshold is plotted as a function of the time delay from the masker onset. The noise had a spectral power of 25 dB SPL. The tone signal and the masking noise were passed through the same filter. [From Zwicker (1965b). By permission of the Acoustical Society of America.]

Closely related to the question of temporal masking changes is the question of temporal constancy of auditory critical bands. In early experiments on the subject, Scholl (1962a,b) and Elliot (1967) were thought to have found evidence for a gradual narrowing of critical bands with the delay from the masker onset. They found that the masking overshoot was greater when the masking and test sounds were in different frequency regions than when they were in the same region, more specifically, the same critical band. Interpolation of their data leads to the conclusion that the masking effect of a narrow-band masker extends over a wider frequency range at the masker onset than after a time delay. Since the frequency distribution of steady-state masking was used routinely as a measure of critical bandwidths, it appears straightforward to interpret Scholl and Elliot's results as a widening of critical bands at the masker onset. However, this conclusion appears to be inconsistent with the temporal constancy of neural tuning curves of VIIIth nerve units (Kiang, 1965), with temporal changes of loudness, which are the same for pure tones and wide-band noise (Zwicker, 1965a,b), and with central masking data, to be discussed in a later section (Zwislocki, Buining, & Glantz, 1968). In view of Zwicker's masking experiments (1965a,b) and Green's (1969) suggestion that spectral energy splatter due to switching transients could have affected the transient masking effects found by him and Elliot, the conclusion of temporally variable critical bands seems no longer tenable.

B. Forward Masking

When a sound stimulus is turned off, it leaves a trace of aftereffects that die out gradually. Aftereffects that disappear within less than .5 sec are now subsumed under the operational term of *forward masking*. Forward masking is measured in essentially the same way as simultaneous masking, that is, by means of changes in detectability of a test stimulus.

The first systematic measurements of forward masking were conducted by Lüscher and Zwislocki (1946, 1947, 1949) and by Gardner (1947) and Munson and Gardner (1950). Both groups used essentially the same stimulus paradigm, which has become standard for forward-masking experiments. A masking sound burst is followed by a short test tone, which is adjusted to a given criterion of detectability. The masker threshold measured in this way is compared to the threshold measured in the absence of the masking sound, and the resulting threshold difference in decibels is taken as the masking effect.

In the early experiments, the masking stimulus was usually at least 400 msec long, a duration that permitted the auditory system to approach a steady-state response. Both the masking and test bursts were turned on and off with onset and decay times on the order of 10 msec to avoid audible transients. For the same reason, the test burst was made at least 20 msec long. The time delay was usually specified in terms of the time interval between the offset of the masking stimulus and the offset of the test stimulus. As later experiments showed, this specification was the correct one.

The experiments of Lüscher and Zwislocki have shown that forward masking increases with the masker intensity and decays with the time delay. The decay is more rapid for higher masker intensities, so that the masking practically disappears within the same time interval of about 300 msec (Lüscher & Zwislocki, 1947, 1949). This finding, established for pure tones (Zwislocki, 1960a), was later confirmed by Stein (1960) for wide-band noise. Lüscher and Zwislocki (1947) also found that forward masking did not depend on sound frequency when the masker was kept at a constant SL and the sound frequency of the test tone was the same as that of the masker.

Gardner (1947) and Munson and Gardner (1950) focused their attention on the frequency distribution of forward masking and on effects of the masker intensity. They established that, at low and moderate intensities, the masking was maximum at the masker frequency. It decayed gradually toward higher frequencies, and more rapidly toward the low ones. At high intensities, the maximum shifted to about .5 octave above the masker frequency. According to Zwislocki and Pirodda (1952), the maximum is not shifted gradually toward higher frequencies but, rather, a secondary maximum arises when the SL of the masker exceeds 80 dB. These results obtained on three listeners at a masker frequency of 3150 Hz and two SPLs of 60 and 100 dB, respectively, are shown in Fig. 19.

Zwislocki and Pirodda suggested that the physiological mechanism underlying the secondary maximum is different from that of the primary

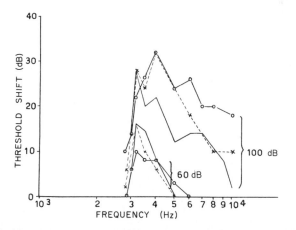

FIG. 19. Individual frequency distributions of forward masking for a masker frequency of 3150 Hz and two masker SPLs. The masker had a duration of .4 sec, and the test burst of 30-msec duration was delayed by 150 msec from the masker offset. [From Zwislocki and Pirodda (1952). By permission of *Experientia*.]

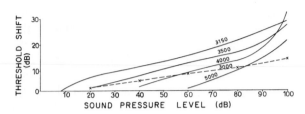

FIG. 20. Forward masking as a function of masker SPL for several test frequencies. The masker has a frequency of 3150 Hz and was .4 sec long. The test tone of 30-msec duration was delayed by 150 msec. [From Zwislocki and Pirodda (1952). By permission of *Experientia*.]

maximum. This is indicated by two related phenomena. At the frequency of this maximum, the masking begins to grow faster than at other frequencies when the masker intensity increases above about 80 dB SPL. This is evident in Fig. 20 for the 4000-Hz curve. When this happens, the masking decay becomes slower, so that some residual effect is still left after .5 sec from the end of the masking burst. The location of the secondary maximum and the slow recovery resemble characteristics of the temporary threshold shift (TTS) that is found after long exposures to intense sound (Zwislocki, 1960a).

Munson and Gardner (1950) found that the growth of forward masking with the masker intensity seems to go through three phases when the masker and test frequencies approximately coincide, and the time delay is not too short. As can be seen in Fig. 21 for two listeners, the masking curve rises at low masker levels, reaches a plateau at moderate ones, and accelerates again at high levels. They suggested that the flat transition at moderate levels may coincide with saturation of firing rate in nerve fibers ending at the outer hair cells, and that the subsequent acceleration could be produced by the response of the inner hair cells. Currently, interaction between outer and inner hair cells is under intense anatomical and physiological investigation. Its nature is not yet clear, but it is unlikely to be a simple summation. In line with this expectation, Zwislocki, Pirodda, and Rubin (1959) found that the form of the intensity functions of forward masking depends not only on the frequency relationship between the masking and test tones and on the time delay from the masker offset, but also on the masker duration. Their investigation revealed four more fundamental features of forward masking.

In a first experimental series, they used 1000-Hz masking and test tones, turned on and off with sufficient time constants to avoid audible transients. The masker was at 85 dB SL and had a duration of .5 sec. The test burst was either 20 msec long and was begun at a variable time delay from the masker offset, or the time delay was kept constant at 20 msec, and the duration of the test burst was varied. In either event, the time interval between the offsets of the masking and test stimuli served as the independent variable. Figure 22 shows the results for two listeners, which are approximated by the

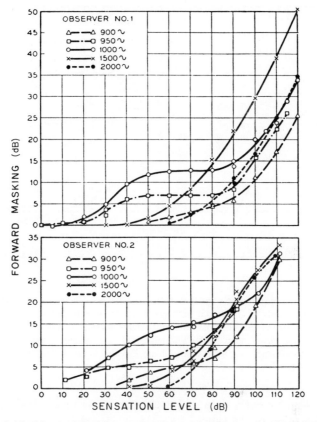

FIG. 21. Individual forward masking as a function masker SL for several test frequencies. The masker had a frequency of 1000 Hz and a duration of .4 sec. The test tone had a duration of 70 msec, and its offset was delayed by 98 msec from the masker offset. [From Munson and Gardner (1950). By permission of the Acoustical Society of America.]

smooth curves. The filled symbols and continuous line belong to the variable interval; the unfilled symbols and dashed line, to the variable test-tone duration. Note that, for time delays smaller than 200 msec, both variables produced essentially the same result, which appears to be uniquely determined by the time delay of the test-tone offset. This finding was later confirmed by Elliot (1962b). At time intervals greater than 200 msec, making the test stimulus longer produces a lower threshold than delaying a short stimulus. This result is not surprising in view of the well-known effect of temporal summation (for review and analysis, see Zwislocki, 1960b). Why temporal summation does not manifest itself at shorter time intervals is not clear, but the slope of the masking function could be responsible.

Figure 22 also shows that forward masking does not decay exponentially,

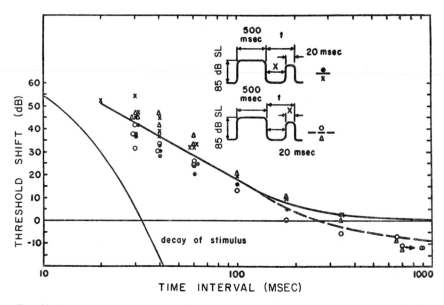

FIG. 22. Forward masking as a function of the time interval between the masker offset and test-tone offset. Means of individual data produced by two listeners are approximated by smooth curves. Filled circles and crosses correspond to a variable interval between the masker offset and test-tone onset; open circles and triangles, to a variable duration of the test tone. Masker and test frequency was at 1000 Hz. [From Zwislocki *et al.* (1959). By permission of the Acoustical Society of America.]

as was implied by early data of Lüscher and Zwislocki (1947) but, rather, follows a function of the type

$$y = A/(1 - e^{-\alpha x})^\beta , \tag{20}$$

which becomes

$$10 \log y \simeq 10 \log A - 10\beta \log \alpha x \tag{21}$$

for $\alpha x \ll 1$. Similar decay functions were obtained by Stein (1960) and by Elliot (1962a,b).

In a second experimental series, the duration and the frequency spectrum of the masking stimulus were variable. The remaining stimulus parameters were fixed—masker SL at 80 and 60 dB, test-tone frequency at 1000 Hz, test-burst duration at 20 msec, and the time delay between the masker offset and test-burst onset at 40 msec. The test tone was turned on and off without audible transients. In a first experiment, the masker consisted of a 1000-Hz sinusoid turned on and off either without audible transients or abruptly. Surprisingly, the two different modes of turning the masker on and off produced distinctly different results for durations shorter than 100 msec, as can be seen in Fig. 23. While in the absence of audible switching transients the masking appears to be the same for 5- and 1000-msec durations, with an extended minimum in between, the abrupt cutoff of the masker almost completely abolishes the masking effect for short durations. In the latter situation, the masking curve rises monotonically with the masker duration. The relationships look as if the audible transient eliminated one component of the masking effect. This is confirmed introspectively. When no switching transients can be heard, the tone sensation seems to outlast the masker, and the test tone is detected as an increment in the persisting sensation. Audible transients seem to abolish the persisting tone sensation. It is possible that forward masking has two components, one arising from persistence of sensation, and another, from decreased sensitivity of the auditory system. The first would be more like simultaneous masking, the second more like sensory adaptation (Lüscher & Zwislocki, 1947; Zwislocki, 1960a; Zwislocki & Pirodda, 1952).

To check whether the effect of the audible transient was equivalent to that of its spectral bandwidth, the pure-tone masker was replaced by random noise of appropriate bandwidth. The masking burst was turned on and off gradually. Despite the gradual offset, the masking effect as a function of masker duration followed a course parallel to the lower curve of Fig. 23. Thus, the conclusion could be reached that broadening the frequency spectrum even for a very short duration abolished one component of forward masking.

In a third series, forward masking was investigated as a function of masker duration for several masker SLs. Both the masker and test stimuli consisted of bursts of a 1000-Hz sinusoid turned on and off without audible transients.

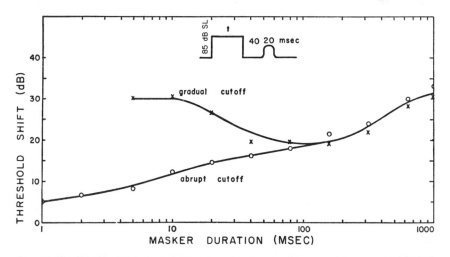

FIG. 23. Forward masking as a function of masker duration for a sound frequency of 1000 Hz. Crosses correspond to a gradual and circles to an abrupt masker cutoff. [From Zwislocki *et al.* (1959). By permission of the Acoustical Society of America.]

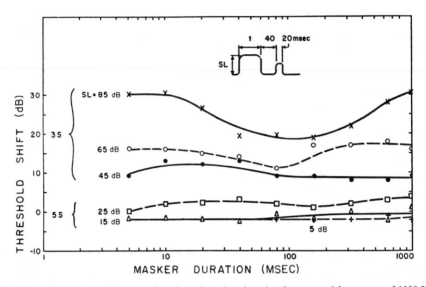

FIG. 24. Forward masking as a function of masker duration for a sound frequency of 1000 Hz and several masker SLs. [From Zwislocki *et al.* (1959). By permission of the Acoustical Society of America.]

The test-burst duration and the interburst interval were fixed at 20 and 40 msec, respectively. Under these conditions, both masking components intervened, as is evident in Fig. 24. A new feature in this figure is the lowering of the threshold for masker SLs of 5 and 15 dB. Whether this sensitization is related to one or the other component of forward masking or is the result of an additional process, could not be ascertained thus far. The phenomenon itself was confirmed extensively by Rubin (1960).

The experimental results just described indicate that the so-called forward masking involves at least three processes. One seems to refer to changes in sensitivity of short duration, a second to changes in sensitivity of longer duration, and a third to persistence of excitation. On the basis of published experimental constants, it appears that most experiments dealt with the first process and only very few touched upon the remaining two.

C. Backward Masking

When a test stimulus precedes another stimulus, a threshold elevation can be found. This elevation in threshold is called *backward masking*. This apparently paradoxical phenomenon implies that an effect can precede its cause. As a rational explanation, a difference in neural latencies between the responses to the masking and test stimuli was proposed. The response to the stronger masking stimulus should have a smaller latency and could "catch up with" the response to the test stimulus. However, the argument is strained, since the difference between the masking and test intensities is small under some conditions, and substantial backward masking may precede the masker onset by as much as 30 msec. The known temporal scatter of neural responses may help the latency argument somewhat. It would increase the overlap between the neural activity elicited by the test stimulus and that produced by the masker. Whether this help is sufficient, will have to remain for future research to decide.

Some early work on backward masking was done by Samoilova (1959) who used sinusoidal stimuli, and by Chistovich and Ivanova (1959) who used clicks. The latter were also used by Raab (1961). Osman and Raab (1963) and later Robinson and Pollack (1971) masked clicks by random broad-band noise. In his experiments, Pickett (1959) replaced clicks by a sinusoidal test stimulus, as did Elliot (1962a,b). In general, it was found that, when clicks or random noise masked clicks, backward masking extended over a shorter duration than when the test stimulus consisted of tone bursts. Part of this difference could be due to a necessarily longer duration of the tone stimuli. However, it is also possible that a process related to the effect of spectral bandwidth on forward masking (Zwislocki et al., 1959) intervened.

From the point of view of time definition, backward masking experiments with pairs of clicks are the most accurate, and Fig. 25 shows the results of Raab (1961) for one listener. Even for 85 dB SL of the masking click, the major portion of the effect disappears in about 10 msec. Other listeners produced similar results. For masking of clicks by random noise, the data of Robinson and Pollack (1971) may be regarded as representative. Some of them are shown in Fig. 26. The large number of time intervals brings out the details of the backward-masking curves. Over a time span of about 4 msec, the backward masking remains constant. At larger time intervals, it decreases steeply at a decelerating rate. At lower masker levels, the masking

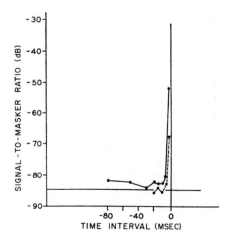

FIG. 25. Individual backward masking of a click by a following click, as a function of the interclick time interval. The masking click had sensation levels of 70 and 85 dB. [From Raab (1961). By permission of the Acoustical Society of America.]

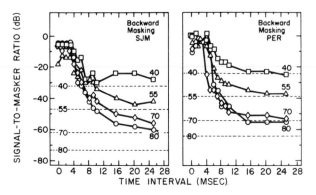

FIG. 26. Two sets of individual backward-masking curves for several SPLs of the masker. The masker consisted of broad-band random noise, the test stimulus, of a click. [From Robinson and Pollack (1971). By permission of the Acoustical Society of America.]

practically vanishes within 10 msec; at higher levels, some effect remains even after 25 msec.

The measurement of backward masking of tones by tones, or more generally, by stimuli with narrow-band spectra appears the most difficult because of the conflict between time definition and bandwidth. At medium audible sound frequencies, tone bursts shorter than 10 msec cannot be tolerated if the main portion of their frequency spectrum is to be held within one critical band. For the same reason, they cannot be turned on and off abruptly. The difficulty was partially overcome by Wright (1964a,b) through the use of long test stimuli, which partially overlapped the masker in time. The masker consisted of a 600-msec burst of critical-band noise centered at 1000 Hz and turned on and off with rise and decay times of 10 msec. The test tone was always turned off 100 msec ahead of the masker offset. By varying its duration, Wright could manipulate the time interval between its onset and that of the masker. He assumed that the audibility of the test tone was determined by the combined effects of masking and temporal summation. This assumption is related to the finding of Zwislocki *et al*. (1959) that the audibility of a tone of variable duration following another tone is determined by forward masking and temporal summation. If no backward masking were present, the summation interval would be equal to the time interval between the test-tone and masker onsets. In the presence of backward masking, the summation interval should be reduced. Wright's raw data obtained on three listeners are shown in Fig. 27. The open symbols correspond to the situation where the test-tone onset precedes the masker onset; the filled symbols, to the situation where the test-tone onset lags the masker onset. The dichotomy between the two situations is clearly evident. Wright normalized the data by referring them to the threshold at the test-tone duration of 1000 msec, which corresponds to a time interval between the onsets of the masking and test stimuli

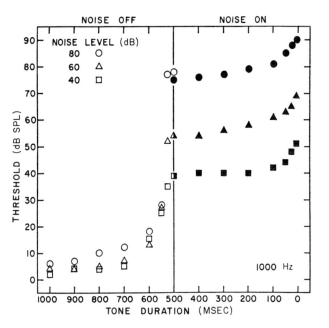

FIG. 27. Backward and simultaneous masking of a 1000-Hz tone by a narrow-band noise as a function of test-tone duration. The masker was 600 msec long, and the test tone terminated 100 msec before the masker did. The onsets and offsets of both stimuli were gradual. [From Wright (1964a). By permission of the Acoustical Society of America.]

of 500 msec. Subsequently, he applied the correction for temporal summation. This correction was computed from the diagram shown in Fig. 28, which contains two curves: One for temporal summation in quiet or in the presence of a steady-state masking noise; the other, for the normalized data of Fig. 27 plotted as a function of the time interval between the stimulus onsets. On the assumption that equal summation intervals produce equal threshold shifts, it is possible to assign to each point of the experimental curve an effective stimulus duration, as indicated by the dashed lines and arrows. For instance, to an interval of 100 msec between the stimulus onsets, there corresponds an effective summation time of 15 msec. When the experimental data are plotted as a function of the effective durations, the values plotted in Fig. 29 are obtained. They show a strong effect of backward masking, which extends over a much longer time interval than for clicks and broad-band noise. Over an interval of about 30 msec, the backward masking is nearly constant and approximately equal to simultaneous masking. Around 50 msec, it decays almost abruptly to a small residual value, which slowly decays over another 100 msec. It should be noted that, within the time interval during which the masking is substantial, its magnitude depends strongly on the intensity level of the masker. Beyond the sharp masking

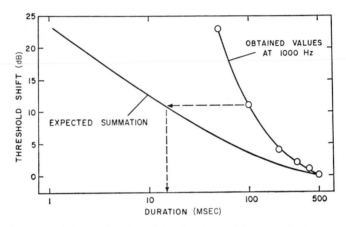

FIG. 28. Threshold shift as a function of the time interval between the test-tone onset and masker onset, derived from Fig. 27, and threshold shifts that should have taken place if there were no backward masking. It is assumed that the expected threshold shifts are due to temporal summation. [From Wright (1964a). By permission of the Acoustical Society of America.]

cutoff, the threshold is unaffected by the masker level. It seems that two different processes control the detectability in the two intervals.

In order to check the validity of the correction for temporal summation, Wright repeated his backward-masking measurements, using tone bursts of 10-msec duration. Data obtained in this way were found to be consistent with the computed ones.

A comparison of the data produced by stimuli having narrow-band spectra with the data produced by stimuli having broad-band spectra leads to the conclusion that backward masking, like forward masking, depends on the

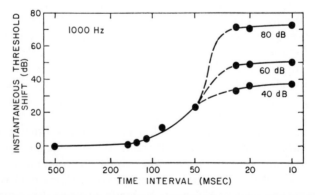

FIG. 29. Instantaneous backward masking of a pure tone by a narrow-band noise, computed with the help of Figs. 27 and 28. [From Wright (1964a). By permission of the Acoustical Society of America.]

spectral bandwidth. The nature of this dependence remains to be determined.

D. Central Masking

Central masking seems to have been discovered by Wegel and Lane (1924) on the occasion of their classic experiments on monaural masking. They found the effect to be extremely small, which probably delayed its systematic investigation for several decades. Hughes (1940) found a slightly larger effect between 4 and 10 dB. Ingham (1957, 1959) could obtain contralateral threshold shifts on the order of 10 dB when the sound frequencies of the test and masking stimuli were similar. He found a sharp frequency selectivity. Finally, Scherrick and Albernaz (1961) made the observation, later confirmed by Dirks and Malmquist (1965), that central masking was relatively large when both the masking and test stimuli were either continuous or simultaneously pulsed, and was very small when the masker was continuous and the test tone pulsed.

Systematic experiments on central masking did not begin until the midsixties (Zwislocki et al., 1968; Zwislocki, Damianopoulos, Buining, & Glantz, 1967). They were facilitated considerably by the development of earphone systems providing an interaural sound attenuation of 80 dB or more (Zwislocki, 1953). The experiments brought to light several features of central masking and showed that its major portion was transient. The threshold shift produced at the onset of the masker was always substantially larger than after a time delay. Two distinct processes of temporal decay were uncovered. One, more substantial, occurring with a time constant of 50 to 60 msec, and another, smaller, manifesting itself over a duration of several minutes. A strong frequency selectivity was also found, in agreement with Ingham's results.

A typical stimulus paradigm and corresponding individual data are shown in Fig. 30. The masking stimulus of 250-msec duration was presented to one ear, the test stimulus with a Gaussian envelope and 10-msec duration at half-power points, to the other. The test burst had a variable sound frequency, and its onset was delayed with respect to the masker onset by 20 msec. The masker had a frequency of 1000 Hz and a 60 dB SL. The data points and the smooth curves drawn through them by eye show two individual frequency distributions of the masking effect. Note the substantial difference in the amount of masking between the two listeners. Of some interest may be the fact that the main peak has a bandwidth of one critical band and that this bandwidth is found at a time delay of only 20 msec from the masker onset. This does not support the notion that auditory frequency selectivity develops gradually with the delay from the stimulus onset.

The fast temporal decay of central masking is shown in Fig. 31 for several masker SLs. The masker consisted of a critical-band noise centered at 1000

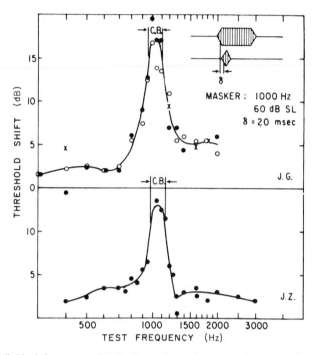

FIG. 30. Individual frequency distributions of transient central masking for the stimulus paradigm shown in the inset. The masker duration amounted to 250 msec; the test-tone duration to 10 msec. C.B. indicates the critical bandwidth. [From Zwislocki *et al.* (1967). By permission of *Perception and Psychophysics.*]

Hz, and the Gaussian test bursts had a carrier frequency of 1000 Hz. The data points represent medians of six listeners, and the curves obey the empirical equation

$$S_t/S_\infty = 1 + (S_1/S_\infty)e^{-\beta t}, \tag{22}$$

where S_t/S_∞ is the linear expression for the threshold shift relative to the asymptotic level, and $1/\beta$ is the time constant on the order of 50 msec. Note that the amount of decay decreases with the SL of the masker and practically completely disappears at about 20 dB, but the basic course of the decay remains the same.

The slow decay of central masking appears to be more unstable than the fast decay. It does not seem to occur when the masker consists of a broadband noise or its frequency is substantially different from that of the test stimulus. Several possible results are shown for one listener in Fig. 32. The test bursts were cut out of a 1000-Hz sinusoid and their onsets coincide with the onsets of 250-msec masking bursts repeated once per second. The data show that the masking effect decreased by 4 dB over a period of 5–6 min

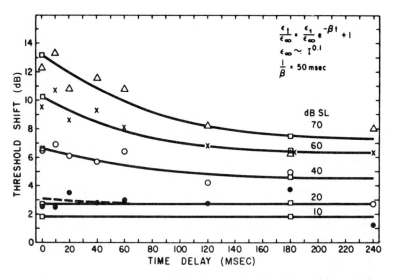

FIG. 31. Temporal decay of central masking as a function of time interval from masker onset. The masker consisted of a critical-band random noise at several SLs; the test-tone frequency was at 1000 Hz, the center of the noise band. Equations in the upper right-hand corner describe the decay pattern, the vertical distances among the curves, and the decay time constant. [From Zwislocki (1970). By permission from A. W. Sijthoff.]

when the masker consisted of a 950-Hz sinusoid. When its frequency was changed to 600 Hz, the decay disappeared. The same happened when the pure-tone masker was replaced by a noise masker with a broad frequency spectrum. There is no ready explanation for these differences in the slow masking decay, but at least some of them appear to manifest themselves in

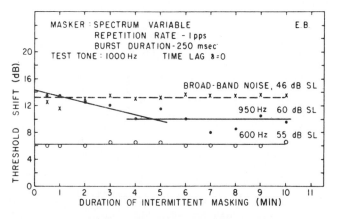

FIG. 32. Slow decay of central masking during repetitive exposure to various maskers: broad-band noise, 950-Hz, and 600-Hz tones. Individual data. [From Zwislocki et al. (1967). By permission of *Perception and Psychophysics*.]

other experiments on the auditory system. For instance, it is well known in audiology that the acoustic muscle reflex in the middle ear slowly disappears with time when it is produced by a pure tone but remains approximately constant when the stimulus consists of broad-band noise. Both the slow and the fast decay can be observed in the responses of single units in the auditory nerve (Kiang, 1965).

The slow decay of central masking produces difficulties in experiments in which the masker frequency has to be kept constant for prolonged periods of time. For this and other reasons which will become apparent later on, it is convenient to determine frequency distributions of central masking by keeping the frequency of the test tone constant and varying the frequency of the masker. The distributions obtained in this way roughly approximate the mirror image of distributions determined with a constant masking frequency and a variable test-tone frequency (Fig. 30), when plotted on a logarithmic frequency scale. This is so because of the logarithmic relationship of the location of the vibration maximum in the cochlea and sound frequency. An example of typical individual masking distributions for a test frequency of 1000 Hz and a zero time delay is shown in Fig. 33. Each curve was obtained at a different SL, and the smooth curves were fitted to the data points by eye. Several features may be noted. The distributions tend to be bimodal; at low masker SLs, even trimodal. The relative maximum at high frequencies

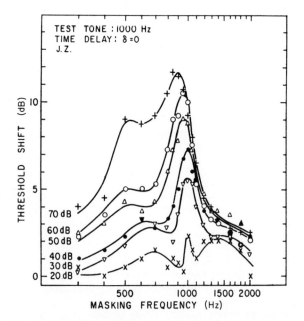

Fig. 33. Individual frequency distributions of central masking for a test tone of 1000 Hz and a variable masker frequency. Masker SL was varied stepwise. [From Zwislocki *et al.* (1968). By permission of the Acoustical Society of America.]

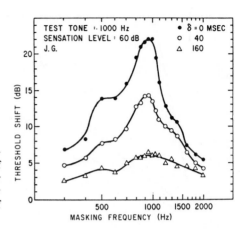

FIG. 34. Individual frequency distributions of central masking for a test tone of 1000 Hz and 3 time delays from the masker onset. [From Zwislocki *et al.* (1968). By permission of the Acoustical Society of America.]

seems to disappear as the masker level increases. On the other hand, the relative maximum at low frequencies becomes more prominent. Its position moves away from the test frequency. The same is true, although to a lesser extent, for the principal maximum, which is centered at the test frequency for sufficiently small masker levels. It is possible that this shift is produced by the same process that causes a slight pitch change as tone intensity increases (Stevens, 1935).

The secondary maxima cannot be accounted for by the interaction of distortion products of the masking stimulus with the test stimulus, as this was done by Greenwood (1971) for monaural masking, since no physical interaction between them takes place. A simple effect of distortion products is excluded by the inharmonic relationship between the frequencies of the maxima.

Because of implications for mechanisms of auditory frequency analysis, changes in frequency distribution of central masking, which occur as the time delay from the masker onset increases, are of considerable interest. An example of such changes is given in Fig. 34, which shows individual frequency distribution curves for three time delays: 0, 40, and 160 msec. Clearly, the principal maximum does not become more pronounced as time passes. On the contrary, the distribution becomes flatter. This results from the positive coupling between the magnitude of the initial masking effect and its temporal decay (Zwislocki *et al.,* 1968).

Also of considerable theoretical interest is the dependence of central masking on masker intensity. As shown in Fig. 35 by means of median data (Zwislocki, 1970, and unpublished), the relationship depends quite critically on temporal conditions. The open circles refer to the masking effect measured at the onset of a narrow-band masker by means of 10-msec test bursts; the filled circles refer to a time delay of 20 msec. The crosses indicate the steady-state effect obtained by means of a continuous pure tone masking 250-msec test bursts of nearly the same sound frequency. For comparison,

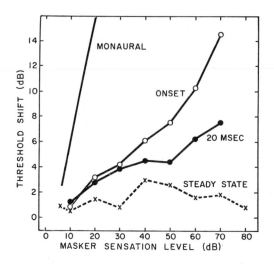

Fig. 35. Central masking at 1000 Hz as a function of masker SL for three temporal conditions: at the onset of masker bursts, at a delay of 20 msec, and for a continuous masker. In the first two instances the test signal consisted of 10-msec bursts; in the last one, of 250-msec bursts. The slope of monaural masking curve is drawn in for comparison.

the uppermost curve shows the slope of steady-state monaural masking when both the masker and test stimuli are at similar sound frequencies. Four features of central masking are evident in the graph. First, even the onset curve has a much smaller slope than the monaural masking curve, which has a slope of one. Consequently, the central masking effect is nonlinearly related to masker intensity. Second, the curve for a 20-msec delay shows a plateau at medium SLs. Third, the steady-state curve has a smaller slope than the onset curve at all masker levels above 10 dB SL. Fourth, the steady-state masking curve is nonmonotonic. The maximum masking effect is reached at about 40 dB SL. At higher levels the threshold shift decreases. This surprising phenomenon was seen in several experimental series, and its existence appears to be firmly established. It may be of some interest to point out that steady-state intensity characteristics of many VIIIth nerve units show a similar nonmonotonic course (Kiang, 1965).

Psychophysiological relationships concerning central masking are discussed in the last section of this chapter. Here it should be emphasized that central masking characteristics differ radically from the characteristics of monaural masking. In particular, they show quite unequivocally the nonlinear, time-dependent nature of the auditory system, whereas numerous characteristics of monaural masking can be described in linear, time-invariant terms.

III. SOME THEORETICAL CONSIDERATIONS

A. General Considerations

Although our knowledge of the masking phenomenon is not sufficient for a general theory of masking processes, certain relationships seem sufficiently well established for a theoretical treatment. In psychophysical theorizing, we may inquire about relationships among psychophysical characteristics or about psychophysiological relationships. Both approaches appear worthwhile, provided the accepted theoretical postulates do not contradict existing empirical knowledge. Otherwise, the theories suffer a stillbirth.

In the following two subsections, both psychophysical and psychophysiological relationships are discussed. Because of space limitations, only a few selected problems can be treated. We begin with the problem of the signal-to-noise ratio in monaural masking, and discuss some of the consequences of its constancy and its variability. We inquire into the relationships of monaural masking to the loudness function and to the auditory frequency analysis, and, furthermore, into the relationships between monaural masking and central masking, and between central masking and neural activity associated with it. On the basis of experimental evidence and mathematical derivations, it is shown that central masking tells us more about the mechanisms of hearing than does monaural masking.

All the arguments are based on the proposition accepted in signal detection theory (Green & Swets, 1966) that detectability is determined by random fluctuation of the masker or of the neural response it produces. The assumption is made that the aspect of this fluctuation that determines detection is directly proportional to the masker intensity at least to the first order of approximation. Furthermore, it is assumed that, in the absence of an extrinsic masker, detectability is determined by the internal noise of the organism, and that the effective aspect of this noise is added arithmetically to the effective aspect of the extrinsic noise. For simplicity, we discuss the system as if it were an energy detector (Green & Swets, 1966), but such restriction is not otherwise necessary, and the conclusions reached do not become automatically invalid if it is not satisfied in reality.

Under the assumption of an energy detector, it is possible to state that the effective equivalent energy of the internal noise is added arithmetically to the energy of the extrinsic masker. In other words, the intrinsic noise is so transformed that it acts like the extrinsic noise. The meaning and validity of these assumptions should become more evident in the following subsections concerning more specifically certain effects of monaural and central masking.

B. Monaural Masking

It is well known that the ratio of signal power to noise power remains constant for constant detectability and constant signal duration, when the masker consists of either a broad-band, random noise, or a narrow-band, random noise centered at the frequency of the test stimulus. If the auditory system were a linear energy detector, this would be expected. The question is: Does the auditory system have to be a linear detector to satisfy the requirement of a constant signal-to-noise ratio? In order to answer this question, we should realize that the decision process involved in detection of sound does not operate directly on acoustic stimuli but, rather, on the neural responses they produce. As a consequence, a possibility exists that a constant signal-to-noise ratio in the stimulus domain is transformed into a variable signal-to-noise ratio in the neural domain. Assumption of such a transformation would not be parsimonious, however, and we reject it on a trial basis. We now have the condition that a constant signal-to-noise ratio in the stimulus domain should be preserved in the neural domain.

Let us assume that the neural response to noise obeys the function $F(N)$, where N means the noise power, and the response to noise plus signal, the function $F(N + S)$, where S means the signal power. For $S \ll N$, as is approximately true at what is usually accepted as the masked threshold of audibility, it is possible to write approximately

$$F(N + S) \simeq F(N) + SF'(N). \tag{23}$$

The requirement of constant signal-to-noise ratio in the physiological domain leads to

$$F(N + S)/F(N) \simeq 1 + SF'(N)/F(N) = C, \tag{24}$$

with C constant. The relation can be satisfied only for $F'(N) = kF(N)$, with k constant. This is true for all power functions

$$F(N) = AN^\theta , \tag{25}$$

where A and θ can take any constant values. This result is not unexpected, but it needs to be emphasized. The assumption that the constant signal-to-noise ratio encountered in monaural-masking experiments is contingent upon a constant signal-to-noise ratio in the neural domain leads to a power function transformation that is consistent with S. S. Stevens' (1955) demonstration that the loudness function approximates a power function of stimulus intensity. Accordingly, the assumption that a constant signal-to-noise ratio in the stimulus domain leads to a constant signal-to-noise ratio in the neural domain is strengthened.

Since any power-function transformation satisfies simultaneously constant signal-to-noise ratios in the stimulus and neural domains, the monaural masking results tell us very little about the internal characteristics of the auditory system. As an example, let us consider the frequency distribution of the masking effect produced by a narrow band of random noise. If we were interested in the sharpness of auditory filters, we could define it in terms of the ratio of masking effects between two test frequencies, f_1 and f_2. We would determine the signal power necessary for criterion detection as a function of frequency, $S(f)$. Because of the postulate of constant signal-to-noise ratio, we could write for the effective noise power at the frequency f

$$N_{\mathrm{M}}(f) = k_{\mathrm{M}}S(f), \tag{26}$$

where k_M is a constant. The ratio of the effective noise powers between frequencies f_1 and f_2 would follow the equation

$$N_M(f_2)/N_M(f_1) = S(f_2)/S(f_1), \tag{27}$$

which determines the filter sharpness as it appears in the stimulus domain. If we now accepted the optimistic assumption that the same power-function transformation applies to all test frequencies, irrespective of the amount of masking, we could attempt to calculate the filter sharpness in the neural domain. Applying Eq. (25) to the left side of Eq. (27), we would obtain

$$F[N_M(f_2)]/F[N_M(f_1)] = \{N_M(f_2)/N_M(f_1)\}^\theta. \tag{28}$$

This equation defines the filter sharpness in the neural domain as a function of the filter sharpness in the stimulus domain. Unfortunately, the value of θ is not known, so that the numerical relationship turns out to be indeterminate.

If the auditory nonlinearity consisted of a single power-function transformation with a known exponent, the numerical conclusions derived from masking experiments could be corrected accordingly. Unfortunately, the situation seems to be much more complicated. Single unit responses do not approximate simple power functions; however, their sum does (Stevens, 1970; Zwislocki, 1965). The effect of these transformations on frequency selectivity must depend on their location relative to the filtering action. Some filtering takes place in the mechanical part of the cochlea, prior to nonlinear transformations. However, the distribution of neural activity appears to be more peaked than the mechanical amplitude distribution. Accordingly, further filtering must be assumed in the nonlinear part of the auditory system.

In agreement with these suspected relationships, the monaural masking characteristics look more complicated than was assumed in connection with the power-function transformation. A glance at masking curves produced at various test frequencies by a narrow-band masker of constant frequency shows that the constancy of the signal-to-noise ratio in the stimulus domain is preserved only within the noise band. Outside it, the ratio varies with the masker level. As an example, Fig. 36 shows steady-state masking results obtained by Egan and Hake (1950) with the help of a random noise of 90-Hz bandwidth centered at 410 Hz. When the test frequency was at 430 Hz, the masking increments were equal to the increments in masker intensity but, at higher frequencies, the masking curves became steeper, indicating an increasing signal-to-noise ratio. From other results it is known that the ratio decreases as the masker intensity increases, when the test frequency is below the masker frequency band (see, e.g., Wegel & Lane, 1924).

On the basis of the preceding arguments, we have to conclude that monaural masking does not give us straightforward numerical information about the internal characteristics of the auditory system.

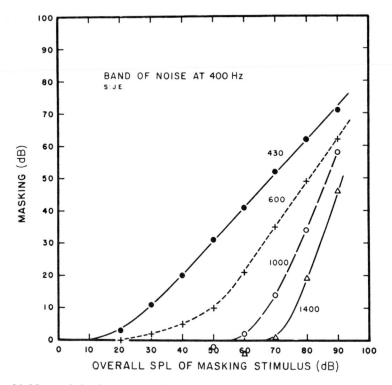

FIG. 36. Monaural simultaneous masking of pure tones at various frequencies by a narrow band of random noise centered at 400 Hz. Threshold shift as a function of masker SPL. [From Egan and Hake (1950). By permission of the Acoustical Society of America.]

C. Central Masking

The statement that central masking can tell us more about the mechanisms of hearing than can monaural masking may appear surprising. However, experimental evidence in support of this statement is rapidly accumulating.

The sharp frequency selectivity of central masking is not contaminated by distortion products of the masking and test stimuli, as is monaural masking. This means that the binaural interaction responsible for central masking is subject to a highly developed tonotopic organization. As a consequence, the masking effect exerted on a pure-tone test stimulus reflects processes limited to a small group of neural units that are excited simultaneously by the masking and test stimuli. Since the usually much stronger masker excites a much larger number of units than does the test tone, the threshold shift of which rarely exceeds 10 dB, the group of units controlling central masking must be effectively determined by the test frequency. In this sense, the test tone picks out a group of units in a way somewhat analogous to a microelectrode selecting one or several units. At the end of this section the proposition that the small groups of neurons controlling central masking are homogeneous enough to parallel closely the characteristics of single-unit responses is validated by means of psychophysiological comparisons.

The following psychophysical analysis of central masking rests upon three postulates, for which there is substantial empirical evidence independent of central masking (Zwislocki, 1972).

1. The detectability of the test stimulus is determined by the signal-to-noise ratio in the neural domain. That is, the signal-to-noise ratio is constant when the detectability is constant. The assumption holds for extrinsic as well as intrinsic noise and, in view of the statements already made with respect to frequency selectivity, it should be applied to the group of neurons maximally excited by the test stimulus.
2. Neural inputs from the two ears are linearly summated in a binaural adding stage.
3. At low sound intensity levels, the driven neural firing rate is directly proportional to sound intensity.

The first postulate is a simple extension of the postulate made in conjunction with monaural masking. The second postulate results from general neurophysiological evidence and, more specifically, from the experiments performed by Goldberg and Brown (1969) on the medial superior olive. The superior olive appears to be the lowest nuclear complex of the auditory system where the afferent innervations of both ears interact. As a consequence, it may be the sight that controls central masking. The third postulate follows directly from an analysis of the intensity characteristics of single-auditory units (Zwislocki, 1970). A more extensive documentation can be found in an original paper (Zwislocki, 1972).

In order to apply the three postulates to a numerical calculation, the following symbols are introduced.

E_Q	output of the binaural adding stage in the absence of extrinsic noise
E_M	output of the adding stage in the presence of extrinsic noise
E_I	contribution of spontaneous activity of one ear
E_{SQ}	contribution of the activity produced by the signal in the absence of extrinsic noise
E_{SM}	contribution of the activity produced by the signal in the presence of masking noise
E_N	contribution of the activity produced by the extrinsic masking noise
M	portion of the activity produced by the masker ear, which interacts with the activity produced by the test ear
S_Q	signal intensity at criterion detection level in the absence of masking noise
S_M	signal intensity at criterion detection level in the presence of masking noise

In the absence of extrinsic masking noise, the postulate on binaural summation (2 above) leads to the equation

$$E_Q = E_{SQ} + E_I + ME_I,\tag{29}$$

where ME_I indicates the contribution of the spontaneous activity of the masker ear. In the presence of extrinsic masking noise, the second postulate calls for

$$E_M = E_{SM} + E_I + M(E_N + E_I).\tag{30}$$

In the first equation, E_{SQ} has the meaning of a signal, $E_I + ME_I$, of noise; in the second, the same is true for E_{SM} and $E_I + M(E_N + E_I)$, respectively. Because of the requirement of a constant signal-to-noise ratio, we must have

$$E_{SM}/[E_I + M(E_N + E_I)] = E_{SQ}/(E_I + ME_I),\tag{31}$$

or, after appropriate transformation,

$$E_{SM}/E_{SQ} = 1 + [M/(1 + M)](E_N/E_I).\tag{32}$$

According to the third postulate,

$$E_{SM}/E_{SQ} = S_M/S_Q,\tag{33}$$

so that, substituting from Eq. (33) in Eq. (32), we obtain

$$S_M/S_Q = 1 + [M/(1 + M)](E_N/E_I).\tag{34}$$

The ratio S_M/S_Q is the linear expression for the threshold shift $TS = 10 \log S_M/S_Q$, and the equation describes a direct relationship between it and the ratio of driven and spontaneous neural activities. At sufficiently high levels of driven activity, the equation can be approximated by

$$S_M/S_Q \simeq [M/(1 + M)](E_N/E_I)\tag{35}$$

or, in the logarithmic form,

$$TS \simeq 10 \log[M/(1 + M)] + 10 \log(E_N/E_I).\tag{36}$$

If we remember that E_N increases much more slowly than the masker intensity, we can see why central masking increases more slowly with the masker intensity than does monaural masking. The rate is decreased even further by the addition of the constant 1 in the complete equation.

Equation (34) can be transformed into

$$E_N/E_I = [(1 + M)/M][(S_M/S_Q) - 1],\tag{37}$$

a form that, according to the theory, makes it possible to calculate neural activities from threshold shifts. However, Eq. (37) has the flaw that the numerical values of the constants E_I and M are not well known. To eliminate it, we limit the calculations to ratios of driven activities. In other words, we normalize all the values with respect to a convenient reference. Let us assume that $10 \log(S_{M0}/S_Q)$ is a reference threshold shift in decibels, and E_{N0}/E_I the corresponding ratio of driven and spontaneous activities. Then, by introducing the reference values into Eq. (37) and dividing the general equation [Eq. (37)] by the specific equation, we obtain

$$\frac{E_N}{E_{N0}} = \frac{(S_M/S_Q) - 1}{(S_{M0}/S_Q) - 1}.$$

(38)

The latter expression has no free constants and establishes a unique relationship between psychophysically measured threshold shifts and neural responses at the binaural adding stage. These theoretical responses can be compared with appropriate recordings of single-unit activity (Zwislocki, 1972).

The quantitative theory just described applies directly to the binaural adding stage, which we suspect to be located in the superior olive. Consequently, recordings from superior-olive units should be used for psychophysiological comparisons. However, it could be shown that at least some neural populations of the superior olive have basically the same normalized characteristics as the VIIIth nerve units (Zwislocki, 1972), so that the theory may be applied indirectly to the latter. This is of great advantage, since much more extensive empirical data become available.

The first comparison, illustrated in Fig. 37, refers to the fast decay of firing rate that seems to be exhibited to the same degree by all VIIIth nerve units,

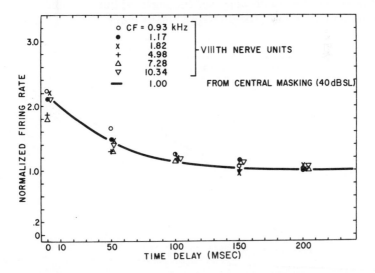

FIG. 37. Temporal decay of driven firing rate in 6 units of the VIIIth nerve, as a function of the time delay from the stimulus onset. The curve has been calculated from central masking for a comparable stimulus intensity level. [From Zwislocki (1972). By permission of the Acoustical Society of America.]

independent of their characteristic frequency (CF). The various symbols in the figure indicate empirical data computed from poststimulus time (PST) histograms (Kiang, 1965). The curve has been calculated from central masking by means of Eq. (38) for a corresponding stimulus intensity.

In Fig. 38 the empirical intensity characteristics of five VIIIth nerve units obtained with 40-msec tone bursts (Wiederhold, 1967) are compared with an approximately corresponding curve calculated from central masking. The correspondence was achieved by measuring the threshold shifts with a time delay of 20 msec from the masker onset. It should be pointed out that the normalized characteristic is not sensitive to time delay. The theoretical curve agrees almost exactly with the empirical data up to 50 dB. At higher levels, it takes a deviant course. This is the only instance of disagreement between the theory and corresponding empirical data found thus far. Apparently, at SLs of over 50 dB, transient processes are at work that have not been included in the theory (for a more extensive discussion of the discrepancy, see Zwislocki, 1972).

Finally, Fig. 39 compares empirical tuning curves obtained on two VIIIth nerve neurons by means of 50-msec tone bursts (Kiang, Watanabe, Thomas, & Clark, 1962) and steady-state tones (Kiang, 1965), respectively, with theoretical tuning curves obtained from Fig. 33 by intersecting the masking curves with horizontal lines at various threshold-shift values. The low threshold shifts correspond to the low levels of neural activity at which the empirical curves were obtained. Note that, according to the empirical results, the form of the tuning curves is the same for transient and steady-state conditions and, therefore, should be practically independent of the time delay

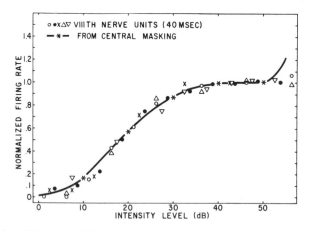

Fig. 38. Driven firing rate of five VIIIth nerve units, as a function of the intensity level of 40-msec tone bursts. The curve has been calculated from central-masking data from comparable stimulus conditions. [From Zwislocki (1972). By permission of the Acoustical Society of America.]

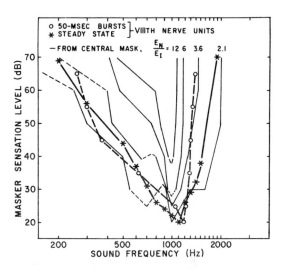

FIG. 39. Tuning curves of two VIIIth nerve units with CFs around 1000 Hz (heavy lines), and tuning curves derived from central masking for various theoretical ratios between the driven and spontaneous firing rates. [From Zwislocki (1972). By permission of the Acoustical Society of America.]

from the stimulus onset. The empirical curves were brought to coincidence with the lowest theoretical one by placing their minima at a masker sensation level of 20 dB. It should be evident that both sets of curves have all the main features in common: approximately the same slopes at the low- and high-frequency sides and the same spread.

Many more psychophysiological comparisons relevant to the theory of central masking are possible (Zwislocki, 1970–1972). Thus far, no fundamental discrepancy between the theoretical and empirical results has been found, except the one of Fig. 38. It seems that, at least up to moderate intensity levels, central masking is related in a simple way to neural activity in certain neural populations at the peripheral and low central levels of the auditory system.

References

Békésy, G. von. Zur Theorie des Hörens; die Schwingungsform der Basilarmembran. *Physikalische Zeitschrift,* 1928, **29,** 793–810.

Békésy, G. von. Ueber die Resonanzkurve und die Abklingzeit der verschiedenen Stellen der Schneckentrennwand. *Akustische Zeitschrift,* 1943, **8,** 66–76.

Békésy, G. von. *Experiments in hearing.* New York: McGraw-Hill, 1960. (a)

Békésy, G. von. Neural inhibitory units of the eye and skin. Quantitative description of contrast phenomena. *Journal of the Optical Society of America,* 1960, **50,** 1060–1070. (b)

Bos, C. E., & de Boer, E. Masking and discrimination. *Journal of the Acoustical Society of America,* 1966, **39,** 708–715.

Carterette, E. C., Friedman, M. P., & Lovell, J. D. Mach bands in auditory perception. In R. Plomp & G. F. Smoorenburg (Eds.), *Frequency analysis and periodicity detection in hearing.* Leiden: A. W. Sijthoff, 1970.

Chistovich, L. A., & Ivanova, V. A. Mutual masking of short sound pulses. *Biofizika,* 1959, **4,** 170–180.

Dirks, D. D., & Malmquist, C. Shifts in air conduction thresholds produced by pulsed and continuous contralateral masking. *Journal of the Acoustical Society of America*, 1965, **37**, 631–637.

Egan, J. P., & Hake, H. W. On the masking pattern of a simple auditory stimulus. *Journal of the Acoustical Society of America*, 1950, **22**, 622–630.

Elliot, L. L. Backward masking: monotic and dichotic conditions. *Journal of the Acoustical Society of America*, 1962, **34**, 1108–1115. (a)

Elliot, L. L. Backward and forward masking of probe tones of different frequencies. *Journal of the Acoustical Society of America*, 1962, **34**, 1116–1117. (b)

Elliot, L. L. Changes in the simultaneous masked threshold of brief tones. *Journal of the Acoustical Society of America*, 1965, **38**, 738–746.

Elliot, L. L. Development of auditory narrow-band frequency contours. *Journal of the Acoustical Society of America*, 1967, **42**, 143–153.

Feldtkeller, R., & Zwicker, E. *Das Ohr als Nachrichtenempfänger*. Stuttgart: S. Hirzel, 1956.

Fletcher, H. Auditory patterns. *Review of Modern Physics*, 1940, **12**, 47–65.

Gardner, M. B. Short duration auditory fatigue as a method of classifying hearing impairment. *Journal of the Acoustical Society of America*, 1947, **19**, 178–190.

Goldberg, J. M., & Brown, P. B. Response of binaural neurons of dog superior olivary complex to dichotic tonal stimuli: Some physiological mechanisms of sound localization. *Journal of Neurophysiology*, 1969, **32**, 613–628.

Goldstein, J. L. Auditory nonlinearity. *Journal of the Acoustical Society of America*, 1967, **41**, 676–689.

Green, D. M. Masking with continuous and pulsed sinusoids. *Journal of the Acoustical Society of America*, 1969, **46**, 939–946.

Green, D. M., & Swets, J. A. *Signal detection theory and psychophysics*. New York: Wiley, 1966.

Greenwood, D. D. Auditory masking and the critical band. *Journal of the Acoustical Society of America*, 1961, **33**, 484–502.

Greenwood, D. D. Aural combination tones and auditory masking. *Journal of the Acoustical Society of America*, 1971, **50**, 502–543.

Hamilton, P. M. Noise masked thresholds as a function of tonal duration and masking noise band width. *Journal of the Acoustical Society of America*, 1957, **29**, 506–511.

Hawkins, J. E., Jr., & Stevens, S. S. The masking of pure tones and of speech by white noise. *Journal of the Acoustical Society of America*, 1950, **22**, 6–13.

Hughes, J. W. The monaural threshold: The effect of subliminal and audible contralateral and ipsilateral stimuli. *Proceedings of the Royal Society*, 1940, **128B**, 144–152.

Ingham, J. G. The effect upon monaural sensitivity of continuous stimulation of the opposite ear. *Quarterly Journal of Experimental Psychology*, 1957, **9**, 52–60.

Ingham, J. G. Variation in cross masking with frequency. *Journal of Experimental Psychology*, 1959, **58**, 199–205.

Kiang, N. Y.-S. Discharge patterns of single fibers in the cat's auditory nerve. *M.I.T. Research Monograph No. 35*. Cambridge, Massachusetts: M.I.T. Press, 1965.

Kiang, N. Y.-S., Watanabe, T., Thomas, E. C., & Clark, L. F. Stimulus coding in the cat's auditory nerve. *Annals of Otology, Rhinology and Laryngology*, 1962, **71**, 1009–1027.

Leshowitz, B., & Wightman, F. L. On-frequency masking with continuous sinusoids. *Journal of the Acoustical Society of America*, 1971, **49**, 1180–1190.

Lüscher, E., & Zwislocki, J. Ueber Abklingvorgänge des Ohres. *Practica Oto-rhino-laryngologica*, 1946, **8**, 531–533.

Lüscher, E., & Zwislocki, J. The decay of sensation and the remainder of adaptation after short pure-tone impulses on the ear. *Acta Otolaryngologica*, 1947, **35**, 428–445.

Lüscher, E., & Zwislocki, J. Adaptation of the ear to sound stimuli. *Journal of the Acoustical Society of America*, 1949, **21**, 135–139.

Miller, G. A. Sensitivity to changes in the intensity of white noise and its relation to masking and loudness. *Journal of the Acoustical Society of America*, 1947, **19**, 609–619.

Munson, W. A., & Gardner, M. B. Loudness patterns—a new approach. *Journal of the Acoustical Society of America*, 1950, **22**, 177–190.

Osman, E., & Raab, D. H. Temporal masking of clicks by noise bursts. *Journal of the Acoustical Society of America*, 1963, **35**, 1939–1941.

Pickett, J. M. Backward masking. *Journal of the Acoustical Society of America*, 1959, **31**, 1613–1615.

Raab, D. H. Forward and backward masking between acoustic clicks. *Journal of the Acoustical Society of America*, 1961, **33**, 137–139.

Ratliff, F. *Mach bands*. San Francisco: Holden-Day, 1965.

Robinson, C. E., & Pollack, I. Forward and backward masking: Testing a descrete perceptual-moment hypothesis in audition. *Journal of the Acoustical Society of America*, 1971, **50**, 1512–1519.

Rubin, H. Auditory facilitation following stimulation at low intensities. *Journal of the Acoustical Society of America*, 1960, **32**, 670–681.

Sachs, M. B., & Kiang, N. Y.-S. Two-tone inhibition in auditory-nerve fibers. *Journal of the Acoustical Society of America*, 1968, **43**, 1120–1128.

Samoilova, I. K. Masking of short tone signals as a function of the time interval between masked and masking sounds. *Biofizika*, 1959, **4**, 550–558.

Schafer, T. H., Gales, R. S., Shewmaker, C. A., & Thompson, P. O. The frequency selectivity of the ear as determined by masking experiments. *Journal of the Acoustical Society of America*, 1950, **22**, 490–496.

Scharf, B. Loudness of complex sounds as a function of the number of components. *Journal of the Acoustical Society of America*, 1959, **31**, 783–785.

Scherrick, C. E., Jr., & Mangabeira-Albernaz, P. L. Auditory threshold shifts produced by simultaneously pulsed contralateral stimuli. *Journal of the Acoustical Society of America*, 1961, **33**, 1381–1385.

Scholl, H. Ueber die Bildung der Hörschwellen und Mithörschwellen von Impulsen. *Acustica*, 1962, **12**, 91–101. (a)

Scholl, H. Das dynamische Verhalten des Gehörs bei der Unterteilung des Schallspektrums in Frequenzgruppen. *Acustica*, 1962, **12**, 101–107. (b)

Smith, R. L., & Zwislocki, J. J. Response of some neurons of the cochlear nucleus to tone-intensity increments. *Journal of the Acoustical Society of America*, 1971, **50**, 1520–1525.

Stein, H. J. Das Absinken der Mithörschwelle nach dem Abschalten von weissem Rauschen. *Acustica*, 1960, **10**, 116–119.

Stevens, S. S. The relation of pitch to intensity. *Journal of the Acoustical Society of America*, 1935, **6**, 150–154.

Stevens, S. S. The measurement of loudness. *Journal of the Acoustical Society of America*, 1955, **27**, 815–829.

Stevens, S. S. The surprising simplicity of sensory metrics. *American Psychologist*, 1962, **17**, 29–39.

Stevens, S. S. Neural events and the psychophysical law. *Science*, 1970, **170**, 1043–1050.

Tonndorf, J. Dimensional analysis of cochlear models. *Journal of the Acoustical Society of America*, 1960, **32**, 493–497.

Wegel, R. L., & Lane, C. E. The auditory masking of one pure tone by another and its probable relation to the dynamics of the inner ear. *Physical Review*, 1924, **23**, ser. 2, 266–285.

Wever, E. G. *Theory of hearing*. New York: John Wiley and Sons, 1949.

Wiederhold, M. L. A study of efferent inhibition of auditory nerve activity. Unpublished Ph.D. dissertation, M.I.T., Cambridge, Massachusetts, 1967.

Wightman, F. L. Detection of binaural tones as a function of masker bandwidth. *Journal of the Acoustical Society of America*, 1971, **50**, 623–636.

Wright, H. N. Temporal summation and backward masking. *Journal of the Acoustical Society of America,* 1964, **36**, 927–932. (a)

Wright, H. N. Backward masking for tones in narrow-band noise. *Journal of the Acoustical Society of America,* 1964, **36**, 2217–2221. (b)

Zwicker, E. Die Verdeckung von Schmalbandgeräuschen durch Sinustöne. *Acustica,* 1954, **4**, 415–420.

Zwicker, E. Temporal effects in simultaneous masking by white-noise bursts. *Journal of the Acoustical Society of America,* 1965, **37**, 653–663. (a)

Zwicker, E. Temporal effects in simultaneous masking and loudness. *Journal of the Acoustical Society of America,* 1965, **38**, 132–141. (b)

Zwicker, E., & Feldtkeller, R. *Das Ohr als Nachrichtenempfänger.* Stuttgart: S. Hirzel, 1967.

Zwicker, E., Flottorp, G., & Stevens, S. S. Critical band width in loudness summation. *Journal of the Acoustical Society of America,* 1957, **29**, 548–557.

Zwislocki, J. Theorie der Schneckenmechanik. *Acta Oto-Laryngologica,* 1948, Suppl. 72.

Zwislocki, J. J. Acoustic attenuation between the ears. *Journal of the Acoustical Society of America,* 1953, **25**, 752–759.

Zwislocki, J. Relation of adaptation to fatigue, masking and recruitment. *International Society of Audiology,* 1960, *5th Congress,* 279–285. (a)

Zwislocki, J. Theory of temporal auditory summation. *Journal of the Acoustical Society of America,* 1960, **32**, 1046–1060. (b)

Zwislocki, J. Analysis of some auditory characteristics. In R. D. Luce, R. R. Bush, & E. Galanter (Eds.), *Handbook of mathematical psychology.* vol. 3. New York: Wiley, 1965. Pp. 1–97.

Zwislocki, J. J. Central masking and auditory frequency selectivity. In R. Plomp & G. F. Smoorenburg (Eds.), *Frequency analysis and periodicity detection in hearing.* Leiden: A. W. Sijthoff, 1970.

Zwislocki, J. J. Central masking and neural activity in the cochlear nucleus. *Audiology,* 1971, **10**, 48–59.

Zwislocki, J. J. A theory of central auditory masking and its partial validation. *Journal of the Acoustical Society of America,* 1972, **52**, 644–659.

Zwislocki, J. J., Buining, E., & Glantz, J. Frequency distribution of central masking. *Journal of the Acoustical Society of America,* 1968, **43**, 1267–1271.

Zwislocki, J. J., Damianopoulos, E. N., Buining, E., & Glantz, J. Central masking: Some steady-state and transient effects. *Perception and Psychophysics,* 1967, **2**, 59–64.

Zwislocki, J., & Pirodda, E. On the adaptation, fatigue and acoustic trauma of the ear. *Experientia,* 1952, **8**, 279–284.

Zwislocki, J., Pirodda, E., & Rubin, H. On some poststimulatory effects at the threshold of audibility. *Journal of the Acoustical Society of America,* 1959, **31**, 9–14.

Chapter 9

AUDITORY MASKING

ROY D. PATTERSON AND DAVID M. GREEN

I. INTRODUCTION

When one sound makes another difficult or impossible to hear, *masking* has occurred. This phenomenon does not seem surprising: If one sound is intense and another weak, it seems natural that the louder sound should mask the softer. Masking is not, however, simply a question of relative intensities. The occurrence of masking depends as much on the frequency composition of the two sounds as it does on their relative intensities. For example, an 80-dB, 500-Hz sinusoid will not mask a 20-dB, 3000-Hz sinusoid despite the fact that the 500-Hz sinusoid has 1 million times the power of the 3000-Hz sinusoid. It is primarily the relation between masking and frequency that will be the concern of this chapter.

The early work in audition emphasized frequency analysis, the ability of the observer to separate a complex musical sound into its constituents and to

HANDBOOK OF PERCEPTION, VOL. IV

appreciate, at least to a limited extent, the individual components of the complex. Masking is an interaction between two stimuli that demonstrates a frequency-analysis failure. Masking data provide quantitative information about the extent and limits of frequency analysis. And thus the two phenomena reflect different aspects of the same process.

The intense sound of modern-day machinery, such as the roar of jet air-craft, makes masking a common occurrence. But despite the importance of the phenomenon, it is a comparatively recent topic in the study of hearing. The reasons for this neglect are simple: Before the advent of modern elec-tronics, it was virtually impossible to control and measure the intensity of a sound field with precision. Helmholtz had a diaphragm that he mounted at the end of his resonator. By controlling the size of the opening in the dia-phragm, he could regulate the intensity of a sinusoidal wave over a limited range. But systematic study of the topic of masking had to await the development of convenient apparatus. For example, Mayer (1876) com-mented, on the basis of observations made while listening to an organ, that he believed low-frequency sounds to be better maskers of high-frequency sounds than the reverse. The amount of this asymmetry, in power terms, can be as much as 10^{10}, which shows just how uncertain earlier investigators were about the exact intensity of their sounds.

Once the equipment necessary to perform controlled experiments on masking became available, a sustained research effort in this area began. In this chapter we shall review this empirical effort and try to summarize the main findings. But our primary goal will be not so much an exhaustive review of the many studies as an attempt to relate a subset of the data to theory about the hearing mechanism, and particularly to current thinking about frequency analysis. Therefore, we emphasize integration rather than comprehensiveness. We shall have to omit several important and interesting areas of research; such as contralateral masking and speech interference. These omissions are unfortunate, but some of the topics are covered in other chapters.

We have also omitted a rather sizable body of theory in that we shall treat masking in terms of signal-to-noise-ratio analysis and completely ignore statistical fluctuation. The use of fluctuation statistics and its application to masking may be found in a number of articles (Green, 1960; Green & McGill, 1970; Jeffress, 1964; Marill, 1956; McGill, 1967; Pfafflin & Mathews, 1962; Siebert, 1965; Tanner, Swets, & Green, 1956). We may justify this omission to some extent by arguing that the signal-to-noise-ratio analysis given in this chapter is a good first approximation. Consideration of statistical fluctuation might change some of the details but not the major conclusions of our arguments (Patterson & Henning, 1977).

Historically, the first modern study of masking was a study of sinusoidal masking by Wegel and Lane (1924). We shall begin with noise masking, however, since the results are somewhat simpler and easier to summarize.

II. NOISE MASKING

A. Broad Band Noise

In these experiments the masker is a noise, and for the initial studies, it is broad band or "white" noise. The signal that the observer is trying to detect is a sinusoid. The signal is sometimes called a *maskee* but to distinguish between "masker" and "maskee" on the basis of the last letter in six seems to put an undue burden on the reader. We use the words "masker" and "signal" for these two elements.

1. MASKING AND NOISE LEVEL

In one of the most basic masking experiments, signal threshold (that is, the minimum power the sinusoid must have to be just detectable in the noise), is determined as a function of the level of the noise. This relation was first measured by Fletcher (1940) and a decade later by Hawkins and Stevens (1950). Figure 1 shows Hawkins and Stevens's data for three frequencies, 1000, 2800, and 5600 Hz. The results of this experiment are extremely sim-

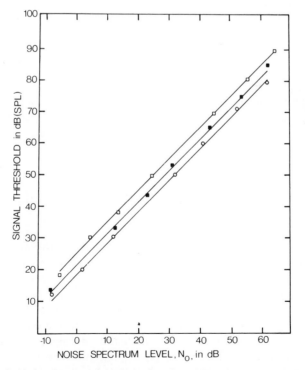

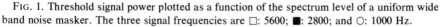

FIG. 1. Threshold signal power plotted as a function of the spectrum level of a uniform wide band noise masker. The three signal frequencies are □: 5600; ■: 2800; and ○: 1000 Hz.

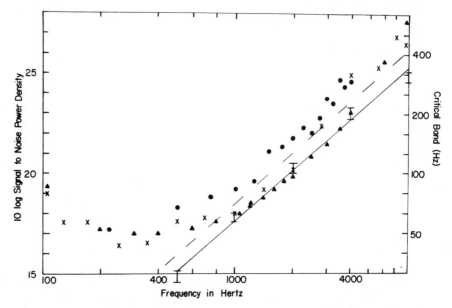

Fig. 2. Threshold signal-to-noise ratio plotted as a function of signal frequency. The masker is a uniform wide band noise. ▲: Data from Fletcher (1953, Table 16); ●: data from Green, McKey, and Licklider (1959); ×: data from Hawkins and Stevens (1950, Fig. 6).

ple: The power of the signal at threshold is directly proportional to the power of the noise, provided the noise is intense enough to raise the sinusoid a few decibels over its absolute threshold. If P_s is the threshold signal power, N_0 is the spectrum level of the noise, that is, the noise power in a 1-Hz band, and $P_0(f)$ is the absolute threshold of the signal, that is, its threshold value with the noise turned off ($N_0 = 0$), then

$$P_s = k(f)N_0 + P_0(f), \qquad (1)$$

where $k(f)$ is a constant that depends on the frequency of the sinusoid.

2. Masking and Signal Frequency

The vertical displacement of the lines in Fig. 1 shows that $k(f)$ is an increasing function of f. In other words, threshold is an increasing function of frequency when the noise level is held constant. A more detailed view of this relationship is presented in Fig. 2, a plot of threshold signal-to-noise ratio versus frequency. In the earlier experiments shown in Fig. 2, those of Fletcher (1953) and Hawkins and Stevens (1950), an unlimited signal duration was used. The subject simply adjusted the signal power until the sinusoid was just detectable in the noise. The more recent experiment by Green, McKey, and Licklider (1959) employed a $\frac{1}{10}$-sec signal duration and two-alternative forced-choice procedure. Consequently, for any specific frequency, the signal power at threshold is somewhat greater than that found in the other studies. Nevertheless, the relation of signal level and frequency does not seem to depend markedly on signal duration.

Next we turn to a compelling interpretation of the masking results, namely, a filter interpretation, and some direct tests of this hypothesis.

III. AUDITORY FILTERING

A. Rectangular Filtering

When the noise level is high enough to raise signal threshold, P_s, 10 dB or more above absolute threshold, $P_0(f)$, then Eq. (1) reduces to

$$P_s = k(f)N_0, \tag{2}$$

since $P_0(f)$ becomes negligible with respect to $k(f)N_0$. The relation summarized in Eq. (2), the fact that the signal power at threshold is proportional to the noise power, has a simple and convenient interpretation that was first suggested by Fletcher (1940). Suppose the observer, in attempting to detect the signal, listens to only those frequencies in a narrow band about the signal frequency. If we assume (*1*) that all noise outside this listening band is rejected and all noise within the band passes unaffected, that is, the transfer function of the observer's auditory filter, $H(f)$, has the form

$$H(f) = \begin{cases} 1, & f_1 < f < f_u \\ 0, & \text{otherwise} \end{cases} \tag{3}$$

(f_1 and f_u are the lower and upper limits of the listening band) and (*2*) that the signal is just detectable when the signal power is equal to the total noise power coming through the filter, that is,

$$P_s = \int_0^\infty N_0 |H(f)|^2 \, df, \tag{4}$$

and if we substitute for $H(f)$ in Eq. (4) to get

$$P_s = \int_{f_1}^{f_u} N_0 \, df, \tag{5}$$

or

$$P_s = (f_u - f_1)N_0, \tag{6}$$

then we are led by the similarity of Eqs. (2) and (6) to the conclusion that the proportionality constant $k(f)$ in Eq. (2) is simply the width of the listening band $(f_u - f_1)$. The fact that $k(f)$ increases with frequency is interpreted to suggest that the bandwidth of the filter increases with center frequency, a most reasonable relationship, since many physical filter systems have a bandwidth that increases with center frequency. Zwicker, Flottorp, and Stevens (1957) have suggested that this method of determining the width of the listening band be called the critical-ratio method; and it is, in fact, one of the means used to estimate what is called the width of the critical band. Notice that this procedure involves two assumptions: *(1)* that the listening band is rectangular, and *(2)* that the threshold of the signal occurs when the signal power is equal to the total effective noise, or the total noise power coming through the critical band. These assumptions can be partially checked in other, independent, experiments to verify their accuracy. We shall turn to these experiments next.

The important point in summarizing the relationship just discussed is to note that there is almost perfect linearity over a rather large range of noise powers between the noise level and the signal level at threshold. If Weber's law is interpreted to mean that the signal is just detectable when it causes a certain percentage increase in the background, then the data on sinusoids masked by noise are consistent with Weber's law over practically the entire range of the masking stimulus. As we shall see, however, Weber's law is not as accurate a summary of data using sinusoidal maskers.

B. A Direct Test of the Filter Hypothesis

One of the most direct tests of the assumption that the observer is listening to only a narrow range of frequencies about the signal frequency was carried out by Fletcher (1940). This is the original critical-band study; and since it antedates other related experiments by almost a decade, it seems regrettable that this direct method of measurement is not cited as often as the critical-ratio method. He first determined the threshold of a 1000-Hz sinusoid presented in a reasonably loud, wide-band noise. Next, the power of the noise was reduced by narrowing its bandwidth, retaining at its original level only the noise in a 500-Hz-wide band centered at 1000 Hz, and then the signal threshold was determined again. Surprisingly, he found the same threshold as that measured using wide-band noise. This is especially startling if we listen to the two maskers, since the wide band masker is considerably louder than the narrow band masker. He continued the experiment by progressively decreasing the width of the masker, always keeping the masker band centered at the signal frequency. Finally, when the noise bandwidth became very narrow, the signal became easier to hear; its threshold decreased. This break in the function relating masker bandwidth and signal threshold is a measure of the critical listening interval or critical bandwidth. Fletcher suggested that as the masker bandwidth is decreased beyond this critical point, signal threshold varies linearly with the width of the noise band. This relation, if true, supports the assumptions listed in connection with the critical-ratio approach. Fletcher performed this experiment repeatedly with different signal frequencies. The data appear in Fig. 3.

These results show that the width of the listening band, the break points in the figure, increase with increasing signal frequency. The width is approxi-

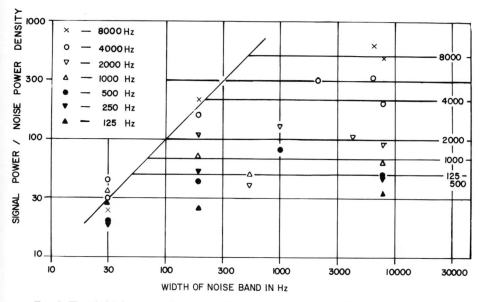

FIG. 3. Threshold signal-to-noise ratio plotted as a function of the width of a band of uniform noise centered at the signal frequency. ×:8000; ○:4000, ∇:2000; △:1000; ●:500; ▼:250; ▲: 125 Hz.

mately 40 Hz in the 250-Hz region, about 60 Hz at 1000 Hz, and about 150 Hz near 4000 Hz. To the extent that the data cluster on the line with unit slope at the left of the figure they support the assumption that at threshold, the power of the signal is exactly equal to the total noise power coming through the listener's band as the critical-ratio method would have it.

The basic assumption of the critical-ratio method, namely, that a constant signal-to-noise ratio within the critical band yields constant detectability, is reasonably compelling. However, the assumption that the proportionality constant relating signal power and noise power is unity at threshold requires some justification. Fletcher's critical-band experiment indicates that this assumption is a good first approximation; the constant would appear to be between .3 and 3. Since the ratio method depends on a single threshold determination and does not involve measuring the break point in a function, it is apparent that Fletcher relied more heavily on the critical-ratio method in estimating the size of the critical band. Nevertheless, the direct method was explored by Fletcher and the data collected in 1940.

C. Refinements of the Critical-Band Study

When the masker is a broad-band stimulus, such as noise, the exact shape of the auditory filter is usually unimportant. However, when the masker and the signal both have relatively restricted spectral loci, the shape of the filter can be crucial.

Schafer, Gales, Shewmaker, and Thompson (1950) were the first to try to estimate the shape of the auditory filter in more detail. Their experiment was essentially a repeat of Fletcher's original critical-band experiment, except that their masker had nearly a rectangular spectrum and they took more measurements of the increase in the detectability of the signal as the band was narrowed. The noise they used was constructed by dubbing a large number of closely spaced sinusoids on a film track. Thus, except for non-linear effects, the spectrum of the masking "noise" was contained within the boundaries of the many added sinusoids. Their data showed a gradual decrease in the threshold of the signal—a sinusoid placed in the middle of their masking noise—as the bandwidth of the noise decreased. Thus, their results indicated that the ear's filter is not rectangular but has a gradual attenuation characteristic outside the pass-band. In fact, they found that their data could be fit fairly well if they assumed that the ear's filter was a single-tuned system. The transfer function for a single-tuned system is

$$H(f) = \frac{1}{1 + \{[(f_l f_u)^{1/2}/(f_u - f_l)][f/f_0 - f_0/f]\}^2},$$

where f_0 is the center frequency of the filter, f_l is the frequency below f_0 at which the filter reduces input power by half, and f_u is the frequency above f_0 at which input power is reduced by half. It is common practice to describe filters in terms of their "half-power" bandwidth. The "half-power" bandwidth or the "3-dB" bandwidth of a filter is the distance between its half-power points. Estimates by Schafer et al. of half-power bandwidth for the single-tuned filters that best fit their data were 65 Hz at both 200 and 800 Hz and 240 Hz at 3200 Hz, which is fairly close to Fletcher's estimates.*

Somewhat smaller bandwidths were estimated by still another replication of Fletcher's direct measurement of the ear's bandwidth in a study by Swets, Green, and Tanner (1962). They used a simple-tuned filter to filter the noise and a single signal frequency, 1000 Hz. If the external filter is a single-tuned filter and the ear's filter is the same, then the effective noise spectrum can be calculated by computing the product of the two in series. As the external filter's bandwidth decreases, the effective noise power decreases, and an estimate of the internal filter's bandwidth can be made. Estimates made on this assumption of an internal single-tuned filter were smaller and more consistent than estimates based on several other assumptions. The estimated bandwidth was about 40 Hz at 1000 Hz for three observers.

These critical-band studies provide considerable evidence in favor of an auditory filter. Additional support is provided by an experiment by Webster, Miller, Thompson, and Davenport (1952). Their experiment is the logical

* In the case of the rectangular filter, the half-power bandwidth is clearly just the distance between the lower and upper cutoffs of the filter.

converse of the original critical-band experiment. Instead of using a narrow band of noise as a masker, they used a wide-band noise with an octave band filtered out of it. They measured thresholds for sinusoids in the region of the gap and, as might be anticipated, they found that the signal is most easily heard when it is near the center of the gap and becomes progressively harder to hear as it approaches the sides of the gap. Like Schafer *et al.*, they found that their data supported the assumption of a single-tuned rather than a rectangular filter shape.

D. Direct Determination of Auditory Filter Shape

Patterson (1974) has attempted to measure the auditory filter characteristic in greater detail, especially the skirts of the filter. Patterson's experiment is conceptually very simple. He repeatedly determined the threshold for the signal, a sinusoid of constant frequency, as the cutoff of a low-pass filtered noise was varied from well below to somewhat above the frequency of the signal. As would be anticipated, signal threshold increased monotonically as the low-pass filtered noise approached the signal. Deriving the shape of the auditory filter from this experiment depends on two assumptions: *(1)* that the noise cutoff is very sharp and *(2)* that the auditory filter is centered on the signal. If these conditions are met, then the auditory filter's amplitude characteristic is simply the derivative of the curve relating signal power at threshold to the cutoff of the noise.

The argument is most easily understood in terms of power spectra; Fig. 4 contains the idealized power spectra of the signal and the low-pass filtered noise masker in addition to the squared transfer function of the hypothetical auditory filter. The shaded area, where the power spectrum of the noise and

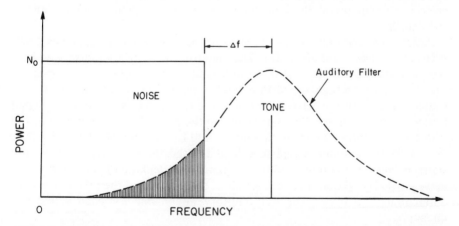

Fig. 4. Schematic representation of a tone, a low-pass filtered uniform noise, and the hypothetical auditory filter. The shaded area where the noise spectrum and filter characteristic overlap represents the noise that is effective in masking the tone.

the squared transfer function of the filter overlap, represents the amount of input noise that passes through the auditory filter and hence is effective in masking the tone. The level of the effective noise increases, obviously, as the upper frequency edge of the noise increases. So long as the ratio of the height of the tone to the shaded area is large enough, the tone is heard. If we let the power spectra of the signal and noise be P_s and $N(f)$ and the transfer function of the filter be $H(f)$, then the model is represented mathematically by

$$P_s = K \int_0^\infty N(f) |H(f)|^2 \, df. \tag{7}$$

That is, the minimum power P_s that a sinusoid must have to be heard in a noise $N(f)$ is some constant proportion K of the integral of the noise spectrum, weighted by the square of the transfer function of the filter. We now proceed to determine how the transfer function of the auditory filter can be obtained from the curve relating tone threshold to the cutoff of the low-pass noise. If the spectrum level of the noise is constant at N_0 below the cutoff W, and constant at 0 above W, that is, the cutoff of the low-pass filter is very sharp, then Eq. (7) becomes

$$P_s = KN_0 \int_0^W |H(f)|^2 \, df. \tag{8}$$

If, in addition, we assume first that the auditory filter is centered on the tone and second that K and $H(f)$ remain constant as W is varied, then we may differentiate both sides of Eq. (8) and obtain

$$\frac{d}{dW}[P_s] = KN_0 \frac{d}{dW}\left[\int_0^W |H(f)|^2 \, df\right] = KN_0 |H(W)|^2. \tag{9}$$

That is, the derivative of the curve relating tone threshold to the cutoff of the noise is the square of the transfer function of the auditory filter times a constant KN_0.

Patterson's experiment was conducted at five signal frequencies (500, 1000, 2000, 4000, and 8000 Hz). The spectrum level of the noise was held constant at 40 dB SPL. The data, averaged for three observers, appear in Fig. 5a where average signal threshold is plotted as a function of Δf, the frequency separation between the upper edge of the noise and the signal frequency (see Fig. 4). The parameter on the curve is the frequency of the signal in kilohertz. Thus, for example in Fig. 5a, the point at $\Delta f = 300$, $P_s = 26$ is the average signal threshold for the three observers when the signal is 1000 Hz (as indicated by the parameter) and the upper cutoff of the noise is 700 Hz. Smooth curves are fit to these data and then the curves are differentiated to obtain the five auditory filters, one for each signal frequency.

The curves in Fig. 5a provide a sensitive measure of the lower half of the corresponding auditory filter. However, a low-pass noise does not lead to a reliable estimate of the upper half of the filter. When the noise cutoff is above

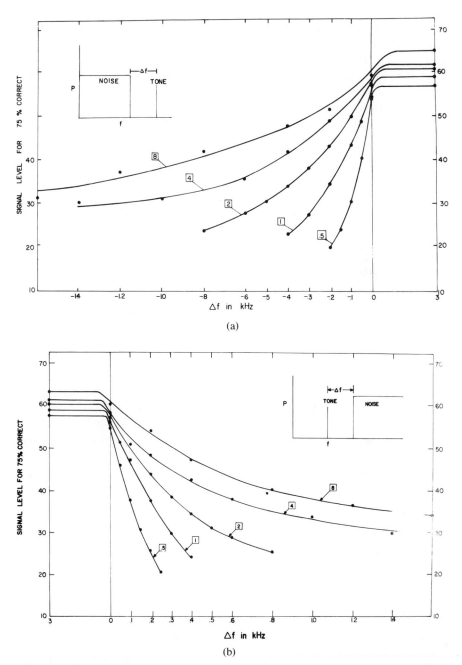

FIG. 5. (a) Threshold signal power plotted as a function of the distance between the signal and the edge of a *low-pass* filtered noise. (b) Threshold signal power plotted as a function of the distance between the signal and the edge of a *high-pass* filtered noise. The five curves show the data obtained at five different signal frequencies, .5, 1, 2, 4, and 8 kHz.

the signal frequency, large changes in cutoff frequency result in little or no change in tone threshold. To obtain reliable estimates of the upper halves of the filters, the basic experiment is repeated varying the cutoff of a high-pass noise. The data from this half of the experiment appear in Fig. 5b. Using these data and the same procedures, Fig. 5b provides a sensitive estimate of the upper skirts of the auditory filters.

The five transfer functions have the following properties:

1. The bandwidths of the filters increase with signal frequency.
2. The center-frequency to bandwidth ratio of these filters increases with center frequency (it is not a "constant Q" system).
3. The filters are nearly symmetric on a linear frequency scale. This was not anticipated because previous data had supported the assumption that the filter was similar to a single-tuned filter, which is not symmetric on a linear frequency scale.
4. The attenuation rate of the filter skirts is very high; it rises with signal frequency from around 65 dB/oct at 500 Hz to over 100 dB/oct at 8000 Hz. This is in contrast to the 6 dB/oct of the skirts of the single-tuned filter.

Patterson found that a simple mathematical expression could describe the filter characteristics quite well. The expression is

$$|H(f)|^2 = [(\Delta f/\alpha)^2 + 1]^{-2}, \tag{10}$$

where 1.29α is the 3-dB bandwidth of the filter and Δf is the deviation from center frequency, $\Delta f = f - f_0$. The bandwidth estimates obtained by fitting Eq. (10) to the derived filters increase from about 30 to 320 Hz as center frequency increases from 500 to 8000 Hz.* This transfer function is symmetric on a linear frequency scale. For purposes of identification, this filter is referred to as the *symmetric filter* in the sections that follow.

IV. PREDICTING TONE-IN-NOISE DATA

The test of a model is its ability to predict data that were not used in its creation. In this section, we briefly review attempts to use this symmetric filter form to predict masking results from a variety of studies.

In general, Fletcher's auditory-filter model predicts that tone threshold is some constant proportion of the integral of the noise-spectrum, filter-characteristic product [Eq. (7)]. On substituting the symmetric filter charac-

---

* Since this chapter was written a number of papers on auditory filter shape have appeared, some of which conclude that the filter is broader than indicated here. The most relevant papers are de Boer (1973), Evans and Wilson (1973), Houtgast (1974), Margolis and Small (1975), Patterson (1976), and Patterson and Henning (1977).

teristic shown in Eq. (10) into the general equation for tone threshold, Eq. (7), we find

$$P_s = K \int_0^\infty \frac{N(f)}{[(\Delta f/\alpha)^2 + 1]^2} \, df. \tag{11}$$

This expression is used throughout this section to predict tone threshold P_s. Note that it is assumed that the filter is centered on the signal, i.e., $\Delta f = f - f_s$.

The value of K depends on such variables as the signal duration, the criterion of detectability used to measure the signal threshold, and other factors. It is of interest, however, that in Patterson's experiment using a $\frac{1}{10}$-sec signal, the value of K is near unity, which is consistent with Fletcher's original assumption. In the discussions that follow, we use K as a fitting parameter, although in all of the different experiments K never changes by more than a factor of two.

A. Wide Band Noise

When the masker is a uniform wide band noise, $N(f)$ is a constant N_0, and Eq. (11) becomes

$$P_s = KN_0 \int_0^\infty \frac{1}{[(\Delta f/\alpha)^2 + 1]^2} \, df, \tag{12}$$

which reduces to

$$P_s = KN_0(\pi/2)\alpha, \tag{13}$$

since the integral of the symmetric filter is $(\pi/2)\alpha$. Consequently, if we assume $K = 1$, it follows that the symmetric filter predicts that the signal-to-noise ratio at threshold, P_s/N_0, will be $(\pi/2)\alpha$; or since the 3-dB bandwidth of the symmetric filter is 1.29α we have

$$P_s/N_0 = 1.22BW, \tag{14}$$

where BW is the 3-dB bandwidth of the filter.

In Fig. 2, Patterson's estimates of the width of the 3-dB bandwidth for the symmetric filter are plotted as a function of center frequency. At each signal frequency there are two estimates of bandwidth, one associated with the low-pass noise (Fig. 5a) and one associated with the high-pass noise (Fig. 5b). The former estimate was always smaller than the latter. The solid line in Fig. 2 shows the bandwidth estimates used in predicting the data that follow. The line has the form $10 \log P_s/N_0 = 8.34 \log f - 7.37$. The values on the dashed line in Fig. 2 are 1.22 times the values on the solid line and, therefore, the dashed line embodies the predicted tone-in-wide-band-noise thresholds.

B. Notched Noise

The data from one condition in the Webster *et al.* experiment, mentioned earlier, appear in Fig. 6. The dotted line shows the thresholds that would be predicted with the assumption of a rectangular filter. The dashed line shows the predictions associated with a single-tuned filter having a 65 Hz 3-dB bandwidth. The solid line shows the predictions associated with the symmetric filter characteristic [Eq. (10)]. In the 650- to 750-Hz range the predictions using the rectangular assumption are too low and those from the single-tuned assumption are too high, indicating that the attenuation rates of these filters are too high and too low, respectively. The symmetric filter has an attenuation rate between that of the rectangular and single-tuned filters and, as might be anticipated, the predictions using this filter are closer to the data.

C. Bandpass Noise

1. GREENWOOD

Greenwood (1961a,b) carried out an extensive investigation of the way in which bandpass noise masks tones. Greenwood's masker had extremely

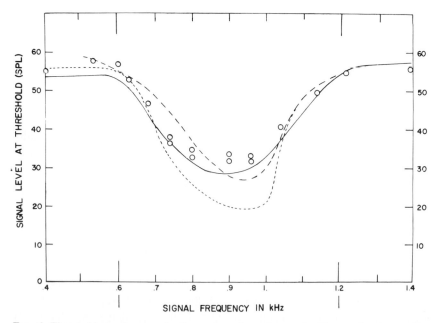

FIG. 6. Threshold signal power in the region of a noise notch. The masker is a uniform wide-band noise with a spectrum level of 38 dB that has had one octave band (600–1200 Hz) filtered out. The data are from Webster *et al.* (1952). The dotted, dashed, and solid lines represent the thresholds predicted by the rectangular, single-tuned, and symmetric filter characteristics, respectively.

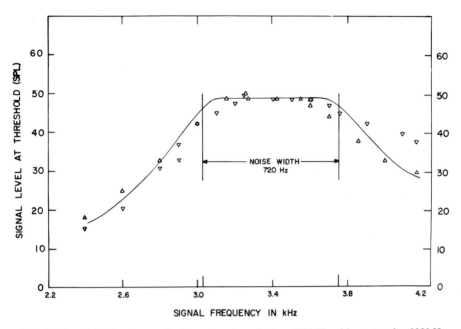

FIG. 7. Threshold signal power in the region of a noise band 720 Hz wide centered at 3390 Hz. The spectrum level of the noise in the pass-band is 31 dB SPL. The data are from Greenwood (1961a).

sharp skirts; the attenuation rates were between 200 and 500 dB/oct. Greenwood studied three center frequencies—approximately 400, 1000, and 3000 Hz. At each center frequency, he varied the bandwidth of the noise, for example, at 3000 Hz he used noise widths of 100, 175, 238, 435, 720, and 1270 Hz. For each noise width, he measured tone threshold in the vicinity of the noise; for example, at 3000 Hz he measured thresholds for tones between 2400 and 4600 Hz in about 100-Hz steps. Data for two observers appear in Fig. 7. The data are for the condition in which the width of the noiseband was 720 Hz and it was centered at 3390 Hz. The trapezoidal form of these data is typical of those experimental conditions where the width of the noise is large relative to the center frequency of the band. When the noise width is decreased, with center frequency held constant, the width of the top of the trapezoid decreases but the sides of the trapezoid maintain essentially the same shape. Eventually, decreasing the width of the noise causes the data to fall into a triangular shape. Greenwood proposes that the noise width at which the trapezoid changes to a triangle is, in fact, a measure of the critical band, since widening the width of the noise beyond this point does not further elevate tone-threshold in the center of the band. With this procedure Greenwood measures critical bandwidths that are about 2.5 to 3.0 times larger than the bandwidths that appear in Fig. 2. For example, at 3400 Hz,

Greenwood estimates a bandwidth of around 450 Hz. Greenwood's masking experiment is not the only study that leads to critical-band estimates greater than those shown in Fig. 2. A series of experiments using a variety of different techniques have estimated larger critical bands. For a review of these experiments, the articles by Scharf (1961, 1966) and Zwicker *et al.* (1957) are recommended.

Patterson calculated the tone thresholds that the symmetric-filter model [Eq. (10)] would predict, given Greenwood's noise maskers. The solid line in Fig. 7 is the predicted tone threshold curve. The 3-dB bandwidth of the symmetric filter in this frequency region is about 150 Hz ($K \approx \frac{1}{2}$). Despite the fact that this bandwidth estimate is one-third that of Greenwood's, the fit of the model to the data is very good.

2. EGAN AND HAKE

Wegel and Lane's study of tonal masking showed asymmetric masking patterns, that is, a particular tone masks a tone above it better than a tone below it. Similarly, Egan and Hake (1950) found that a narrow band of noise masks tones above it much better than the tones below it. At first, this result would appear to rule out a symmetric filter, such as Eq. (10), since the data appear to indicate that the attenuation rate of the upper skirt of the assumed filter is greater than that of the lower skirt. However, the symmetric filter predicts an asymmetric masking curve, because the bandwidth of the filter increases with center frequency. Egan and Hake's data for two observers are plotted in Fig. 8. The solid line is the symmetric-filter prediction when a K of 1 is assumed. To understand better why the symmetric filter leads to an asymmetric masking curve, consider the thresholds at 300 and 520 Hz in Fig. 8. The assumed filter bandwidth at 300 Hz, which is 110 Hz below the center of the noise, is 20 Hz. The filter bandwidth a similar distance above the noise center (520 Hz) is 33 Hz. According to the model, the threshold at 300 is lower than that at 520, not because of asymmetry in the filter, but because a narrower filter, which is better able to attenuate the noise, is used at the lower frequency.

In Fig. 8, Egan and Hake's data are plotted in SPL units (dB *re* .0002 dynes cm^{-2}). In their original paper, Egan and Hake plotted their data in terms of the amount of masking that the masker caused, that is, decibels *re* absolute threshold at that frequency. Much of the asymmetry in Egan and Hake's original graphs arises from this method of plotting the data. At low frequencies (below 800 Hz) absolute threshold decreases rapidly as frequency increases. When this curve, with its negative slope, is subtracted from the curve of masked thresholds in SPL units, it makes the masking function below the masker steeper and the masking function above the masker shallower, thus enhancing any asymmetry in the masked audiogram. The symmetric filter predicts Egan and Hake's data quite well, provided the noise spectrum level is below 45 dB.

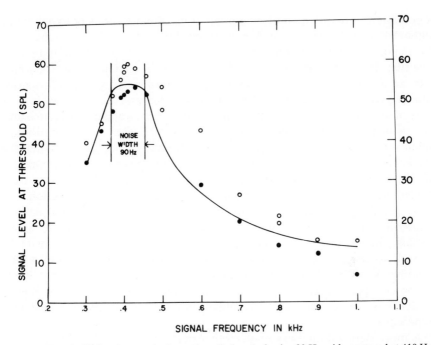

FIG. 8. Threshold signal power in the region of a band of noise 90 Hz wide centered at 410 Hz. The spectrum level of the noise in the pass-band is 40 dB SPL. The data are from Egan and Hake (1950).

It is important to emphasize before leaving this section that the auditory filter is only symmetric when the spectrum level of the noise is below about 45 dB. Patterson (1971) reran his experiment on auditory filter shape using spectrum levels of 25 and 55 dB in an effort to determine the effect of amplitude on bandwidth. He found that lowering the spectrum level had virtually no effect on bandwidth, but that increasing the spectrum level from 40 to 55 dB produced a marked increase in bandwidth. This increase in bandwidth was entirely due to a flattening of the lower skirt, that is, a decrease in the off-band attenuation rate on the low side of the filter. This result is in agreement with the observation that at high levels, low frequencies mask high frequencies better than the reverse.

V. SINUSOIDAL MASKING

A. General Considerations

The preceding analysis of noise masking has, we hope, indicated the advantages of a filter analogy. Once the shape of the auditory filter is known, it is possible to provide quantitative predictions about a series of experiments without having to estimate new parameters for each set of data. Obviously the analogy is an oversimplification, and, at the very least, we should recognize that the cochlea must be likened to a series of elements, each of which acts as a tuned filter. Detection is then determined by the information gathered over the entire set of elements. In our analysis of noise masking, we were able to assume a single filter tuned to the signal frequency because only the elements located in the vicinity of signal frequency were contributing much information about the presence or absence of the signal. When the masker is a band-limited process, such as a continuous sinusoid, the analysis of the detection process is much more complicated, because it is usually difficult to determine the elements that are responsible for the detection. The basic problem is that a seemingly insignificant amount of signal energy, located in some remote portion of the spectrum, is often detectable simply because there is no masker energy in that region. This is precisely why it is so difficult to mask a gated sinusoid, having a wide band spectrum with a continuous sinusoid having essentially a line spectrum (Green, 1969). Leshowitz and Wightman (1971) have marshalled considerable experimental evidence in support of this view, which they call the *off frequency* listening hypothesis.

A more detailed analysis of detection performance in the presence of a band-limited masker requires the calculation of signal-to-noise-power ratio for each element along the cochlea. The crucial factor in this calculation is often the shape of the skirt of the filter element, that is, one's assumption about how the excitation pattern changes as one moves away from the maximum of excitation. For wide band noise maskers, the crucial parameter of the auditory system is the width and shape of the excitation pattern in the vicinity of the signal. This is the region where the signal-to-noise ratio is a maximum and, therefore, the region primarily responsible for the detection performance. For sinusoidal maskers, however, the crucial area for detection performance may be a remote region of the spectrum, where, in absolute amount, little energy is located, but where the signal-to-masker ratio is large. When predicting data for sinusoidal maskers, the width of the critical band is not nearly so important as the detailed shape of the filter, especially the skirt of the filter since this determines the signal-to-noise ratio at remote frequencies.

Band-limited maskers were used in several of the experiments reported in the preceding sections. Data from Egan and Hake (1950), Greenwood (1961a), Patterson (1974), and Webster *et al.* (1952) were all explained in Section IV on the basis of a simple filter model and the possibility of off-frequency listening was not mentioned. This problem was ignored because in these experiments profitable off-frequency listening was precluded; in each case the experimenter had restricted the signal spectrum to a narrow band about the signal frequency and consequently the maximum signal-to-noise-power ratio occurred at or near the signal frequency. In Patterson's experiment the signal was square-gated but it was passed through a filter with a 50-Hz bandwidth and very sharp skirts before it was presented to the observer. In the experiments of Webster *et al.*, Egan *et al.*, and Greenwood the signals were turned on and off slowly. This procedure, which is traditionally used to eliminate gating transients, is simply the time-domain equivalent of filtering.

A corollary of the off-frequency-listening theory is that amplitude distortion becomes increasingly important in sinusoidal masking, because amplitudes 60 and 90 dB below the peak amplitudes of the masker may be responsible for detection. Over these ranges it is unlikely that the ear is completely free of distortion and, therefore, the assumptions one makes about the nature and amount of this distortion become crucial. Greenwood (1971) has considered a number of masking situations in which the masker occupies a narrow frequency region. His discussion of these data emphasizes both the critical band and simple amplitude distortion. Neither our analysis nor Greenwood's is sufficiently precise to allow us to say whether these explanations are exactly similar, but certainly the general lines of attack are very much alike.*

For these reasons, we shall not attempt to extend the filter analogy to the data of sinusoidal masking but content ourselves with a brief recitation of the most pertinent data.

B. Frequency Relations

The basic data on sinusoidal masking were first collected by Wegel and Lane (1924) in the first controlled masking experiment. They employed six different sinusoids as maskers—200, 400, 800, 1200, 2400, and 3500 Hz. At each masker frequency, a sinusoidal signal was presented at various frequencies both above and below the masker and the signal threshold was determined. The level of the masker was also systematically varied in 20-dB steps so that the masking produced by six different frequencies at five widely spaced levels can be determined from Wegel and Lane's data. Because of the scope of the study and its theoretical interest the data have been widely reproduced in secondary sources, see for example, Fletcher (1953) and Stevens and Davis (1938). For low masking levels, the masker 20 or 40 dB above threshold, the masking patterns measured by Wegel and Lane are fairly symmetric, showing the maximum threshold shift in the vicinity of the masking frequency and less effect at remote frequency regions. Wegel and Lane presented the masker and signal simultaneously for a long duration and, therefore, beats between the two became evident at the appropriate frequen-

---

* In Section IV, it was not necessary to consider the question of amplitude distortion since the signal powers involved are all below the level at which appreciable distortion is thought to occur.

cies and appear as local minima in their data. Except for these local minima, the masking patterns at the lower levels are nearly symmetric on a linear frequency scale and monotonic decreasing as the signal frequency moves away from the masker frequency. At higher levels the data are quite different. The masking pattern becomes distinctly asymmetric; for example, at 1200 Hz, a masker of 80 dB SL produces a threshold shift of 42 dB for a signal of 1600 Hz and only 15 dB for an 800-Hz signal. In addition to this asymmetry, other anomalies appear. At these higher levels, local minima occur near the second and third harmonics of the masker, presumably representing beats between the signal frequency and the second and third harmonics of the masker. The exact source of these harmonics is difficult to assess although some are undoubtedly caused by distortion in the equipment used in this pioneering study.

In 1959, 25 years after Wegel and Lane's original experiment, the topic of sinusoidal masking received attention in two papers, Ehmer (1959) and Small (1959). Both of these studies confirm the main findings of the earlier study, namely, at low masking levels the masking curve is roughly symmetric with a maximum at the signal frequency, whereas at higher masker levels marked asymmetries occur, with low tones masking higher ones much more than the reverse. The major discrepancies between the early and later studies concern the location and probable cause of the local irregularities attributed to distortion in the Wegel and Lane study. Both Ehmer and Small find marked irregularities in the masking function when the ratio of signal frequency to masker frequency is 1.2–1.5. For such ratios, it is impossible that simple amplitude distortion is the cause of the irregularities, and thus the theory that the irregularities in the masking pattern are the results of beats between the harmonics of the masker and the signal must be revised. Greenwood (1971) has confirmed the nonharmonic values of these irregularities but relates them to the width of the critical band and certain interactions between signal and distortion products of the masker.

C. Intensity Relations

1. MASKER AND SIGNAL AT DIFFERENT FREQUENCIES

Thus far, we have discussed how masking depends on the frequency relation between masker and signal. Of equal importance is the question of how the amount of masking depends on the level of the masker, given a fixed frequency relation between signal and masker. Such data can of course be constructed from the three studies just discussed, and the relations are quite different from those encountered in noise masking. For broad band noise, as we have seen, the relation is extremely simple. The masker and signal level required for some constant level of detectability is constant once the signal is a few decibels above threshold, see Fig. 1. For sinusoidal maskers the relationships are extremely complicated. First consider a signal frequency an octave or two above the masker frequency. If the masker is raised in level by 10 dB, the signal has to be increased by as much as 30 dB to maintain it at a just detectable level. If the signal is much below the masker frequency, then a reverse situation holds; increasing the masker by 10 dB may necessitate only 3–5 dB increase in the signal level. This asymmetry is only another reflection of the frequency asymmetry at higher level, which was discussed earlier. As the masker level increases, it is increasingly true that lower frequencies mask higher frequencies better than the reverse.

This lack of a proportional relation between masker level and signal level is, of course, completely inconsistent with a simple fixed-frequency filter model such as the type suggested earlier. It is not, however, difficult to adapt the filter model to give a qualitative account of these data. In essence, the idea is that the optimum frequency for detection changes as a function of level, and thus, the data reflect not only changes in the signal-to-noise ratio at the output of the filter but also changes in filter locations as well. To understand this explanation, let us take a simple example. Consider a 1200-Hz masker and a 2000-Hz signal. As we increase the masker from a very low to very high level the 2000-Hz signal is at first unaffected, only the internal noise is limiting the detection of the signal and undoubtedly the maximum signal-to-noise ratio is at the region of the cochlea associated with the 2000 Hz signal. As the masker increases, however, more and more masker energy spreads into the 2000-Hz region and the optimum signal-to-noise ratio shifts to a higher frequency, say 2500 or even 3000 Hz. The result is a small rise in the threshold of the signal, say 2 or 3 dB, for a 10 dB increase in masker level. Finally, when the masker reaches a level of 50–60 dB SL, significant amounts of distortion are generated at the harmonics of 1200 Hz. This distortion increases disproprotionately with respect to the energy at the fundamental and, therefore, the next increase of 10 dB of the masker increases the effective masker energy by 20 dB. The signal energy must, therefore, also be increased disproportionately, and the highly nonlinear relation between signal and masker level is explained. On the other hand, when the signal frequency is below that of the masker, little or no subharmonic distortion occurs. As the masker increases, more energy might leak into filters situated below the masker and hence the optimum signal-to-masker ratio might occur at somewhat lower frequencies. The small increase in signal level for large changes in masker level could then be explained. The difficulty with this model in addition to its being ad hoc, is that it is only qualitative. Obviously filter shapes and amplitude distortion characteristics could be constructed to account for some of the data, but a complete consistent treatment is lacking.

2. MASKER AND SIGNAL AT THE SAME FREQUENCY

Probably the easiest situation to begin quantitative analysis of sinusoid masking is the situation in which the signal and masker frequency are the same. In this case, the detection task is simply to discriminate an increase in the amplitude of a sinusoid. The ratio of increment energy to base energy is called the Weber fraction. Weber's law is the assertion that the Weber fraction is constant and independent of the intensity of the original sinusoid. For the case of a sinusoid masked by noise, we have seen that this law is true once the sinusoid is a few decibels above its absolute threshold. For the case of a sinusoidal masker, it is almost true but systematic and consistent discrepancies have been noted by many authors (Braida & Durlach, 1972; Campbell & Lasky, 1967; Dimmick & Olson, 1941; Green, 1967; McGill & Goldberg, 1968a; Reisz, 1928; Wegel & Lane, 1924). The nature of this discrepancy is quite simple: $\Delta I/I$ decreases as I increases.

Probably the most influential treatment of this problem is McGill and Goldberg (1968a,b). They relate the "near miss" to Weber's law, as they call it, to a Poisson model and show that this near miss implies that the growth of loudness with intensity is a power function with an exponent in the range .15–.30. A treatment of this problem by Viemeister (1972) suggests another explanation, one consistent with the qualitative account given earlier. Basically, Viemeister assumes that detection is determined at high levels of I by the following ratio

$$d' = \frac{(I + \Delta I)^{P_i} - I^{P_i}}{I^{P_i}} = \left(1 + \frac{\Delta I}{I}\right)^{P_i} - 1,$$

where P_i is the exponent relating the growth of intensity at the ith frequency location. Thus, at the fundamental $P_1 = 1.0$, at the second or third harmonic, the growth is nonlinear, i.e., $P_2 = 2.0, P_3 = 3.0$. For small $\Delta I/I$, using a power series approximation, we have

$$d' = P_i(\Delta I/I),$$

and if I is intense enough, the discrimination is determined by the second or third harmonic of the fundamental. Since a 1-dB increase at the fundamental produces a 2-dB increase at the first harmonic and a 3-dB increase at the third, smaller and smaller values of $\Delta I/I$ are required as I increases and these harmonics become audible. Viemeister has shown that $\Delta I/I$ is nearly constant, independent of I, if high-frequency masking noise is used to obscure the harmonics of the sinusoid.

VI. SUMMARY

In summary, we have reviewed the major empirical results in the area of auditory masking. The utility of the concept of an auditory filter or critical band is apparent in our review of noise masking. Here a great deal of data can be simply summarized in terms of a single attenuation curve, the bandwidth of which depends on center frequency. With sinusoidal maskers, the situation is not as simple. First, the maximum signal-to-noise ratio may not occur at or near the signal frequency as it does in the noise masking case. Calculation of where the maximum does occur may be difficult, since it depends to some extent on the width but more critically on the exact shape of the attenuation characteristic 40–50 dB down from the peak. Second, there is the problem of nonlinear distortion and the possibility that these effects are playing a large role in sinusoidal masking. The simplest case occurs when the signal and masker are the same frequency and the study of Weber's fraction is discussed in terms of two current models.

Acknowledgments

This research was supported by the National Institutes of Health, Public Health Service, U.S. Department of Health, Education and Welfare; by a research grant awarded to the Center for Human Information Processing; and by the Defence and Civil Institute of Environmental Medicine, Toronto, Ontario, Canada. We also wish to acknowledge the following people who read a previous draft of this chapter: Irwin Pollack, Neal F. Viemeister, and M. J. Penner.

References

de Boer, E. On the principle of specific coding. *Journal of Dynamic Systems, Measurement, and Control,* Sept. 1973.

Braida, L. D., & Durlach, N. I. Intensity perception. II. Resolution in one-interval paradigms. *Journal of the Acoustical Society of America,* 1972, **51,** 483–502.

Campbell, R. A., & Lasky, E. Z. Masker level and sinusoidal-signal detection. *Journal of the Acoustical Society of America,* 1967, **42,** 972–976.

Dimmick, F., & Olson, R. M. The intensive difference limen in audition. *Journal of the Acoustical Society of America,* 1941, **12,** 517–525.

Egan, J. P., & Hake, H. W. On the masking pattern of a simple auditory stimulus. *Journal of the Acoustical Society of America,* 1950, **22,** 622–630.

Ehmer, R. H. Masking patterns of tone. *Journal of the Acoustical Society of America,* 1959, **31,** 1115–1120.

Evans, E. F., & Wilson, J. P. Frequency selectivity of the cochlea. In A. R. Møller (Ed.), *Basic mechanisms of hearing.* New York: Academic Press, 1973. Pp. 519–551.

Fletcher, H. Auditory patterns. *Review of Modern Physics,* 1940, **12,** 47–65.

Fletcher, H. *Speech and hearing in communication.* (2nd ed.) New York: D. Van Nostrand, 1953.

Green, D. M. Auditory detection of a noise signal. *Journal of the Acoustical Society of America,* 1960, **32,** 121–131.

Green, D. M. Additivity of masking. *Journal of the Acoustical Society of America,* 1967, **41,** 1517–1525.

Green, D. M. Masking with continuous and pulsed sinusoids. *Journal of the Acoustical Society of America,* 1969, **46,** 939–946.

Green, D. M., & McGill, W. J. On the equivalence of detection probabilities and well-known statistical quantities. *Psychological Review,* 1970, **77(4),** 294–301.

Green, D. M., McKey, M. J., & Licklider, J. C. R. Detection of a pulsed sinusoid in noise as a function of frequency. *Journal of the Acoustical Society of America,* 1959, **31,** 1446–1452.

Greenwood, D. D. Auditory masking and the critical band. *Journal of the Acoustical Society of America,* 1961, **33,** 484–502. (a)

Greenwood, D. D. Critical bandwidth and the frequency coordinates of the basilar membrane. *Journal of the Acoustical Society of America*, 1961, **33**, 1344–1356. (b)

Greenwood, D. D. Aural combination tones and auditory masking. *Journal of the Acoustical Society of America*, 1971, **50**, 502–543.

Hawkins, J. E., Jr., & Stevens, S. S. The masking of pure tones and of speech by white noise. *Journal of the Acoustical Society of America*, 1950, **22**, 6–13.

Houtgast, T. Lateral suppression in hearing. Doctoral dissertation, University of Amsterdam, The Netherlands, 1974.

Jeffress, L. A. Stimulus-oriented approach to detection. *Journal of the Acoustical Society of America*, 1964, **36**, 766–774.

Leshowitz, B., & Wightman, F. L. On-frequency masking with continuous sinusoids. *Journal of the Acoustical Society of America*, 1971, **49**, 1180–1190.

Margolis, R. H., & Small, A. M. The measurement of critical masking bands. *Journal of Speech and Hearing Research*, 1975, **18**, 571–587.

Marill, T. M. Detection theory and psychophysics. *MIT: Research Laboratories of Electronics, Technical Report No. 319*, 1956.

Mayer, A. M. Research in acoustics. *Philosophical Magazine*, 1876, **11**, 500–507.

McGill, W. J. Neural counting mechanisms and energy detection in audition. *Journal of Mathematical Psychology*, 1967, **4**, 351–376.

McGill, W. J., & Goldberg, J. P. A study of the near-miss involving Weber's law and pure-tone intensity discrimination. *Perception and Psychophysics*, 1968, **4**, 105–109. (a)

McGill, W. J., & Goldberg, J. P. Pure-tone intensity discrimination and energy detection. *Journal of the Acoustical Society of America*, 1968, **44**, 576–581. (b)

Patterson, R. D. Effect of amplitude on auditory filter shape. *Journal of the Acoustical Society of America*, 1971, **49**, 81(A).

Patterson, R. D. Auditory filter shape. *Journal of the Acoustical Society of America*, 1974, **55**, 802–809.

Patterson, R. D. Auditory filter shapes derived with noise stimuli. *Journal of the Acoustical Society of America*, 1976, **59**, 640–654.

Patterson, R. D., & Henning, G. B. Stimulus variability and auditory filter shape. *Journal of the Acoustical Society of America*, 1977, **62**, 649–664.

Pfafflin, S. M., & Mathews, M. V. Energy detection model for monaural auditory detection. *Journal of the Acoustical Society of America*, 1962, **34**, 1842–1852.

Reisz, R. R. Differential intensity sensitivity of the ear for pure tones. *Physical Review*, 1928, **31**, 867–875.

Schafer, T. H., Gales, R. S., Shewmaker, C. A., & Thompson, P. O. The frequency selectivity of the ear as determined by masking experiments. *Journal of the Acoustical Society of America*, 1950, **22**, 490–496.

Scharf, B. Complex sounds and critical bands. *Psychological Bulletin*, 1961, **58**, 205–217.

Scharf, B. Critical bands. *Laboratory of Sensory Communication (LSC-S-3)*, 1966, Syracuse Univ., Syracuse, N.Y.

Siebert, W. M. Some implications of the stochastic behavior of primary auditory neurons. *Kybernetik*, 1965, **2**, 206–215.

Small, A. M., Jr. Pure tone masking. *Journal of the Acoustical Society of America*, 1959, **31**, 1619–1625.

Stevens, S. S., & Davis, H. *Hearing: Its psychology and physiology*. New York: Wiley, 1938.

Swets, J. A., Green, D. M., & Tanner, W. P., Jr. On the width of critical bands. *Journal of the Acoustical Society of America*, 1962, **34**, 108–113.

Tanner, W. P., Jr., Swets, J. A., & Green, D. M. Some general properties of the hearing mechanism. *University of Michigan: Electronic Defense Group, Technical Report No. 30*, 1956.

Viemeister, N. F. Intensity discrimination of pulsed sinusoids: The effects of filtered noise. *Journal of the Acoustical Society of America,* 1972, **51,** 1265–1269.

Webster, J. C., Miller, P. H., Thompson, P. O., & Davenport, E. W. Masking and pitch shifts of pure tones near abrupt changes in a thermal noise spectrum. *Journal of the Acoustical Society of America,* 1952, **24,** 147–152.

Wegel, R. L., & Lane, C. E. The auditory masking of one pure tone by another and its probable relation to the dynamics of the inner ear. *Physical Review,* 1924, **23,** Series 2, 266–285.

Zwicker, E., Flottorp, G., & Stevens, S. S. Critical band width in loudness summation. *Journal of the Acoustical Society of America,* 1957, **29,** 548–557.

Part IV
Binaural and Spatial Hearing

Chapter 10

BINAURAL PHENOMENA

NATHANIEL I. DURLACH AND H. STEVEN COLBURN

I. INTRODUCTION

Most people who are fortunate enough to have good hearing in both ears are unaware of the advantages afforded by the second ear. Unlike the visual sense, in which one can play at being one-eyed by shutting an eyelid, it is very difficult to shut one ear. (The fact that nature did not provide us with earlids is probably due to the physical difficulties involved in constructing earlids that are effective at low frequencies and to the use of the acoustical channel for warning signals, a function to which it is exceptionally well matched.) For normal-hearing subjects, a dramatic opportunity for appreciating the advantages of two ears is provided by a comparison of binaural and monaural tape recordings of complex acoustical environments (e.g., a large, noisy, cocktail party in a reverberant room) constructed with the use of microphones positioned in the listener's ear canals, and then presented to the listener through earphones. In the binaural presentation, the perception is reasonably faithful in the sense that the different sound sources appear to be located in roughly the same positions relative to the listener's head as they were when the recording was made, and the listener is able to concentrate on one source to the exclusion of others (the so-called "cocktail party effect"). In the monaural presentation, however, the different sources become overlayed, all the sounds appear to originate at the stimulated ear, and it is difficult to concentrate on a single source. In other words, both the localization of signals in auditory space and the detection of signals in backgrounds of interference are severely degraded when the stimulus is restricted to one ear. For people suffering from severe unilateral impairments, these degradations are experienced directly and continuously, and are sufficiently severe to lead to avoidance of complex acoustical environments.

From an evolutionary viewpoint, it is clear that the existence of more than one ear is a very basic property of the auditory system. Not only are the functions served by the additional ear extremely important to survival (e.g., a prey that cannot localize the sound of a predator is likely to be in serious trouble), but the existence of spatially distributed sensing elements in order to achieve these functions occurs throughout all phyla of the animal kingdom and all sense modalities. (Even the trail-following behavior of ants has been shown to involve the use of such a system.) In speculating about evolution, it is perhaps less reasonable to ask "Why does man have two ears?" than to ask "Why does man have *only* two ears?"

In order to appreciate the feats that are normally achieved by the use of the binaural system, consider the schematic diagram of an auditory stimulus impinging on a two-eared listener shown in Fig. 1. Each ear not only receives signals from many sources, but it receives the signal from a given source over many paths because of reflections. Somehow, the listener transforms this hodgepodge of a stimulus into a clear and distinct perception of the various sources, each of which can be identified and localized in space, as well as a perception of various acoustic properties of the room in which the sources are located. Although a portion of this transformation could certainly be accomplished by the monaural auditory system, much of it represents the results of binaural interaction. The attempt to characterize and understand this interaction constitutes a primary focus of the research on binaural hearing.

In this chapter, we attempt to familiarize the reader with a wide variety of binaural hearing phenomena. We make no attempt to interpret these phenomena in terms of models of binaural interaction or to relate them to physiological results. (A survey of models of binaural interaction, for which the present chapter provides background, is presented in the next chapter.) Also, we focus upon results obtained from experiments that are directed primarily toward improved understanding of the auditory system rather than toward applications (such as sound reproduction). In most of the experiments considered, the stimuli are presented through earphones and are relatively simple and well controlled. In many cases, these stimuli have been chosen for analytic purposes and are strongly unnatural.

The material is divided into three major sections. In Section II, we comment upon the feature of binaural stimulation that is most central to binaural perception, namely, interaural differences. In Section III, we discuss various

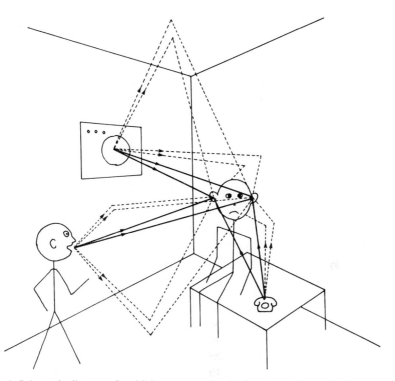

Fig. 1. Schematic diagram of multiple-source and multiple-path problems. Each ear receives signals from many sources and over many paths simultaneously. Through auditory processing, much of which involves binaural interaction, the listener is capable of perceiving and localizing each source and of simultaneously perceiving certain acoustic properties of the room.

perceptual attributes of the binaural image. In Section IV, we examine the binaural system's sensitivity. (No concluding remarks are presented because of the continued discussion of binaural hearing in the next chapter.)

Despite the fact that we consider a wide variety of phenomena in this chapter, there are some important ones that have been entirely omitted. Perhaps the most important are those associated with *(1)* perception of competing messages in the two ears and the differences obtained in this perception for verbal and nonverbal stimuli (often discussed under the headings of "dichotic listening," "binaural message competition," "selective attention," "two-channel listening," or "cerebral asymmetries"), and *(2)* binaural perception in the hearing-impaired. We have not discussed these topics in this chapter because of space limitations and because we believe that they are most usefully studied after the material surveyed in this (and the following) chapter has been studied. Material concerning these areas can be found in the literature on speech perception and hearing impairments.

II. INTERAURAL DIFFERENCES

The component of binaural perception that is most uniquely binaural, as opposed to monaural, is the perception of differences between the stimuli presented to the two ears. In a natural environment, these differences result from differences in the propagation paths to the two ears and include, for each source in the environment, the differential effects on the two signals of the listener's body, head, and pinna, as well as of other objects in the environment. It is precisely the perception of these differences that underlies the improved performance in localization and detection that occurs when two ears are used in place of a single ear. (A binaural stimulus in which there are no interaural differences is referred to as *diotic*, and a stimulus that is not diotic as *dichotic*.)

Despite the fundamental role played by interaural differences, it is obvious that in most cases the perception of these differences constitutes only one component of the overall perception. For example, the perceived location of a source depends not only on the perceived interaural differences, but also on the perceived position and orientation of the listener's head (normally constructed from proprioceptive, kinesthetic, and vestibular cues), on localization information obtained monaurally or through the visual sense, and on the listener's expectation of where the source is located. Exactly how these different components are combined depends on the specific situation.

Experimentally, the binaural stimulus and the associated interaural differences (which can be monitored by the use of probe tubes or microphones placed inside the ear canals) can be generated and controlled in a variety of ways. One common method is to place the listener inside an anechoic chamber, present the signals through a loudspeaker, and manipulate the interaural differences by controlling the geometry (including, perhaps, using a clamp or a "bite plate" to fix the position of the listener's head). A second common method is to place the listener inside a soundproof room, present the signals through earphones, and manipulate the stimulus and its interaural differences electronically. Other methods include the use of multiple-speaker configurations, reverberent rooms, and pseudophones or artifical heads.

The suitability of a particular method for presenting the binaural stimulus and controlling the interaural differences depends on the objectives of the experiment and on the available equipment. If one requires a stimulus situation that does not involve elaborate instrumentation and that is relatively natural with respect to the interaural relations, the effects of the body, head, and pinna, and the way in which the stimulation varies as a function of the listener's movements, it makes sense to present the signals through loudspeakers and to have listeners perceive these signals directly through their own ears. If, on the other hand, one's approach is more analytic, and one needs a configuration that is flexible, that is capable of producing unnatural stimuli, and that permits one to manipulate the various components of the stimulus situation independently in order to determine how each of the various components contributes to the overall perception, then it is useful to present the signals through earphones and to be able to interpose a variety of devices between the signal generator and the earphones. The ideal configuration from this point of view (and one which is likely to be available in the near future) would not only be computer-controlled and include the capability of creating a wide variety of binaural stimuli and interaural differences, but also a system for monitoring the listener's movements and automatically adjusting the stimulus to match these movements in a precise and continuous manner, and thus for simulating the effects of movements (of either the source or the listener) in a natural environment. Many of the configurations actually used are intermediate between these two extremes. Loudspeakers and an artificial head with microphones located in the artificial ears and with the listener stimulated through earphones in a separate room allow one to decouple the listener's movements from the acoustic stimulation, to eliminate nonauditory cues, to effectively shut off one ear for monaural–binaural comparisons, and to explore the effects of artificial pinnae. Loudspeakers and a system of microphones and earphones mounted on the listener's head allow one to distort the binaural stimulation while preserving the coupling between changes in this stimulation and the listener's movements, and have been used to explore the role of sensory–motor feedback in adaptation to atypical stimuli. Multiple-speaker configurations have been used for presenting unrelated signals from different points in space (e.g., to study the cocktail-party effect) and for creating a variety of effects with a common signal or with closely related signals where the relations are carefully controlled. A significant portion of the work using the latter type of presentation has been oriented toward the development of improved sound systems for lecture halls and music reproduction, and has led to a variety of "illusions" (e.g., those involved in stereophonic listening). Although some of these illusions depend upon important perceptual phenomena, and thus are of interest from the perceptual point of view, others are based almost exclusively on purely physical considerations and are obvious once the actual stimuli (specifically, the interaural differences) have been computed.

Independent of how the interaural differences are created, they can be usefully specified in terms of the ratio of the complex spectra of the acoustical signals at fixed and symmetric reference points in the two ear canals. For each frequency, this ratio specifies both the ratio of the amplitudes at the two points (the absolute value of the ratio) and the interaural phase difference at the two points (the phase of the ratio). The amplitude ratio can be replaced by the power, intensity, or energy ratio, and the interaural phase difference by the interaural time delay. When the binaural stimulus is composed of a number of distinct and identifiable sources, it is sometimes useful to specify also the ratio of the complex spectra for each of the sources taken individually.

For a configuration in which the observer is listening with his naked ears to the signal produced by a single point source, it is often useful to represent the complex spectrum of the signal at a given ear as a product of the following components: the spectrum of the signal emitted by the source, the transfer function describing the transformation associated with the propagation of the signal from the source to the subject, and the transfer function describing the transformation produced by the listener's body, head, and pinnae. For multiple-point sources (corresponding to the use of more than one loudspeaker or to the existence of reflections), such a factorization can be carried out for each point separately, and the total signal at the ear represented as the sum of the individual signals.

The principal problems associated with the specification of interaural differences are those concerned with the actual measurements of the signals in the ear canals. To the extent that the head is perfectly symmetric and the interaural differences are obtained directly from measurements at the two ears, the only problem is that of the symmetry of the reference points. Changes in the position of the common reference point between measurements have no effect on the interaural differences. However, if the interaural differences for a fixed spatial configuration are estimated from two measurements in a single ear (by simulating the results that would be obtained in the other ear through the use of the given ear and the complementary geometry), then changes in the position of the reference point between measurements for different spatial configurations will introduce an artifact. One fact that helps to reduce the complexity of this measurement problem is that the transformation of the signal that occurs in going from one reference point to another within the ear canal is, in many cases, relatively independent of the angle of the source. On the other hand, it is clear that the head is not perfectly symmetric and, therefore, that the assumption of symmetric reference points, or the technique of using only one ear, can provide only a rough approximation.

One concept of considerable importance in studying the perception of interaural differences is that of "natural differences," whereby "natural" we mean those differences that the listener is likely to have experienced previously in his "everyday life" and the perception of which is likely to have been correlated through normal developmental and learning processes with perceptual components derived through other sensory inputs. For a binaural stimulus in which the differences are natural, the perception is obviously going to be consistent with the class of natural environments that actually produce such differences. Thus, for example, it is no surprise that binaural stimuli in which the interaural differences are zero always appear to originate at some point in the median plane, and that if a listener suffers a sudden hearing loss in one ear that makes the effective interaural differences nonzero, he will at first perceive a stimulus with zero interaural differences as being located off the median plane, but will soon tend to adapt and come again to perceive it as lying on the median plane.

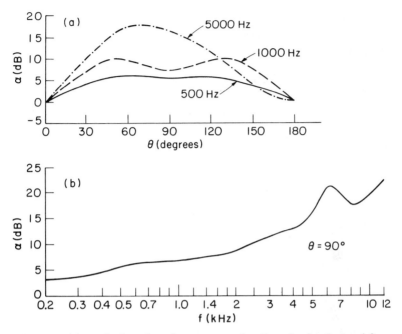

FIG. 2. Interaural amplitude ratio α for tones as a function of azimuth θ and frequency f (Shaw, 1974a,b). (a) Dependence of α on θ for f = 500, 1000, and 5000 Hz; (b) Dependence of α on f for θ = 90°. Curves were obtained from Shaw's synthesis of a wide variety of experimental data. The average source distance in the experiment was 1.5 m and the subjects were always seated.

Some results on interaural differences obtained with a single source in a more-or-less anechoic environment are shown in Figs. 2 and 3 [derived from the summary of data that has been provided by Shaw (1974a,b)]. Figure 2 shows how the interaural amplitude ratio α for tonal stimuli depends on the azimuth θ and the tone frequency f (where the source is always confined to the horizontal plane and θ = 0° corresponds to a source directly in front of the listener). As one would expect, the amplitude ratio tends to increase as the source is moved to the side and as the frequency is increased. Note, however, that the dependencies are not strictly monotonic: In certain regions of θ and f, α decreases as the source is moved further to the side or as the frequency increases. Figure 3 shows how the interaural time delay τ depends on the angle θ for tones and clicks. The results for tones were derived from interaural phase measurements made on artificial heads (Firestone, 1930; Mills, 1958; Nordlund, 1962). Note that the delay is not completely independent of frequency, but tends to increase as the frequency is lowered. Note also that since α and τ depend on frequency, when the stimulus is a click the waveforms at the two ears will not be identical and the estimate of delay can vary with the feature of the waveform selected for measurement. Although the feature selected for the click measurements shown in Fig. 3, which were

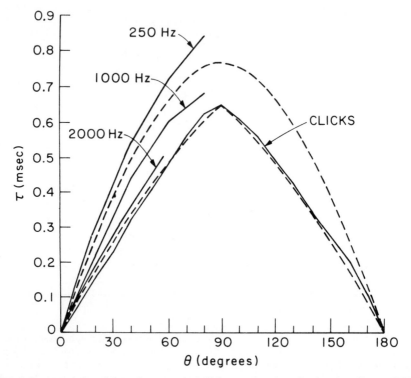

FIG. 3. Interaural time delay τ for tones and clicks as a function of azimuth θ (Shaw, 1974b). Solid lines represent data and dashed lines theoretical results. The solid lines representing the results for tones were derived from the summary of phase measurements presented by Shaw (obtained by Firestone, 1930; Mills, 1958; and Nordlund, 1962). The click data were obtained by Feddersen *et al.* (1957). The lower dashed curve (essentially identical to the curve for clicks) is derived from the formula $\tau = (r/c)(\theta + \sin \theta)$ and the upper dashed curve from the formula $\tau = (r/c)(3 \sin \theta)$, where $r = 8.75$ cm and $c = 344$ m/sec (see text for details).

made on real subjects with microphones located at the entrance to the ear canals, was not specified in detail in the original report concerning these measurements (Feddersen, Sandel, Teas, & Jeffress, 1957), it appears that the time of arrival of the click was specified by the time at which the signal first exceeded some fixed threshold. Click results obtained with an artifical head that are essentially the same as those shown, and in which τ was estimated by observing the times of arrival of the first peak in the waveforms, are available in Nordlund (1962). For most reasonable definitions of the time of arrival of the click waveform, the results on the function $\tau(\theta)$ for clicks is approximately the same as for high-frequency tones. The theoretical curves shown in Fig. 3 are derived from a model in which the head is assumed to be a hard sphere and the ears are assumed to be located on a diameter of the sphere. The lower curve is derived from the formula

$\tau = (r/c)(\theta + \sin \theta)$ and the upper curve from the formula $\tau = (r/c)(3 \sin \theta)$, where r is the radius of the sphere (assumed to be 8.75 cm) and c is the velocity of sound (assumed to be 344 m sec^{-1}). The first formula (Woodworth, 1938) is based on simple geometric considerations and the second (Rayleigh, 1945) represents the limiting case of diffraction theory as the frequency goes to zero. If the assumed radius of the sphere were increased, both curves would be raised proportionately. Extensive summaries of material related to the interaural differences that arise with single sources in anechoic environments are available in Shaw (1974a,b) and Blauert (1974). (Blauert's summary includes the results of attempts to determine amplitude and phase differences by measurements of the impulse response.)

Finally, it is important to note that the measurements of interaural differences that are currently available do not constitute an adequate description of natural differences for the purposes of perceptual theory. Aside from technical measurement difficulties and the insufficiently large sample of source locations (in both angle and distance) that have been tested, practically no consideration has been given to the interaural differences that arise in environments that are not anechoic. Although the problem of characterizing interaural differences in reverberant environments is extremely complex (because there are so many different reverberant environments) and the characterization would undoubtedly have to be expressed in probabilistic terms, some such characterization is necessary if one hopes to take serious account of how an individual's previous experience influences the perception of binaural stimuli.

III. PERCEPTUAL ATTRIBUTES OF THE BINAURAL IMAGE SPACE

The relation between the perceptual attributes of a sound generated from a binaural stimulus and those of a sound generated from the component monaural stimuli depends strongly on the particular attributes and stimuli considered. In this section, we consider a variety of attributes and stimuli for which binaural interaction plays a significant role in the determination of the attributes. In Section III,A, we consider attributes concerned with spatial organization, attributes that are often discussed under the heading "directional hearing" or "localization." In Section III,B we consider two of the most fundamental nonspatial attributes—loudness and pitch.

A. Spatial Attributes

The study of the spatial attributes of sounds constitutes a fundamental, rich, and provocative area of binaural hearing research. Indeed, Békésy (1960) has written "In no other field of science known to the writer does a stimulus produce so many different sensations as in the area of directional hearing [p. 272].''

The phenomena in this area will be considered in terms of externalization, fusion and lateralization, head movements, and monaural localization. In Section III,A,1, we make some brief introductory remarks on these topics. In Section III,A,2, we discuss fusion and lateralization in detail. Of the topics mentioned, fusion and lateralization have been studied most intensively and are the most relevant to models of binaural interaction.

1. GENERAL REMARKS

When a listener is stimulated in a natural way by a source that is located outside his body, the sound image is usually localized in space in the vicinity of the source. This implies, among other things, that the image is fused and externalized. An image is said to be *fused* when it is spatially compact and unitary, and *externalized* when it is located outside the head. Also implied is the fact that the presence of other sounds (such as the echoes caused by reflections), as well as changes in stimulation caused by movements of the listener, do not seriously alter the preceived location of the source.

When a binaural stimulus is presented through earphones, the sound usually will not be externalized, but will appear to originate within the listener's head. The degree of externalization that can be achieved under such conditions depends on a complex interaction of many factors and is difficult to predict (or even describe) with precision. Clearly, however, it increases as the stimulation approximates more closely stimulation that is natural. In particular, it can be increased by presenting signals that have natural spectral characteristics and interaural differences (i.e., by simulating the effects of the listeners head and pinna on an impinging stimulus) or that vary in a natural way with the listener's movements. The fact that substantial externalization can be achieved without taking account of movements is proved by results obtained with dummy heads. Despite the fact that there is no coupling between the binaural stimulus and the movements of the person listening through the earphones (so that, for example, the source appears to move in absolute coordinates whenever the listener rotates his head), if the stimulus is carefully constructed, the image will be externalized. Exactly what components of the transformation of the incoming signal imposed by the interaction with the dummy head are the most important in achieving externalization or, equivalently, how the externalization varies with different types of dummy heads, depends on the character of the signal and has not yet been worked out in detail. The idea that in-head images might be caused by factors related directly to the use of earphones is disproved not only by the fact that one can achieve externalized images with earphones, but also by the fact that in-head images can be achieved with multiple speakers in an anechoic chamber (e.g., Gardner, 1969b; Hanson & Kock, 1957; Jeffress, 1957; Leakey, 1957; Toole, 1970). A comprehensive review of the externalization problem, which includes the natural generalization to the problem of distance perception (e.g., Coleman, 1962, 1963, 1968; Gardner, 1969a; Laws, 1972; Molino, 1973) can be found in Blauert (1974). As one would expect on the basis of purely physical considerations, if one eliminates the cues arising from changes in loudness and changes in reverberent structure, the binaural system is exceedingly poor at determining the distance of a source.

Even if a stimulus configuration is sufficiently unnatural to produce a sound image inside the head, the image may still resemble that generated by a point source outside the body in that it is well-fused and localizable. Under such conditions, the image can be moved around within the head (just as an externalized image can be moved around outside the head) by manipulating the interaural differences. Inasmuch as a major portion of this in-head movement is usually perceived to occur along the interaural axis, the position of the in-head image is usually specified in terms of its *lateralization*. Descriptions of the spatial character of the images elicited by earphone stimulation that include dimensions beyond that of mere lateralization can be found in Békésy (1960) and Blauert (1974).

The extent to which a binaural stimulus produces a single fused image (either inside or outside the head) depends on the interaural differences and, it is reasonable to assume, on the extent to which such differences approximate those that occur naturally with a point source. Situations where fusion breaks down, either because the image spreads out and loses its compactness and localizability or because it splits up into a number of subimages, each with a different location, can be created with multiple-speaker configurations or with earphones. Aside from the obvious cases of multiple or broadened images that can be achieved merely by presenting binaural stimuli that are composed of summations of binaural stimuli from unrelated sources at different locations (actual or simulated), fusion can be destroyed by employing strongly abnormal interaural differences. Thus, for example, it can be destroyed by presenting signals that are unusually different with respect to frequency or time of arrival, that are statistically independent, or that involve abnormal combinations of interaural time delay and interaural amplitude difference.

If there are no interaural differences, the image will be well fused and lateralized in the median plane. As the interaural amplitude ratio varies from unity, the image will move toward the ear receiving the more intense signal. If, instead, the interaural time delay is varied, and the signal provides low-frequency timing information (either from the low-frequency components directly or from the envelope of high-frequency components within a single critical band), the image will move toward the ear receiving the leading signal. An interesting demonstration of the image movement with time delay can be achieved by using a low-frequency tone and inserting a slight interaural frequency difference (which is mathematically equivalent for the tone to a time-varying interaural phase or time shift). Under these conditions, the image will move back and forth across the median plane periodically and evidence the phenomenon known as *binaural beats*.

If the signal provides low-frequency timing information so that its lateralization is influenced by both interaural amplitude ratio and interaural time difference, there exists a variety of combinations of these two parameters that produce the same lateralization, a phenomenon that is referred to as *time–intensity trading*. Similarly, if a signal is decomposed into its envelope and microstructure, and the interaural time delay is dissected into an envelope delay and a microstructure delay, there exists a variety of combinations of these two delay parameters that produce the same lateralization, a phenomenon that could be referred to as *envelope–microstructure trading*. In all such trading situations, however, there is a tendency for the image to diffuse as the relation between the two parameters involved becomes strongly unnatural. Thus, for example, if time and intensity are put in opposition (i.e., the signal is more intense in one ear and leads in the other ear) and the values of the parameters are adjusted to produce an image in the median plane, the image will be less fused than that produced by a signal with no interaural differences.

Another important phenomenon involving lateralization and fusion (that has been exploited in the design of multichannel reproduction systems) is related to the perception of sound sources in reverberant rooms. Provided the differences in the lengths of the various paths to a given ear are not too large, the multiple pairs of signals received at the two ears from a single source in such a room are perceived not as a collection of distinct, temporally ordered, images at different locations, but rather as a single image at roughly the correct location with a special quality associated with the room acoustics. Although most listeners are not fully aware of the echoes in such situations, they can be made aware of them by eliminating the echoes (i.e., using an anechoic chamber) or by recording an impulsive sound in a reverberant room and then reproducing it reversed in time (so that the echoes of the sound come before the direct sound). For naive listeners, both these experiences are extremely striking. The fact that the localization of a source in a reverberant room is dominated by the first pair of signals to reach the two ears is referred to as the *precedence effect*. Further discussion of this phenomenon, as well as many of those mentioned in the preceding paragraphs, is contained in the next section, where we consider lateralization and fusion in greater detail.

In all the preceding remarks, we have ignored the obvious fact that in a natural environment the listener is capable of localizing a source not only with respect to a coordinate system that is fixed relative to the position and orientation of the listener's head, but also relative to a coordinate system that is fixed relative to the local environment. Thus, for example, if a listener turns his head while listening to a stationary source, the sound image remains fixed in the environmental coordinate system, despite the changing pattern of interaural differences. This ability to separate out and correctly interpret source position (or movement) and head position (or movement) depends on proprioceptive, kinesthetic, and vestibular cues for head position and on a comparison of these cues with the auditory cues. This ability serves not only to preserve "localization constancy" but also to resolve the localization ambiguities that occur when the head is held fixed. Although a precise description of these ambiguities is relatively complex and depends on a variety of details concerning the specific experimental configuration, insight can be gained by examining the ambiguities that would necessarily occur under the assumptions that reflections from the listener's body can be ignored, that the listener's head is a perfect, pinnaless sphere, that the interaural axis constitutes a diameter of the sphere, and that the only cues available for localization are interaural differences. Under these assumptions, any cone whose apex is at the center of the head and whose axis is collinear with the interaural axis constitutes a surface of ambiguity (i.e., all points on such a surface produce the same pattern of interaural differences). The two limiting cases of these surfaces are the median plane, corresponding to an angle of 180° at the apex, and the line through the two ears, corresponding to an angle of 0° at the apex. In general, these ambiguities (either the ones specified by this simplified model or the actual ones, which tend to be a subset of the former) can be resolved by relatively small rotations of the head. Furthermore, if one monitors head position and moves the source in a way that is correlated with head position, one can create a variety of spatial illusions. For example, if the head is constrained to rotations around the vertical axis, and the source is moved in such a way as always to be directly in front of the listener (so that the interaural differences are always zero), the source will appear to be located on the vertical axis (Wallach, 1940). Inasmuch as points on this axis are the only ones for which a fixed source would lead to zero interaural differences independent of the amount of rotation, this result is not surprising. In addition to the role head movements play in resolving ambiguities, they play a central role in the listener's ability to adapt his localization perception to artificial transformations imposed on the incoming signals by the use of pseudophones. For example, it has been shown that the ability to adapt to the atypical stimuli produced by a pseudophone which effectively rotates the interaural axis about the vertical axis (so that the interaural axis is no longer perpendicular to the median plane) depends crucially on active head movements (Held, 1955). Such movements and sensory–motor feedback are also clearly important for the development of normal localization perception and for adaptation to asymmetric hearing impairments.

Finally, it should be noted that the ability to localize cannot be explained entirely on the basis of interaural differences. Some localization ability is also present (primarily for signals that contain high-frequency components) when the stimulus is perceived through a single ear (e.g., Angell & Fite, 1901a,b;

Batteau, 1967, 1968; Butler, 1969; Freedman & Fisher, 1968; Harris & Sergeant, 1970; Perrott & Elfner, 1968). Theoretically, if one assumes that the listener knows the acoustic receptivity pattern of his ear, monaural localization can be achieved for signals with high-frequency components either through head movements or through the use of a priori information on the transmitted signal (so that the influence on the received signal of the transmitted signal and of the receptivity pattern can be properly factored). Unfortunately, so far as we know, there is no study available in which the a priori information on the transmitted signal has been carefully controlled and systematically varied in order to obtain a clear picture of monaural localization capabilities with a fixed head. It should also be noted that the ability to localize in the median plane (e.g., Blauert, 1969, 1971; Butler, 1969; Gardner & Gardner, 1973; Roffler & Butler, 1968a,b) can only be regarded as equivalent to monaural localization ability in the same plane under the assumption that the head is perfectly symmetric (so that all interaural differences are zero). To the extent that the receptivity patterns of the two ears are asymmetric, the ability to localize in the median plane, like the ability to localize in the horizontal plane, may involve sensitivity to interaural differences (e.g., Searle, 1973).

An excellent summary of auditory localization is available in Mills (1972), and a comprehensive and detailed review of this topic (with an enormous number of references) can be found in the book by Blauert (1974).

2. Fusion and Lateralization

The discussion in this section is subdivided into five subsections: *(a)* response structures and pointing techniques; *(b)* pure interaural amplitude differences, *(c)* pure interaural time differences; *(d)* combinations of interaural time and amplitude differences; and *(e)* other interaural differences. The last subsection includes discussion of binaural beats, envelope versus microstructure, and the precedence effect. Fusion and lateralization phenomena that arise in connection with masking are considered both in this subsection and Section IV.

a. Response structures and pointing techniques. One of the main problems in designing experiments to explore the spatial attributes of the binaural image space is the selection of an appropriate set of available responses to enable the listener to communicate his perception of this space to the experimenter. In most cases, these sets have been chosen to be compatible primarily with position properties rather than fusion properties, in the sense that they focus on the "centroid" of the image rather than its spatial extent. Also, since the primary change in image position as the interaural parameters are changed is a change in lateralization, the response sets have usually been chosen to be compatible with lateralization.

The techniques that have been employed for these "pointers" (i.e., image-location indicators) vary greatly with respect to their resolution and the sense modalities and motor systems involved, as well as the degree of compatibility with the perceptual phenomena. Depending on the specific technique, the listener may be required to indicate whether the image position is left or right of center (e.g., Sayers & Cherry, 1957), to match a point on a visual scale or the position of a mechanical lever with the lateralization of the image (e.g., Hafter, Bourbon, Blocker, & Tucker, 1969; Sayers, 1964; Teas, 1962), to match the position of a sensation produced by a tactual stimulus on the head with the position of the sound image (e.g., Békésy, 1960), or to match the lateralization of two different sound images (e.g., Whitworth & Jeffress, 1961). The fusion properties of the image are usually derived merely from qualitative verbal reports about the breadth of the image, or from results of lateralization experiments that indicate multiple or split images (i.e., lateralization ambiguities), or from measurements of sensitivity to changes in the stimulus parameters that determine the lateralization. In the last case, it is implicitly assumed that the listener's ability to detect changes in lateralization increase proportionately with the compactness of the image. That this assumption may not be correct, however, is suggested by the fact that broad-band signals such as clicks or white noise produce images that appear considerably more compact than those produced by certain narrow-band low-frequency signals—such as a 500-Hz tone—despite the approximate equivalence of these two classes of signals with respect to interaural time sensitivity (see Section IV). The only method of which we are aware that has been used to describe the spatial extent of an image directly (beyond qualitative verbal statements) is that in which the perception is matched with a two-dimensional drawing (e.g., Blauert, 1974; Licklider, 1948). In general, it is clear that the development of improved experimental techniques for the measurement of spatial properties of the image other than the position of its centroid would be highly useful.

b. PURE INTERAURAL AMPLITUDE DIFFERENCES. It is well known that the effect of introducing an interaural amplitude ratio $\alpha \neq 1$ into signals that are otherwise identical is to move the image away from the median plane toward the ear receiving the more intense signal, and that when the deviation of α from unity is sufficiently large, the image will closely approximate the image produced by stimulation of that ear alone. However, the quantitative details of the image behavior are not yet clear. With few exceptions, the effect of α on lateralization and fusion has been studied only qualitatively or in terms of its interaction with the effect of interaural time (discussed in Section III,A,2,d). Some studies suggest that the dependence of the image on α is independent of the type of signal employed and that the image will be completely lateralized when α is roughly 10 dB. For example, the lateralization at a given α has been reported to be approximately the same for tones above 3000 Hz, for noise, and for clicks (Békésy, 1960). Similarly, the α required for a noise burst to be lateralized at one ear has been reported to be roughly 10 dB independent of the level and duration of the burst (Pinheiro &

Tobin, 1969). The independence of level and the value 10 dB for complete lateralization has also been found for a click train of 100 pps (Békésy, 1959). Other studies, however, suggest that this picture is, at best, oversimplified. For example, some reports suggest that clicks are completely lateralized before α reaches 10 dB (e.g., Flanagan, David, & Watson, 1964). Similarly, some results for tones and clicks obtained in studies designed to explore the interaction of interaural amplitude and interaural time indicate that the value of α required for complete lateralization when the interaural delay $\tau = 0$ is much greater than 10 dB (e.g., Guttman, 1962a; Moushegian & Jeffress, 1959; Sayers, 1964; Whitworth & Jeffress, 1961) and that the lateralization for a given α with $\tau = 0$ depends upon the frequency of the signal (Moushegian & Jeffress, 1959). Moreover, it is not yet clear how the fusion of the image depends upon α. On the one hand, when $\alpha = 1$ or ∞, the image is well fused. On the other hand, some results indicate that the image diffuses or splits up when α becomes large (Békésy, 1960; Harris, 1960; Sayers, 1964; Sayers & Lynn, 1968; Whitworth & Jeffress, 1961).

The extent to which the lack of consistency among the various descriptions of the effects of α on fusion and lateralization is due to the different stimuli employed in the different experiments and the extent to which it is due to variations in subjective criteria is uncertain. It appears obvious, however that the latter factor is important.

c. PURE INTERAURAL TIME DIFFERENCES. Unlike the case of pure amplitude differences, the case of pure time differences has been studied extensively. The greater attention paid to time appears to be the result of two basic facts. First, the nature of the signal plays a more important role in the dependence of lateralization and fusion on pure time differences than on pure amplitude differences. Second, interaural time has played a more crucial role than interaural amplitude in the development of theories of binaural interaction. In the following paragraphs, we review the effect of interaural time for various types of signals.

For pure tones, the behavior of the image is (of necessity) periodic in the interaural delay τ with a period equal to the period T of the tone. For frequencies substantially above 1500 Hz, this periodicity is degenerate because the image is totally insensitive to interaural delay and remains centered for all τ. For the lower frequencies, as the delay is increased from 0 to T, the image will first be well fused and move toward the lead ear (in the region $0 \leq \tau < T/2$); then diffuse and be difficult to lateralize (in the vicinity of $T/2$); and then finally be re-fused and return to the center from the lag ear (in the region $T/2 < \tau \leq T$). In general, the perception in the vicinity of the "antiphasic" point $T/2$ (corresponding to a phase shift of π radians) is complex and labile. Most reports, however, can be well understood by assuming that the image splits into two parts positioned symmetrically about the center. Under this assumption, one would not only expect direct reports of such a perception, but also reports that the image is diffused and lateralized on the midline, that the image is well fused and far to the left, or that the image is well fused and far to the right (all of which have actually been obtained). The maximum lateralization that is obtained over τ occurs in the vicinity of $T/2$ and depends on the frequency of the tone, higher frequencies tending to produce smaller maximum lateralizations. Roughly, the maximum lateralization is all the way to the side when $T/2 > .7$ msec (i.e., when the frequency f of the tone is below approximately 700 Hz); approaches the center monotonically as $T/2$ decreases below .7 msec; and is at the center for $T/2 < .3$ msec (i.e., when f is significantly greater than 1500 Hz). The critical delay $\tau = .7$ msec is often referred to as the Hornbostel–Wertheimer constant (Békésy, 1960; Hornbostel & Wertheimer, 1920) and is roughly equal to the headwidth delay (i.e., the delay that occurs in a free field when the source is 90° to the side). Note also that this critical delay is equal to the period T of the critical frequency $f = 1500$ Hz, above which the binaural system is insensitive to interaural delay for tones. Whether this relationship is significant and remains valid for animals of different head-widths (so that animals with smaller heads are sensitive to phase shifts of tones at higher frequencies), or whether it is merely an example of "psychoacoustic numerology" is uncertain. Most physiologists appear to believe the latter. Also, one should not conclude from the fact that the system is insensitive to interaural delay for high-frequency tones that it is insensitive to this parameter for all high-frequency signals. Provided the high-frequency signal has an envelope with low-frequency time structure, a change in delay will produce a change in lateralization. This point is considered further in later sections.

Illustrative experimental results on the lateralization of tone signals as a function of interaural delay are shown in Figs. 4 and 5. The results in Fig. 4 (Sayers & Cherry, 1957) are derived from an experiment in which the listener is required to judge whether the image is to the left or right of center, and are sometimes referred to as "binaural coherence curves." For frequencies significantly greater than those shown, the curves are horizontal lines at 50%. The results in Fig. 5 (Sayers, 1964) are derived from an experiment in

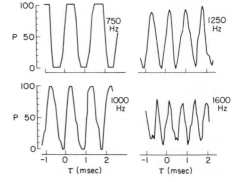

FIG. 4. Binaural coherence curves for tones of different frequency. P denotes the percentage of judgments "to the left," and positive τ corresponds to the left ear leading. [Adapted from Sayers and Cherry (1957).]

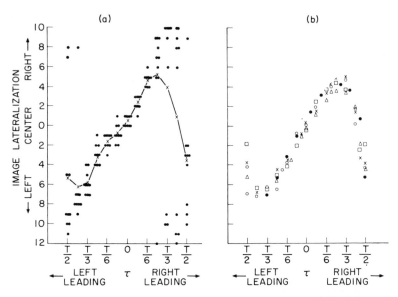

FIG. 5. Lateralization data for tones. T denotes the period of the tone and the ordinate gives the tone's lateralization as determined with the aid of a visual scale. (a) Individual responses and average-response curve for one subject at 600 Hz; (b) results averaged over both judgments and subjects for a variety of frequencies between 200 and 1200 Hz. See text for details. [Adapted from Sayers (1964).]

which the listener is required to assign a position to the sound image with the aid of a visual scale. Figure 5a shows the results for one subject and one frequency, without any averaging. The large dispersion of the points for large $|\tau|$ reflects the ambiguities in lateralization in the vicinity of the antiphasic point. Figure 5b shows the results averaged over both judgments and subjects for a variety of frequencies between 200 and 1200 Hz. The curves for different listeners exhibited different magnitudes of image position, but suitable linear expansions of the judgment scale were found to compensate for such differences, and these expansions were performed before averaging. Of greater interest is the fact that no such scaling was required to compensate for the results obtained by one listener at different frequencies. Superficially, this would appear to contradict the statement that the maximum lateralization tends to decrease with increasing frequency. An alternative explanation, however, is that the listener adjusts his judgment scale to cover a convenient range, independent of frequency. This explanation was confirmed by additional experiments in which different frequencies were interlaced within a single experimental run, and in which it was shown that under these conditions the maximum lateralization tended to decrease with increasing frequency.

If the signal is continuous broad-band noise, the results are similar to those for low-frequency tones, except that the perception does not vary periodically with τ and the breakdown of fusion at large $|\tau|$ occurs differently. Specifically, as τ increases beyond the value at which the image is lateralized to one side (again, of the order of 1 msec), the image remains at the leading ear but begins to lose its compactness. Eventually, the image becomes so diffuse that it fills the whole head and is indistinguishable from the image produced by statistically independent noise at the two ears. (If, instead of decorrelating the noise signals through the introduction of an interaural delay, they are decorrelated by adding statistically independent noise at the two ears while decreasing the level of the noise common to both ears so that the overall levels at the two ears remain fixed, then the image will remain centered, but will increasingly fill the head as the proportion of independent noise is increased.) Although apparently no experiment has been performed to determine the ability to discriminate between time-delayed noise and statistically independent noise as a function of the time delay, a variety of experiments indicate that the time-delay threshold for this discrimination, which is a measure of the interaural memory for the details of the noise waveform, would be in the region $10 \leq \tau \leq 30$ msec. This estimate is based on the results of experiments on the ability to judge sidedness of time-delayed noise (Blodgett, Wilbanks, & Jeffress, 1956); on the ability to discriminate noise correlation (Pollack & Trittipoe, 1959a,b) and to center noise as a function of the noise correlation (Jeffress, Blodgett, & Deatherage, 1962a); and on the ability to detect signals in noise as a function of the interaural delay in the noise and the interaural correlation of the noise (Dolan & Robinson, 1967; Jeffress, Blodgett, & Deatherage, 1952, 1962b; Langford & Jeffress, 1964; Rabiner, Laurence, & Durlach, 1966; Robinson & Jeffress, 1963; Wilbanks, 1971). Most of these results on discrimination and detection are considered further under sensitivity in Section IV. In view of the above-mentioned basic phenomena on fusion and lateralization of broad-band noise, it is clear that the binaural coherence curve for such a signal would rapidly increase from 50% to 100% as τ is increased from zero, remain at 100% over a large region of τ, and then slowly return to 50%, where it would remain as τ is further increased. Coherence curves with forms intermediate between the curves for broad-band noise and the curves for tones can obviously be generated by filtering the noise. For example, the coherence curve for narrow-band low-frequency noise would be a damped version of the periodic curve for a tone at the center frequency of the band, with the damping factor determined by the bandwidth. A further phenomenon that occurs with interaurally delayed noise, namely, the appearance of a weak secondary image whose pitch, but not position, depends on the delay, is discussed in Section III,B in connection with binaural pitch phenomena.

If the signal is a broad-band click, the results are roughly similar to those for broad-band noise, except for the way in which fusion breaks down as τ is increased beyond approximately 1 msec. In the vicinity of $\tau = 0$, there is a single fused image whose position depends on τ. As τ is increased beyond the value for which the click is well lateralized to one side, the image splits into two images, one on the lead-ear side followed by one on the lag-ear side. As τ is further increased, the lateralization of these images increases slightly, until finally they are located at the two ears and there is no further interaction with respect to lateralization. The appearance of the two distinct images occurs in the region $1 \le \tau \le 5$ msec (Babkoff & Sutton, 1966; Guttman, 1962a; Teas, 1962), and the point at which the lateralization interaction totally disappears is of the order of $\tau = 15$ msec (Guttman, 1962a). Although Guttman, based on a very brief experiment, reports that the value of τ for noise corresponding to the value $\tau = 15$ msec for clicks is only 5 msec, it should be noted that the value $\tau = 15$ msec is roughly comparable to the delay at which broad-band noise no longer evidences sidedness or can be distinguished from statistically independent noise, and the delay at which a speech signal no longer evidences sidedness (Cherry & Taylor, 1954). In other words, there appears to be a second critical time constant (besides the 1-msec constant associated with the headwidth delay), which reflects a limitation on interaural "memory" for lateralization. It should also be noted that, at least for clicks, there are interactions at delays longer than the point at which fusion breaks down for variables other than lateralization. Specifically, both loudness judgments and temporal-order judgments (i.e., judging which ear received the first click) are influenced by τ at these longer delays (Babkoff & Sutton, 1963; Hirsh & Sherrick, 1961). Finally, it should be noted that multiple images can arise with single diotic clicks. In addition to the main image, weak secondary images (as revealed by multimodal distributions of the delay required to center the image) may appear on either side of the main image (Harris, Flanagan, & Watson, 1963). This phenomenon is considered further in a later section.

The influence of intensity and spectral content of the click on the dependence of fusion and lateralization on τ cannot be easily summarized. Most studies indicate that an increase in intensity causes τ to have a more potent effect (e.g., Babkoff & Sutton, 1966; Guttman, 1962a; Teas, 1962), but some studies indicate that intensity has no effect (Mickunas, 1963) or that the effect is in the opposite direction (Békésy, 1960). Similarly, although most studies suggest that τ is more potent for low-frequency clicks than for high-frequency clicks (e.g., Teas, 1962), other studies indicate the opposite (e.g., Babkoff & Sutton, 1966). The results to be considered in the next section on time–intensity trading are consistent with the idea that τ becomes more potent as the intensity is increased or the frequency content lowered. If the click is bandpass filtered, then, as with noise, the lateralization and fusion results must approach those for tones as the bandwidth decreases.

Illustrative data on lateralization of a broad-band click in the region $0 \le \tau \le 3.5$ msec at various intensity levels obtained in an experiment in which the listeners were required to indicate the lateral position of the image on a sheet of graph paper on which the center, ear, and eye were used as

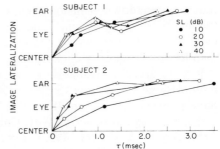

FIG. 6. Lateralization data for a broad-band click. The ordinate gives the click's lateralization as determined with the aid of graph paper on which the ear, eye, and center of the head were located as reference points. [Adapted from Teas (1962).]

reference points are shown in Fig. 6 (Teas, 1962). Note that interaural time becomes more effective in producing lateralization as the intensity of the click is increased. The slight shift toward center at roughly 1.5 msec evidenced in the results of subject 1 becomes much more pronounced (and may lead to points on the other side of center) if the click is low-pass filtered. Moreover, the value of τ at which the dip occurs is closely related to the cutoff frequency (Teas, 1962). Clearly, if the click were bandpass filtered, the graph would approach that for bandpassed noise and exhibit damped oscillatory behavior. Thus these shifts can probably be interpreted in terms of dominant frequency regions. Illustrative data on the value τ_0 of τ at which the perception changes from one click to two clicks (the "two-click threshold") as a function of level and for two different bandpass-filtered clicks are shown in Fig. 7 (Babkoff & Sutton, 1966). Aside from supporting the statements

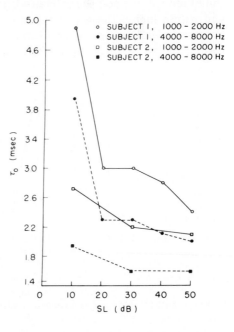

FIG. 7. Data on the two-click threshold τ_0 as a function of the sensation level of the click for two different bandpass-filtered clicks. [Adapted from Babkoff and Sutton (1966).]

that the breakdown of fusion occurs in the region $1 \leq \tau \leq 5$ msec and that the interaural delay becomes more potent at higher levels, these data indicate that the breakdown occurs at smaller delays for high-frequency clicks than for low-frequency clicks.

Results are also available on the dependence of lateralization on τ for multiple-tone complexes (Sayers, 1964; Sayers & Cherry, 1957; Toole & Sayers, 1965a), click trains (Sayers & Toole, 1964; Toole & Sayers, 1965a,b), and speech signals (Cherry, 1961; Cherry & Sayers, 1956; Cherry & Taylor, 1954; Sayers & Cherry, 1957). For speech (which is quasi-random), the lateralization judgments and coherence curves are similar to those for broad-band noise. For multiple-tone complexes and periodic click trains, sophisticated listeners can often identify a variety of images and trajectories as τ is varied. Thus, for example, with multiple-tone complexes, such listeners can lateralize each component separately. Similarly, with click trains, such listeners can track not only the main impulsive image, but also tonal images corresponding to the harmonics of the pulse train. An illustration of the trajectories obtained for the dominant impulsive image and the second and fifth harmonic images from a pulse train with a repetition period of 6 msec is shown in Fig. 8 (Toole & Sayers, 1965a). The lateralization curves obtained in experiments in which only one lateralization output is required are interpreted in terms of dominant images or weighted averages.

d. Combinations of interaural time differences and interaural amplitude differences. As discussed in the previous two subsections, the lateralization of a sound image can be influenced by both the interaural amplitude ratio α and the interaural time difference τ. To a certain extent, and within limits, these two types of interaural difference are tradable in the sense that the same lateralization can be achieved with various combinations of the two variables. For example, one can move the image away

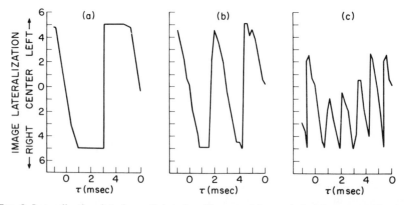

Fig. 8. Lateralization data for a click train with a repetition period of 6 msec. (a) The image corresponding to the fundamental; (b) the image corresponding to the second harmonic; (c) the image corresponding to the fifth harmonic. [Adapted from Toole and Sayers (1965a).]

from the center by introducing an amplitude shift or a time shift, and then return it to the center with a compensating time shift or amplitude shift (the "centering" method). Similarly, one can achieve roughly the same off-center position with an amplitude shift or time shift (the "equilaterality" method). This ability to match positions with different combinations of time and intensity is referred to as *time–intensity trading* and the rate at which the two variables are traded as the *time–intensity trading ratio* (usually specified in microseconds per decibel). This ratio constitutes a measure of the relative potency of the two interaural parameters with respect to the attribute lateralization. A substantial portion of the work on time–intensity trading has been motivated by (or stimulated) concern with the physiological mechanisms underlying the lateralization perception.

The values that have been reported for the trading ratio cover more than two orders of magnitude and range all the way from 1 to 300 μsec dB^{-1}. This wide range of variation is the result of systematic dependencies of the trading ratio on the region of (τ, α) in which it is estimated, the properties of the signal, and the method used to determine the ratio, as well as of large intersubject differences. It appears that some of the disparities among different subjects can be ascribed to the breakdown of fusion (broadened or multiple images) in these experiments and by variations in the strategy used by the subjects to describe the position of the diffused image (Hafter & Jeffress, 1968; Harris, 1960; Sayers & Lynn, 1968; Whitworth & Jeffress, 1961). Also, for a given individual the measured trading ratio may vary as a function of exposure time due to adaptation effects. In particular, it has been shown that the value of τ required to compensate for a given α decreases with time (Bertrand, 1972). Finally, it should be noted that, since stimuli can be constructed for which the sensitivity of the auditory system to τ becomes vanishingly small, the upper bound on the reported trading ratios is more a function of the configurations chosen for study than of the auditory system.

Many results on clicks using the centering method show that the time–intensity trading ratio τ/α tends to decrease as the overall intensity increases (David, Guttman, & van Bergeijk, 1959; Deatherage & Hirsh, 1959; Hafter & Jeffress, 1968; Harris, 1960) and as the frequency content of the click is lowered (e.g., Harris, 1960). In other words, the delay τ becomes more potent relative to the amplitude difference α as the intensity increases or the frequency content is lowered. Data illustrating these results are shown in Figs. 9 through 11. Figure 9 (Harris, 1960) shows the τ, α combinations required for centering a click for a variety of low-pass and high-pass clicks at low intensity and for two subjects. (The abrupt change in the curves in the neighborhood of 1500 Hz occurred only at low levels and was less pronounced for other subjects.) Figure 10 (Harris, 1960) shows the results on the trading ratio τ/α for the various clicks at various levels obtained by estimating the average slope of the curves and averaging over subjects. Note that the strongest dependence on level occurs for low-pass clicks with cutoff

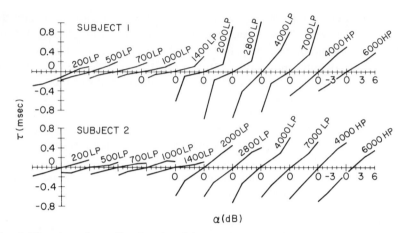

FIG. 9. Time–intensity trading data for clicks as a function of the click cutoff frequency. LP denotes low pass and HP high pass. The overall level of the clicks was 20 dB SL, and the data were obtained using the centering method. [Adapted from Harris (1960).]

frequencies above 1500 Hz, and that there is essentially no dependence on level for low-pass clicks with low cutoff frequencies. The result that the trading ratio is independent of level for low-pass clicks with cutoffs below 1500 Hz, but decreases with level for low-pass clicks with cutoffs above 1500 Hz, is also consistent with a number of other studies (e.g., David, Guttman, & van Bergeijk, 1958; Deatherage & Hirsh, 1959; Sayers & Lynn, 1968). It should also be noted that the curve relating τ to log α from which the trading ratio is estimated is often significantly nonlinear (and tends to be of the form shown by Subject 1 in Fig. 9 at a low-pass cutoff of 2000 Hz) and that the precise form of this curve, as well as its average slope, depends on both level and frequency content (David et al., 1958; Deatherage & Hirsh, 1959). Additional data on the effect of level for high-pass clicks (2 kHz cutoff) are shown in Fig. 11 (David et al., 1959). Results on the influence of interaural amplitude ratio α on the dependence of the click-image position on τ, and on the value τ_0 at which two click images first appear, are available in the click studies cited previously (Guttman, 1962a; Babkoff & Sutton, 1966). A

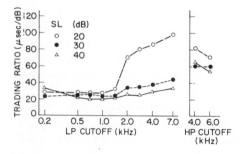

FIG. 10. Data on the time–intensity trading ratio for clicks as a function of the click cutoff frequency and sensation level. [Adapted from Harris (1960).]

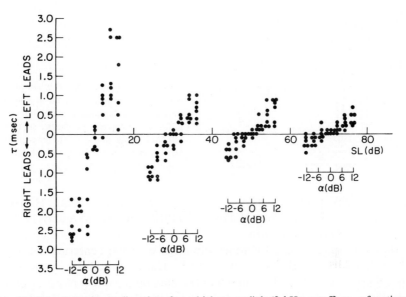

FIG. 11. Time–intensity trading data for a high-pass click (2 kHz cutoff) as a function of sensation level. Data were obtained from one subject, using the centering method. [Adapted from David *et al.* (1959).]

schematic illustration of the click-image position as a function of τ for a broad-band click and various α is shown in Fig. 12 (Guttman, 1962a). For intermediate α, the fused image may or may not reach the center, depending upon the exact value of α. Note also that when the signal in one ear is so weak that it is not heard for any τ, it may still influence the position of the image when τ is small. The occurrence of broadened or multiple images for

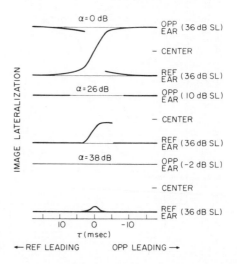

FIG. 12. Schematic illustration of click-image position as a function of τ and α for a broad-band click. Heavy lines represent the path of the click image as τ is varied, and multiple paths represent multiple images. [Adapted from Guttman (1962a).]

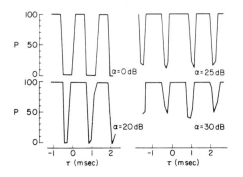

FIG. 13. Dependence of binaural coherence curve on α for a tone at 800 Hz. P denotes the percentage of judgments "to the left," $\tau > 0$ corresponds to the signal in the left ear leading, and $\alpha > 1$ to the signal in the left ear being more intense. [Adapted from Sayers and Cherry (1957).]

clicks or click trains is discussed in Flanagan *et al.* (1964), Hafter and Jeffress (1968), Harris (1960), Harris *et al.* (1963), and Sayers and Lynn (1968), as well as in Guttman (1962a).

Although some results for tones obtained with the centering method are also available (e.g., Banister, 1926, 1927; Hafter & Jeffress, 1968; Harris, 1960; Shaxby & Gage, 1932), much of the data on the effect of time–intensity combinations for tones has been obtained with other methods. Results showing the effect of an interaural amplitude ratio α on the coherence curve for a tone at frequency $f = 800$ Hz and on the lateralization curve obtained with the use of a visual scale for a tone at $f = 600$ Hz are shown in Figs. 13 (Sayers & Cherry, 1957) and 14 (Sayers, 1964). Both sets of results are consistent with the idea that as α deviates from 0 dB, the region of lateralization covered by variations in τ moves toward the ear receiving the greater intensity and decreases in extent. Since the data for the limiting case of monaural

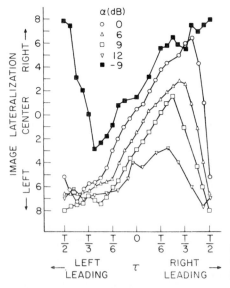

FIG. 14. Dependence of lateralization curve on α for a tone at 600 Hz. $\alpha > 1$ corresponds to the signal in the left ear being more intense. [Adapted from Sayers (1964).]

stimulation ($|\log \alpha| = \infty$) must lie on a horizontal line at an extreme of the ordinate range, these results are not surprising.

One of the most extensive studies of the dependence of lateralization on τ and α for tones (Moushegian & Jeffress, 1959) employed a broad-band noise source with a variable delay τ_p as a pointer. The results of this study, in which the listener was required to match the lateralization of the tone with the lateralization of the noise by adjusting τ_p (and in which the data depended strongly on the subject), are shown in Fig. 15. Various combinations of τ and α leading to the same lateralization are determined by the intersection points of the empirical curves with a horizontal straight line. The extent to which a pure time delay produces the same lateralization for the tone as for the noise is measured by the extent to which the ordinate values τ_p of the points at $\alpha = 0$ dB for the different values of τ are equal to these values of τ. According to the data, this equivalence is reasonably well satisfied at 500 Hz, but breaks down at the high frequencies for Subjects 2 and 3. The degradation of this equivalence at higher frequencies is qualitatively consistent with the results stated in the previous section concerning maximum lateralization over τ as a function of frequency. The extent to which the effect of α can be interpreted in terms of a simple trade from amplitude to time ($\tau_\alpha = k \log \alpha$, k constant) is measured by the extent to which all the curves for a fixed f are related merely by horizontal translations and the extent to which the magnitudes of the translations between successive curves (parametrized by

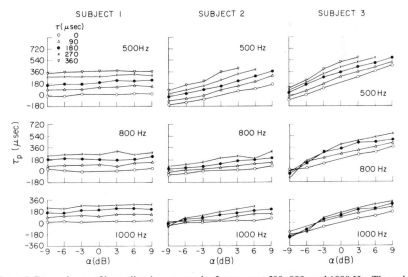

FIG. 15. Dependence of lateralization on τ and α for tones at 500, 800, and 1000 Hz. The values of α are given on the abscissa and the values of τ by the code in the upper left-hand corner of the figure. The ordinate τ_p gives the interaural delay of a broad-band-noise pointer whose lateral position matches that of the tone. [Adapted from Moushegian and Jeffress (1959).]

equal steps in τ) are all the same. Under such conditions, the time–intensity trading ratio (determined by k) would be measured by comparing the change in α (the magnitude of the translation) to the change in τ (the difference in the curve parameter). Clearly, however, the results for Subjects 2 and 3 do not satisfy these conditions. Also, for the same two subjects (who had high-frequency hearing losses), it is clear from the fact that the curves for different values of τ tend to exhibit greater horizontal separation for larger values of α, that the effect of τ relative to α increases with α. In particular, this effect is smaller when τ and α are antilateral (i.e., in opposition) than when they are collateral (i.e., in concert). The range of values of the trading ratios measured locally are essentially unbounded: Whereas for Subject 1 the ratio in most regions is exceedingly close to 0, for Subjects 2 and 3 at the higher frequencies and small α it is essentially infinite. In this connection, note that the trading ratios should not generally be computed (as was done in the original study) by estimating the slopes of the empirical curves, since these curves involve the transformation from the lateralization function of the tone to the lateralization function of the noise. This involvement also implies that the simple trading hypothesis $\tau_\alpha = k \log \alpha$ could be valid without the curves being linear. In general, the trading relation $\tau_\alpha = g(\alpha)$ (where g is some unknown fixed function) is valid if and only if the curves, when plotted with $g(\alpha)$ as the abscissa, are equally spaced horizontal translates. Finally, it should be noted that the results for Subject 2 at 1000 Hz and Subject 3 at 800 and 1000 Hz are extremely puzzling and contradict a variety of other data. Specifically, these results imply that when $\alpha = -9$ dB, the tone is lateralized close to the center, independent of τ. According to other studies, one would expect that when $\tau = 0$ the image would be lateralized further to the side (or if not, would be significantly influenced by τ). Data on the interaction of time and intensity in the lateralization of narrow-band noise signals from experiments in which the listener is required merely to judge left or right of center and in which the results are again strongly subject-dependent are also available (Jeffress & McFadden, 1971; McFadden, Jeffress, & Ermey, 1971; McFadden, Jeffress, & Lakey, 1972; McFadden, Jeffress, & Russell, 1973).

As indicated previously, part of the reason for the lack of clarity in the results on the interaction of time and intensity may be caused by the presence of multiple images and variations in how the subjects respond to the perception of such images when the experiment is structured as though there were only one image. Some results from experiments that reflect the existence of multiple images are shown in Figs. 16 and 17. The data in Fig. 16 (Whitworth & Jeffress, 1961) were obtained for a tone pulse with $f = 500$ Hz and in a manner similar to those shown in Fig. 15, except that the pointer was a 500-Hz tone pulse (like the signal) rather than broad-band noise. After preliminary practice sessions, all the subjects with normal hearing (but not those with substantial high-frequency losses) reported two distinct images, one of which—the "time image"—depended almost totally on τ for its laterali-

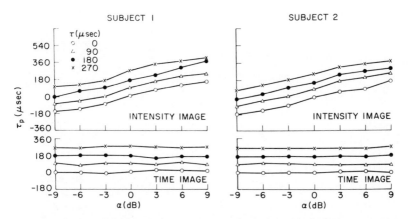

FIG. 16. Multiple-image lateralization data. Upper graphs present results for one image and lower graphs for another image. Both the signal and the pointer were 500-Hz tones with a duration of 800 msec and an overall level of 52 dB SPL. [Adapted from Whitworth and Jeffress (1961).]

zation; the other—the "intensity image"—depended on both τ and α. The data in Fig. 16 are those produced by two of the normal subjects. Note that the curves for the time image are essentially identical to those for Subject 1 in Fig. 15. Note also that since the pointer and signal are identical, the interpretation of the curves in Fig. 16 is much simpler than those in Fig. 15. In general, these curves are consistent with the statement that, for each image, there is a simple trade of the form $\tau_\alpha = k \log \alpha$. Moreover, the trading ratio can be estimated directly from the slopes of the empirical curves. These slopes were found to be in the ranges .4–2.5 μsec dB^{-1} (time image) and 20–26 μsec dB^{-1} (intensity image). The subjects with high-frequency losses perceived only one image, produced curves that were similar in form (parallel, equally spaced lines) to those of the normal subjects, but not to those of the subjects with high-frequency losses in the previous study (Moushegian & Jeffress, 1959), and produced trading ratios in the region 9–23 μsec dB^{-1} (roughly comparable to the ratios for the intensity image of the normal subjects). The data in Fig. 17 (Hafter & Jeffress, 1968) are obtained from a study that was motivated in part by the question of whether two images can also be formed for click stimuli. In this study, which employed a constant α of 9 dB and a variation of the centering method (so that time and amplitude were antilateral), two experiments were conducted. In the first, trading ratios were estimated for a 500-Hz tone pulse as a function of tone duration and rise–decay time (all pulses were low-pass filtered at 850 Hz). The results of this experiment (averaged over subjects) are shown in Fig. 17a. In the second, trading ratios were estimated for a broad-band click as a function of click level. The results of this experiment are shown in Fig. 17b. Note that the trading ratio for both images of the broad-band click is reduced as the intensity is increased. The results of both these experiments strongly support

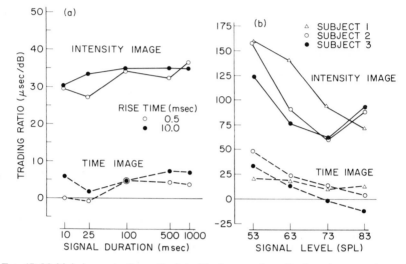

FIG. 17. Multiple-image trading-ratio data. The interaural amplitude ratio α was always 9 dB and the data were collected using a variation of the centering method. In (a) the signal was a 500-Hz tone pulse (low-pass filtered at 850 Hz) and the overall level was 52 dB SPL. In (b) the signal was a broad-band click. [Adapted from Hafter and Jeffress (1968).]

the notion that the two-image phenomenon occurs for clicks as well as for tones. It should be noted, however, that this phenomenon is rather subtle and usually requires considerable training (as well as a suitable experimental format and instructions) in order to perceive it. Also, it is not clear that the experiments conducted on this phenomenon have always been sufficiently sharp to distinguish between the existence of two separate images and the existence of a single broad image. Certain of the data might be interpreted equally well by assuming that the two images are merely the edges of a single broad image whose width, as well as centroid, depends upon the signal parameters.

e. OTHER INTERAURAL DIFFERENCES. Aside from the few comments contained in Section III,C concerning the effects of decorrelating noise signals by the addition of independent sources, the previous discussion has been restricted exclusively to the effects of introducing an overall amplitude shift and/or an overall time delay. In this section, we consider briefly some of the effects that occur with other interaural differences. In particular, we consider the effects on fusion and lateralization of interaural frequency differences (including the binaural-beat effect), of differentially delaying the envelope and microstructure of a signal, of adding a masking signal, and of presenting multiple-click stimuli in which the number of clicks in the two ears are different or the temporal patterns of the clicks in the two ears are different (including the precedence effect).

(i). INTERAURAL FREQUENCY DIFFERENCES. Consider first the case in which the stimulus consists of a tone of frequency f below 1500 Hz to one ear and a tone of the same amplitude and of frequency $f + \Delta f$ to the other ear. If $\Delta f = 0$, then the stimulus will produce an image whose lateralization and fusion depend on the interaural delay (or phase) in the manner that we have already discussed. If Δf is slightly different than zero, then the image will move back and forth across the head with a frequency equal to Δf. (This result is to be expected, since a small interaural frequency difference is mathematically equivalent to a slowly varying interaural phase.) As $|\Delta f|$ is made larger, the periodic fluctuation will become more rapid, the image will tend to become more diffuse, and the perceptual dimension in which the fluctuation is occurring will change from lateralization to loudness. As $|\Delta f|$ is increased still further, the ability to perceive the individual fluctuations will vanish and the diffused tonal image will exhibit a quality of "roughness." Eventually, when $|\Delta f|$ is sufficiently large, the image will split into two distinct, smooth, images of different pitch, one at each ear. During this transition, there may appear an intermediate stage at which the image appears partially split, with both parts somewhat rough. Also, the images may appear relatively distinct in both lateralization and pitch, but still exhibit some lateralization interaction in the sense that the location of each image is pulled slightly toward the center by the presence of the contralateral signal. Although the precise regions in which the different perceptions associated with Δf occur depend on the value of f and the intensity of the signals, as well as on what the listeners are expecting (determined by previous listening experience and instructions), it has been estimated that the perception of lateralization fluctuation dominates when $|\Delta f|$ is less than approximately 2 Hz, loudness fluctuation when $|\Delta f|$ is in the region 2–10 Hz, and roughness when $|\Delta f|$ exceeds 20 Hz but is less than the value at which the smooth bitonal image is heard (Licklider, Webster, & Hedlun, 1950). Results showing the value $(\Delta f)_0$ of Δf at which the transition occurs between roughness and smoothness as a function of f and intensity are shown in Fig. 18 (Licklider *et al.*, 1950). As these authors point out, the data above 1000 Hz must be interpreted with caution, since $(\Delta f)_0$ was recorded as zero on all trials in which no beats were perceived, where a beat was defined as a fluctuation in lateralization or loudness, or a roughness. Results showing the percentage of beat responses, where a beat was defined as a fluctuation in loudness (and the signal level was 12 sones), are shown in Fig. 19 (Perrott & Nelson, 1969). When these data were reprocessed in a manner like that used to derive the results shown in Fig. 18, the two sets of results were found to be consistent (Perrott & Nelson, 1969). If instead of choosing $f < 1500$ Hz, one chooses $f > 1500$ Hz, then, since the auditory system is insensitive to interaural phase above 1500 Hz, as $|\Delta f|$ is increased from zero, the fluctuation stages of the perception will be skipped over and the single fused image in the center that

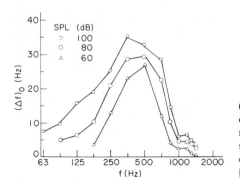

FIG. 18. Threshold frequency difference $(\Delta f)_0$ for binaural beat detection as a function of the reference frequency f. Subjective criterion was the transition from roughness to smoothness. $(\Delta f)_0$ was recorded as zero in all cases for which no beats were perceived. [Adapted from Licklider *et al.* (1950).]

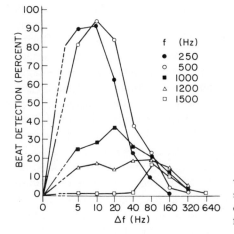

FIG. 19. Beat detection as a function of Δf for various tone frequencies f. Tone duration was 1 sec and loudness level was 12 sones. Subjective criterion was a fluctuation in loudness. [Adapted from Perrott and Nelson (1969).]

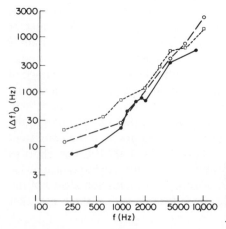

FIG. 20. Threshold frequency $(\Delta f)_0$ for separation of tonal images as a function of the reference frequency f (O: Thurlow & Bernstein, 1957; □: Thurlow & Elfner, 1959; ●: Perrott & Barry, 1969). See text for specification of subjective criteria.

occurs when $\Delta f = 0$ will transform directly into the smooth, spatially separated, bitonal image. Figure 20 summarizes results from three studies on how $(\Delta f)_0$ depends on f, where $(\Delta f)_0$ is defined in a manner that applies equally well to all frequencies. In the first study (Thurlow & Bernstein, 1957), $(\Delta f)_0$ was defined in terms of the perception of two pitches. In the second (Thurlow & Elfner, 1959), $(\Delta f)_0$ was defined in terms of whether any change took place in the apparent location of either tone when the contralateral tone was turned on. In the third (Perrott & Barry, 1969), $(\Delta f)_0$ was defined in terms of the perception of more than one tone. According to the first study, $(\Delta f)_0$ is independent of level in the region 10–50 dB SL. (The second and third studies were conducted at 30 dB SL and 12 sones, respectively). Also, according to the first study, the results are essentially the same when the two tones are presented together monaurally. Clearly, the $(\Delta f)_0$ shown in Fig. 20 is closely related to the critical bandwidth. Finally, it should be noted that binaural beats can be detected at low frequencies even when there is a large interaural amplitude difference (Tobias, 1963) or when the two frequencies constitute a mistuned octave (Thurlow & Bernstein, 1957), and that the ability of women to hear beats is significantly different from that of men and depends on the phase of the menstrual cycle (Oster, 1973; Tobias, 1963). Data concerning the influence of signal duration and rise time on the value of Δf at which more than one tone is heard is available in the study by Perrott, Briggs, and Perrott (1970).

Consider next the case in which the basic stimulus is a click rather than a tone and in which the interaural frequency differences are created by filtering the clicks differentially before they are presented to the two ears. In this case, the well-fused image that exists when there are no frequency differences (and the interaural delay τ is reasonably small) will tend both to diffuse and to change its lateralization, and, if the frequency content of the two clicks is sufficiently large, break up into multiple images. Data showing the values of τ required to center the images produced by a 250- to 500-Hz bandpass click to one ear and a higher-frequency bandpass click to the other ear as a function of the intensity of the clicks and of the frequency content of the higher-frequency click are shown in Fig. 21 (Deatherage, 1961). Note that when the higher-frequency click is confined to frequencies below 4.0 kHz, only one image appears and the higher-frequency click must lag the low-frequency click in order for the image to be centered (Fig. 21a). If the frequency content of the higher-frequency click is further increased, then two distinct images appear (Fig. 21b). For one of the images, the high-frequency click must lag the 250- to 500-Hz click, and for the other, it must lead it. The image that was centered by delaying the high-frequency click was judged to be lower both in pitch and in position within the vertical plane than the second image. When a 250- to 500-Hz click was paired with a 19- to 6000-Hz click, or a 19- to 500-Hz click was paired with a 19- to 6000-Hz click, there were again two images, but for both these images the higher-frequency

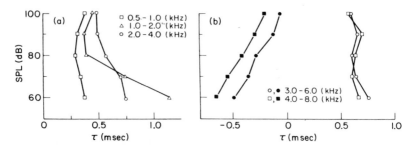

FIG. 21. Values of τ required to center images of clicks containing interaural frequency differences. All stimuli were bandpassed clicks, and the passband for one ear was always 250–500 Hz. The passbands for the other ear are indicated on the figure. (a) Results obtained for passbands of 0.5–1.0, 1.0–2.0, and 2.0–4.0 kHz; (b) Results obtained for passbands of 3.0–6.0 and 4.0–8.0 kHz. The zero time reference for each signal was chosen to be the first rarefaction maximum in the output of the filter, and $\tau > 0$ corresponds to the 250–500 Hz click leading. The two curves for each passband in (b) correspond to the presence of two images with distinct lateralizations. [Adapted from Deatherage (1961).]

click had to be delayed in order to center the image (Deatherage, 1961). An interpretation of some of these results in terms of a cochlear model is available in Flanagan *et al.*, 1964. Further data relevant to the interaction of signals of different frequency content (although they are not always discussed in these terms) are available in Butler and Naunton (1964), Deatherage (1966), Toole and Sayers (1965b), Ebata, Sone, and Nimura (1968a), Scharf (1969), and Dunn (1971).

(ii). ENVELOPE VERSUS MICROSTRUCTURE. As indicated previously, the lateralization of high-frequency signals is influenced by interaural time delay, provided the high-frequency signal produces a low-frequency envelope at the output of a critical-band filter. Although the sensitivity to delay for such signals (discussed further in Section IV) has often been found to be less than for low-frequency or broad-band signals, some degree of sensitivity has been demonstrated for high-frequency noise, high-frequency clicks, and amplitude modulated high-frequency tones (e.g., Békésy, 1960; Cronin, 1973; David *et al.*, 1958, 1959; Harris, 1960; Henning, 1974a; Klumpp & Eady, 1956; Leakey, Sayers, & Cherry, 1958; Licklider & Webster, 1950; Yost, Wightman, & Green, 1971). Moreover, some of these experiments have demonstrated that the perception of fusion and lateralization for such stimuli depends principally on the interaural relations of the envelope, not the microstructure. For example, the coherence curve for 4-kHz tone modulated by 500-Hz low-pass random noise (with the interaural delay inserted only in the modulation) is essentially the same as the coherence curve for the noise alone (Leakey *et al.*, 1958). Similarly, fused images and lateralization effects can be achieved with high-frequency noise pulses even when the two noise

signals are statistically independent and the lateralization is controlled by delaying the pulse envelopes (e.g., David *et al.,* 1959).

In view of the important role played by the envelope for high-frequency signals and by the microstructure for low-frequency signals (such as a low-frequency tone), the question naturally arises as to the relative strengths of these two factors for signals having both a low-frequency envelope and low-frequency microstructure. Tobias and Schubert (1959), in a study motivated primarily by concern with the precedence effect, examined the relative potency of envelope delay and microstructure delay by using stimuli consisting of pulsed broad-band noise, inserting an interaural time delay in the envelope (the transient disparity), and requiring the subject to center the image by appropriately adjusting the interaural time delay in the noise (the ongoing disparity). Data obtained from this study of "envelope–microstructure trading" for a variety of values of stimulus duration are shown in Fig. 22. According to these results, the ongoing disparity completely dominates the transient disparity when the duration of the noise burst is at least 300 msec. When the duration is only 10 msec, the trading ratio (i.e., the slope of the line) is roughly .2. In a further study concerned with envelope versus microstructure, Schubert and Wernick (1969) used carriers consisting of tones or noise, an envelope that approximated a triangle, and stimulus durations of 20, 50, and 100 msec (corresponding to rise/fall times of 10, 25, and 50 msec). Interaural time delays were applied only to the envelope and the subjects were required to judge whether or not a single fused image appeared. The noise was either high-passed or low-passed with a cutoff of 1000 Hz, and either interaurally identical or statistically independent. The results for each of these four cases and for the durations 20 and 100 msec (obtained by averaging over many subjects, with each subject making a relatively small number of judgments) are shown in Fig. 23. According to these results, fusion is maintained for larger envelope delays when the duration is increased. Also, with respect to the four types of microstructure considered, fusion is always relatively good for low-pass identical noise and relatively bad for high-pass independent noise. The relative degree of fusion

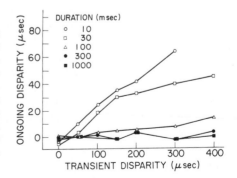

FIG. 22. Envelope–microstructure trading data for broad-band noise pulses of various durations. For each duration, the data points show the combinations of delay in the pulse envelope (transient disparity) and the delay in the broad-band noise (ongoing disparity) that result in a centered image. The signal level was adjusted as a function of duration to maintain constant loudness and was 65 dB SPL for the durations 100, 300, and 1000 msec. [Adapted from Tobias and Schubert (1959).]

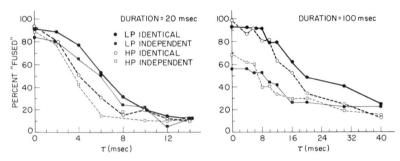

FIG. 23. Dependence of fusion on interaural delay of envelope for signal durations of 20 and 100 msec and various types of microstructure. The envelope was triangular with a rise–decay time equal to one-half the duration, and the microstructure was either low-pass noise (1000-Hz cutoff) or high-pass noise (1000-Hz cutoff) and either interaurally identical or statistically independent. Results are averaged over sensation levels of 20, 40, and 60 dB. [Adapted from Schubert and Wernick (1969).]

for the other two cases depends upon the duration. Whereas for 20 msec, the fusion for the low-pass independent noise is better than for the high-pass identical noise and almost as good as the low-pass identical noise, for 100 msec the fusion for the low-pass independent noise is worse than for the high-pass identical noise and as bad as for the high-pass independent noise. In view of the arbitrary nature of the subjective criteria that must have been used by the subjects to decide whether or not to report a fused image in these experiments (and the fact that these criteria are likely to be context-dependent), it is difficult to make meaningful comparisons between the delays required for the breakdown of fusion in these experiments with the delays required for the breakdown of fusion in other experiments.

(iii). MASKING. A wide variety of experiments have demonstrated that the fusion and lateralization of a signal can be substantially altered by the introduction of a masking signal. In one class of experiments, many of which have been motivated by concern with cochlear function, efforts have been made to determine the effects of masking noise on the lateralization of clicks. Data showing the effect of unilateral high-pass noise with a cutoff frequency of 4000 Hz on the interaural delay required to center identical 2400-Hz low-pass clicks are shown in Fig. 24 (Deatherage & Hirsh, 1959). According to these results, as the noise level is increased, the click in the ear with the noise must be presented earlier in order for the click image to be centered. In other words, the presence of the unilateral high-pass noise tends to push the click image away from the ear receiving the noise. It has also been shown (Schubert & Elpern, 1959) that if a binaural broad-band click is partially masked by binaural high-pass statistically independent noise with different cutoff frequencies in the two ears, the image of the click will be pushed toward the ear with the higher cutoff (and that the amount of interaural delay

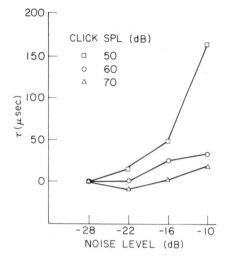

FIG. 24. Effect of unilateral highpass masking noise on the lateralization of a low-pass click. Results show the value of interaural delay τ required to center the click image as a function of the noise level for three click levels. The click was low-pass filtered at 2400 Hz and the noise was high-pass filtered at 4000 Hz. The noise level is referenced to the level required to just mask the 50 dB click (roughly 80 dB SPL). $\tau > 0$ corresponds to the masked click leading. [Adapted from Deatherage and Hirsh (1959).]

required to center the click image can be used to estimate the velocity of propagation down the cochlea). Important and extensive results on the effect of symmetrical high-pass noise, symmetrical low-pass noise, and asymmetrical noise, on the interaural delay required to center both cophasic and antiphasic broad-band clicks, and comparisons of these results with a detailed model for the operation of the cochlea, are available in Flanagan *et al.* (1964). Results from an experiment using a broad-band click and broad-band unilateral masking noise, in which the effect of the noise on lateralization was measured by adjusting the interaural amplitude ratio of the click rather than the interaural delay, are shown in Fig. 25 (Raab & Osman, 1962). Also included for comparison purposes are data showing the relations between the levels of the masked and unmasked clicks required to make the clicks sound equally loud when the loudness balancing is achieved using a sequential

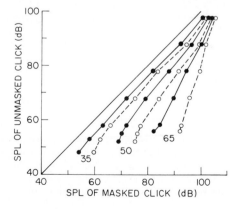

FIG. 25. Effect of unilateral broad-band masking noise on the lateralization and loudness of a broad-band click. Solid curves show the combinations of levels for the masked and unmasked clicks that result in a centered image. Dashed curves show the combinations that result in equal loudness (using a sequential monaural presentation). The numbers associated with the pairs of curves give the SPL in decibels of the unilateral masking noise. [Adapted from Raab and Osman (1962).]

monaural presentation. According to these results, the effect of the unilateral noise is again to push the binaural image of the click away from the ear receiving the noise, and for a given level of the masking noise and a given level of the unmasked click, the level of the masked click required to center the binaural image is less than the level required to achieve a monaural loudness balance. Results on the effect of both monaural and binaural noise on the interaural delay for which the single click image breaks up into two click images (the "two-click threshold") are available in Babkoff and Sutton (1966).

Further results on the effect of unilateral masking signals on fusion, lateralization, and localization of signals have been reported by Cherry and Sayers (1956), Sayers and Cherry (1957), Cherry (1961), Butler and Naunton (1962, 1964), Dunn and Parfitt (1967), and Dunn (1971). The effect of unilateral noise on the binaural coherence curve of speech is shown in Fig. 26 (Sayers & Cherry, 1957). According to these results, when the unmasked signal is leading in time, the signal is well lateralized on the side of the unmasked signal; however, when the unmasked signal is lagging in time, the judgment varies strongly with delay. The same phenomenon has been shown to occur for a wide variety of signals other than speech (including tone complexes and broad-band noise), and for signals that are corrupted by distortion as well as unilateral masking noise (Cherry, 1961; Cherry & Sayers, 1956; Sayers & Cherry, 1957). In the work by Butler and Naunton, subjects were required to determine the direction of a signal emanating from a concealed loudspeaker while an interfering signal was presented monaurally through an earphone (which also, of course, attenuated the signal from the loudspeaker to that ear). In most cases, the presence of the earphone signal caused the subjects to localize the loudspeaker signal closer to the ear receiving the earphone signal than when the earphone signal was absent. This "pulling effect" of the earphone signal is illustrated in Fig. 27 for the case in which both signals are tones (Butler & Naunton, 1964). These results, as might be expected, are similar to results on the frequency selectivity of the ear. For example, the pulling is greatest when the frequencies are identical, and the pulling is greater when the frequency of the earphone signal is below

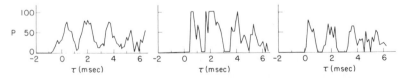

FIG. 26. Effect of unilateral masking noise on the binaural coherence curve of speech. The noise was presented to the left ear, P denotes percentage of judgments "to the left," and $\tau > 0$ corresponds to the masked speech leading. The levels of the speech signals in the two ears were adjusted so that the masked and unmasked speech were equally loud. The three graphs present the results for three subjects. [Adapted from Sayers and Cherry (1957).]

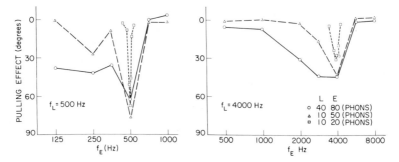

FIG. 27. Dependence of "pulling effect" on the frequency f_E of the tone presented through the earphone. f_L denotes the frequency of the tone presented through the loudspeaker. The loudness levels of the loudspeaker and earphone signals are indicated in the lower right-hand portion of the figure. The earphone was mounted in a Noise-Foe Mark II cushion which attenuated the signal from the loudspeaker by 19 dB at 500 Hz and 38 dB at 4000 Hz. [Adapted from Butler and Naunton (1964).]

that of the loudspeaker signal than when it is above it. Exactly why these data are so often discussed in terms of interference effects rather than in terms of the interaction of the earphone signal in one ear with the loudspeaker signal in the other is not clear. So far as we have been able to determine, many of the results would be essentially the same if the attenuation of the loudspeaker signal provided by the earphone were infinite.

Results on masking and lateralization that have been obtained in connection with studies of signal detection in backgrounds of noise are considered in Section IV.

(iv). MULTIPLE CLICKS. In the previous discussion of fusion and lateralization of clicks, the click stimuli have always consisted either of merely one click to each ear or a periodic train of such stimuli. We now mention briefly some of the phenomena, including the precedence effect, that arise when other stimulus configurations are employed.

In a variety of studies, fusion and lateralization have been examined for stimuli composed of one click to one ear and two to the other or of periodic trains of such stimuli (e.g., Guttman, 1965; Guttman, van Bergeijk, & David, 1960; Harris *et al.*, 1963; Sayers & Toole, 1964; Toole & Sayers, 1965a). In the study by Guttman *et al.* (1960), the binaural interactions were used to deduce information on monaural temporal masking. The single click was visualized as a probe, and the listeners were required to center the images they encountered by adjusting the overall delay between this probe and the doublet. When the clicks comprising the doublet were far apart, a distinct centered image could be obtained by aligning the probe with either member of the doublet (the other member leading to a background sound in the ear with the doublet). When the clicks comprising the doublet were close together, however, only one distinct centered image could be obtained. The critical monaural time interval at which the transition between one and two images occurs, as well as the values of interaural delay required for centering, were measured as a function of the levels of the clicks and the repetition rate at which the whole binaural stimulus was presented. According to these experiments, the critical monaural interval decreases with an increase in repetition rate, and changes from roughly 6 msec at 8 pps to roughly 3 msec at 125 pps. The study by Harris et al. (1963) was motivated by a comparison of the values obtained for this critical monaural interval and the value of 1 msec associated with the distance between the peaks of multimodal distributions of centering values that had occasionally been observed when only one click was presented to each ear ("multiple-image lateralizations"). Some results of this study are shown in Fig. 28. This figure shows histograms of the interaural delays (between the single click A and the first click B of the doublet) chosen by subjects to center the images that they encountered as they swept through the delay variable. Figure 28a gives the results for the case in which all three pulses are rarefaction pulses and Fig. 28b for the case in which the polarity of the second pulse C in the doublet is reversed. Each horizontal block gives the results for a different delay between the two pulses B and C in the doublet. The histograms combine the data from four subjects

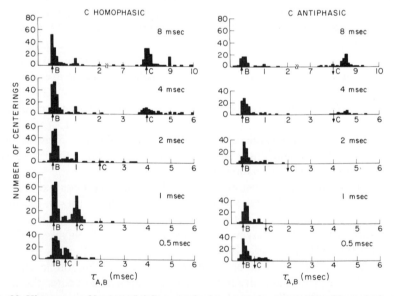

FIG. 28. Histograms of interaural delays required to center images produced by a single click (A) to one ear and a double click (B followed by C) to the other ear. Clicks A and B were always rarefaction pulses, whereas click C was either a rarefaction pulse (C homophasic) or a condensation pulse (C antiphasic). The abscissa gives the interaural delay $\tau_{A,B}$ between clicks A and B and the ordinate gives the number of centering responses. Different horizontal blocks correspond to different delays between clicks B and C. The level of all three clicks was 40 dB above the binaural threshold for single clicks, and the histograms combine data from four subjects and three repetition rates (2, 10, and 50 pps). [Adapted from Harris et al. (1963).]

and three repetition rates (2, 10, and 50 pps). Among the features to be noted in the histograms for the case in which C is homophasic are the disappearance of the peak corresponding to a temporal match between A and C as the delay between B and C is decreased from 8 to 2 msec (corresponding to the loss of separable distinct fusions for B and C), and the existence in certain cases of secondary peaks 1 msec behind the main peaks (corresponding to multiple-image lateralizations). The fact that the secondary peaks, presumed to be associated with cochlear function, occur only after the main peaks and not before them is due to the asymmetry between the stimuli to the two ears; if only one click is presented to each ear, secondary peaks occur both before and after. When B and C are separated by 1 msec, the secondary peak that would be associated with the AB interaction and the primary peak that would correspond to the AC interaction if B and C were resolved coincide. According to the authors, at this separation only one image is actually heard, despite the fact that the histogram is bimodal (and that bimodal histograms were obtained for each subject individually). The bimodal aspects of the histogram for .5 msec were due primarily to the results of one subject. When click C is antiphasic, the peak corresponding to the AC interaction occurs when A is roughly .6 msec behind C (corresponding to the notion of a dominant frequency region in the vicinity of 800 Hz), and the secondary peaks tend to disappear. In attempting to explain the results of this experiment, the authors make use of a model of basilar membrane motion, a neural refractory period, and the notion of a neural gate located peripherally to the place of binaural interaction (the latter two elements being introduced to interpret the results for separations of 1 and 2 msec). Further results on fusion and lateralization phenomena that arise with three-click stimuli are available in Guttman (1965), Sayers and Toole (1964), and Toole and Sayers (1965a).

Studies of fusion and lateralization phenomena involving four-click stimuli have often been conducted in connection with an exploration of the effects of reverberations and of the precedence effect. These effects not only have important implications for auditory theory, but they are of great practical significance in the design of concert halls and multichannel sound-reproduction systems.

In the analytic portion of the classical study of the precedence effect by Wallach, Newman, and Rosenzweig (1949), the listener was stimulated with two successive pairs of equal-level 1-msec clicks in which the interaural delay τ_A for the first pair (A_L, A_R) differed from the interaural delay τ_B for the second pair (B_L, B_R), the delay between the first click to the left ear (A_L) and the second click to the right ear (B_R) was 2 msec (so that the two pairs of clicks produced a single fused image), and the listeners were required to judge the lateralization of the image. Data showing the pairs of values (τ_A, τ_B) that produced a centered image for τ_B in the interval $|\tau_B| \leq .6$ msec are shown in Fig. 29a. Clearly, the delay τ_A of the first pair dominates the lateralization (the precedence effect). In the interval $|\tau_B| \leq .4$ msec, the

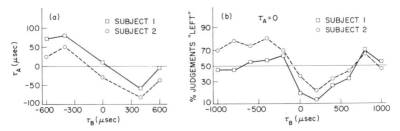

FIG. 29. Data on the precedence effect. The stimulus consisted of two dichotic clicks [(A$_L$, A$_R$) followed by (B$_L$, B$_R$)]. All clicks were 1 msec in duration and presented at the same level, and the delay between the first click in the left ear (A$_L$) and the second click in the right ear (B$_R$) was 2 msec. (a) Shows the value of the interaural delay τ_A of the first dichotic click required to center the total image of the two dichotic clicks as a function of the interaural delay τ_B of the second dichotic click. (b) Shows the percentage of judgments "to the left" as a function of τ_B for the case $\tau_A = 0$. [Adapted from Wallach, Newman, and Rosenzweig (1949), *American Journal of Psychology*. Copyright 1949 by the University of Illinois Press. Used by permission of the University of Illinois Press.]

trading ratio (the slope of the line) is roughly 1/6. Note also that smaller values of $|\tau_A|$ are required to compensate for $|\tau_B|$ when $|\tau_B| = .6$ msec than when $|\tau_B| = .4$ msec, and that at $|\tau_B| = .6$ msec the trading ratio is only approximately 1/16. In an experiment designed to explore further this reversal at .4 msec (in which the 2 msec spacing between A$_L$ and B$_R$ was maintained), τ_A was set equal to zero and the range of τ_B was extended to 1 msec. The percentage of responses indicating that the resultant image appeared on the left is shown in Fig. 29b. Apparently, by the time $|\tau_B|$ reached 1 msec, the image returned almost completely to the center. In a further experiment, it was shown that as the interaural delay between A$_L$ and B$_R$ is increased from 2 to 10 msec, the image splits into two parts, and each part can be lateralized independently.

In general, the effects of reverberations (or their simulation) on the spatial attributes of sound are exceedingly complex and depend upon a wide variety of parameters, including the type of signal that is employed, the number of echoes, the amplitude and time structure of the echoes, and the spectral composition of the echoes. For example, the trade between τ_A and τ_B shown in Fig. 29 depends strongly on the separation between A$_L$ and B$_R$; if this separation is substantially reduced, the trade is significantly altered and the precedence effect no longer occurs. Similarly, the maximum value of this separation for which the precedence effect can be demonstrated is substantially increased if the pulses are replaced by complex long-duration sounds such as music or speech. A summary of the historical background of the precedence effect can be found in Gardner (1968a) and an up-to-date summary of the experimental work on this effect, as well as a variety of other effects related to the perception of sounds in reverberant environments, can be found in Blauert (1974).

B. Loudness and Pitch

Two of the most obvious and most studied subjective attributes of the binaural image, beyond the spatial ones, are loudness and pitch. As in the rest of this chapter, our comments on these two topics are restricted to phenomena that involve binaural interaction.

1. BINAURAL LOUDNESS SUMMATION

In general, the loudness of a binaural stimulus is greater than that of either of the monaural components, i.e., there is binaural summation of loudness. Studies of this phenomena have employed a variety of techniques, but the one that is most direct and has been employed most widely, is that of loudness matching. In this technique, the loudness of the binaural sound is matched to the loudness of a monaural component by adjusting the intensity of one of the two sounds being matched, and the results are presented in terms of the intensities required for equal loudness. The amount of binaural summation varies between 0 and 12 dB, depending upon the types of signals, the levels of the signals, and the interaural differences in the signals. Data illustrating the dependence of binaural loudness summation on the overall level of the stimulation for the case of a diotic stimulus and various types of waveforms are shown in Fig. 30 (Reynolds & Stevens, 1960). Whereas at low levels the monaural signal has to be increased by only about 3 dB to match the loudness of the diotic signal, at high levels the required increase is approximately 12 dB. Moreover, according to this study, the results are roughly independent of the signal characteristics (e.g., of frequency and bandwidth), and roughly consistent with results obtained by a comparison of binaural and monaural loudness functions determined by loudness scaling techniques such as magnitude estimation. According to later studies (Scharf, 1968, 1969), however, the dependence of binaural summation on level depends on the signal bandwidth: For broad-band stimuli, binaural loudness

FIG. 30. Dependence of binaural loudness summation on level for a diotic stimulus. Data points show the level of the diotic stimulus required to match its loudness to that of the equivalent monotic stimulus as a function of the level of the monotic stimulus. The diagonal line represents the results that would be obtained if there were no binaural summation. The circles and squares represent data for noise stimuli obtained by Reynolds and Stevens. The other symbols represent data for tone stimuli at a variety of frequencies obtained from previous experiments by other investigators and summarized by Reynolds and Stevens. [Adapted from Reynolds and Stevens (1960).]

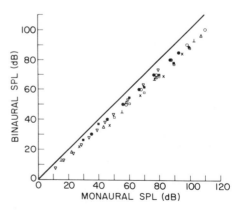

summation increases with level; for narrow-band stimuli, it first increases and then decreases slightly. Data illustrating this bandwidth effect are shown in Fig. 31 (Scharf, 1968).

Data illustrating how the intensities in the two ears can be traded in order to maintain a constant loudness are shown in Figs. 32 and 33 (Irwin, 1965; Keen, 1972). If one takes the diotic stimulus as a reference to specify the equal loudness contour, and raises the intensity a small amount in one ear, the decrease required in the other ear to maintain the same loudness will be symmetric in decibels. When the intensity increase is substantial, however, the situation becomes asymmetric and the required decrease becomes greater than the increase. For sufficiently large increases (i.e., greater than the amount of binaural summation obtained for the diotic reference stimulus), there is no decrease that will maintain equal loudness; even if the signal to the other ear is turned off, the loudness will exceed that of the diotic reference. An interesting theoretical analysis of Irwin's data is included in the study by Treisman and Irwin (1967). Further results on binaural loudness summation involving unequal intensities at the two ears (as well as the application of simultaneous conjoint measurement theory) can be found in Levelt, Riemersma, and Bunt (1972).

Studies have also been conducted on the effects of interaural time or phase and the effects of interaural frequency differences on loudness. For tone stimuli, loudness is roughly independent of interaural phase provided the tone stimulus is sufficiently far above its threshold (Hirsh & Pollack, 1948; Townsend & Goldstein, 1972). Near threshold, however, an antiphasic tone appears slightly louder than a homophasic tone [a fact that can be deduced from the difference in thresholds for these two configurations (Diercks & Jeffress, 1962)]. Also, if the tone is presented in a background of interaurally identical noise and is near its masked threshold, the effect of the interaural phase of the tone on its loudness can be substantial (Hirsh & Pollack, 1948; Townsend & Goldstein, 1972). This effect is closely tied to the dependence of the masked threshold itself on phase, a dependence that is considered in

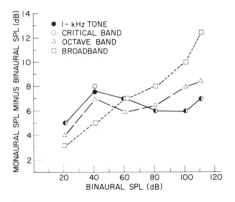

FIG. 31. Influence of signal bandwidth on the dependence of binaural loudness summation on level. Data show the amount by which the SPL of the monaural stimulus must exceed the SPL of the binaural stimulus in order to produce equal loudness. The stimuli were a 1-kHz tone and noise signals of various bandwidths centered on 1 kHz. [Adapted from Scharf (1968).]

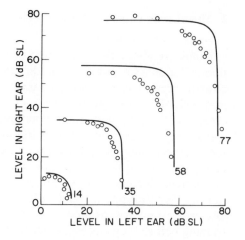

FIG. 32. Contours of constant loudness for different overall levels. The numbers associated with the contours give the sensation level in decibels of the equally loud monaural stimulus. The solid curves are contours of constant total power. The signal was broadband random noise. [Adapted from Irwin (1965), *American Journal of Psychology*. Copyright 1965 by the University of Illinois Press. Used by permission of the University of Illinois Press.]

detail in Section IV. For click stimuli, it has been shown that loudness effects can occur at delays greater than those producing fusion or lateralization effects (e.g., Babkoff & Sutton, 1963; Békésy, 1960; Guttman, 1962a). In the study by Babkoff and Sutton (1963), results were obtained on the relation of loudness judgments to temporal-order judgments (Hirsh & Sherrick, 1961) as a function of the interaural time delay of equally intense clicks in the region $2 \leq \tau \leq 40$ msec. Apparently, the loudness of the click in one ear relative to the loudness of the click in the other ear, which depends on the delay, constitutes an important perceptual cue for determining which ear received the first click. The effect of interaural frequency differences on binaural loudness summation for tones has been examined by Porsolt and Irwin (1967) and Scharf (1969). According to these studies, binaural loudness summation (unlike monaural loudness summation of different-frequency tones) is independent of the frequency separation Δf between the tones.

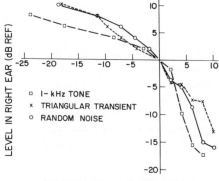

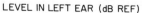

FIG. 33. Contour of constant loudness for different types of signals. The loudness level in all cases was 70 phons. [Adapted from Keen (1972).]

2. Binaural Creation of Pitch

Under the assumption that the monaural components of a binaural stimulus are above their detection thresholds, the effect of binaural interaction on loudness is merely to modify the magnitude of a perceptual attribute already present in the two monaural components. For the attribute *pitch,* however, it is possible to construct stimuli in which a pitch sensation is created entirely by binaural interaction, in the sense that the pitch sensation cannot be perceived in either of the monaural components, independent of the listener's monaural sensitivity. Depending upon the specific stimulus configuration and specific author, the names that have been used for such phenomena include, "binaural creation of pitch," "binaural subjective tones," "central pitch," and "dichotic repetition pitch." Although binaurally created pitch sensations are often very weak and require considerable training before they can be detected reliably, they provide further important constraints for theories of binaural interaction.

One of the first-discovered and most easily perceived pitches of this type arises when a listener is presented with a binaural stimulus in which the signal to one ear consists of white Gaussian noise and the signal to the other ear consists of the same noise except for a narrow-band phase shift at relatively low frequencies. Under these conditions, the listener hears a weak signal in addition to the noise (Cramer & Huggins, 1958; Guttman, 1962b; Licklider, 1959). Moreover, this signal sounds like a narrow-band noise whose pitch corresponds to the region of phase shift. Since phase-shifted white Gaussian noise is still white Gaussian noise, there is no possibility of hearing this signal monaurally. The ability to perceive this pitch, or to detect changes in pitch caused by translating the region of phase shift, decreases with increasing frequency and with decreasing noise level. Also, it decreases as the bandwidth of the phase shift becomes either very small or very large. Data illustrating the decrease in the detectability of the pitch with increasing bandwidth and increasing frequency are shown in Fig. 34 (Cramer & Huggins, 1958).

A relatively weak sensation of pitch can also be elicited with noise sources using full-band interaural time delays τ in the region $.5 \le \tau \le 15$ msec (Bilsen & Goldstein, 1974; Fourcin, 1962a,b, 1970). According to Fourcin, the creation of such a sensation depends on the existence of at least two noise sources, each having a different delay. According to the more recent work of Bilsen and Goldstein (1974), however, the sensation can be elicited with merely one source and one delay (although it may be somewhat weaker). In both sets of studies, it was found that the pitch image is completely distinct from the lateralized noise images, and that it is impossible to hear the pitch if one focuses attention on the noise images. Also, at least in the case of a single source, the pitch image appears to be lateralized in the median plane (independent of the delay τ) and requires considerable training to detect. The

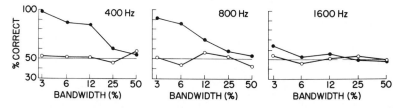

Fig. 34. Ability to detect a change in the binaural subjective pitch associated with a narrow-band interaural phase shift in broad-band noise as a function of the center frequency and bandwidth of the phase-shift frequency band. For each center frequency and bandwidth, the interaural phase increased from 0° to 360° with increasing frequency and was 180° at the center frequency. The bandwidth numbers on the abscissa specify the percent increase in frequency required to change the interaural phase from 180° to 270° and provide a measure of the half-bandwidth. The subject's task was to discriminate a 10% shift in the center frequency of the phase-shift frequency band. The filled circles present the results of the discrimination task when the interaural phase shift was included, and the open circles present the results of a control experiment in which the phase shift was omitted. Chance performance corresponds to 50% correct. [Adapted from Cramer and Huggins (1958).]

value of the pitch has generally been measured by the use of matching procedures, and the parameters that have been studied include, aside from the number of sources and the associated delays τ, the bandwidth and interaural phase shifts of the sources. For the case in which there are two sources, one with a fixed delay of zero ($\tau_1 = 0$) and one with a variable delay τ_2, the elicited pitch corresponds to the pitch of a tone of frequency f according to the relation $f = 3/4\tau_2$ when both sources have 0° or 180° phase shifts and $f = 1/\tau_2$ when one source has 0° phase shift and the other has 180° phase shift (Fourcin, 1970). Moreover, the pitch appears to be determined by the relative delay $\tau_1 - \tau_2$ rather than the absolute delay. Thus, for example, if $\tau_1 = 3$ msec rather than $\tau_1 = 0$, and Source 1 has a 180° phase shift while Source 2 is in-phase, then the pitch is given by $f = 1/(\tau_1 - \tau_2)$. For the case in which there is only one noise source with an interaural delay τ_b, and in which the matching stimulus is the sum of the two noise signals presented monaurally with a delay τ_m (which according to Bilsen and Ritsma, 1969, elicits a pitch sensation of value $1/\tau_m$), pitch matches have been made over the region $3 \le \tau_b \le 12$ msec (Bilsen & Goldstein, 1974). Data showing the results of these matches for an in-phase low-passed (2000-Hz cutoff) noise signal at 25 dB SL are shown in Fig. 35a. Clearly, the pitch value of the binaural case is essentially identical to that for the monaural case (i.e., the pitch of the binaural stimulus is $1/\tau_b = 1/\tau_m$). Data showing the results obtained with the same monaural matching stimulus when the phase is inverted for the binaural presentation are shown in Fig. 35b. For this case, two pitches can be perceived, one a little higher and one a little lower than $1/\tau_b$. Further results of this study (using multiple noise sources, as well as narrow-band sources) suggest that the pitch phenomena obtained with one

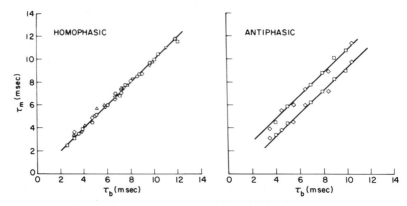

FIG. 35. Results of pitch-matching experiments for time-delayed noise. The noise was low pass (2000-Hz cutoff) and low level (25 dB SL). The monaural stimulus consisted of this noise added to itself after a delay τ_m. The binaural stimulus consisted of this noise with an interaural delay τ_b (homophasic) or with both an interaural delay τ_b and an interaural phase shift of 180° (antiphasic). In both cases, the subjects' task was to adjust τ_m to match the pitch of the monaural stimulus to the pitch of the binaural stimulus. The different symbols in the graphs refer to different subjects. [Adapted from Bilsen and Goldstein (1974).]

source are essentially the same as those obtained with more than one source and that the dominant frequency region in creating the pitch sensation is centered about approximately 600 Hz (which is roughly the same region as that in which optimum binaural beats are obtained).

Another study of binaurally created pitch (Houtsma & Goldstein, 1972), which was conducted prior to the study of Bilsen and Goldstein (1974) and helped to motivate that study, as well as the recent theoretical work on central pitch by Goldstein (1973), involves the use of harmonic tone complexes and the classical phenomenon of the "missing fundamental" (i.e., the ability to perceive the fundamental of an harmonic tone complex even when there is no energy in the stimulus at the fundamental). In this study, it was shown that if signals are composed of two low-intensity randomly chosen successive harmonics n and $n + 1$ (with n randomly chosen from three successive integers $\bar{n} - 1$, $\bar{n}$, and $\bar{n} + 1$) and the listener is required to identify the melody conveyed by a sequence of such signals (and defined by the corresponding sequence of fundamental frequencies), the identification performance is essentially the same (and, in most cases, well above chance) if the two harmonics comprising each signal are presented to the same ear or one harmonic is presented to one ear and the other harmonic to the other ear. All melodies had identical time structure and began with the same note, and performance was studied as a function of the middle of the lower harmonic number range $\bar{n}$ and the fundamental frequency f_0 of the first note. Data illustrating the equivalence at low intensities for the case in which the listener was required to identify on each trial which of eight known two-note

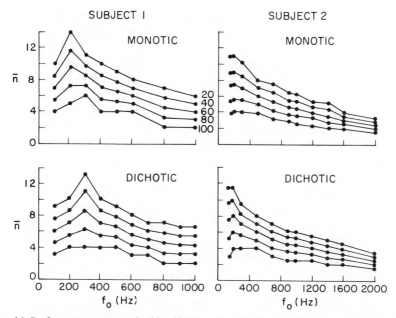

FIG. 36. Performance contours for identification of musical intervals constructed from stimuli devoid of energy at the fundamental frequency. Stimuli were composed of randomly chosen successive harmonics n and $n + 1$ with n chosen randomly from three successive integers $\bar{n} - 1$, $\bar{n}$, and $\bar{n} + 1$. f_0 denotes the fundamental frequency of the first note. In the monotic presentation, both harmonics were presented to a single ear. In the dichotic presentation, one harmonic was presented to each ear. The numbers associated with the contours specify the performance levels in percent-correct (change performance corresponds to $12\frac{1}{2}\%$ correct). All stimuli were presented at 20 dB SL. [Adapted from Houtsma and Goldstein (1973).]

melodies (i.e., musical intervals) was presented are shown in Fig. 36. At higher intensities, it was found that the monotic presentation led to superior performance. However, additional experiments indicated that this divergence was caused primarily by monaural combination-tone phenomena. In general, these results demonstrate that the ability to extract the fundamental from harmonic tone complexes that have no energy at the fundamental is based on central processing and does not require interaction of the harmonics at the periphery.

IV. SENSITIVITY

As in any area of perception or psychophysics, one of the main tasks in the study of binaural hearing consists of determining the system's sensitivity to differences among stimuli. Such a determination provides a measure of the extent to which differences in the external world are mirrored by differences in the perceptual world, and the extent to which different physical stimuli are transformed into a single common sensation by the sensing and perceiving mechanisms. These sensations (which, except for the random elements in human responses, can be defined as equivalence classes of physical stimuli) constitute the basic stuff out of which the organism constructs its perceptual space.

Moreover, since the essential difference between binaural and monaural hearing concerns the perception of interaural differences, and the sensitivity of the binaural system when the signals to the two ears are identical (diotic stimulation) is, at best, only marginally improved over that obtained with the monaural system, the principal focus of research on binaural sensitivity has been the study of sensitivity to changes in interaural differences (or in other parameters of the stimulus as a function of these differences).

In this section, sensitivity is usually discussed in terms of detection "thresholds" and "just-noticeable differences" (jnds) in stimuli. It should be understood, however, that this practice is employed merely for simplicity, that the thresholds and jnds are merely points on psychometric functions for which the subject's performance reached some reasonable criterion (such as 75% correct or a sensitivity index d' of unity), and that, ideally, it is necessary to consider these functions in their entirety. Also, the discussion is dominated by concern with stimuli involving tone pulses (as opposed, for example, to clicks or speech). This choice is based on our belief that an understanding of sensitivity for such stimuli is a prerequisite to further work in this area and on the fact that most previous quantitative research has been devoted to such stimuli (and that many theoretical models of binaural interaction have been strongly influenced by this research).

The material on sensitivity is divided into five subsections: (a) spatial resolution, (b) interaural jnds, (c) binaural unmasking and masking-level differences (MLDs), and (d) related phenomena. The last subsection includes comments on central masking, monaural detection with a contralateral cue (MDCC), binaural discrimination with interaural differences, and the relation between lateralization and MLDs. Results obtained in connection with coherent masking studies (i.e., masking studies in which the target and masker are derived from the same source and are coherently related) are considered in every subsection but the first.

A. Spatial Resolution

Much of the work on the sensitivity of the binaural system has been an outgrowth of questions concerning spatial resolution, such as "How well can one detect a change in the location of a sound source?" or "How well can one detect the presence of a target signal originating at one location in the presence of a noise signal originating at another location?" Furthermore, since the spatial dimension along which variations generally produce the

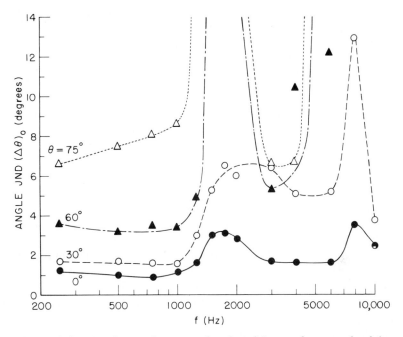

FIG. 37. Angle jnd $(\Delta\theta)_0$ for tone bursts as a function of the tone frequency f and the angle θ between the sound source and the median plane (Mills, 1958, 1972). In those regions of θ and f for which the curves exceed the maximum ordinate value of 14° (e.g., $\theta \geq 60°$ and $1500 \leq f \leq 2000$ Hz), the jnd was found to be indeterminably large. [Adapted from Mills (1958).]

greatest change in interaural differences is azimuth (as opposed to elevation or distance), the principal focus of spatial-resolution studies concerned with binaural sensitivity has been azimuth.

Results of two experiments (conducted in anechoic chambers with the listener's head constrained to prevent movements) that illustrate the binaural system's resolution in azimuth are shown in Figs. 37 and 38. The results in

FIG. 38. Dependence of detection threshold of a 500-Hz tone produced by one loudspeaker in the presence of broad-band masking noise produced by another loudspeaker as a function of the angle between the two loudspeakers. The ordinate specifies the decrease in the tone threshold below the threshold obtained when the two speakers are collinear. The angle between the target and masker was varied by changing the angle of the masker and the data represent the average of the results obtained with the target straight ahead and with the target 90° to the side. [Adapted from Moter (1964).]

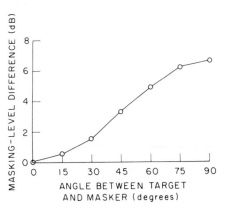

Fig. 37 (Mills, 1958, 1972) show that the jnd in azimuth, often referred to as the "minimum audible angle" in azimuth, can be as small as 1°, that it increases as the source moves away from the median plane, and that in certain regions it depends strongly on the frequency of the signal. The results in Fig. 38 (Moter, 1964) illustrate the fact that one's ability to detect signals in backgrounds of noise depends strongly on the angular separation between the signal and noise. As will become evident in Section IV,C, where we consider detection of signals in noise using earphone stimulation, the crucial element in the "unmasking" of the signal as the angular separation is increased is the increase in the difference between the interaural differences for the signal and the interaural differences for the noise.

Further results on spatial resolution can be found in Kock (1950); Sandel, Teas, Feddersen, and Jeffress (1955); Coleman (1962, 1963, 1968); Pollack and Rose (1967); Ebata, Sone, and Nimura (1968b); Perrott (1969); Perrott and Elfner (1968); Roffler and Butler (1968a,b); Gardner (1968b, 1969a); Harris and Sergeant (1970); Harris (1972); Mills (1972); Molino (1973); Banks and Green (1973); and Blauert (1969, 1971, 1974). These results not only include data for various types of signals, but also data on elevation and distance as well as azimuth, on the effects of head or source movement, and on the differences between binaural and monaural listening. As indicated in Section III, the failure in most experiments concerned with monaural localization (or localization in the median plane) to take adequate account of the role played by a priori information on the spectrum of the target signal makes the results of these experiments difficult to interpret.

B. Interaural jnds

Sensitivity to changes in interaural differences depends upon the specific parameters changed, upon the region of interaural differences in which sensitivity is examined, and upon the level and type of signal employed. Our discussion of this topic is divided into three subsections: *(1)* pure interaural time and interaural amplitude jnds; *(2)* jnds involving increments in both interaural time and interaural amplitude (combination jnds); and *(3)* further jnd results. Included in the last subsection is a consideration of the jnd in interaural correlation.

1. PURE INTERAURAL TIME AND INTERAURAL AMPLITUDE jnds

Results for tone pulses on the interaural time jnd $(\Delta\tau)_0$ [or, equivalently, interaural phase jnd $(\Delta\phi)_0$] and the interaural amplitude jnd $(\Delta\alpha)_0$ are shown in Figs. 39, 40, and 41 (based on data from Klumpp & Eady, 1956; Zwislocki & Feldman, 1956; Mills, 1960; Hershkowitz & Durlach, 1969a; and Domnitz, 1973). Figure 39 shows results for the jnds $(\Delta\tau)_0$ and $(\Delta\alpha)_0$ as a function of the frequency of the tone pulse in the region of the interaural-time-interaural-amplitude plane $[\tau,\alpha(dB)]$ about the origin (where the binaural image is rela-

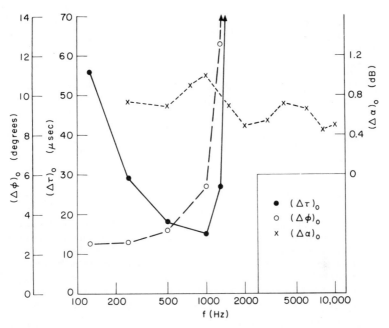

FIG. 39. Interaural time jnd $(\Delta\tau)_0$ and interaural amplitude jnd $(\Delta\alpha)_0$ for tone bursts as a function of the tone frequency f. [The data on $(\Delta\tau)_0$ are from Durlach's (1972) summary of the data of Klumpp and Eady (1956) and Zwislocki and Feldman (1956), and the data on $(\Delta\alpha)_0$ are from Mills (1960).] These data are for the interaural reference conditions $\tau = 0$ and $\alpha = 1$ and for tone bursts of roughly 1-sec duration and 50 dB SL. The interaural phase jnd $(\Delta\phi)_0$ corresponding to $(\Delta\tau)_0$ is also plotted. Discrimination of interaural time, or, equivalently, interaural phase, was found to be impossible above roughly 1400 Hz.

tively compact and located on the midline). Figure 40 shows results for both $(\Delta\tau)_0$ and $(\Delta\alpha)_0$ for a 500-Hz tone pulse in regions along the axes of the $[\tau,\alpha(\mathrm{dB})]$ plane (as well as for the dependence of the two jnds on the overall level A at the origin of the plane). Figure 41 shows results for $(\Delta\tau)_0$ for a 500-Hz tone pulse in regions off the axes of the $[\tau,\alpha(\mathrm{dB})]$ plane.

These results illustrate a number of important facts about sensitivity to interaural amplitude and interaural time. First, sensitivity to interaural amplitude is roughly the same as monaural amplitude sensitivity. Second, the interaural time jnd $(\Delta\tau)_0$ can be as small as a few microseconds, and is substantially smaller than any result on time resolution that has been obtained monaurally. Third, $(\Delta\tau)_0$ has a minimum at roughly 1000 Hz and becomes unbounded above approximately 1500 Hz. Fourth, for a given $\alpha \neq 1$, $(\Delta\tau)_0$ tends to be smaller when τ and α are collateral than when they are antilateral, and the minimum value of $(\Delta\tau)_0$ (minimized over τ) is roughly equal to the value of $(\Delta\tau)_0$ when $\tau = 0$ and $\alpha = 1$.

These results can also be examined with respect to their relations to the subjective phenomena of lateralization and time–intensity trading. For

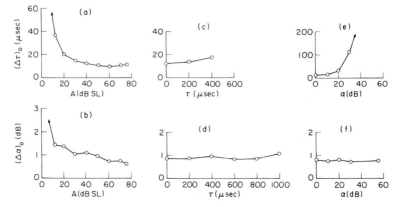

FIG. 40. Interaural time jnd $(\Delta\tau)_0$ and interaural amplitude jnd $(\Delta\alpha)_0$ for a 500-Hz tone burst as a function of the level A, the interaural time delay τ, and the interaural amplitude ratio α. The tone burst had a duration of 300 msec and a rise–fall time of 50 msec. In graphs (a) and (b), $\tau = 0$ and $\alpha = 1$; in (c) and (d), $\alpha = 1$ and $A = 50$ dB SL; in (e) and (f), the tone in the left ear always had a level of 50 dB SL and the different values of $\alpha = A_L/A_R$ were obtained by lowering the level in the right ear. The increment $\Delta\alpha$ was always constructed by lowering the level in one ear and raising it in the other by the same amount (in decibels). [Adapted from Hershkowitz and Durlach (1969a).]

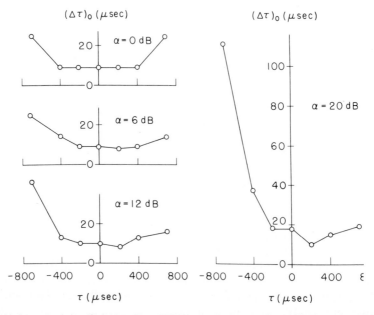

FIG. 41. Interaural time jnd $(\Delta\tau)_0$ for a 500-Hz tone burst as a function of τ and α. The burst duration and rise–fall time were the same as in Fig. 40. $\tau > 0$ and $\alpha > 1$ correspond to collateral configurations, and $\tau < 0$ and $\alpha > 1$ to antilateral configurations. The signal to the right ear always had a level of 55 dB SPL, and nonunity values of α were achieved by attenuating the signal to the left ear. [Adapted from Domnitz (1973).]

example, the fact that the ratio $(\Delta\tau)_0/(\Delta\alpha)_0$ in the vicinity of the origin of the $[\tau,\alpha(\mathrm{dB})]$ plane (roughly 10–20 μsec dB^{-1} for levels greater than 10 dB SL according to Fig. 40) is approximately the same as the time–intensity trading ratio obtained in corresponding lateralization matching experiments is consistent with the hypothesis that the effects of interaural time and interaural amplitude can be described primarily in terms of a common unidimensional lateralization sensation and that the perceptual cue used in these jnd experiments is derived primarily from this sensation. On the other hand, the fact cited in item four above (illustrated in Fig. 41) that $(\Delta\tau)_0$ is smaller when τ and α are collateral (and the image is lateralized off to the side) than when they are antilateral (and the image is lateralized near the midline), combined with the fact (again illustrated in Fig. 41) that $(\Delta\tau)_0$ tends to increase with τ when $\alpha = 1$, implies that this hypothesis cannot be valid in general.

Results illustrating the idea that sensitivity to azimuth can at least be roughly explained in terms of sensitivity to these interaural parameters are shown in Fig. 42 (Mills, 1960, 1972). According to these results, the sensitivity to azimuth about the median plane can be explained by sensitivity to interaural time (or phase) for frequencies below approximately 1500 Hz, and by sensitivity to interaural amplitude between roughly 1500 Hz and 6000 Hz. (It is uncertain whether the result that sensitivity to azimuth above 6000 Hz is less than would be predicted on the basis of sensitivity to interaural amplitude is due to faulty measurements or to some other factor.) Although an equivalent comparison for azimuths off the median plane has not been carried out in detail, the results obtained by comparing the data in Fig. 37 with those in Fig. 40 indicate an equivalent consistency at points off the median plane for the frequency 500 Hz (Hershkowitz & Durlach, 1969a). The idea that localization of tones is determined primarily by interaural time at low frequencies and by interaural amplitude at high frequencies is, of

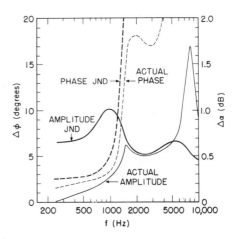

FIG. 42. Comparison of interaural phase jnd $(\Delta\phi)_0$ and interaural amplitude jnd $(\Delta\alpha)_0$ for $\tau = 0$ and $\alpha = 1$ with the changes $\Delta\phi$ and $\Delta\alpha$ that occur when an actual source is moved a jnd $(\Delta\theta)_0$ in angle from the median plane. The curves for the phase and amplitude jnds represent the data shown in Fig. 39. The fact that the two phase curves coincide below roughly 1500 Hz (but not above 1500 Hz) and that the two amplitude curves coincide between 1500 and 6000 Hz (but not outside this region) indicates that the localization of tone pulses is determined by sensitivity to interaural phase below 1500 Hz and by sensitivity to interaural amplitude in the region 1500–6000 Hz. The results above 6000 Hz are not well understood. [Adapted from Mills (1960, 1972).]

course, supported by a wide variety of other data. Aside from all the data on lateralization obtained in experiments using earphone stimulation that are consistent with this idea, there is a substantial amount of supporting data obtained from experiments conducted with loudspeakers in anechoic chambers (e.g., Sandel et al., 1955). It should also be noted that the use of time at low frequencies and amplitude at high frequencies is exactly what one would predict from a consideration of natural interaural differences: At low frequencies, natural interaural amplitude differences are small; at high frequencies, natural interaural time delays involve a multiplicity of phase ambiguities.

In considering the fact that the binaural system is totally insensitive to interaural time for high-frequency tones, one should not conclude that it is insensitive to interaural time for all high-frequency signals. As mentioned in Section III, some degree of sensitivity to interaural time has been demonstrated for high-frequency noise, high-frequency clicks, and amplitude-modulated high-frequency tones (e.g., Békésy, 1960; Cronin, 1973; David et al., 1958; Harris, 1960; Henning, 1974a,b; Klumpp & Eady, 1956; Leakey et al., 1958; Licklider & Webster, 1950; Yost et al., 1971). According to Klumpp and Eady, the value of $(\Delta\tau)_0$ for bandpass noise with frequencies in the region 3050–3340 Hz is roughly 60 μsec. According to Yost, Wightman, and Green, the sensitivity to high-pass clicks falls off sharply as the cutoff frequency is raised above 1500 Hz, but some sensitivity remains for cutoff frequencies as great as 5000 Hz [for a 5000-Hz cutoff, $(\Delta\tau)_0$ is reported to be a few hundred microseconds]. According to Henning, the value of $(\Delta\tau)_0$ for a sinusoidally amplitude-modulated high-frequency tone can be as small as the value of $(\Delta\tau)_0$ for a pure low-frequency tone at the modulation frequency [e.g., the value of $(\Delta\tau)_0$ for a 3900-Hz carrier modulated by a 300-Hz sine wave was found to be approximately the same as the value of $(\Delta\tau)_0$ for a 300-Hz tone]. In many of these experiments, (e.g., Cronin, 1973; Henning, 1974a,b; Licklider & Webster, 1950; Yost et al., 1971), masking noise was used to mask some of the low-frequency distortion products, and the results (particularly those of Henning) strongly suggest that timing information carried solely by auditory-nerve fibers with high characteristic frequencies can be used to discriminate interaural time delay in high-frequency signals.

Results on the effect of signal duration on $(\Delta\tau)_0$ for $\tau = 0$ and $\alpha = 1$ and a signal consisting of pulsed noise are shown in Fig. 43 (Tobias & Zerlin, 1959). According to these results, $(\Delta\tau)_0$ decreases by roughly 2 μsec for every doubling of duration until the duration reaches approximately 500 msec, whereupon it levels off in the region 6–8 μsec. We know of no reliable data indicating that stimuli can be constructed for which the interaural time jnd is significantly less than 6 μsec. Results on the effect of duration on $(\Delta\tau)_0$, as well as on $(\Delta\alpha)_0$, for a signal consisting of narrow-band (50–Hz wide) noise centered at 500 Hz, can be found in McFadden and Sharpley (1972). Further results for tones on the value of $(\Delta\tau)_0$ as a function of τ for $\alpha = 1$ and for a

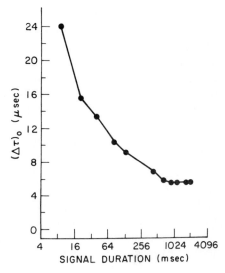

FIG. 43. Interaural time jnd $(\Delta\tau)_0$ for pulsed noise as a function of the pulse duration. The noise was low passed at 5000 Hz, had a level of 65 dB SPL at the longer durations, and was adjusted to maintain constant loudness at the shorter durations. The interaural amplitude ratio α was unity and the reference interaural delay τ was zero. [Adapted from Tobias and Zerlin (1959).]

variety of frequencies in the region 250–2000 Hz have been reported by Yost (1974).

Additional results on interaural amplitude jnds are available in Chocholle (1957), Sorkin (1966), Elfner and Perrott (1967), Rowland and Tobias (1967), and Babkoff and Sutton (1969). In most of these studies (unlike the ones discussed previously) the amplitude increment to be detected was inserted in only one ear so that the perceptual cue used for discrimination was likely to have an appreciable loudness component as well as a lateralization component. In the studies cited previously, the increment was always constructed by lowering the level in one ear and raising it in the other by the same amount (in decibels). This procedure eliminates the loudness cue for values of α near unity but not for other values of α. So far no experiment on interaural amplitude sensitivity has yet been reported in which the loudness cue was effectively eliminated for all α.

In a study motivated by the observation that the insertion of an interaural delay into a diotic stimulus necessarily results in momentary interaural amplitude differences, Elfner and Tomsic (1968) explored the effect of the rise time of tone pulses on interaural time sensitivity and examined the hypothesis that this sensitivity is determined primarily by the momentary amplitude differences associated with the delay rather than by the delay itself.

A summary of the values of the interaural time and amplitude jnds that can be estimated from binaural detection experiments in which the target and masker are coherently related is available in Robinson, Langford, and Yost (1974).

2. Combination jnds

In the preceding discussion of sensitivity to changes in interaural differences, we considered the listener's ability to discriminate between two stimuli that differed either by an interaural time increment or an interaural amplitude increment, but not by both simultaneously. Results on the ability to discriminate simultaneous changes in these parameters are available in studies concerned with the tradability of interaural time and interaural intensity (Babkoff, Sutton, & Barris, 1973; Gilliom & Sorkin, 1972; Hafter & Carrier, 1972; Hershkowitz & Durlach, 1969b) or with the detection of a target signal in the presence of a masking signal that is coherently related to the target signal (Hafter & Carrier, 1970; Jeffress & McFadden, 1971; McFadden et al., 1971, 1972a; McFadden & Sharpley, 1972; Rilling & Jeffress, 1965; Robinson et al., 1974; Wightman, 1969, 1971; Yost, 1972). The central question with regard to the first concern has been to determine the extent to which the tradability evident in the results of conventional time–intensity trading experiments is complete in the sense that listeners are not only capable of matching the lateralizations produced by different combinations of interaural time and interaural intensity, but are incapable of discriminating between such combinations. Studies of detection with coherent maskers have occurred primarily as an outgrowth of interest in the general area of binaural unmasking (see Section IV,C) and in the relation of binaural unmasking to lateralization.

Illustrative data on the ability to discriminate between stimuli that differ in both interaural time τ and interaural amplitude α are shown in Figs. 44 through 47. Figure 44 (Hafter & Carrier, 1972) shows data for a 500-Hz tone

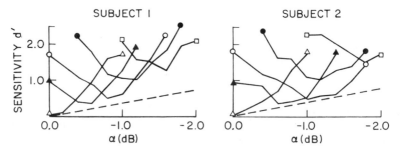

FIG. 44. Sensitivity to the difference between a diotic tone burst and a tone burst that contains both a small interaural time difference τ and a small interaural amplitude difference α as a function of both τ and α. The ordinate gives the sensitivity index d' of decision theory, and $d' = 0$ corresponds to chance performance. The different curves correspond to different values of τ ($\triangle$: $\tau = 0$; $\blacktriangle$: $\tau = 10$ μsec; $\bigcirc$: $\tau = 20$ μsec; $\bullet$: $\tau = 30$ μsec; $\square$: $\tau = 40$ μsec). $\tau > 0$ and $\alpha < 1$ corresponds to the antilateral condition. The signal was a 500-Hz 125-msec tone burst at 70 dB SL, and nonunity α's were achieved by raising the level in one ear and lowering it in the other by equal amounts. The dashed lines represent the observed monaural amplitude discrimination performance. [Adapted from Hafter and Carrier (1972).]

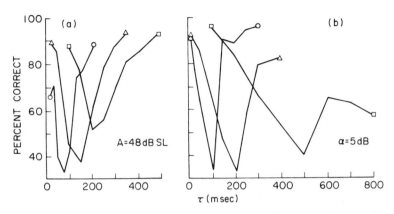

FIG. 45. Sensitivity to the difference between an interaural delay τ ($\alpha = 1$) and an interaural amplitude difference α ($\tau = 0$) for a broad-band click stimulus as a function of τ, α, and the level A. Chance performance corresponds to 33% correct. (a) shows results for fixed A and various α (○: $\alpha = 4$ dB; △: $\alpha = 6$ dB; □: $\alpha = 9$ dB) and (b) shows results for fixed α and various A (○: $A = 54$ dB SL; △: $A = 39$ dB SL; □: $A = 24$ dB SL). $\tau > 0$ and $\alpha > 1$ corresponds to the collateral condition. In each case, the summed sensation level of the α-stimulus was matched to the summed sensation level of the τ-stimulus. [Adapted from Babkoff et al. (1973).]

burst on the ability to discriminate between a diotic stimulus and a stimulus that contains both a small interaural delay τ and a small interaural amplitude difference α, where τ and α are antilateral. Figure 45 (Babkoff et al., 1973) shows data for a broad-band click on the ability to discriminate between a stimulus that contains a delay τ (with $\alpha = 1$) and a stimulus that contains an amplitude difference α (with $\tau = 0$), where τ and α are collateral. In both figures, the extent to which τ and α are completely tradable is measured by the extent to which the performance values at the minima of the curves correspond to pure chance. Also, to the extent that the primary perceptual cue in these discrimination tasks is lateralization, the abscissa values of the minima can be used to estimate the time–intensity trading ratio for lateraliza-tion. As one would expect, the extent to which τ and α are completely tradable decreases (i.e., the performance at the minimum increases) as τ or α increases. For large τ or α, these variables are clearly not completely trad-able and there must exist perceptual cues other than a simple, unitary, lateralization difference. Note also that the results in Fig. 45 indicate greater tradability than those in Fig. 44. Whether this difference is due to the differ-ence between colateral and antilateral conditions (e.g., the greater tendency for multiple images to appear in the antilateral condition), the difference in the basic stimulus, or to other factors in the experiments, is uncertain. Roughly speaking, the values of the time–intensity trading ratio derived from these data are consistent with those derived from lateralization matching experiments. An analysis of the antilateral tone data in terms of multiple images is contained in Hafter and Carrier (1972).

Figure 46 shows combinations of τ and α that correspond to constant detection performance in experiments on coherent masking (Hafter & Carrier, 1970; Jeffress & McFadden, 1971; McFadden *et al.*, 1971, 1972a). In these experiments, the same basic signal plays the role of both target and masker so that one can control the phase ψ of the target relative to the masker as well as the interaural phases of the target and masker. The data shown in Fig. 46 are derived from experiments in which the masker was diotic and the target had an interaural phase shift of 180°. By varying the phase ψ, the interaural differences in the total signal (target plus masker) can be made to consist of pure amplitude differences ($\psi = 0$), pure time differences ($\psi = 90°$), or a combination of time and amplitude differences. Furthermore, since the threshold target-to-masker ratios in these experiments are usually sufficiently small to prevent overall loudness from becoming a significant cue, one can regard the detection task as a task of discriminating between a diotic stimulus and a stimulus containing interaural time and/or amplitude differences. In Fig. 46, each connected set of data points corresponds to a fixed level of detection performance and the values of τ and α are computed from the target-to-masker ratio that produced this performance and the value of ψ that was used in the stimulus presentation. If time and intensity were completely tradable according to a linear trading relation ($\tau = k \log \alpha$), each contour of constant detection performance would be

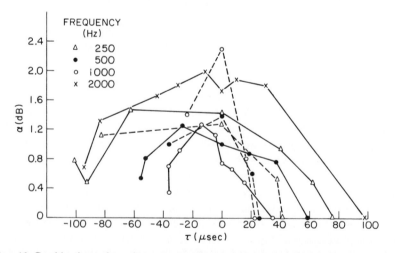

FIG. 46. Combinations of τ and α corresponding to constant detection performance in coherent masking experiments. Dashed curves are for tone signals (Hafter & Carrier, 1970) and solid curves are for narrow-band noise signals (Jeffress & McFadden, 1971; McFadden *et al.*, 1971, 1972a). The stimuli had levels in the region 65–80 dB SPL and durations in the region 100–200 msec. The bandwidth of the narrow-band noise signals was roughly 50 Hz. $\tau > 0$ corresponds to collateral and $\tau < 0$ to antilateral. The points have been joined by straight lines merely for clarity; the resulting curves do not necessarily provide a good approximation to the contours that would be obtained if the data points were much more dense (see text).

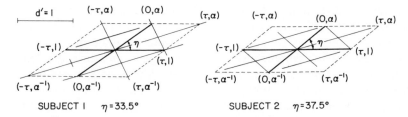

FIG. 47. Geometric representation of τ,α discrimination space. For each subject, the values of τ and α were constant, and the representation summarizes the results of eight discrimination experiments: $(-\tau, 1)$ vs $(\tau, 1)$, (O, α) vs (O, α^{-1}), (τ, α) vs $(-\tau, \alpha^{-1})$, $(-\tau, \alpha)$ vs (τ, α^{-1}), $(-\tau, 1)$ vs (O, α), (O, α) vs $(\tau, 1)$, $(\tau, 1)$ vs (O, α^{-1}), and (O, α^{-1}) vs $(-\tau, 1)$. The lengths of the lines (dark solid or light solid) give the measured sensitivity indices derived from these experiments. The angle η between the lines that represent sensitivity to pure time delay and pure amplitude difference (the dark solid lines) was chosen to give a best fit to the remaining data (the light solid lines). The goodness of the fit is measured by the extent to which the light solid lines terminate on the outside parallelogram (dashed lines). The extent to which time and intensity are completely tradable is measured by the angle η: $\eta = 0°$ corresponds to complete tradability and $\eta = 90°$ to complete independence. The signal was a 500-Hz tone burst with a duration of 800 msec, a rise-fall time of 20 msec, and a level of 60 dB SPL. The value of α was always 1 dB and τ was roughly 15 μsec. [Adapted from Gilliom and Sorkin (1972).]

composed of two parallel lines (corresponding to lateralization shifts to the right and to the left of the centered image produced by the masker alone) with equal negative slopes (corresponding to the time–intensity trading ratio) and with intercepts on the abscissa positioned symmetrically about $\tau = 0$. If τ and α were completely independent, each contour would be perfectly symmetric about the $\tau = 0$ line. Although in most of the curves shown in Fig. 46 the points are not sufficiently dense to permit one to regard these curves as good approximations to the actual contours, it is clear that these data (particularly some of those for the antilateral condition $\tau < 0$) are not consistent with the notion of complete linear tradability. (A similar but slightly generalized argument shows that these data are inconsistent with the notion of complete tradability even if the trading relation is not constrained to be linear.) According to the studies of Jeffress, McFadden, and their associates, which included measurements of lateralization as well as detection, it is possible in certain cases to discriminate between a diotic stimulus and a stimulus containing both time and amplitude differences without being able to judge reliably whether the latter image is to the left or right of the former. One possible interpretation of this phenomenon is based on the idea that the latter stimulus leads to multiple images. It should also be noted that the values of τ at $\alpha = 1$ and the values of α at $\tau = 0$ in Fig. 46 provide additional data on the pure interaural time and amplitude jnds. The reason for the relatively large values of these jnds in these experiments (particularly those for $f = 500$ and 1000 Hz) is not clear.

Figure 47 (Gilliom & Sorkin, 1972) shows data for a 500-Hz tone burst on the ability to discriminate between different combinations of τ and α for small fixed values of τ and α. The lengths of the lines in these diagrams show the values of the sensitivity index d' that were obtained in discriminating between the various combinations, and the angle η measures the degree of correlation between the sensation associated with the delay τ and the sensation associated with the amplitude difference α. The condition $\eta = 0°$ corresponds to complete tradability and the condition $\eta = 90°$ to complete independence. The range of η obtained over the four subjects tested was $11.5°$–$37.5°$ and the average was $28.3°$ (corresponding to a correlation of roughly .88). According to this experiment, a large proportion of the total sensation associated with interaural time is combined (adds to or subtracts from) with the total sensation associated with interaural amplitude; however, there is a significant residual component for which this is not the case. Moreover, this residual component can be detected even when the deviations of τ from 0 and of α from 1 are very small and in the vicinity of the pure time and amplitude jnds.

In general, the results discussed in this section tend to support the idea that time and intensity are not completely tradable even for relatively small values of τ and α. It should be noted, however, that an underestimation of tradability can result from the existence of spurious loudness cues or from random variations during the course of the testing in the coupling of the earphones to the head (Hershkowitz & Durlach, 1969b). Unlike experiments on the pure time and amplitude jnds, a subject can significantly improve his performance in many of these experimental paradigms by adjusting his earphones when the discrimination task becomes difficult. To date, no experiments have been conducted on these combination jnds in which the acoustical signals actually delivered to the ears are monitored.

3. FURTHER jnd RESULTS

Results of the jnd $(\Delta\rho)_0$ in the interaural correlation ρ of noise signals have been obtained by Pollack and Trittipoe (1959a,b). In these experiments, ρ was controlled by using three statistically identical and statistically independent noise sources (one to both ears, one to the left ear, and one to the right ear) and adjusting the level of the common source relative to the level of the two independent sources. Unlike the experiments on pure time and amplitude jnds, in which the primary subjective cue is the lateralization of the image, in these experiments the subjective cue is the fusion or compactness of the image. Sensitivity to changes in ρ was explored as a function of ρ, noiseburst duration, noise level, spectral content of the noise, and interaural amplitude difference α of the noise. Data showing the dependence of $(\Delta\rho)_0$ on ρ for a long-duration, high-level broad-band noise burst with equal amplitudes in the two ears, are shown in Fig. 48. At $\rho = 1$, the jnd is roughly .04. Results for the dependence of $(\Delta\rho)_0$ on the other parameters indicate that $(\Delta\rho)_0$ increases with decreasing duration (particularly between 100 and

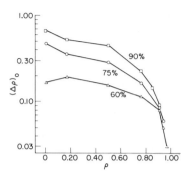

FIG. 48. Interaural correlation jnd $(\Delta\rho)_0$ as a function of the interaural correlation ρ. The stimulus consisted of a noise burst with a duration of 1 sec, a level of 90 dB SPL, a frequency range of 100–7000 Hz, and equal amplitudes in the two ears. The different curves correspond to different criteria for defining the jnd (60, 75, and 90% correct, where change performance corresponds to 50% correct). [Adapted from Pollack and Trittipoe (1959a).]

30 msec); is relatively independent of level at intermediate levels, but increases at either low or high levels (particularly when ρ is close to unity); increases as the bandwidth is narrowed (by low-passing or high-passing the noise) in a manner that depends on ρ; and increases as the interaural amplitude ratio α deviates from unity over a wide range. It was also shown that sensitivity to changes in ρ is roughly the same for negative ρ as for positive ρ (where negative values of ρ were achieved by inverting the phase of the common source at one ear). In view of these results on $(\Delta\rho)_0$, one would expect that the task of discriminating between $\rho = 1$ and $\rho = -1$ for broad-band noise signals would be trivial. There exist data, however, which indicate that this expectation may not be correct (Pollack and Trittipoe, 1959a; McFadden, 1967). Results on sensitivity to interaural correlation for pulse trains are available in Pollack (1971).

Results on the accuracy with which subjects can center the image of a noise signal by adjusting interaural delay τ for various values of ρ (where again ρ was controlled by the use of three independent sources) are available in Jeffress *et al.* (1962a). According to these results, the standard deviation of the τ-adjustments doubles by a factor of roughly 2 as ρ decreases from 1 to .2, and then increases rapidly to the value corresponding to chance performance as ρ decreases from .2 to 0. Although the absolute values of the results obtained in this experiment are substantially larger than those that would be obtained in precise jnd experiments (e.g., the standard deviation at $\rho = 1$ was roughly 50 μsec), the form of the dependence on ρ is probably similar. Although no experiment has been conducted to determine the maximum value of τ for which one can distinguish between pure time-delayed noise (i.e., $\rho = 1$ at $\tau = 0$) and statistically independent noise, as pointed out in Section III, there are a variety of experiments which suggest that this value is in the region $10 \le \tau \le 30$ msec.

Results on the interaural time jnd $(\Delta\tau)_0$ at $\tau = 0$ and $\alpha = 1$ for a bandpassed noise signal having a center frequency at 500 Hz and a bandwidth of one octave, in the presence of a statistically independent and statistically identical masking noise with an interaural delay of 400 μsec (so that the image of the masking noise is off to the side), are shown in Fig. 49 (Houtgast & Plomp, 1968). This figure illustrates the effects on $(\Delta\tau)_0$ of both signal-to-masker ratio and signal duration. (The data plotted at $S/M = \infty$ are consistent with those of Tobias and Zerlin plotted in Fig. 43). Houtgast and Plomp attempt to relate these results to both the precedence effect and binaural detection phenomena.

Finally, it should be noted that although we are not aware of any comprehensive study of sensitivity to interaural frequency differences, certain features of this sensitivity are obvious. In particular, since an interaural frequency difference for tone pulses can be regarded as a time-varying interaural time delay (or phase shift), the ability to discriminate between a stimulus with a small frequency difference and one with no frequency difference will be closely tied to the ability to discriminate interaural delay. At low frequencies (i.e., below 1500 Hz), it should be possible to detect an arbitrarily small frequency difference (even if the interaural phase is zero at the beginning of the pulse), provided the duration of the pulse is sufficiently long. Note also that under such conditions the listener can detect the existence of an interaural frequency difference without being able to specify which ear is receiving the higher frequency. For signals in which the coding of frequency does not include temporal information, such as high-frequency tones, interaural sensitivity to frequency differences should be roughly the same as monaural sensitivity to these differences (provided, of course, that in the monaural case the frequencies are presented sequentially to avoid monaural beats).

C. Binaural Unmasking and MLDs

The ability to detect a target signal in a background of masking signal, like the ability to localize sound sources, is substantially improved by the use of two ears. Moreover, the experimental results on this ability have played an

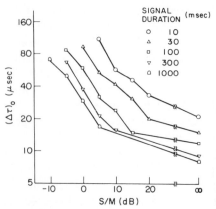

FIG. 49. Interaural time jnd $(\Delta\tau)_0$ as a function of signal-to-masker ratio and signal duration. The signal and masker were statistically independent and statistically identical noise signals with a center frequency of 500 Hz and a bandwidth of one octave. For the signal, $\tau = 0$ and $\alpha = 1$; for the masker, $\tau = 400 \mu\text{sec}$ and $\alpha = 1$. The level of the signal was held at a constant SPL that corresponded to 50 dB SL at the longer durations. The masker was presented continuously. [Adapted from Houtgast and Plomp (1968).]

exceptionally important role in the development of theoretical models of binaural interaction. In general, this ability depends upon the characteristics of the target and masker and upon the interaural differences in the target and masker. This ability has been studied for tones masked by tones, noise masked by noise, speech masked by speech, tones masked by noise, narrow-band noise masked by broad-band noise, clicks masked by noise, and speech masked by noise; and as a function of the levels, frequency contents (center frequency and bandwidth), and temporal aspects (time of occurrence and duration) of the target and masker, as well as of the correlation between the target and masker. Included among the interaural parameters that have been studied are time, phase, amplitude, and correlation. Under optimum conditions, the amount of "binaural unmasking," i.e., the improvement in the detection threshold for binaural listening as compared with monaural listening, will exceed 25 dB.

Our discussion of this topic is divided into two subsections: (1) tones in broad-band noise and (2) other configurations. In the first subsection, we consider the effects of variations in the interaural parameters of the tone and noise and in the tone frequency and noise level. The second subsection contains comments on the effects of varying the frequency content of the noise, on coherent masking, on temporal aspects of binaural unmasking, and on binaural unmasking for other types of signals and maskers.

1. TONES IN BROAD-BAND NOISE

Some insight into the characteristics of binaural unmasking can be gained by considering the detection of a 500-Hz tone pulse in continuous broad-band noise at a noise spectrum level of approximately 50 dB SPL per cycle in the following sequence of experiments. First, determine the tone threshold level for the tone and noise presented monaurally to the same ear [denoted $T(M|M)$]. Second, add exactly the same noise to the second ear so that there are no interaural differences in the noise, but the tone is still presented monaurally, and determine the threshold level for this case [denoted $T(M|0)$]. A comparison of $T(M|M)$ and $T(M|0)$ will show that the ratio $T(M|M)/T(M|0)$ (referred to as a masking level difference or MLD) is approximately 6 dB. In other words, adding the noise to the second ear makes the tone presented to the first ear easier to hear and lowers its threshold by roughly 6 dB. Third, add exactly the same tone to the second ear so that there are no interaural differences in either the tone or the noise and measure the threshold level for this case [denoted $T(0|0)$]. A comparison of this threshold with the first will show that $T(M|M) \approx T(0|0)$. In other words, adding the tone to the noise in the second ear and making the total signals in the two ears identical makes the tone harder to hear and raises its threshold back to the level for the purely monaural case. Fourth, keep the tone and noise in both ears, but reverse the polarity of the tone in one ear (equivalent to a phase shift of magnitude π) and measure the threshold level for this case [denoted $T(\pi|0)$]. The results of this experiment will show that $T(\text{M}|\text{M})/$ $T(\pi|0) \approx T(0|0)/T(\pi|0) \approx 12$ dB. In other words, the antiphasic presentation $(\pi|0)$ makes the tone more detectable than the monaural $(\text{M}|\text{M})$ or homophasic $(0|0)$ presentation by roughly 12 dB. (If one inserts a slight frequency difference Δf into the tone signal so that the interaural phase of the tone varies slowly as a function of time, the detectability of the tone will vary periodically with a period equal to $1/\Delta f$—another version of the binaural beat phenomenon.) Fifth, and finally, reverse also the polarity of the noise in one ear and measure the threshold level for this case [denoted $T(\pi|\pi)$]. The results of this last experiment will show that $T(\pi|\pi) \approx T(0|0) \approx T(\text{M}|\text{M})$. In other words, reversing the polarity of both the tone and the noise (so that the interaural differences for the noise are identical to those for the tone) again raises the threshold back to the level for the monaural case. The fact that the three thresholds $T(\text{M}|\text{M})$, $T(0|0)$, and $T(\pi|\pi)$ are all approximately the same is a general one and holds for all types of signals and maskers, provided only that the level of the masker is not too close to absolute threshold. Similarly, the fact that the antiphasic presentation $(\pi|0)$ provides the greatest amount of binaural unmasking is a general one. The precise amount of unmasking depends, of course, on the characteristics of the signal and masker. Note also that the threshold level for the ideal receiver in the cases $(\text{M}|0)$ and $(\pi|0)$ is zero (i.e., the ideal receiver need merely subtract the total signal in one ear from that in the other in order to completely eliminate the noise). Finally, it should be noted that since most data indicate that the form of the psychometric function is independent of the values of the interaural parameters (e.g., Egan, 1965; Egan, Lindner, & McFadden, 1969; Green, 1966), the values of the various MLDs are independent of the level of performance that is chosen to define the threshold.

A variety of data on MLDs for tones in broad-band noise is shown in Figs. 50–62. Unless stated otherwise, these data satisfy the following three constraints: The tonal signal has a relatively long duration (duration ≥ 100 msec); the masking noise has a relatively large bandwidth (power spectrum flat across the critical band centered on the tone); the masking noise has a relatively high level (spectrum level between 45 and 60 dB SPL per cycle). In most cases, the MLD is referenced to the case $(0|0)$ or $(\text{M}|\text{M})$. [Since $T(0|0) \approx T(\text{M}|\text{M}) \approx T(\pi|\pi)$ except when the level of the masking noise is near threshold, at moderate and high levels the MLD is independent of which of these three conditions is selected for the reference. A summary of data on the equivalence of these three thresholds is available in Durlach (1972).] We have chosen the configurations $(0|0)$ or $(\text{M}|\text{M})$ as references because almost all experiments contain a measurement of $T(0|0)$ or $T(\text{M}|\text{M})$ and because the MLDs then provide a direct measurement of the amount of binaural unmasking. It should be noted, however, that the dependence of the data on various stimulus parameters (such as tone frequency, noise level, and noise bandwidth), as well as on the experimental procedure and individual listener, is simplified if a nontrivial binaural configuration (i.e., one which evidences binaural unmasking) such as $(\pi\,|\,0)$ is used as the reference. In other words, a substantial portion of the variation in MLDs that is observed when $(0\,|\,0)$ or $(M\,|\,M)$ is used as the reference arises from variations in the threshold for $(0\,|\,0)$ or $(M\,|\,M)$, not from variations in the threshold for the configuration with which $(0\,|\,0)$ or $(M\,|\,M)$ is compared. This point will be considered further below (see Fig. 65).

In citing the various sources from which we have obtained data, the following code will be used: BJT (Blodgett, Jeffress, & Taylor, 1958), BJW (Blodgett, Jeffress, & Whitworth, 1962), CD (Colburn & Durlach, 1965), D (Durlach, 1963), DJ (Diercks & Jeffress, 1962), DO (Dolan, 1968), DR (Dolan & Robinson, 1967), E (Egan, 1965), G (Green, 1966), H (Hirsh, 1948), HB (Hirsh & Burgeat, 1958), HW (Hirsh & Webster, 1949), JBD (Jeffress, Blodgett, & Deatherage, 1952, 1962b), JBSW (Jeffress, Blodgett, Sandel, & Wood, 1956), LJ (Langford & Jeffress, 1964), M (McFadden, 1968), RD (Robinson & Dolan, 1972), RIJ (Rilling & Jeffress, 1965), RJ (Robinson & Jeffress, 1963), RLD (Rabiner, Laurence, & Durlach, 1966), S (Schenkel, 1964), SG (Sondhi & Guttman, 1966), W (Webster, 1951), WM (Weston & Miller, 1965), WW (Wilbanks & Whitmore, 1968). Except for the data obtained after 1966, the summaries of the data that we present are essentially the same as those presented in Durlach (1972).

Figures 50–53 show the dependence of binaural unmasking on the frequency f of the tone and on the interaural phase shift ϕ_s and interaural amplitude ratio α_s of the tone for the case in which the masking noise is identical in the two ears. Figure 50 shows the dependence of the MLD $T(0\,|\,0)/T(\pi\,|\,0)$ on frequency. According to these results, this MLD is roughly

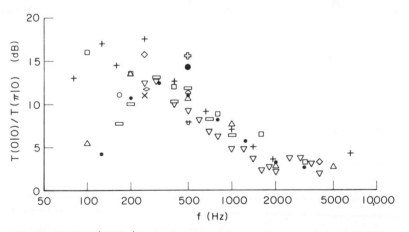

FIG. 50. The MLD $T(0\,|\,0)/T(\pi\,|\,0)$ as a function of the tone frequency f ($\triangle$: H; $\bigtriangledown$: HB; +: w; ×: HW; $\bigcirc$: JBD; ϕ: JBSW; $\diamondsuit$: G; $\uplus$: SG; •: S; $\square$: D; $\bigcirc$: CD; $\square$: RLD; ●: JBD, RJ, BJT, LJ, RIJ, E).

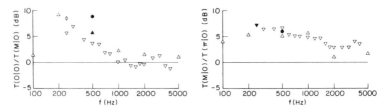

FIG. 51. The MLDs $T(0|0)/T(M|0)$ and $T(M|0)/T(\pi|0)$ as functions of the tone frequency f ($\triangle$: H; $\triangledown$: HB; $\blacktriangle$: H, CD, WM; $\diamond$: G; $\blacktriangledown$: HB, G; $\bullet$: BJT, BJW, E, CD).

3 dB at frequencies above the critical frequency 1500 Hz, increases to roughly 15 dB as the frequency is lowered to a few hundred hertz, and then tends to remain constant as the frequency is lowered still further. The increased scatter at the very low frequencies is due to an increased dependence of the MLD on the precise noise level at these moderately high noise levels and low frequencies and also, perhaps, to an increased dependence of the MLD on the amount of training at these low frequencies. The dependence of MLDs on noise level is considered further below. Note also that the existence of a positive MLD at frequencies above 1500 Hz does not contradict the fact that the binaural system is insensitive to the interaural phase of tones at these frequencies. The task of the listener in these experiments is to distinguish between noise-alone and tone-plus-noise, and the presentation of the antiphasic tone introduces fluctuations in the instantaneous interaural amplitude ratio of the stimulus that are absent when a homophasic noise alone is presented (Durlach, 1964). Figure 51 shows data on the MLDs $T(0|0)/T(M|0)$ and $T(M|0)/T(\pi|0)$ as functions of f. According to these results, the amount of binaural unmasking for $(M|0)$ is roughly 6 dB less than for $(\pi|0)$ below 1500 Hz and 3 dB less (i.e., zero) above 1500 Hz. Figure 52

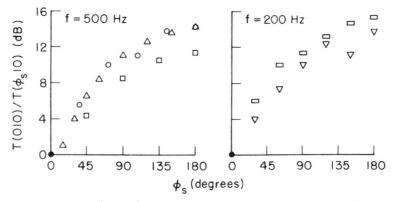

FIG. 52. The MLD $T(0|0)/T(\phi_s|0)$ as a function of the interaural phase ϕ_s of the tone ($\bigcirc$: JBD; $\triangle$: RIJ; $\square$: CD; $\triangledown$: H; $\square$: D).

shows the dependence of the MLD $T(0|0)/T(\phi_s|0)$ on the interaural phase ϕ_s of the tone. These results serve to interpolate between the thresholds $T(0|0)$ and $T(\pi|0)$. Results for the case in which the tone signal contains a frequency difference Δf rather than a phase shift ϕ_s (Robinson, 1971) suggest that the threshold for this case always lies between the thresholds $T(\pi|0)$ and $T(M|0)$ for the best of the two frequencies and converges to $T(M|0)$ for the best frequency as Δf becomes large. Figure 53 shows the dependence of the MLD $T(0|0)/T(\alpha_s, \phi_s|0)$ on the interaural phase shift ϕ_s and amplitude ratio α_s in the tone. The symmetry relation $T(\alpha_s, \phi_s|0) = T(1/\alpha_s, \phi_s|0)$ evident in the data of Colburn and Durlach (which was substantiated by additional experiments), combined with the assumption of bilateral symmetry, implies that the threshold $T(\alpha_s, \phi_s|0)$ is independent of the signs of both ϕ_s and log α_s [i.e., that $T(\alpha_s, \phi_s|0) = T(\alpha_s, -\phi_s|0) = T(1/\alpha_s, \phi_s|0) = T(1/\alpha_s, -\phi_s|0)$]. Further data on this MLD (similar to those plotted from Egan's experiment) are available in McFadden (1969) and Schenkel (1967b).

Figures 54–58 show the effects of introducing interaural phase shifts or time delays in the masking noise. Figure 54 shows the dependence of the MLDs $T(0|\pi)/T(\pi|0)$ and $T(M|\pi)/T(M|0)$ on the tone frequency f. According to these results, these two MLDs are roughly the same at all frequencies. Whereas at the higher frequencies $T(0|\pi) \approx T(\pi|0)$ and $T(M|\pi) \approx T(M|0)$, as

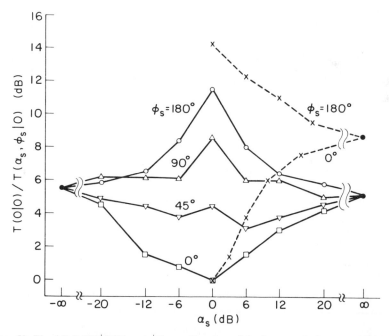

FIG. 53. The MLD $T(0|0)/T(\alpha_s, \phi_s|0)$ as a function of the interaural phase ϕ_s and interaural amplitude ratio α_s of a 500-Hz tone ($\bigcirc$, $\triangle$, ∇, $\square$: CD; $\times$, $+$: E). When $\alpha_s \neq 1$, the threshold signal-to-noise ratio is defined by the larger of the two monaural ratios.

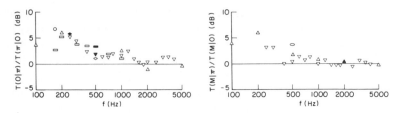

Fig. 54. The MLDs $T(0|\pi)/T(\pi|0)$ and $T(M|0)$ as functions of the tone frequency f ($\triangle$: H; $\triangledown$: HB; $\bigcirc$: JBD; $\bigcirc$: E; $\square$: RLD; $\diamondsuit$: SG; $\blacktriangle$: H, HB; $\blacktriangledown$: H, HB, JBD, RJ; $\blacklozenge$:SG, HW; $\blacksquare$: RLD, BJT).

the frequency is decreased below 500 Hz the configurations involving phase shifts in the noise lead to significantly larger thresholds (i.e., less binaural unmasking) than their noise-in-phase counterparts. Results on the MLDs $T(0|0)/T(0|\pi)$ and $T(0|0)/T(M|\pi)$ can be obtained by comparing Fig. 54 with Figs. 50 and 51. Figure 55 shows the dependence of $T(0|0)/T(\phi_s|\phi_n)$ on simultaneous phase shifts ϕ_s in the signal and ϕ_n in the noise. To a rough approximation, these results suggest that $T(\phi_s|\phi_n)$ depends only on the difference $\phi_s - \phi_n$ rather than on the individual values of ϕ_s and ϕ_n. This simplification is approximately valid for $f \geq 500$ Hz, but, as indicated by the data on $T(0|\pi)/T(\pi|0)$ in Fig. 54, is invalid for lower frequencies. The MLD $T(0|0)/T(\pi|\pi)$, however, is roughly 0 dB at all frequencies (Durlach, 1972). Figure 56 illustrates the dependence of $T(0|0)/T(0|\phi_n)$ on ϕ_n for $f < 500$ Hz and serves to interpolate between $T(0|0)$ and $T(0|\pi)$. Also included in this figure is a curve representing the dependence of $T(0|0)/T(\phi_s|0)$ on ϕ_s. A comparison of the data with this curve shows that the functions $T(0|0)/$

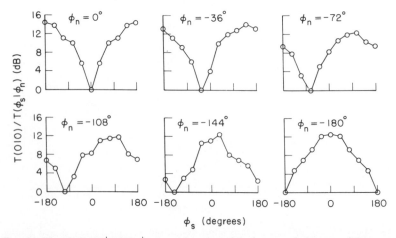

Fig. 55. The MLD $T(0|0)/T(\phi_s|\phi_n)$ as a function of the interaural phase ϕ_s of the tone and the interaural phase ϕ_n of the noise for a 500-Hz tone. [Adapted from Jeffress et al., (1952).]

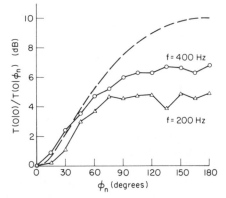

FIG. 56. The MLD $T(0|0)/T(0|\phi_n)$ as a function of the interaural phase ϕ_n of the noise for tone frequencies below 500 Hz. The values of $T(0|0)/T(\pi|0)$ obtained in the same experiment were 10 dB (200 Hz) and 10.2 dB (400 Hz). The dashed curve represents the dependence of $T(0|0)/T(\phi_s|0)$ on ϕ_s when $T(0|0)/T(\pi|0) \approx$ 10 dB. [Adapted from Rabiner et al. (1966).]

$T(0|\phi_n)$ and $T(0|0)/T(\phi_s|0)$ have different shapes at low frequencies. Specifically, the former function has a much flatter top than the latter. It is precisely this flattening that leads to the discrepancy between $T(0|\pi)$ and $T(\pi|0)$ at low frequencies. Figure 57 shows the dependence of $T(0|0)/T(0|\tau_n)$ and $T(0|0)/T(\pi|\tau_n)$ on the interaural time delay τ_n of the noise. The damped oscillatory behavior of these dependencies is a consequence of the critical-band filtering performed by the auditory system: The periodicity of the func-

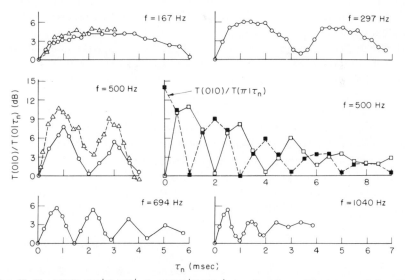

FIG. 57. The MLDs $T(0|0)/T(0|\tau_n)$ and $T(0|0)/T(\pi|\tau_n)$ as functions of the interaural time delay τ_n of the noise and the frequency f of the tone ($\bigcirc$: RLD; $\triangle$: JBD; $\square$, $\blacksquare$: LJ). Open symbols give data for $T(0|\tau_n)$ and filled symbols for $T(\pi|\tau_n)$. The values of $T(0|0)/T(\pi|0)$ obtained in the same experiments were : 6.7 dB (167 Hz, RLD), 10.9 dB (297 Hz, RLD), 11.3 dB (500 Hz, RLD), 7.8 dB (694 Hz, RLD), 5 dB (RLD, 1040 Hz), 11 dB (167 Hz, JBD), and 14.3 dB (500 Hz, JBD). The corresponding value for the LJ data at 500 Hz is given by the filled square at $\tau_n = 0$.

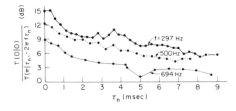

FIG. 58. The MLD $T(0|0)/T(\pi|\tau_n, -2\pi f\tau_n)$ as a function of the interaural delay τ_n of the noise and the tone frequency f. [Adapted from Rabiner *et al.* (1966).]

tions corresponds to the center frequency of the filtered noise and the damping to the bandwidth of the filtered noise. For very long delays τ_n, these oscillations are completely damped out and the MLDs asymptote to their values for statistically independent noise (discussed below). Note also that the shapes of the individual cycles are not independent of tone frequency, but, as with the dependence on ϕ_n, exhibit flatter tops at the lower frequencies. If the noise is both time-delayed by an amount τ_n and phase-shifted by an amount $-2\pi f\tau_n$ (so that the interaural differences in the noise are zero at the frequency of the tone), then the oscillatory behavior will be eliminated and the MLDs will exhibit only the damping behavior. Results on this MLD, denoted $T(0|0)/T(\pi|\tau_n, -2\pi f\tau_n)$, are shown in Fig. 58.

Figures 59 and 60 illustrate the effects of decorrelating the noise signals presented to the two ears by the use of statistically independent noise sources. Figure 59 shows that the MLDs $T(0|0)/T(0|U)$ and $T(0|0)/T(\pi|U)$ (where U denotes statistically independent noise) as a function of the tone frequency f. These MLDs [which are equivalent to the MLDs $T(0|0)/T(0|\tau_n)$ and $T(0|0)/T(\pi|\tau_n)$ as τ_n approaches ∞] are both approximately 4 dB for $f < 1500$ Hz; however, the data suggest that the MLD $T(0|0)/T(0|U)$ decreases at higher frequencies. [No data are available for $T(0|0)/T(\pi|U)$ at the higher frequencies.] Figure 60 shows the MLDs $T(0|0)/T(0|\rho_n)$, $T(0|0)/T(\pi|\rho_n)$, and $T(M|M)/T(M|\rho_n)$ as functions of the interaural correlation ρ_n of the noise for a 500-Hz tone (where ρ_n is controlled by the use of statistically independent noise sources). Data on the dependence of $T(M|M)/T(M|\rho_n)$ on ρ_n for frequencies ranging from 150 to 4000 Hz are available in Wilbanks and Whitmore (1968). Roughly speaking, the form of the dependence on ρ_n is independent of frequency: All the curves coincide if they are normalized by the magnitude of the MLD for $\rho_n = 1$.

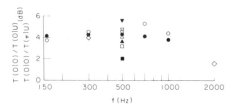

FIG. 59. The MLDs $T(0|0)/T(0|U)$ and $T(0|0)/T(\pi|U)$ as functions of the tone frequency f ($\bigcirc$, $\bullet$: RLD; $\square$, $\blacksquare$: RJ; $\triangle$, $\blacktriangle$: BJT; $\triangledown$, $\blacktriangledown$: JBSW; $\diamondsuit$: RD). Open symbols give $T(0|0)/T(0|U)$ and filled symbols give $T(0|0)/T(\pi|U)$. [The RD MLDs were actually referenced to $T(M|M)$ rather than $T(0|0)$, but we have assumed $T(M|M) = T(0|0)$].

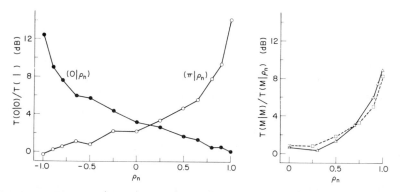

FIG. 60. The MLDs $T(0|0)/T(0|\rho_n)$, $T(0|0)/T(\pi|\rho_n)$, and $T(M|M)/T(M|\rho_n)$ as functions of the interaural correlation ρ_n of the noise (O, ●: RJ; △: DR; □: WW). The frequency of the tone was 500 Hz. (The spectral level of the noise for the WW data was 33 dB SPL per cycle.)

Figure 61 illustrates the dependence of MLDs on the overall spectral level of the noise. In general, MLDs tend to decrease as the level is lowered. Note, however, that the MLDs do not go to zero even when the masking noise is turned off; there exist small differences in the absolute threshold of the tone depending upon whether it is presented monaurally or binaurally, and binaurally in-phase or out-of-phase. Note also that according to the Hirsh data in Fig. 61, the dependence on N_0 of $T(0|0)/T(\pi|0)$ and $T(0|0)/T(M|0)$ are similar, and the dependence on N_0 of $T(0|0)/T(0|\pi)$ and $T(0|0)/T(M|\pi)$ are similar, but that there exist significant differences between the two pairs. In addition, note that the Hirsh data suggest that the MLDs at 200 Hz increase steadily with N_0 over a range of at least 70 dB. According to a

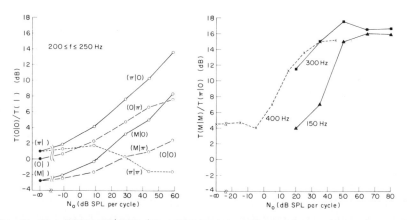

FIG. 61. The MLDs $T(0|0)/T(\pi|0)$, $T(0|0)/T(0|\pi)$, $T(0|0)/T(M|0)$, $T(0|0)/T(M|\pi)$, $T(0|0)/T(\pi|\pi)$, and $T(M|M)/T(\pi|0)$ as functions of the spectral level N_0 of the noise (O: 200 Hz, H; ●: 250 Hz, DJ; ×: 400 Hz, M; ■: 300 Hz, DO; ▲: 150 Hz, DO).

variety of more recent data (for example, the 400-Hz data of McFadden and the 150-Hz data of Dolan in Fig. 61), the range of N_0 over which the magnitude of the MLDs change significantly is confined to roughly 40 dB. The slow and steady increase in the 200-Hz Hirsh data also seem to contradict a variety of studies in which the effect of tone frequency on the level dependence has been considered (Dolan, 1968; Schenkel, 1964; Townsend & Goldstein, 1972; Wilbanks & Cornelius, 1969; Wilbanks & Whitmore, 1968; Wilbanks, Cornelius, & Houff, 1970). One illustration of this effect, which suggests that the level dependence becomes steeper in the region around $N_0 = 40$ dB as the frequency is lowered is obtained by comparing the Dolan data at 300 Hz with the Dolan data at 150 Hz in Fig. 61. According to the studies of Wilbanks, Cornelius, and Houff, and of Townsend and Goldstein, the curves for the MLD $T(0|0)/T(\pi|0)$ at 250 and 500 Hz cross each other as N_0 increases from 10 to 55 dB SPL. For example, the latter study shows that the MLD for 500 Hz is roughly 5 dB greater than the MLD for 250 Hz at $N_0 = 10$ dB, but that it is roughly 3 dB smaller at $N_0 = 55$ dB. At 150 Hz, Wilbanks $et\ al.$ state that the MLD increases by 15 dB as N_0 increases from 10 to 55 dB. In general, the fact that the region of SPL in which the MLDs increase rapidly with SPL is higher for the very low frequencies than for 500 Hz is to be expected on the basis of the absolute threshold curve for tones in this frequency region. However, the absolute threshold curve is insufficient to explain the observed changes in the form of the level dependence as a function of frequency.

Figure 62 illustrates the dependence of MLDs on the interaural amplitude ratio α_n of the noise. In the configuration $(M|\alpha_n, 0)$, the tone is presented monaurally and the noise is presented binaurally in-phase with an interaural amplitude imbalance α_n. For $\alpha_n \leq 1$, the data on $T(M|\alpha_n, 0)$ serve to interpolate between $T(M|0)$ (corresponding to $\alpha_n = 1$) and $T(M|M)$ (corresponding to $\alpha_n = 0$). In the configuration $(\alpha_s = \alpha_n, \pi|\alpha_n, 0)$, the tone is presented binaurally out-of-phase, the noise is presented binaurally in-phase, and both the tone and noise are presented with the same amplitude imbalance (so that the signal-to-noise ratio in the two ears is identical, independent of α_n). For $\alpha_n \leq 1$, the data on $T(\alpha_s = \alpha_n, \pi|\alpha_n, 0)$ serve to interpolate between $T(\pi|0)$ (corresponding to $\alpha_n = 1$) and $T(M|M)$ (corresponding to $\alpha_n = 0$). According to the results shown in Fig. 62, detectability for $(M|\alpha_n, 0)$ is best when the noise in the ear not receiving the tone is at the same level as in the ear with the tone; it decreases as the noise level in the nonsignal ear becomes either smaller $(\alpha_n < 1)$ or greater $(\alpha_n > 1)$ than the noise level in the signal ear. Provided the noise level in the signal ear is sufficiently great, the presence of the noise in the opposite ear causes a significant improvement in detection performance even when it is more than 30 dB below the level in the signal ear. Note also that according to these data, performance for $(M|\alpha_n, 0)$ appears to be roughly independent of overall level when the noise level in the opposite ear is greater than in the signal ear $(\alpha_n > 1)$.

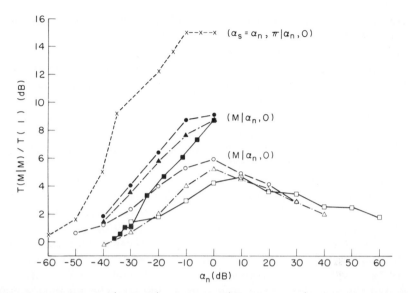

FIG. 62. The MLDs $T(\text{M}|\text{M})/T(\text{M}|\alpha_n,0)$ and $T(\text{M}|\text{M})/T(\alpha_s = \alpha_n,\pi|\alpha_n,0)$ as functions of the interaural amplitude ratio α_n of the noise for tone frequencies in the region $400 \leqslant f \leqslant 500$ Hz ($\times$: M; $\bullet$: DR; $\blacktriangle$: E; $\blacksquare$: BJW; $\bigcirc$, $\triangle$, $\square$: WM). In all cases, α_n was varied by holding the spectral level N_0 in one ear constant and varying the level in the other ear. For $(\text{M}|\alpha_n,0)$, $\alpha_n < 1$ corresponds to stimuli in which the noise level is lower in the ear not receiving the tone. For $(\alpha_s = \alpha_n,\pi|\alpha_n,0)$, the signal-to-noise ratio is always the same in both ears. When $\alpha_n = -\infty$ dB, all the MLDs reduce to 0 dB, by definition. For $\times$, $\bullet$, $\blacktriangle$, $\blacksquare$, and $\bigcirc$, the spectral level N_0 of the fixed-level noise was in the region 40–45 dB SPL per cycle. For $\triangle$ and $\square$, it was 26 and 11 dB, respectively.

2. FURTHER MLD RESULTS

In the preceding subsection, attention has been confined to tones masked by broad-band noise and, aside from the interaural parameters of the tone and noise, to the parameters tone frequency and noise level. As indicated previously, studies have been conducted for a wide variety of signals, and on the effects of a wide variety of parameters. In this subsection, we consider bandwidth effects, coherent masking, temporal effects, and other types of signals.

a. BANDWIDTH EFFECTS. Results relevant to the dependence of binaural unmasking of tones masked by noise on the bandwidth of the noise have been obtained in a variety of studies (e.g., Bourbon & Jeffress, 1965; Langford & Jeffress, 1964; Metz, von Bismark, & Durlach, 1968; Rabiner *et al.*, 1966; Sondhi & Guttman, 1966; Wightman, 1971; Wightman & Houtgast, 1972). In general, binaural unmasking tends to increase as the bandwidth is narrowed and, under optimum conditions and for a sufficiently narrow bandwidth, may exceed 30 dB.

According to Bourbon and Jeffress (1965), who showed that as the bandwidth of the noise is narrowed (while the spectral level is kept constant) the improvement in detection performance for the antiphasic configuration $(\pi\,|\,0)$ occurs earlier and more rapidly than for the homophasic configuration $(0\,|\,0)$, the effective bandwidth of the masker for $(\pi\,|\,0)$ is greater than for $(0\,|\,0)$. In the experiment by Sondhi and Guttman (1966), the width of the spectrum that is effective in binaural unmasking was studied by employing a broad-band noise masker in which an inner band of frequencies of width B centered on the tone had an interaural phase shift of 0 or π while the remaining noise (at higher and lower frequencies) had an interaural phase shift of π or 0 (denoted π–0–π and 0–π–0, respectively), and determining the amount of binaural unmasking as a function of B. The results of this experiment are shown in Fig. 63. By definition, when $B = 0$ the configurations $(0\,|\,0–\pi–0)$, $(\pi\,|\,\pi–0–\pi)$, $(\pi\,|\,0–\pi–0)$ and $(0\,|\,\pi–0–\pi)$ reduce to $(0\,|\,0)$, $(\pi\,|\,\pi)$, $(\pi\,|\,0)$, and $(0\,|\,\pi)$, respectively, and when $B = W$ (the full range of frequencies), these configurations reduce to $(0\,|\,\pi)$, $(\pi\,|\,0)$, $(\pi\,|\,\pi)$, and $(0\,|\,0)$, respectively. Note that the amount of unmasking for $(\pi\,|\,0–\pi–0)$ and $(0\,|\,\pi–0–\pi)$ decreases rapidly to zero as B increases from 0 to 50–100 Hz, whereas the amount of unmasking for $(\pi\,|\,\pi–0–\pi)$ and $(0\,|\,0–\pi–0)$ increases steadily as B increases from 0 to 150–300 Hz.

In the experiment by Metz *et al.* (1968), the masking noise was narrowed while maintaining a constant overall power level, and the effect of different total bandwidths W on the binaural unmasking function $T(0\,|\,0)/T(\phi_s\,|\,\phi_n)$ was studied. Some results of this experiment are shown in Fig. 64. In addition to showing the effect of decreasing W from 250 to 4.2 Hz, this figure again illustrates the fact that $T(\phi_s\,|\,\phi_n)$ cannot be regarded as a function of $\phi_s - \phi_n$ at low frequencies. In particular, note the difference between the results for $(\phi_s\,|\,0)$ and $(0\,|\,\phi_n)$, that is, the flattening phenomenon. Note also the change in

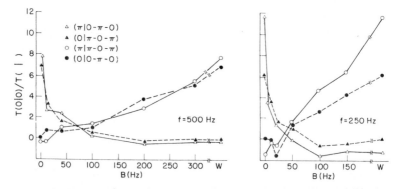

FIG. 63. The MLDs $T(0\,|\,0)/T(0\,|\,\pi - 0 - \pi)$, $T(0\,|\,0)/T(\pi\,|\,\pi - 0 - \pi)$, $T(0\,|\,0)/T(0\,|\,0 - \pi - 0)$, and $T(0\,|\,0)/T(\pi\,|\,0 - \pi - 0)$ as functions of the bandwidth B of the inner band of noise for the tone frequencies 250 and 500 Hz. The total bandwidth W of the noise was 2500 Hz and the spectrum level of the noise was 57 dB SPL per cycle. [Adapted from Sondhi and Guttman (1966).]

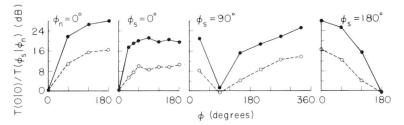

FIG. 64. The MLD $T(0|0)/T(\phi_s|\phi_n)$ as a function of the interaural phases ϕ_s and ϕ_n and the noise bandwidth W. $\bigcirc$: $W = 250$ Hz; $\bullet$: $W = 4.2$ Hz. For $\phi_n = 0°$, the abscissa ϕ denotes ϕ_s. For $\phi_s = 0°$, $90°$, and $180°$, ϕ denotes ϕ_n. The signal was a 500-msec, 250-Hz tone plus with a rise–decay time of 25 msec. The total noise power was 85 dB SPL for both values of W. [Adapted from Metz *et al.* (1968).]

form of the curve between $(0|\phi_n)$ and $(\pi|\phi_n)$ and the asymmetry in $(\pi/2|\phi_n)$ about $\phi_n = \pi/2$. The bandwidth effect in these data is accurately summarized by noting that the difference in the MLDs for the two bandwidths is always approximately 10 dB except when $\phi_s = \phi_n$, where there is no binaural unmasking for either bandwidth. According to the results obtained in this experiment for the thresholds themselves, the bandwidth has essentially no effect on detection for cases in which $\phi_s \neq \phi_n$ (i.e., in which there is binaural unmasking); the effect of bandwidth on binaural unmasking results principally from its effect on detection for the homophasic case $\phi_s = \phi_n$. Also, the results obtained in this study indicate that the tendency for MLDs to increase with a decrease in bandwidth occurs at all frequencies, not only low ones.

A replotting of the data on $(\phi_s|0)$ for the two bandwidths, in which the reference configuration is chosen to be $(\pi|0)$ rather than $(0|0)$, is shown in Fig. 65. This figure also includes a similar replotting of the data on $(\phi_s|0)$ shown previously in Fig. 52. This figure provides a dramatic illustration of the extent to which variations in MLDs that appear when $(0|0)$ is used as the reference condition and that result from changes in the parameters of the

FIG. 65. The MLD $T(\phi_s|0)/T(\pi|0)$ as a function of ϕ_s for a variety of frequencies and bandwidths. Data points obtained from Figs. 52 and 64. (The data from Fig. 64 are replotted using the symbols $+$ and $\times$ rather than $\bullet$ and $\bigcirc$; the data from Fig. 52 are replotted using the same symbols as in Fig. 52.)

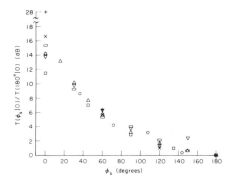

stimulus (such as bandwidth) or from changes in experimental subjects or experimental procedures tend to disappear when the reference condition is chosen to be one in which there is substantial binaural unmasking. All the data on $T(\phi_s|0)/T(\pi|0)$ from the different experiments coincide rather precisely except for the case $\phi_s = 0$. An extensive summary of MLDs in which $(\pi|0)$ is used as the reference condition is available in Colburn (1977).

Further results on the effect of noise bandwidth, which include data for the limiting case of a tonal masker at the same frequency as the target tone (coherent tone-on-tone masking) are available in Wightman (1971). In considering this limiting case, it should be noted that although binaural unmasking generally tends to increase as the bandwidth of the masker is narrowed (provided the frequency spectrum of the masker remains centered on the target and the total power in the masker remains constant), this increase does not necessarily continue to the limit. Even if the phase ψ of the target relative to the masker in the tone-on-tone masking is chosen to optimize the amount of unmasking, this amount may be less than the amount that can be achieved with narrow-band noise. Basically, this is due to the fact that the homophasic threshold $T(0|0)$ [or monaural threshold $T(M|M)$] for a noise masker can be made exceedingly large by choosing the bandwidth of the noise and the duration of the target so that the amplitude fluctuations in the masker occur at a rate that effectively obscures the change in amplitude caused by the addition of the target signal. (In this connection, note that for the narrow-band noise results shown in Fig. 64, the duration of the target signal and the reciprocal of the noise bandwidth differed by only a factor of 2.) Results on coherent tone-on-tone masking are considered in the next subsection. Results from detection experiments in which the frequency of the target tone is not covered by the frequency spectrum of the masker (remote masking) are available in Hirsh and Burgeat (1958) and McFadden, Russell, and Pulliam (1972).

b. COHERENT MASKING. When a tone is masked by noise, the phase ψ of the target signal relative to the phase of the effective masking signal (i.e., the masking signal at the output of the peripheral filter) varies randomly in time. However, when the target and masker are derived from the same source (coherent masking), the phase ψ can be controlled and varied systematically as an experimental parameter. Also, as discussed previously in connection with combination jnds (Section IV,B,2), by varying the phase ψ in the configuration $(\pi|0)$, the interaural differences in the total signal (target plus masker) can be made to be pure amplitude differences ($\psi = 0°$), pure time or phase differences ($\psi = 90°$), or a combination of the two. Coherent masking experiments in which the effect of ψ has been explored have been conducted with tone signals, narrow-band noise signals, and broad-band noise signals (Hafter & Carrier, 1970; Jeffress & McFadden, 1971; McFadden et al., 1971, 1972a; McFadden & Sharpley, 1972; Rilling & Jeffress, 1965; Robinson et al., 1974; Wightman, 1969, 1971; Yost, 1972). Some of the results on detection for the $(\pi\,|\,0)$ configuration have been presented previously (Fig. 46) in terms of the values of the interaural time delay τ and amplitude ratio α that occur at threshold for various values of ψ.

Figure 66 illustrates the dependence of the signal-to-masker ratio at threshold on ψ for low-frequency tones and for the configurations $(\pi\,|\,0)$ and $(0\,|\,0)$ (Hafter & Carrier, 1970; Robinson et al., 1974; Wightman, 1971). The values plotted for $(\pi\,|\,0)$ from the experiment by Hafter and Carrier are the same as those used to derive the $(\tau,\,\alpha)$ plots for 250 and 500 Hz from this experiment in Fig. 46. For $(0\,|\,0)$ the addition of the target merely causes an increment (or decrement) in the total energy, and the results merely reflect the transformation from ψ to a constant threshold increment (or decrement). If one defines the MLD by the difference between the thresholds for $(0\,|\,0)$ and $(\pi\,|\,0)$ at the same value of ψ, then the MLD is seen to grow rapidly as ψ increases from 0 to 90° and to achieve a rather large value. On the other hand, if one chooses the $(0\,|\,0)$ threshold at $\psi = 0$ as a fixed reference (as done, for example, by Jeffress & McFadden, 1971), then the MLD is much smaller. A summary of many of the coherent-masking results is available in Robinson et al. (1974).

c. TEMPORAL EFFECTS. The temporal aspects of binaural unmasking that have been explored include the dependence of MLDs on the duration of the target signal, the difference between the MLDs obtained with continuous masking noise and with masking noise gated on and off with the signal pulse, and the reduction of MLDs with time separation between the target and masker (nonsimultaneous masking).

Results on the effect of target–signal duration and the effect of gating the masking noise show that MLDs are greater with continuous masking noise than with gated masking noise, that MLDs increase with a decrease in signal duration when the masking noise is continuous, and that MLDs decrease with a decrease in signal duration when the masking noise is gated with the signal (Blodgett et al., 1958; Green, 1966; McFadden, 1966; Robinson & Trahiotis, 1972).

Results on binaural detection for nonsimultaneous masking show that

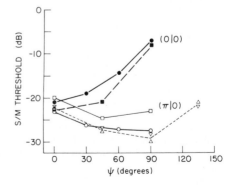

FIG. 66. The signal-to-masker threshold as a function of the phase ψ of the signal relative to the masker for coherent tone-on-tone masking (Hafter & Carrier, 1970; Robinson et al., 1974; Wightman, 1971). Filled symbols are for $(0\,|\,0)$ and open symbols for $(\pi\,|\,0)$. $\bullet$, $\bigcirc$: $F = 262$ Hz, Wightman; $\blacksquare$, $\square$: $f = 250$ Hz, Robinson et al.; $\triangle$, ∇: Hafter and Carrier; $\triangle$: $f = 250$ Hz; ∇: $f = 500$ Hz.

MLDs occur in both forward and backward masking situations (Deatherage & Evans, 1969; Dolan & Trahiotis, 1972; Punch & Carhart, 1973; Small, Boggess, Klich, Kuehn, Thelin, and Wiley, 1972). Illustrative data on the dependence of the MLD $T(0\,|\,0)/T(\pi\,|\,0)$ on the time separation T between the signal and masker (obtained from the last three studies) are shown in Fig. 67. In all three studies, the signal was a tone (250 or 500 Hz), the noise was effectively broad band, the spectral level of the noise was 45–50 dB SPL per cycle, and the rise–decay time of the noise burst was ≤.5 msec. In the study by Small and his associates, the tone burst was 20 msec and was gated on and off at zero crossings, the noise burst was 500 msec, and T refers to the duration of the silent interval between the tone burst and noise burst (with the data at $T = 0$ corresponding to the case in which the tone burst is centered in the noise burst). In the study by Dolan and Trahiotis, the tone burst was 8 msec and had a rise–decay time of 2.5 msec, the noise burst was 75 msec, and T denotes the interval between the onset of the tone burst and the onset of the masker. In the study by Punch and Carhart, the noise burst was 1000 msec, the tone was turned on 250 msec after the noise burst and had a rise–decay time of 5 msec, and the duration of the tone was 750 msec $+ T$, where T denotes the interval from the offset of the noise burst to the offset of the tone burst. According to the results shown in Fig. 67, the MLD $T(0\,|\,0)/T(\pi\,|\,0)$ decreases to roughly half its value at $T = 0$ when T lies in the region 8–16 msec. According to some results obtained by Punch and Carhart not shown in Fig. 67, small MLDs persist for forward masking out to 200 msec.

d. OTHER TYPES OF SIGNALS. In the previous discussion of binaural unmasking and MLDs, attention has been confined primarily to target signals consisting of tones and masking signals consisting of broad-band random noise. (The only exceptions are the stimulus configurations that have been considered in connection with the effect of narrowing the noise bandwidth and with coherent masking.) As mentioned in Section IV,C, there are many other target–masker combinations that have been studied. In particular,

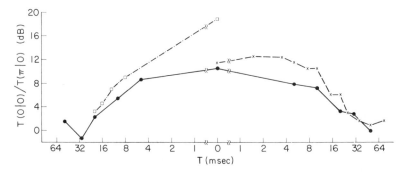

FIG. 67. The MLD $T(0\,|\,0)/T(\pi\,|\,0)$ as a function of the time separation T between the signal and masker (●: Small *et al.*, 1972; □: Dolan & Trahiotis, 1972; ×: Punch & Carhart, 1973). See text for details.

MLDs have been measured for the detection of tones in tones-plus-noise (e.g., Canahl, 1970), of narrow-band noise in broad-band noise (e.g., Henning, 1974b; Rilling & Jeffress, 1965; Webster, 1951; Wilbanks, 1971), of high-frequency amplitude-modulated sinusoids in noise (Henning, 1974b), of clicks or click trains in noise (e.g., Flanagan & Watson, 1966; Pohlmann & Sorkin, 1974; Schenkel, 1967a; Zerlin, 1966), and of speech in noise, or speech in speech, or speech in speech-plus-noise (e.g., Carhart, Tillman, & Dallos, 1968; Carhart, Tillman, & Greetis, 1969a,b; Carhart, Tillman, & Johnson, 1966, 1967, 1968; Kock, 1950; Levitt & Rabiner, 1967a,b; Licklider, 1948; Mosko & House, 1971; Pollack & Pickett, 1958; Schubert, 1956; Schubert & Schultz, 1962; Weston, Miller, & Hirsh, 1965). To a rough approximation, many of these results can be reasonably well predicted from a knowledge of the signal spectra and of the results for tones in noise.

Illustrative data on the binaural unmasking (MLD) of single words in a background of intense broad-band masking noise (with no interaural differences), as well as on the binaural gain in intelligibility (ILD) in the same noise background, are shown in Fig. 68 (Levitt & Rabiner, 1967a). In one portion of this experiment, the results of which are shown in Fig. 68, the frequency spectrum of the speech signal was divided into two regions, one of which was presented without any interaural differences and one of which was phase shifted by magnitude π. In some cases the lower frequencies were in-phase and the higher were out-of-phase (denoted $0-\pi$) and in other cases

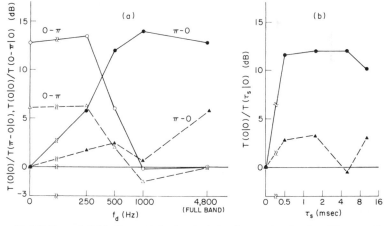

FIG. 68. MLDs and ILDs for speech signals in backgrounds of noise. The speech signal consisted of single words and the masking noise was interaurally identical, bandlimited to 4800 Hz, and presented at a spectrum level of 50 dB SPL per cycle. MLD's are denoted by circles (●, ○) and ILDs (intelligibility-level differences) by triangles (▲, △). (a) shows the dependence of $T(0|0)/T(\pi - 0|0)$ (filled symbols) and $T(0|0)/T(0 - \pi|0)$ (open symbols) on the dividing frequency f_d (see text for details); (b) shows the dependence of $T(0|0)/T(\tau_s|0)$ on the interaural delay τ_s of the speech signal [the dip in the ILD curve in (b) at $\tau_s = 5$ msec was believed to have been the result of experimental error]. [Adapted from Levitt and Rabiner (1967a).]

the lower frequencies were out-of-phase and the higher were in phase (denoted π–0). The detectability and intelligibility of the words were then studied as a function of the frequency f_d dividing the higher and lower regions. By definition, when $f_d = 0$ the configurations $(\pi$–$0|0)$ and $(0$–$\pi|0)$ reduce to $(0|0)$ and $(\pi|0)$, respectively, and when f_d is above the frequency spectrum of speech, they reduce to $(\pi|0)$ and $(0|0)$, respectively. In another portion of this experiment, the results of which are shown in Fig. 68b, the detectability and intelligibility of the words were studied as a function of the interaural time delay τ_s of the speech signal. On the whole, the MLD results are the same as those that would be expected for any target signal having the same frequency spectrum as the speech signals. The fact that the ILDs are substantially smaller than the MLDs [and that the ILD for the configuration $(\pi$–$0|0)$ continues to grow with f_d as f_d is increased above 1000 Hz] is to be expected since intelligibility is more dependent than detectability on high frequencies and since binaural unmasking decreases at high frequencies. A quantitative model for relating these results to MLDs for tones is presented in Levitt and Rabiner (1967b).

D. Related Phenomena

Although the research on sensitivity involving binaural interaction that has been conducted within the context of interaural jnds and binaural MLDs has covered a wide variety of stimulus conditions, interaural configurations, and experimental tasks, it by no means includes all those of importance. Three further topics involving sensitivity and binaural interaction that have received considerable attention are "central" or "cross masking," "monaural detection with a contralateral cue" (MDCC), and the dependence of binaural discrimination of noninteraural parameters on interaural differences. In addition, substantial research has been conducted on the relation of lateralization to MLDs.

1. CENTRAL OR CROSS MASKING

Central masking refers to the reduction in the ability to detect a target signal applied to one ear by the application of a masking signal to the other ear, beyond that associated with direct acoustical interference (caused, for example, by acoustical leakage or bone conduction). In general, the results on central masking indicate that the phenomenon is extremely sensitive to temporal factors and, in particular, to the time delay between the onset of the masker and the onset of the target. Whereas under optimum masking conditions the threshold shift caused by the masking signal is reported to be as large as 10–20 dB, when the masking signal is continuous the shift never exceeds roughly 3 dB. Also, our own unpublished research on central masking suggests that the amount of masking is exceptionally sensitive to the amount of training and degree of concentration of the experimental subjects, as well as the psychophysical method. A detailed discussion of central masking is available in Chapter 8.

2. MONAURAL DETECTION WITH A CONTRALATERAL CUE

The research on MDCC has been motivated primarily by concern with monaural detection and with the decrement in detection performance exhibited by human listeners compared with that which would be exhibited by a mathematically ideal observer operating on the same acoustic stimuli and having complete a priori information on the characteristics of the target signal (i.e., the signal-known-exactly case). Theoretically, this decrement can result from a wide variety of deficiencies in the human listener. The two that have been studied most intensively are the noisy character of the transduction process that transforms the acoustic stimulus into a pattern of impulses on the auditory nerve, and the inability of the listener to make full use of the a priori information on the target signal (usually provided by means of pretest listening or verbal instructions). In the attempt to explore the extent to which the decrement arises from the latter factor, two general approaches have been used. In one approach, the a priori information is reduced through the introduction of target–signal uncertainty, and the decrement in performance is studied as a function of this reduction. In the second approach, an attempt is made to provide the a priori information in a form that is more suitable to the human listener. It is with this second approach in mind that the research on MDCC has been conducted.

In the MDCC paradigm, the listener's objective task is to distinguish between a presentation consisting of masking noise alone to one ear and a presentation consisting of target-signal-plus-masking-noise to the same ear. However, in order to provide the listener with usable a priori information on the target signal, a signal derived from the target signal is presented simultaneously to the contralateral ear on every presentation (i.e., independent of whether the target signal is presented to the ipsilateral ear). Since the contralateral stimulation formally provides no information as to whether the target signal occurs in the presentation to the ipsilateral ear (i.e., the performance of the ideal observer for the signal-known-exactly case is independent of the existence of the contralateral stimulation), the use of the title MDCC is perfectly appropriate for this paradigm. On the other hand, since it is clear from studies of MDCC that the effect of the contralateral cue on detection performance involves properties of binaural interaction that are very similar to those encountered in the study of jnds and MLDs (rather than very central "computational" properties), it is necessary to consider this topic when attempting to develop a theory of binaural interaction.

Among the variables whose effects on detection performance have been studied in the research on MDCC (Sorkin, 1965, 1972; Taylor & Clarke, 1971; Taylor, Clarke, & Smith, 1971; Taylor & Forbes, 1969; Taylor, Smith, & Clarke, 1971) are the nature of the target signal and cue, the degree of coherence between the target signal and cue, the phase shift or time delay between the target signal and cue, and the intensity of the cue. Some of the more interesting results of this research for the case of a tone masked by broad-band random noise are the following. First, with optimum selection of parameters (such as the frequency of the target and cue, and the interaural phase and amplitude of the target and cue), the human listener's performance is much better than that obtained without the cue or by an ideal energy detector, and is within 5 dB of the ideal detector for the signal-known-exactly case. Second, there exist choices of the parameters for which the presence of the cue degrades performance. Third, the dependence of performance on the various relevant parameters is extremely complex, and performance depends strongly on the amount of training. Fourth, although the subjective cue for detection appears in most cases to be that of lateralization, there seems to be no simple relation between lateralization and MDCC. Some illustrative results on MDCC for tones masked by broad-band noise are presented in Fig. 69. Among other things, these results illustrate that under optimum conditions the performance is within 5 dB of the ideal detector for the signal-known-exactly case, that under certain conditions it is worse than when no cue is present, that its dependence on the phase between the target and cue decreases with increasing frequency and decreasing cue intensity, that cues which are more intense than the target tend to decrease performance, and that its dependence on cue intensity is substantially greater at "bad" phases than "good" phases. In addition, note that the interaction of cue intensity and target-cue phase is opposite to that expected from conventional time–intensity trading results in lateralization. Specifically, increasing the cue intensity requires that the cue be advanced in phase to maintain optimum detection performance. In considering these MDCC results, it should be noted that most of the data were obtained using an adaptive procedure (PEST) and that when psychometric functions were obtained using a nonadaptive procedure (without feedback), certain of these functions were nonmonotonic and had minimum values well below chance. Thus, some of the results (particularly those concerning "bad" phases) may be strongly dependent on the detailed measurement procedure.

Further results on detection that involve binaural interaction and that serve to relate MDCC, MLDs, and central masking have been obtained by adding noise to the contralateral ear and varying either the cue-to-noise ratio or the overall level of the stimulation in the contralateral ear while keeping this ratio fixed (Yost, Penner, & Feth, 1972).

3. BINAURAL DISCRIMINATION WITH INTERAURAL DIFFERENCES

The research on the dependence of binaural discrimination of noninteraural parameters on interaural differences is well exemplified by the studies of frequency and amplitude discrimination of tones in backgrounds of noise (Gebhardt, Goldstein, & Robertson, 1972; Henning, 1965, 1973;

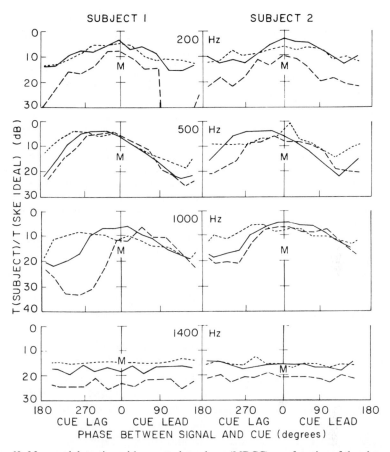

FIG. 69. Monaural detection with a contralateral cue (MDCC) as a function of the phase angle between the signal and cue and the frequency of the signal and cue. The signal was a 140-msec tone burst and the masker was broad-band noise. The signal level was maintained at roughly 40 dB SPL and the threshold signal-to-noise ratio was determined by varying the level of the noise. The cue presented to the contralateral ear was identical to the signal presented to the ipsilateral ear except for phase and amplitude. The ordinate shows the amount by which the subject's threshold signal-to-noise ratio exceeded the threshold of the signal-known-exactly (SKE) ideal observer. The amplitude of the cue relative to the amplitude of the signal was nominally 0 dB (solid curve), 20 dB (dashed curve), and −20 dB (dotted curve). The letter M in the graphs shows the results when no cue is presented (and the stimulus is therefore purely monaural). [Adapted from Taylor, Clarke, and Smith (1971).]

Robertson & Goldstein, 1967). In these studies, the ability to detect a frequency or intensity increment (the same in both ears) of a tone in a background of diotic noise has been examined as a function of the signal-to-noise ratio and the interaural phase (either 0 or π radians) of the tone. Figure 70 (Henning, 1973) shows results for both frequency–discrimination perfor-

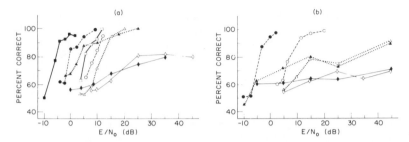

FIG. 70. Binaural discrimination performance of amplitude and frequency for a 250-Hz tone in a background of interaurally identical noise as a function of the signal-to-noise ratio and the interaural phase of the signal. The abscissa E/N_0 is the ratio of signal energy to noise power per cycle (N_0 = 30 dB SPL per cycle). Chance performance corresponds to 50% correct. Open symbols show the results for in-phase signals $(0|0)$ and filled symbols for out-of-phase signals $(\pi|0)$. Graph (a) is for discriminating an increment Δf in frequency f ($\bigcirc$: $\Delta f = 7$ Hz; $\triangle$: $\Delta f = 3$ Hz; $\diamondsuit$: $\Delta f = 1$ Hz) and graph (b) is for discriminating an increment ΔA in amplitude A ($\bigcirc$: $\Delta A = 6$ dB; $\triangle$: $\Delta A = 2$ dB; $\diamondsuit$: $\Delta A = 1$ dB). The corresponding detection results are shown by the squares in graph (a). [Adapted from Henning (1973).]

mance [Graph (a)] and amplitude–discrimination performance [Graph (b)]. As one would expect from the MLD data, performance in the $(\pi|0)$ case is substantially better than in the $(0|0)$ case provided the signal-to-noise ratio is sufficiently small and the increment to be detected is sufficiently large. When the signal-to-noise ratio is large (so that the effect of the noise is negligible) or when the increment is very small (so that discrimination is exceedingly difficult even at high signal-to-noise ratios), then, of course, the results for the two configurations tend to converge. Figure 71 (Gebhardt et al., 1972; Townsend & Goldstein, 1972) shows how the frequency jnd $(\Delta f)_0$ depends on the signal-to-noise ratio for both $(\pi|0)$ and $(0|0)$ [Graph (a)], and also compares the advantage of $(\pi|0)$ over $(0|0)$ with respect to frequency resolution

FIG. 71. Advantage of $(\pi|0)$ over $(0|0)$ with respect to frequency resolution and loudness. (a) frequency jnd $(\Delta f)_0$ as a function of the signal-to-noise ratio E/N_0; (b) difference in signal level between $(\pi|0)$ and $(0|0)$ required for equal performance in frequency discrimination ($\triangle$) and for equal loudness ($\square$) as a function of the sensation level SLM of the signal in $(0|0)$ above its masked threshold. Loudness data are from Townsend and Goldstein (1972). Filled symbols ($\blacktriangle$, $\blacksquare$) in (b) give the results for $T(0|0)/T(\pi|0)$ in the two experiments. The signal was a 500-Hz tone (of duration 275 msec for $\bigcirc$, $\bullet$, $\triangle$, $\blacktriangle$ and 500 msec for $\square$, $\blacksquare$) and the noise was broad band with N_0 = 55 dB SPL per cycle. [Adapted from Gebhardt et al. (1972).]

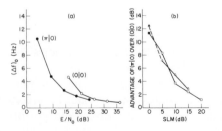

to the advantage of $(\pi \mid 0)$ over $(0 \mid 0)$ with respect to loudness as a function of the level (SLM) of the homophasic tone above its masked threshold [Graph (b)]. According to the latter graph, when the tone levels in $(\pi \mid 0)$ and $(0 \mid 0)$ are adjusted to be equally loud, the frequency jnds $(\Delta f)_0$ in the two cases are equal.

4. Lateralization and MLD

In the attempt to understand the relation of lateralization to binaural unmasking, a variety of studies have been conducted in which lateralization and detection performance are compared for a common stimulus configuration that leads to binaural unmasking.

In one group of studies, the ability to detect a monaurally presented tone in a background of binaurally presented broad-band noise has been compared to the ability to determine which ear received the tone when the ear to which the tone is presented is selected randomly from trial to trial. Illustrative data on this topic are shown in Fig. 72 (Egan & Benson, 1966). Whereas for the case of statistically independent noise $(M \mid U)$, the ability to detect the tone is roughly the same as the ability to determine which ear received it, for the case of diotic noise $(M \mid 0)$, the results are very different. Not only is the lateralization curve displayed towards higher signal-to-noise ratios, but its slope is significantly reduced. In a subsidiary experiment, it was shown that the ability to detect the tone is essentially independent of whether the tone is always presented to the same ear or whether the ear is varied randomly (as in the lateralization paradigm). It has also been shown that as the frequency of the tone is increased, the differences among the curves diminishes (Robinson & Egan, 1974). In particular, at 2000 Hz all four curves have the same slope and are within approximately 4 dB of each other. The result that the lateralization curve is similar to the detection curve for $(M \mid U)$ and that these two curves are similar for $(M \mid 0)$ at high frequencies is not surprising since the amount of binaural unmasking is relatively small under these conditions. In another experiment, in which the ability to detect and lateralize a 400-Hz tone in the $(M \mid 0)$ configuration was studied as a function of tone duration, it has been shown that the difference between detection and lateralization for

FIG. 72. Comparison of lateralization and detection performance for a 500-Hz tone masked by broad-band noise with $N_0 = 45$ dB SPL per cycle. $(M \mid 0)$ denotes monaural signal and interaurally identical noise, $(M \mid U)$ denotes monaural signal and statistically independent noise. D denotes detection and L lateralization. The lateralization task in this experiment was to identify which ear had the signal. [Adapted from Egan and Benson (1966).]

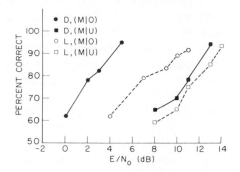

(M|0) is approximately independent of duration in the region 50–800 msec (McFadden & Pulliam, 1971). Finally, if the stimulus is generalized from (M|0) to $(\alpha_s, 0|0)$ or $(\alpha_s, \pi|0)$ (i.e., the tone is presented with an amplitude ratio α_s and either in-phase or out-of-phase) and the lateralization task consists of determining which ear received the more intense signal, then, as α_s decreases from 12 to 0 dB, detection and lateralization become more similar for $(\alpha_s, 0|0)$ and less similar for $(\alpha_s, \pi|0)$ (McFadden, 1969). This result is again consistent with the notion that the extent of the difference between the detection and lateralization curves is directly related to the amount of binaural unmasking.

In a second group of studies, the relation of lateralization to MLDs was explored by obtaining histograms of subjective lateralization responses, computing the sensitivity performance that would be obtained by an ideal receiver with the lateralization response as input, and comparing these results with the measurements of detection performance obtained from the same subjects who produced the lateralization histograms (Hafter, Bourbon, Blocker, & Tucker, 1969; Hafter, Carrier, & Stephan, 1973). In these experiments, the signal was a 100-msec, 500-Hz tone and the noise was broadband with a spectral level of 50 dB SPL per cycle. For the lateralization task, the subjects were provided with a mechanical lever and instructed to respond to each stimulus presentation by setting the lever at the position that best corresponded to the position of the signal image along the line joining the two ears. The histograms were then constructed from the set of lever positions. In the lateralization experiment by Hafter et al. (1969), the tone signal was presented on every trial, the interaural configuration was always $(\pi|0)$, and lateralization histograms were constructed as a function of the signal-to-noise ratio E/N_0 for values in the region $-10 \leq E/N_0 \leq 2$ dB. The histograms thus obtained for one of the subjects tested are shown in Fig. 73a. Whereas for small E/N_0 the lateralization responses cluster around the center (where the noise-alone image is located), for large E/N_0 the histogram shows a bimodal distribution with one peak on either side. A comparison of the average detection performance produced by human subjects with the average detection performance achieved by the ideal observer operating on the lateralization responses (where the averaging is performed over subjects) is shown in Fig. 73b. (In computing the performance of the ideal observer, it was assumed that the lateralization histogram for $E/N_0 = -10$ dB was identical to that which would have been produced by noise alone. Also, the subjects used for the detection task were not the same as those used for the lateralization task.) In the lateralization experiment performed by Hafter et al. (1973), the tone signal was presented on every trial, the stimulus was chosen randomly to be of the form (M|0) or (0|0), and histograms were constructed for both (M|0) and (0|0) as a function of the signal-to-noise ratio E/N_0. In all cases, the values of E/N_0 were adjusted so that the tone was equally detectable in (M|0) and (0|0) [i.e., the level of the tone in (M|0) was

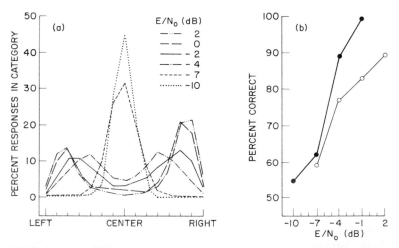

Fig. 73. Comparison of lateralization and detection performance for a 500-Hz tone masked by broad-band noise. (a) Shows histograms for a single subject of lateralization responses obtained with the use of a mechanical lever for the interaural configuration $(\pi \mid 0)$ and for various values of E/N_0; (b) shows the percentage correct obtained in detecting the signal for the configuration $(\pi \mid 0)$ as a function of E/N_0. ($\bullet$: average results of human subjects; $\circ$: average of results obtained by the ideal observer operating on lateralization responses of human subjects under the assumption that the histogram for $E/N_0 = -10$ dB is the same as the histogram for the case in which the noise alone is presented). N_0 was 50 dB SPL per cycle. [Adapted from Hafter et al. (1969).]

set higher than the level of the tone in $(0 \mid 0)$ by an amount equal to the MLD $T(0 \mid 0)/T(M \mid 0)$]. The histograms obtained for both $(0 \mid 0)$ and $(M \mid 0)$ for a single subject and a variety of levels are shown in Fig. 74a. Figure 74b shows the detection results for both $(0 \mid 0)$ and $(M \mid 0)$ for the same subject, as well as the results achieved by the ideal observer in discriminating between $(M \mid 0)$ and $(0 \mid 0)$ using the lateralization responses of the same subject. Inasmuch as the lateralization histogram for $(0 \mid 0)$ is roughly the same as that for noise alone, the results obtained for the ideal observer in discriminating between $(M \mid 0)$ and $(0 \mid 0)$ can be regarded as essentially the same as those describing the ability of the ideal observer to detect the tone in the $(M \mid 0)$ configuration. It should also be noted that the unimodal character of the lateralization histograms for $(M \mid 0)$ in Fig. 74a does not reflect the stimulus configuration but a response bias; half the $(M \mid 0)$ lateralization data were gathered with the tone in the right ear and half with tone in the left ear (the choice between right and left made randomly at the beginning of each session). This response bias, which occurred for all subjects (but usually to the right rather than to the left), was not apparent in the experiment by Egan and Benson (1966) in which the subject's task was to identify which ear received the signal. Comments on the relations among the various results are available in the reports by Hafter and his associates.

In a third group of studies, the relation of lateralization to MLDs has been

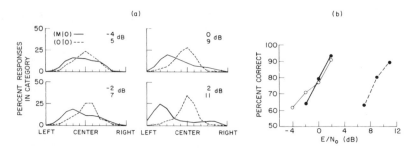

FIG. 74. Comparison of lateralized and detection performance for a 500-Hz tone masked by broad-band noise. (a) Shows histograms for a single subject of lateralization responses obtained with the use of a mechanical lever for the configurations $(0|0)$ and $(M|0)$ and for various signal levels. The decibel values in each graph of (a) specify the values of E/N_0 for $(0|0)$ and $(M|0)$, with the higher level always referring to $(0|0)$. These values were chosen to make the tone equally detectable in the two cases. (b) Shows the detection results for the same subject for both $(M|0)$ (filled circles and solid line) and $(0|0)$ (filled circles and dashed line), as well as the detection results for $(M|0)$ obtained by the ideal observer operating on the lateralization responses (open circles) under the assumption that the histogram for $(0|0)$ is the same as for the case in which noise alone is presented. N_0 was 50 dB SPL per cycle. [Adapted from Hafter *et al.* (1973).]

explored within the context of coherent masking. The detection results in coherent masking situations have already been discussed in previous sections (e.g., see Figs. 46 and 66). In some of these studies, in addition to determining how the detection of the target depends on the phase ψ between the target and masker, experiments have been conducted to explore how lateralization depends upon ψ (Jeffress & McFadden, 1971; McFadden *et al.*, 1971, 1972a). In these lateralization experiments, both the target and masker consist of the same narrow-band noise, the stimulus configuration is of the form $(\pi|0)$, the subject is required to judge whether the sound image appears to the left or right of center, and the percentage of left and right responses is studied as a function of the target-to-masker ratio and the phase ψ. Some data illustrating the dependence on ψ for a narrow-band noise centered on 500 Hz and for a target-to-masker ratio of -19 dB are shown in Fig. 75 (Jeffress & McFadden, 1971). Also included in this figure for some of the ψ values are the values of the interaural amplitude difference α and the interaural time delay τ that correspond to the given value of ψ and the given target-to-masker ratio. When $0 < \psi < 90°$, α and τ are collateral and the image is usually judged to be on the side at which the signal is more intense and leading in time. When $90 < \psi < 180°$, α and τ are antilateral and whether the image is judged to be left or right depends on the relative magnitudes of α and τ. For ψ in the vicinity of $110°$ (the precise value depending upon the subject), the percentage of responses is equally divided between left and right. This uncertainty concerning whether the image is to the left or right of center in this region of ψ, combined with the fact that the amount of binaural unmasking measured in this region of ψ was found to be substantial, suggests that binaural un-

FIG. 75. Lateralization results for $(\pi \mid 0)$ in coherent masking. The signal was a 50-Hz band of noise at 500 Hz with a total power level of roughly 80 dB SPL, and the target-to-masker ratio was −19 dB. The abscissa ψ is the phase of the target relative to the masker and the ordinate gives the percentage of judgments "to the left." The pairs of numbers associated with selected data points (indicated by the large circles) give the values of the interaural amplitude ratio α (upper number) in decibels and the values of the interaural time delay τ (lower number) in microseconds associated with these points. For all ψ, the corresponding detection results were greater than 85% correct. [Adapted from Jeffress and McFadden (1971).]

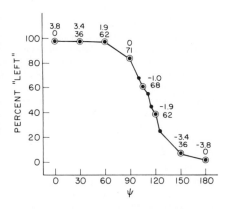

masking cannot be explained purely in terms of a simple lateralization model (i.e., without taking account of image width, multiple images, or some other subjective attribute of the binaural image space).

Finally, it should be noted that in addition to cases for which lateralization is difficult although binaural unmasking is substantial, there appear to be cases for which binaural unmasking is negligible even though lateralization is easy. In particular, it has been reported that complex high-frequency waveforms (narrow bands of noise or high-frequency amplitude-modulated sinusoids) masked by broad-band noise show insignificant amounts of unmasking, despite the fact that these waveforms are well lateralized as a function of interaural delay (Henning, 1974b).

The various models of binaural interaction that have been proposed to interpret results on lateralization and/or binaural detection are discussed in Chapter 11.

Note. This chapter reviews research on binaural phenomena conducted prior to 1974 (the year the chapter was written). Reports of more recent research can be found in the journals cited in the reference list (particularly the *Journal of the Acoustical Society of America*).

Acknowledgments

The authors are indebted to R. Domnitz, N. Guttman, W. M. Rabinowitz, B. McA. Sayers, R. Stern, and W. A. Yost for their useful comments on the original manuscript. Special thanks are due to G. B. Henning and D. McFadden for their detailed reading of the manuscript and their many detailed suggestions. This work was supported by the National Institutes of Health (Grants NIGMS-5-P01-GM14940 and NINCDS-5-R01-NS10916).

References

Angell, J. R., & Fite, W. The monaural localization of sound. *Psychological Review,* 1901, **8,** 225–243. (a)

Angell, J. R., & Fite, W. Further observations on the monaural localization of sound. *Psychological Review*, 1901, **8**, 449–458. (b)

Babkoff, H., & Sutton, S. Perception of temporal order and loudness judgments for dichotic clicks. *Journal of the Acoustical Society of America*, 1963, **35**, 547–577.

Babkoff, H., & Sutton, S. End point of lateralization for dichotic clicks. *Journal of the Acoustical Society of America*, 1966, **39**, 87–102.

Babkoff, H., & Sutton, S. Binaural interaction of transients: Interaural intensity asymmetry. *Journal of the Acoustical Society of America*, 1969, **46**, 887–892.

Babkoff, H., Sutton, S., & Barris, M. Binaural interaction of transients: Interaural time and intensity asymmetry. *Journal of the Acoustical Society of America*, 1973, **53**, 1028–1036.

Banks, M. S., & Green, D. M. Localization of high- and low-frequency transients. *Journal of the Acoustical Society of America*, 1973, **53**, 1432–1433.

Banister, H. Three experiments on the localization of tones. *British Journal of Psychology*, 1926, **16**, 266–279.

Banister, H. Auditory theory: A criticism of Prof. Boring's hypothesis. *American Journal of Psychology*, 1927, **38**, 436–440.

Batteau, D. W. The role of the pinna in human localization. *Proceedings of the Royal Society* (London), Series B, 1967, **168**, 158–180.

Batteau, D. W. Listening with the naked ear. In S. J. Freedman (Ed.), *The neuropsychology of spatially oriented behaviour*, Homewood Illinois: Dorsey Press, 1968. Pp. 109–133.

Békésy, G. von. Neural funneling along the skin and between the inner and outer hair cells of the cochlea. *Journal of the Acoustical Society of America*, 1959, **31**, 1236–1249.

Békésy, G. von. *Experiments in hearing*. New York: McGraw Hill, 1960.

Békésy, G. von. Auditory backward inhibition in concert halls. *Science*, 1971, **171**, 529–536.

Bertrand, M. P. Aspects of binaural experimentation. *Proceedings of the Royal Society of Medicine*, 1972, **65**, No. 9, 807–812.

Bilsen, F. A., & Goldstein, J. L. Pitch of dichotically delayed noise and its possible spectral basis. *Journal of the Acoustical Society of America*, 1974, **55**, 292–296.

Bilsen, F. A., & Ritsma, R. J. Repetition pitch and it's implication for hearing theory. *Acustica*, 1969, **22**, 63–73.

Blauert, J. Sound localization in the median plane. *Acustica*, 1969, **22**, 205–213.

Blauert, J. Localization and the law of the first wavefront in the median plane. *Journal of the Acoustical Society of America*, 1971, **50**, 466–470.

Blauert, J. *Räumliches Hören*. Verlag Stuttgart: S. Hirzel, 1974.

Blodgett, H. C., Jeffress, L. A., & Taylor, R. W. Relation of masked threshold to signal-duration for various interaural phase-combinations. *American Journal of Psychology*, 1958, **71**, 283–290.

Blodgett, H. C., Jeffress, L. A., & Whitworth, R. H. Effect of noise at one ear on the masked threshold for tone at the other. *Journal of the Acoustical Society of America*, 1962, **34**, 979–981.

Blodgett, H. C., Wilbanks, W. A., & Jeffress, L. A. Effect of large interaural time differences upon the judgment of sidedness. *Journal of the Acoustical Society of America*, 1956, **28**, 639–643.

Bourbon, W. T., & Jeffress, L. A. Effect of bandwidth of masking noise on detection of homophasic and antiphasic tonal signals. *Journal of the Acoustical Society of America*, 1965, **37**, 1180 (A).

Butler, R. A. Monaural and binaural localization of noise bursts vertically in the median sagittal plane. *Journal of Auditory Research*, 1969, **3**, 230–235.

Butler, R. A., & Naunton, R. F. Some effects of unilateral auditory masking upon the localization of sound in space. *Journal of the Acoustical Society of America*, 1962, **34**, 1100–1107.

Butler, R. A., & Naunton, R. F. Role of stimulus frequency and duration in the phenomenon of localization shifts. *Journal of the Acoustical Society of America*, 1964, **36**, 917–922.

Canahl, J. A., Jr. Binaural masking of a tone by a tone plus noise. *Journal of the Acoustical Society of America*, 1970, **47**, 476–479.

Carhart, R. Monaural and binaural discrimination against competing sentences. *International Audiology*, 1965, **IV**, 5–10.

Carhart, R., Tillman, T. W., & Dallos, P. Unmasking for pure tones and spondees: Interaural phase and time disparities. *Journal of Speech and Hearing Research*, 1968, **11**, 722–734.

Carhart, R., Tillman, T. W., & Greetis, E. S. Release from multiple maskers: Effect of interaural time disparities. *Journal of the Acoustical Society of America*, 1969, **45**, 411–418. (a)

Carhart, R., Tillman, T. W., & Greetis, E. S. Perceptual masking in multiple sound backgrounds. *Journal of the Acoustical Society of America*, 1969, **45**, 694–703. (b)

Carhart, R., Tillman, T. W., & Johnson, K. R. Binaural masking of speech by periodically modulated noise. *Journal of the Acoustical Society of America*, 1966, **39**, 1037–1050.

Carhart, R., Tillman, T. W., & Johnson, K. R. Release of masking for speech through interaural time delay. *Journal of the Acoustical Society of America*, 1967, **42**, 124–138.

Carhart, R., Tillman, T. W., & Johnson, K. R. Effects of interaural time delays on masking by two competing signals. *Journal of the Acoustical Society of America*, 1968, **43**, 1223–1230.

Cherry, E. C. Two ears–but one world. In W. A. Rosenblith (Ed.), *Sensory Communication.* Cambridge, Massachusetts: M.I.T. Press, 1961. Pp. 99–117.

Cherry, E. C., & Sayers, B. McA. Human cross-correlator—A technique for measuring certain parameters of speech perception. *Journal of the Acoustical Society of America*, 1956, **28**, 889–895.

Cherry, E. C., & Taylor, W. K. Some further experiments upon the recognition of speech, with one and with two ears. *Journal of the Acoustical Society of America*, 1954, **26**, 554–559.

Chocholle, R. La sensibilité auditive différentielle d'intensité en présence d'un son contralátéral de même fréquence. *Acustica*, 1957, **7**, 73–83. [This article also appears in English in J. D. Harris (Ed.), *Forty Germinal papers in human hearing.* Groton, Connecticut: Journal of Auditory Research, 1969.]

Colburn, H. S. Theory of binaural interaction based on auditory nerve data. II. Detection of tones in noise. *Journal of the Acoustical Society of America*, 1977, **61**, 525–533.

Colburn, H. S., & Durlach, N. I. Time-intensity relations in binaural unmasking. *Journal of the Acoustical Society of America*, 1965, **38**, 93–103.

Coleman, P. D. Failure to localize the source distance of an unfamiliar sound. *Journal of the Acoustical Society of America*, 1962, **34**, 345–346.

Coleman, P. D. An analysis of cues to auditory depth perception in free space. *Psychological Bulletin*, 1963, **60**, 302–315.

Coleman, P. D. Dual role of frequency spectrum in determination of auditory distance. *Journal of the Acoustical Society of America*, 1968, **44**, 631–632.

Cramer, E. M., & Huggins, W. H. Creation of pitch through binaural interaction. *Journal of the Acoustical Society of America*, 1958, **30**, 413–417.

Cronin, P. M. A psychoacoustical examination of interaural timing at high frequencies. Unpublished MS thesis, Dept. of Electrical Engineering, MIT, Cambridge, Massachusetts, 1973.

David, E. E., Jr., Guttman, N., & van Bergeijk, W. A. On the mechanism of binaural fusion. *Journal of the Acoustical Society of America*, 1958, **30**, 801–802.

David, E. E., Jr., Guttman, N., & van Bergeijk, W. A. Binaural interaction of high-frequency complex stimuli. *Journal of the Acoustical Society of America*, 1959, **31**, 774–782.

Deatherage, B. H. Binaural interaction of clicks of different frequency content. *Journal of the Acoustical Society of America*, 1961, **33**, 139–145.

Deatherage, B. H. Examination of binaural interaction. *Journal of the Acoustical Society of America*, 1966, **39**, 232–249.

Deatherage, B. H., & Evans, T. R. Binaural masking: Backward, forward, and simultaneous effects. *Journal of the Acoustical Society of America*, 1969, **46**, 362–371.

Deatherage, B. H., & Hirsh, I. J. Auditory localization of clicks. *Journal of the Acoustical Society of America*, 1959, 31, 486–492.

Diercks, K. J., & Jeffress, L. A. Interaural phase and the absolute threshold for tone. *Journal of the Acoustical Society of America*, 1962, 34, 981–984.

Dolan, T. R. Effect of masker spectrum level on masking-level difference at low signal frequencies. *Journal of the Acoustical Society of America*, 1968, 44, 1507–1512.

Dolan, T. R., & Robinson, D. E. Explanation of masking-level differences that result from interaural intensive disparties of noise. *Journal of the Acoustical Society of America*, 1967, 42, 977–981.

Dolan, T. R., & Trahiotis, C. Binaural interaction in backward masking. *Perception and Psychophysics*, 1972, 11, 92–94.

Domnitz, R. The interaural time JND as a simultaneous function of interaural time and interaural amplitude. *Journal of the Acoustical Society of America*, 1973,, 53, 1549–1552.

Dunn, B. E. Effect of masking on the lateralization of binaural pulses. *Journal of the Acoustical Society of America*, 1971, 50, 483–489.

Dunn, B. E., & Parfitt, S. Localization with complete masking in one ear. *Perception and psychophysics*, 1967, 2, 408–410.

Durlach, N. I. Equalization and cancellation theory of binaural masking-level differences. *Journal of the Acoustical Society of America*, 1963, 35, 1206–1218.

Durlach, N. I. Note on binaural masking-level differences at high frequencies: *Journal of the Acoustical Society of America*, 1964, 36, 576–581.

Durlach, N. I. Binaural signal detection: Equalization and cancellation theory. In J. V. Tobias (Ed.), *Foudations of modern auditory theory*, Vol. 2. New York: Academic Press, 1972. Pp. 369–462.

Ebata, M., Nimura, T., & Sone, T. Effects of preceding sound on time-intensity trading ratio. *Seventh International Congress on Acoustics, Budapest*, 1971, 19-H-2, 313–316.

Ebata, M., Sone, T., & Nimura, T. Binaural fusion of tone bursts different in frequency. *Sixth International Congress on Acoustics, Tokyo*, 1968, A-3-7, 33–36. (a)

Ebata, M., Sone, T., & Nimura, T. On the perception of direction of echo. *Journal of the Acoustical Society of America*, 1968, 44, 542–547. (b)

Ebata, M., Sone, T., & Numura, T. Improvement of hearing ability by directional information. *Journal of the Acoustical Society of America*, 1968, 43, 289–297. (c)

Egan, J. P. Masking-level differences as a function of interaural disparities in intensity of signal and of noise. *Journal of the Acoustical Society of America*, 1965, 38, 1043–1049.

Egan, J. P., & Benson, W. Lateralization of a weak signal presented with correlated and uncorrelated noise. *Journal of the Acoustical Society of America*, 1966, 40, 20–26.

Egan, J. P., Lindner, W. A., & McFadden, D. Masking-level differences and the form of the psychometric function. *Perception and Psychophysics*, 1969, 6, 209–215.

Elfner, L. F., & Perrott, D. R. Lateralization and intensity discrimination. *Journal of the Acoustical Society of America*, 1967, 42, 441–444.

Elfner, L. F., & Tomsic, R. T. Temporal and intensive factors in binaural lateralization of auditory transients. *Journal of the Acoustical Society of America*, 1968, 43, 746–751.

Feddersen, W. E., Sandel, T. T., Teas, D. C., & Jeffress, L. A. Localization of high-frequency tones. *Journal of the Acoustical Society of America*, 1957, 29, 988–991.

Firestone, F. A. The phase difference and amplitude ratio at the ears due to a source of pure tone. *Journal of the Acoustical Society of America*, 1930, 2, 260–270.

Flanagan, J. L., David, E. E., Jr., & Watson, B. J. Binaural lateralization of cophasic and antiphasic clicks. *Journal of the Acoustical Society of America*, 1964, 36, 2184–2193.

Flanagan, J. L., & Watson, B. J. Binaural unmasking of complex signals. *Journal of the Acoustical Society of America*, 1966, 40, 456–468.

Fourcin, A. J. Binaural pitch phenomena. *Journal of the Acoustical Society of America*, 1962, 34, 1995 (A). (a)

Fourcin, A. J. An aspect of the perception of pitch. *Proceedings of the Fourth International Congress of Phonetic Science, Helsinki.* The Hague: Mouton, 1962. (b)

Fourcin, A. J. Central pitch and auditory lateralization. In R. Plomp & G. F. Smoorenburg (Eds.), *Frequency analysis and periodicity detection in hearing.* Leiden: Sijthoff, 1970. Pp. 319–328.

Freedman, S. J., & Fisher, H. G. The role of the pinna in auditory localization. In S. J. Freedman (Ed.), *The neuropsychology of spatially oriented behavior.* Homewood, Illinois: Dorsey Press, 1968. Pp. 135–152.

Gardner, M. B. Historical background of the Haas and/or precedence effect. *Journal of the Acoustical Society of America,* 1968, **43**, 1243–1248. (a)

Gardner, M. B. Lateral localization of 0°- or near-0°-oriented speech signals in anechoic space. *Journal of the Acoustical Society of America,* 1968, **44**, 797–802. (b)

Gardner, M. B. Distance estimation of 0° or apparent 0°-oriented speech signals in anechoic space. *Journal of the Acoustical Society of America,* 1969, **45**, 47–53. (a)

Gardner, M. B. Image fusion, broadening, and displacement in sound location. *Journal of the Acoustical Society of America,* 1969, **46**, 339–349. (b)

Gardner, M. B., & Gardner, R. S. Problem of localization in the median plane: Effect of pinnae cavity occlusion. *Journal of the Acoustical Society of America,* 1973, **53**, 400–408.

Gebhardt, C. J., Goldstein, D. P., & Robertson, R. M. Frequency discrimination and the MLD. *Journal of the Acoustical Society of America,* 1972, **51**, 1228–1232.

Gilliom, J. D., & Sorkin, R. D. Discrimination of interaural time and intensity. *Journal of the Acoustical Society of America,* 1972, **52**, 1635–1644.

Goldstein, J. L. An optimum processor theory for the central formation of the pitch of complex tones. *Journal of the Acoustical Society of America,* 1973, **54**, 1496–1516.

Green, D. M. Interaural phase effects in the masking of signals of different durations. *Journal of the Acoustical Society of America,* 1966, **39**, 720–724.

Guttman, N. A mapping of binaural click lateralizations. *Journal of the Acoustical Society of America,* 1962, **34**, 87–92. (a)

Guttman, N. Pitch and loudness of a binaural subjective tone. *Journal of the Acoustical Society of America,* 1962, **33**, 1966. (b)

Guttman, N. Binaural interactions of three clicks. *Journal of the Acoustical Society of America,* 1965, **37**, 145–150.

Guttman, N., van Bergeijk, W. A., & David, E. E. Monaural temporal masking investigated by binaural interaction. *Journal of the Acoustical Society of America,* 1960, **32**, 1329–1336.

Haas, H. H. The influence of a single echo on the audibility of speech. Library communication No. 363, Dept. of Science and Industrial Research, Building Research Station, Garston, Watford, Herts., England, 1949.

Hafter, E. R., Bourbon, W. T., Blocker, A. S., & Tucker, A. A direct comparison between lateralization and detection under conditions of antiphasic masking. *Journal of the Acoustical Society of America,* 1969, **46**, 1452–1457.

Hafter, E. R., & Carrier, S. C. Masking-level differences obtained with a pulsed tonal masker. *Journal of the Acoustical Society of America,* 1970, **47**, 1041–1047.

Hafter, E. R., & Carrier, S. C. Binaural interaction in low-frequency stimuli: The inability to trade time and intensity completely. *Journal of the Acoustical Society of America,* 1972, **51**, 1852–1862.

Hafter, E. R., Carrier, S. C., & Stephan, F. K. Direct comparison of lateralization and the MLD for monaural signals in gated noise. *Journal of the Acoustical Society of America,* 1973, **53**, 1553–1559.

Hafter, E. R., & Jeffress, L. A. Two-image lateralization of tones and clicks. *Journal of the Acoustical Society of America,* 1968, **44**, 563–569.

Hanson, R. L., & Kock, W. E. Interesting effect produced by two loudspeakers under free space conditions. *Journal of the Acoustical Society of America,* 1957, **29**, 145.

Harris, G. G. Binaural interactions of impulsive stimuli and pure tones. *Journal of the Acoustical Society of America*, 1960, **32**, 685–692.

Harris, G. G., Flanagan, J. L., & Watson, B. J. Binaural interaction of a click with a click pair. *Journal of the Acoustical Society of America*, 1963, **35**, 672–678.

Harris, J. D. A florilegium of experiments on directional hearing. *Acta Oto-Laryngologica*, 1972, Suppl. No. **298**, 1–26.

Harris, J. D., & Sergeant, R. L. Sensory behavior of naval personnel: Monaural/binaural minimum audible angle of auditory response. U.S. Naval Submarine Medical Center, Submarine Base, Groton, Conn., Report #607, 1970.

Held, R. Shifts in binaural localization after prolonged exposures to atypical combinations of stimuli. *American Journal of Psychology*, 1955, **68**, 526–548.

Henning, G. B. Binaural masking-level Differences and frequency discrimination. *Journal of the Acoustical Society of America*, 1965, **38**, 929 (A).

Henning, G. B. Effect of interaural phase on frequency and amplitude discrimination. *Journal of the Acoustical Society of America*, 1973, **54**, 1160–1178.

Henning, G. B. Detectability of interaural delay in high-frequency complex waveforms. *Journal of the Acoustical Society of America*, 1974, **55**, 84–90. (a)

Henning, G. B. Lateralization and the binaural masking-level difference. *Journal of the Acoustical Society of America*, 1974, **55**, 1259–1262. (b)

Hershkowitz, R. M., & Durlach, N. I. Interaural time and amplitude JND's for a 500-Hz tone. *Journal of the Acoustical Society of America*, 1969, **46**, 1464–1467. (a)

Hershkowitz, R. M., & Durlach, N. I. An unsuccessful attempt to determine the tradability of interaural time and interaural intensity. *Journal of the Acoustical Society of America*, 1969, **46**, 1583–1584. (b)

Hirsh, I. J. The influence of interaural phase on interaural summation and inhibition. *Journal of the Acoustical Society of America*, 1948, **20**, 536–544.

Hirsh, I. J., & Burgeat, M. Binaural effects in remote masking. *Journal of the Acoustical Society of America*, 1958, **30**, 827–832.

Hirsh, I. J., & Pollack, I. The role of interaural phase in loudness. *Journal of the Acoustical Society of America*, 1948, **20**, 761–766.

Hirsh, I. J., & Sherrick, C. E. Perceived order in different sense modalities. *Journal of Experimental Psychology*, 1961, **62**, 423–432.

Hirsh, I. J., & Webster, F. A. Some determinants of interaural phase effects. *Journal of the Acoustical Society of America*, 1949, **21**, 496–501.

Hornbostel, E. M. von, & Wertheimer, M. Ueber die Wahrnehmung der Schallrichtung. *Sitzungsberichte der Deutschen Akademie der Wissenschaften zu Berlin*, 1920, **15**, 388–396.

Houtgast, T., & Plomp, R. Lateralization threshold of a signal in noise. *Journal of the Acoustical Society of America*, 1968, **44**, 807–812.

Houtsma, A. J. M., & Goldstein, J. L. The central origin of the pitch of complex tones: Evidence from musical interval recognition. *Journal of the Acoustical Society of America*, 1972, **51**, 520–529.

Irwin, R. J. Binaural summation of thermal noise of equal and unequal power in each ear. *American Journal of Psychology*, 1965, **78**, 57–65.

Jeffress, L. A. Note on the 'interesting effect produced by two loudspeakers under free space conditions' by L. R. Hanson and W. E. Kock, *Journal of the Acoustical Society of America*, 1957, **29**, 655.

Jeffress, L. A., Blodgett, H. C., & Deatherage, B. H. The masking of tones by white noise as a function of the interaural phases of both components. I. 500 cycles. *Journal of the Acoustical Society of America*, 1952, **24**, 523–527.

Jeffress, L. A., Blodgett, H. C., & Deatherage, B. H. Effect of interaural correlation on the precision of centering a noise. *Journal of the Acoustical Society of America*, 1962, **34**, 1122–1123. (a)

Jeffress, L. A., Blodgett, H. C., & Deatherage, B. H. Masking and interaural phase. II. 167 cycles. *Journal of the Acoustical Society of America*, 1962, **34**, 1124–1126. (b)

Jeffress, L. A., Blodgett, H. C., Sandel, T. T., & Wood, C. L., III. Masking of tonal signals. *Journal of the Acoustical Society of America*, 1956, **28**, 416–426.

Jeffress, L. A., & McFadden, D. Differences of interaural phase and level in detection and lateralization. *Journal of the Acoustical Society of America*, 1971, **49**, 1169–1179.

Jeffress, L. A., & Taylor, R. W. Lateralization versus localization. *Journal of the Acoustical Society of America*, 1961, **33**, 482–483.

Keen, K. Preservation of constant loudness with interaural amplitude asymmetry. *Journal of the Acoustical Society of America*, 1972, **52**, 1193–1196.

Klumpp, R. G., & Eady, H. R. Some measurements of interaural time difference thresholds. *Journal of the Acoustical Society of America*, 1956, **28**, 859–860.

Kock, W. E. Binaural localization and masking. *Journal of the Acoustical Society of America*, 1950, **22**, 801–804.

Langford, T. L., & Jeffress, L. A. Effect of noise crosscorrelation on binaural signal detection. *Journal of the Acoustical Society of America*, 1964, **36**, 1455–1458.

Laws, P. Untersuchungen zum Entfernungshören und zum Problem der Im-Kopf-Lokalisiertheit von Hörereignissen. Unpublished Ph.D. dissertation, Rheinisch-Westfälischen Technischen Hochschule Aachen, 1972.

Leakey, D. M. Further effects produced by two loudspeakers in echo-free conditions. *Journal of the Acoustical Society of America*, 1957, **29**, 966.

Leakey, D. M., Sayers, B. McA., & Cherry, C. Binaural fusion of low- and high-frequency sounds. *Journal of the Acoustical Society of America*, 1958, **30**, 222.

Levelt, W. J. M., Riemersma, J. B., & Bunt, A. A. Binaural additivity of loudness. *British Journal of Mathematical and Statistical Psychology*, 1972, **25**, 51–68.

Levitt, H., & Rabiner, L. R. Binaural release from masking for speech and gain in intelligibility. *Journal of the Acoustical Society of America*, 1967, **42**, 601–608. (a)

Levitt, H., & Rabiner, L. R. Prediciting binaural gain in intelligibility and release from masking for speech. *Journal of the Acoustical Society of America*, 1967, **42**, 820–829. (b)

Licklider, J. C. R. The influence of interaural phase relations upon the masking of speech by white noise. *Journal of the Acoustical Society of America*, 1948, 20, 150–159.

Licklider, J. C. R. Three auditory theories. In S. Koch (Ed.), *Psychology: A study of a science*. Vol. 1. New York: McGraw-Hill, 1959. Pp. 41–44.

Licklider, J. C. R., & Webster, J. C. The discriminability of interaural phase relations in two-component tones. *Journal of the Acoustical Society of America*, 1950, **22**, 191–195.

Licklider, J. C. R., Webster, J. C., & Hedlun, J. M. On the frequency limits of binaural beats. *Journal of the Acoustical Society of America*, 1950, **22**, 468–473.

McFadden, D. Masking-level differences with continuous and with burst masking noise. *Journal of the Acoustical Society of America*, 1966, **40**, 1414–1419.

McFadden, D. Detection of an in-phase signal with and without uncertainty regarding the interaural phase of the masking noise. *Journal of the Acoustical Society of America*, 1967, **41**, 778–781.

McFadden, D. Masking-level differences determined with and without interaural disparities in masker intensity. *Journal of the Acoustical Society of America*, 1968, **44**, 212–223.

McFadden, D. Lateralization and detection of a tonal signal in noise. *Journal of the Acoustical Society of America*, 1969, **45**, 1505–1509.

McFadden, D., Jeffress, L. A., & Ermey, H. L. Differences of interaural phase and level in detection and lateralization: 250 Hz. *Journal of the Acoustical Society of America*, 1971, **50**, 1484–1493.

McFadden, D., Jeffress, L. A., & Lakey, J. R. Differences of interaural phase and level in detection and lateralization: 1000 and 2000 Hz. *Journal of the Acoustical Society of America*, 1972, **52**, 1197–1206. (a)

McFadden, D., Jeffress, L. A., & Russell, W. E. Individual differences in sensitivity to interaural differences in time and level. *Perceptual and Motor Skills*, 1973, **37**, 755–761.

McFadden, D., & Pulliam, K. A. Lateralization and detection of noise-masked tones of different durations. *Journal of the Acoustical Society of America*, 1971, **49**, 1191–1194.

McFadden, D., Russell, W. E., & Pulliam, K. A. Monaural and binaural masking patterns for a low-frequency tone. *Journal of the Acoustical Society of America*, 1972, **51**, 534–543. (b)

McFadden, D., & Sharpley, A. D. Detectability of interaural time differences and interaural level differences as a function of signal duration. *Journal of the Acoustical Society of America*, 1972, **52**, 574–576.

Metz, P. J., Bismarck, G. von, & Durlach, N. I. Further results on binaural unmasking and the EC model. II. Noise bandwidth and interaural phase. *Journal of the Acoustical Society of America*, 1968, **43**, 1085–1091.

Mickunas, J. Interaural time delay and apparent direction of clicks. *Journal of the Acoustical Society of America*, 1963, **35**, 788 (A).

Mills, A. W. On the minimum audible angle. *Journal of the Acoustical Society of America*, 1958, **30**, 237–246.

Mills, A. W. Lateralization of high-frequency tones. *Journal of the Acoustical Society of America*, 1960, **32**, 132–134.

Mills, A. W. Auditory localization. In J. V. Tobias (Ed.), *Foundations of modern auditory theory*. Vol. 2. New York: Academic Press, 1972. Pp. 303–348.

Molino, J. Perceiving the range of a sound source when the direction is known. *Journal of the Acoustical Society of America*, 1973, **53**, 1301–1304.

Mosko, J. D., & House, A. S. Binaural unmasking of vocalic signals. *Journal of the Acoustical Society of America*, 1971, **49**, 1203–1212.

Moter, J. T. Binaural detection of signal with angular dispersion of masking noise. BS thesis, Dept. of Electrical Engineering, MIT, Cambridge, Massachusetts, 1964.

Moushegian, G., & Jeffress, L. A. Role of interaural time and intensity differences in the lateralization of low-frequency tones. *Journal of the Acoustical Society of America*, 1959, **31**, 1441–1445.

Nordlund, B. Physical factors in angular localization. *Acta Oto-Laryngologica*, 1962, **54**, 75–93.

Oster, G. Auditory beats in the brain. *Scientific American*, 1973, **229**, 94–102.

Perrott, D. R. Rôle of signal onset in sound localization. *Journal of the Acoustical Society of America*, 1969, **45**, 436–445.

Perrott, D. R., & Barry, S. H. Binaural fusion. *Journal of Auditory Research*, 1969, **3**, 263–269.

Perrott, D. R., Briggs, R., & Perrott, S. Binaural fusion: Its limits as defined by signal duration and signal onset. *Journal of the Acoustical Society of America*, 1970, **47**, 565–568.

Perrott, D. R., & Elfner, L. F. Monaural localization. *Journal of Auditory Research*, 1968, **8**, 185–193.

Perrott, D. R., & Nelson, M. A. Limits for the detection of binaural beats. *Journal of the Acoustical Society of America*, 1969, **46**, 1477–1481.

Pinheiro, M. L., & Tobin, H. Interaural intensity differences for intracranial lateralization. *Journal of the Acoustical Society of America*, 1969, **46**, 1482–1487.

Pohlmann, L. D., & Sorkin, R. D. Binaural masking level difference for pulse train signals of differing interaural correlation. *Journal of the Acoustical Society of America*, 1974, **55**, 1293–1298.

Pollack, I. Can the binaural system preserve temporal information for jitter? *Journal of the Acoustical Society of America*, 1968, **44**, 968–972.

Pollack, I. Interaural correlation detection for auditory pulse trains. *Journal of the Acoustical Society of America*, 1971, **49**, 1213–1217.

Pollack, I., & Pickett, J. M. Stereophonic listening and speech intelligibility against voice babble. *Journal of the Acoustical Society of America*, 1958, **30**, 131–133.

Pollack, I., & Rose, M. Effect of head movement on the localization of sounds in the equatorial plane. *Perception and Psychophysics,* 1967, **2,** 591–596.

Pollack, I., & Trittipoe, W. J. Binaural listening and interaural noise cross correlation. *Journal of the Acoustical Society of America,* 1959, **31,** 1250–1252. (a)

Pollack, I., & Trittipoe, W. J. Interaural noise correlations: Examination of variables. *Journal of the Acoustical Society of America,* 1959, **31,** 1616–1618. (b)

Porsolt, R. D., & Irwin, R. J. Binaural summation in loudness of two tones as a function of their bandwidth. *American Journal of Psychology,* 1967, **80,** 384–390.

Punch, J., & Carhart, R. Influence of interaural phase on forward masking. *Journal of the Acoustical Society of America,* 1973, **54,** 897–904.

Raab, D. H., & Osman, E. Effect of masking noise on lateralization and loudness of clicks. *Journal of the Acoustical Society of America,* 1962, **34,** 1620–1624.

Rabiner, L. R., Laurence, C. L., & Durlach, N. I. Further results on binaural unmasking and the EC model. *Journal of the Acoustical Society of America,* 1966, **40,** 62–70.

Rayleigh, J. W. S. *The theory of sound.* Vol. 2. (2nd. ed.) New York: Dover, 1945.

Reynolds, G. S., & Stevens, S. S. Binaural summation of loudness. *Journal of the Acoustical Society of America,* 1960, **32,** 1337–1344.

Rilling, M. E., & Jeffress, L. A. Narrow-band noise and tones as signals in binaural detection. *Journal of the Acoustical Society of America,* 1965, **38,** 202–206.

Robertson, R. M., & Goldstein, D. P. Binaural unmasking and frequency discrimination. *Journal of the Acoustical Society of America,* 1967, **42,** 1180 (A).

Robinson, D. E. The effect of interaural signal-frequency disparity on signal detectability. *Journal of the Acoustical Society of America,* 1971, **50,** 568–571.

Robinson, D. E., & Deatherage, B. H. On the limits of binaural interaction. *Journal of the Acoustical Society of America,* 1964, **36,** 1029 (A).

Robinson, D. E., & Dolan, T. R. Effect of signal frequency on the MLD for uncorrelated noise. *Journal of the Acoustical Society of America,* 1972, **51,** 1945–1946.

Robinson, D. E., & Egan, J. P. Lateralization of an auditory signal in correlated noise and in uncorrelated noise as a function of signal frequency. *Perception and Psychophysics,* 1974, **15,** 281–284.

Robinson, D. E., & Jeffress, L. A. Effect of varying the interaural noise correlation on the detectability of tonal signals. *Journal of the Acoustical Society of America,* 1963, **35,** 1947–1952.

Robinson, D. E., Langford, T. L., & Yost, W. A. Masking of tones by tones and of noise by noise. *Perception and Psychophysics,* 1974, **15,** 159–168.

Robinson, D. E., & Trahiotis, C. Effects of signal duration and masker duration on detectability under diotic and dichotic listening conditions. *Perception and Psychophysics,* 1972, **12,** 333–334.

Roffler, S. K., & Butler, R. A. Localization of tonal stimuli in the vertical plane. *Journal of the Acoustical Society of America,* 1968, **43,** 1260–1266. (a)

Roffler, S. K., & Butler, R. A. Factors that influence the localization of sound in the vertical plane. *Journal of the Acoustical Society of America,* 1968, **43,** 1255–1259. (b)

Rowland, R. C., & Tobias, J. F. Interaural intensity difference limen. *Journal of Speech and Hearing Research,* 1967, **10,** 745–756.

Sandel, T. T., Teas, D. C., Feddersen, W. E., & Jeffress, L. A. Localization of sound from single and paired sources. *Journal of the Acoustical Society of America,* 1955, **27,** 842–852.

Sayers, B. McA. Acoustic-image lateralization judgments with binaural tones. *Journal of the Acoustical Society of America,* 1964, **36,** 923–926.

Sayers, B. McA., & Cherry, E. C. Mechanism of binaural fusion in the hearing of speech. *Journal of the Acoustical Society of America,* 1957, **29,** 973–987.

Sayers, B. McA., & Lynn, P. A. Interaural amplitude effects in binaural hearing. *Journal of the Acoustical Society of America,* 1968, **44,** 973–978.

Sayers, B. McA., & Toole, F. E. Acoustic-image lateralization judgments with binaural transients. *Journal of the Acoustical Society of America*, 1964, **36**, 1199–1205.

Scharf, B. Binaural loudness summation as a function of bandwidth. *Sixth International Congress of Acoustics, Tokyo*, 1968, A-3-5, 25–28.

Scharf, B. Dichotic summation of loudness. *Journal of the Acoustical Society of America*, 1969, **45**, 1193–1205.

Schenkel, K. D. Über die Abhängigkeit der Mithörschwellen von der Interauralen Phasenlage des Testschalls. *Acustica*, 1964, **14**, 337–346.

Schenkel, K. D. Die Abhängigkeit der beidohrigen Mithörschwellen von der Frequenz des Testschalls und vom Pegel des verdeckenden Schalles. *Acustica*, 1966, **17**, 345–356.

Schenkel, K. D. Die biedohrigen Mithörschwellen von Impulsen. *Acustica*, 1967, **16**, 38–46. (a)

Schenkel, K. D. Accumulation theory of binaural-masked thresholds. *Journal of the Acoustical Society of America*, 1967, **41**, 20–30. (b)

Schubert, E. D. Some preliminary experiments on binaural time delay and intelligibility. *Journal of the Acoustical Society of America*, 1956, **28**, 895–901.

Schubert, E. D. Interpretation of the Butler-Naunton localization shifts. *Journal of the Acoustical Society of America*, 1963, **35**, 113.

Schubert, E. D., & Elpern, B. S. Psychophysical estimate of the velocity of the traveling wave. *Journal of the Acoustical Society of America*, 1959, **31**, 990–994.

Schubert, E. D., & Schultz, M. C. Some aspects of binaural signal selection. *Journal of the Acoustical Society of America*, 1962, **34**, 844–849.

Schubert, E. D., & Wernick, J. Envelope versus microstructure in the fusion of dichotic signals. *Journal of the Acoustical Society of America*, 1969, **45**, 1525–1531.

Searle, C. L. Cues required for externalization and vertical localization. *Journal of the Acoustical Society of America*, 1973, **54**, 308 (A).

Shaw, E. A. G. Transformation of sound pressure level from the free field to the eardrum in the horizontal plane. *Journal of the Acoustical Society of America*, 1974, **56**, 1848–1861. (a)

Shaw, E. A. G. The external ear. In W. D. Keidel & W. D. Neff (Eds.), *Handbook of sensory physiology*. Vol. V/1. New York: Springer-Verlag, 1974. (b)

Shaxby, J. H., & Gage, F. H. The localization of sounds in the median plane: An experimental investigation of the physical processes involved. Medical Research Council (Britain), Special Report, 1932, Ser. No. 166, pp. 1–32.

Small, A. M., Boggess, J., Klich, D., Kuehn, D., Thelin, J., & Wiley, T. MLD's in forward and backward masking. *Journal of the Acoustical Society of America*, 1972, **51**, 1365–1367.

Sondhi, M. M., & Guttman, N. Width of the spectrum effective in the binaural release of masking. *Journal of the Acoustical Society of America*, 1966, **40**, 600–606.

Sorkin, R. D. Uncertain signal detection with simultaneous contralateral cues. *Journal of the Acoustical Society of America*, 1965, **38**, 207–212.

Sorkin, R. D. Temporal interference effects in auditory amplitude discrimination. *Perception and Psychophysics*, 1966, **1**, 55–58.

Sorkin, R. D. Monaural detection with partially correlated cues. *Journal of the Acoustical Society of America*, 1972, **51**, 123(A).

Taylor, M. M., & Clarke, D. P. J. Monaural detection with contralateral cue (MDCC). II. Interaural delay of cue and signal. *Journal of the Acoustical Society of America*, 1971, **49**, 1243–1253.

Taylor, M. M., Clarke, D. P. J., & Smith, S. M. Monaural detection with contralateral cue (MDCC). III. Sinusoidal signals at a constant performance level. *Journal of the Acoustical Society of America*, 1971, **49**, 1795–1804.

Taylor, M. M., & Forbes, S. M. Monaural detection with contralateral cue (MDCC). I. Better than energy detector performance by human observers. *Journal of the Acoustical Society of America*, 1969, **46**, 1519–1526.

Taylor, M. M., Smith, S. M., & Clarke, D. P. J. Monaural detection with contralateral cue (MDCC). IV. Psychometric functions with sinusoidal signals. *Journal of the Acoustical Society of America*, 1971, **50**, 1151–1161.

Teas, D. C. Lateralization of acoustic transients. *Journal of the Acoustical Society of America*, 1962, **34**, 1460–1465.

Thurlow, W. R., & Bernstein, S. Simultaneous two-tone pitch discrimination. *Journal of the Acoustical Society of America*, 1957, **29**, 515–519.

Thurlow, W. R., & Elfner, L. F. Pure-tone cross-ear localization effects. *Journal of the Acoustical Society of America*, 1959, **31**, 1606–1608.

Tobias, J. V. Application of a 'relative' procedure to a problem in binaural-beat perception. *Journal of the Acoustical Society of America*, 1963, **35**, 1442–1447.

Tobias, J. V., & Schubert, E. D. Effective onset duration of auditory stimuli. *Journal of the Acoustical Society of America*, 1959, **31**, 1595–1605.

Tobias, J. V., & Zerlin, S. Lateralization threshold as a function of stimulus duration. *Journal of the Acoustical Society of America*, 1959, **31**, 1591–1594.

Toole, F. E. In-head localization of acoustic images. *Journal of the Acoustical Society of America*, 1970, **48**, 943–949.

Toole, F. E., & Sayers, B. McA. Lateralization judgments and the nature of binaural acoustic images. *Journal of the Acoustical Society of America*, 1965, **37**, 319–324. (a)

Toole, F. E., & Sayers, B. McA. Inferences of neural activity associated with binaural acoustics images. *Journal of the Acoustical Society of America*, 1965, **38**, 769–779. (b)

Townsend, T. H., & Goldstein, D. P. Suprathreshold binaural unmasking. *Journal of the Acoustical Society of America*, 1972, **51**, 621–624.

Treisman, M., & Irwin, R. J. Auditory intensity discriminal scale I. Evidence derived from binaural intensity summation. *Journal of the Acoustical Society of America*, 1967, **42**, 586–592.

Wallach, H. On sound localization. *Journal of the Acoustical Society of America*, 1939, **10**, 270–274.

Wallach, H. The role of head movements and vestibular and visual cues in sound localization. *Journal of Experimental Psychology*, 1940, **27**, 339–368.

Wallach, H., Newman, E. B., & Rosenzweig, M. R. The precedence effect in sound localization. *American Journal of Psychology*, 1949, **62**, 315–336.

Webster, F. A. The influence of interaural phase on masked thresholds. I. The role of interaural time-deviation. *Journal of the Acoustical Society of America*, 1951, **23**, 452–462.

Weston, P. B., & Miller, J. D. Use of noise to eliminate one ear from masking experiments. *Journal of the Acoustical Society of America*, 1965, **37**, 638–646.

Weston, P. B., Miller, J. D., & Hirsh, I. J. Release from masking for speech. *Journal of the Acoustical Society of America*, 1965, **38**, 1053–1054.

Whitworth, R. H., & Jeffress, L. A. Time versus intensity in the localization of tones. *Journal of the Acoustical Society of America*, 1961, **33**, 925–929.

Wightman, F. L. Binaural masking with sine-wave masker. *Journal of the Acoustical Society of America*, 1969, **45**, 72–78.

Wightman, F. L. Detection of binaural tones as a function of masker bandwidth. *Journal of the Acoustical Society of America*, 1971, **50**, 623–636.

Wightman, F. L., & Houtgast, T. Binaural critical bandwidth as a function of signal bandwidth. *Journal of the Acoustical Society of America*, 1972, **51**, 124 (A).

Wilbanks, W. A. Detection of a narrow-band noise as a function of the interaural correlation of both signal and masker. *Journal of the Acoustical Society of America*, 1971, **49**, 1814–1817.

Wilbanks, W. A., & Cornelius, P. T. Binaural detection of low-frequency tones as a function of noise level. *Journal of the Acoustical Society of America*, 1969, **46**, 126 (A).

Wilbanks, W. A., Cornelius, P. T., & Houff, C. D. Binaural detection as a function of signal frequency and noise level. *Journal of the Acoustical Society of America*, 1970, **48**, 86 (A).

Wilbanks, W. A., & Whitmore, J. K. Detection of monaural signals as a function of interaural noise correlation and signal frequency. *Journal of the Acoustical Society of America*, 1968, **43**, 785–797.

Woodworth, R. S. *Experimental psychology*. New York: Holt, 1938.

Yost, W. A. Tone-on-tone masking for three listening conditions. *Journal of the Acoustical Society of America*, 1972, **52**, 1234–1237.

Yost, W. A. Discrimination of interaural phase differences. *Journal of the Acoustical Society of America*, 1974, **55**, 1299–1303.

Yost, W. A., Penner, M. J., & Feth, L. L. Signal detection as a function of contralateral sinusoid-to-noise ratio. *Journal of the Acoustical Society of America*, 1972, **51**, 1966–1970.

Yost, W. A., Wightman, F. L., & Green, D. M. Lateralization of filtered clicks. *Journal of the Acoustical Society of America*, 1971, **50**, 1526–1531.

Zerlin, S. Interaural time and intensity difference and the MLD. *Journal of the Acoustical Society of America*, 1966, **39**, 134–137.

Zwislocki, J., & Feldman, R. S. Just noticeable differences in dichotic phase. *Journal of the Acoustical Society of America*, 1956, **28**, 860–864.

Chapter 11

MODELS OF BINAURAL INTERACTION

H. STEVEN COLBURN AND NATHANIEL I. DURLACH

I. INTRODUCTION

In Chapter 10, we discussed a variety of binaural phenomena associated with the perception of interaural differences in the binaural stimulus. In this chapter, we discuss some of the models that have been constructed to explain such phenomena with emphasis on how the two stimulus waveforms are analyzed to make use of these differences. Generally speaking, we have included only those models in which the hypotheses concerning the operations performed on the acoustic inputs are sufficiently well delineated to permit quantitative predictions of psychoacoustic performance. With only minor exceptions, there is no consideration given to the relations between these models and the increasing amount of physiological data showing binaural interaction (see, e.g., the summary by Erulkar, 1972). We have omitted consideration of these relations because of the large amount of other material that requires discussion and because such consideration requires that the models themselves be understood first.

For presentation purposes, the models are divided into five categories, and discussed in following sections. Each section includes outlines of the various models and summaries of the applications of the models to perceptual data. Section II is devoted to "count-comparison models" and includes the work of Békésy, Matzker, van Bergeijk, and Hall; Section III, to "interaural-difference-detector models" and includes the work of Jeffress and his associates, Webster, and Hafter and Carrier; Section IV, to "noise-suppression models" and focuses on the work of Durlach and his associates (and includes a few comments on the work of Schenkel); Section V, to "correlation models" and includes the work of Sayers and his associates, Dolan and Robinson, McFadden, and Osman; and Section VI, to the "auditory-nerve-based model" of Colburn.

In Section VII, we attempt to provide an overview of both the similarities and differences among the models. Included is a discussion of the elements that are common to almost all of the models, as well as a summary of the relations between the models and the data with emphasis on the differences among the models.

II. COUNT-COMPARISON MODELS

In this section, we consider lateralization models in which image position is determined by comparing the activity levels in two neural populations (count-comparison models). On the whole, these models are qualitative, of restricted applicability, do not quantitatively specify internal noise, and have not been applied to binaural phenomena other than lateralization. On the other hand, the mechanism of binaural interaction in these models, especially the way in which lateralization is influenced by an interaural intensity difference, represents an important alternative to the other models. Moreover, the fact that most of the work with these models has been qualitative and concerned only with lateralization does not preclude the development of a more quantitative and general model that incorporates some of the same ideas.

The first model of this type, suggested by Békésy (1930) to describe his own observations of lateralization phenomena, assumed a population of nerve cells that are innervated by fibers from both ears and that become tuned to one of two excited states according to the source of the excitation. Generally speaking, a cell is "tuned left" by an acoustic stimulus if its excitation comes from fibers originating on the left and "tuned right" if its excitation comes from fibers originating on the right. The lateralization of the stimulus is then determined by a comparison of the number of cells "tuned left" with the number of cells "tuned right" (i.e., the image is on the left, at the center, or on the right according to whether the number of cells tuned left is, respectively, greater than, equal to, or less than the number of cells tuned right). For impulsive stimuli, Békésy assumed that the input from each side causes a wave of excitation to sweep through the cell population and that each wave tunes cells according to the source of the wave until the waves from opposite ears meet and extinguish each other. If the binaural stimulus contains no interaural differences, the excitation waves meet in the center of the population and equal numbers of cells are tuned to each direction, resulting in a centered image. If the stimulus contains an interaural time delay, the excitation wave from the delayed component will be extinguished before it has progressed to the center of the cell population, more cells will be tuned to the opposite direction, and thus the image will be localized toward the side whose stimulus arrives earlier. Apparently then, if a cell is not tuned at a particular time, the next input firing from either side will tune it to the appropriate state for some interval of time during which other inputs from the two sides are ignored.

Békésy considered two hypotheses to include the effects of interaural intensity difference. The first, which he rejected, is that neural conduction velocity depends on stimulus intensity. According to this idea (later generalized to include changes in synaptic delays with level, and named the *latency hypothesis*), an interaural intensity difference causes an interaural time difference at the place of interaural comparison. Békésy pointed out, however, that the lateralization of a 3-kHz continuous tone is independent of interaural time (or phase) difference and thus, that in this case the effects of an intensity difference must be caused by some other mechanism. Moreover, since the dependence of lateralization on interaural intensity difference was observed to be the same for the high-frequency tone as for clicks and noise (stimuli whose lateralization does depend upon interaural delay), Békésy concluded that the latency hypothesis is not acceptable. On the basis of these experiments and others with modulated high-frequency tones, Békésy adopted a second hypothesis, namely, that the effect of lateralization caused by interaural intensity difference is determined directly from the relative magnitudes of the excitations at each ear. According to this hypothesis, more cells are tuned by a stronger excitation wave (although the extinction point is independent of the relative strengths), and thus, for a given interaural delay, the number of cells tuned to each side can be manipulated by interaural intensity. In particular, a given time delay can be counteracted by an increase in intensity at the delayed ear, and the model thus predicts qualitatively the subjective phenomenon of time–intensity trading. Figure 1 illustrates the tuned and untuned cells for a centered impulsive image with non-zero interaural time and intensity differences. In order to make a quantitative analysis, or even to make rough predictions for stimuli of longer duration, it is necessary to specify more precisely the nature of the input patterns and the properties of the cell population. There are several difficulties with a direct physiological realization of Békésy's model (particularly the "tunable neurons"), and we turn to extensions of this model that avoid some of these difficulties.

Matzker (1958) suggested a rough outline for a lateralization model that he designed to be consistent with anatomical and electrophysiological data and that is essentially consistent with Békésy's ideas. Both models are based

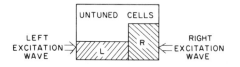

FIG. 1. Schematic illustration of tuned and untuned cells in Békésy's lateralization model. L denotes the cells *tuned left* and R the cells *tuned right*. For the case illustrated, which corresponds to a centered image since the L and R areas are equal, the stimulus to the right ear is more intense, so that the right excitation wave is more effective in tuning cells (vertical extent of R vs L), and the stimulus to the left ear is leading in time, so that the left excitation wave progresses farther than the right wave (horizontal extent of L vs R) before the waves meet and extinguish each other.

upon a comparison of two types of activity, and both reject the latency hypothesis as the fundamental source of time–intensity trading. In Matzker's model, Békésy's population of tunable cells is replaced by two symmetric auditory pathways, each of which is excited by the stimulation at one ear, and lateralization is determined by a comparison between activity levels at some relatively central nucleus. Matzker also assumed that contralateral inhibitory pathways are present so that a firing on an inhibitory fiber blocks the transmission of firings along excitatory fibers for a few milliseconds. The inhibitory mechanism increases the asymmetry of responses on the pathways that is caused by an interaural intensity difference in the stimulus waveforms. By this mechanism, for impulsive stimuli at least, an interaural time delay also results in an asymmetry of responses in the two pathways, since inhibition is increased on the pathway receiving the delayed signal and decreased on the pathway receiving the delayed signal and decreased on the pathway receiving the advanced signal. The influences of time and intensity on activity levels are thus somewhat independent and the effects on lateralization of time and intensity can be made to reinforce or cancel. This model, like Békésy's, is rather vague about detailed structural assumptions, and more detail is required for quantitative testing or for applications to other types of stimuli.

A restatement of Békésy's idea in a form that is both more structurally specific and more physiologically oriented than Békésy's original outline was presented by van Bergeijk (1962). van Bergeijk's model assumes the the binaural interaction occurs at a relatively peripheral pair of nuclei (the accessory nuclei of the superior olive) and that lateralization is determined by a comparison of the number of neural firings in the left nucleus with the number in the right. For each nucleus, ipsilateral inputs are inhibitory and contralateral inputs are excitatory, and the image is lateralized to the side opposite the nucleus with the greater number of firings. Figure 2 illustrates the structure for a single pair of incoming fibers from each side. For a particular neuron in the nucleus, an input firing from an inhibitory fiber blocks the neuron for a few milliseconds so that input firings from an excitatory fiber will not cause the neuron to fire. If input firings from the left and right fibers arrive at the nuclei simultaneously, about half of the neurons in the appropriate row of each nucleus receive the excitatory stimulus before the inhibitory one. Thus, identical inputs result in an equal number of neurons firing in each nucleus, creating a centered image. If the left input leads the right, the excitatory firing will arrive earlier than the inhibitory firing at the right nucleus (and later at the left nucleus), and more neurons will be excited on the right. Thus, a stimulus with the left input leading will create an image to the left. If a firing occurs on a left input fiber and none on the corresponding right fiber, all the neurons in the associated row will be excited in the right nucleus and none in the left nucleus. Thus, a stimulus with the left input more intense will create a band of excited neurons in the right nucleus and a band of inhibited neurons in the left nucleus, and cause the image to be located on the left. A sketch of the distribution of excited cells in each nucleus for various stimulus conditions, including a condition in which time and intensity are traded to result in a centered image, is shown in Fig. 3 (where again the shaded area represents the cells that are excited). In this sketch, it is assumed that the stimuli are impulsive, that each input fiber fires if and only if a threshold intensity for that fiber is exceeded by the corresponding signal, and that the latency is independent of stimulus intensity.

van Bergeijk (1962) pointed out that this model predicts the observed decrease (David, Guttman, & van Bergeijk, 1959) in the time–intensity trading ratio as overall intensity increases if the reasonable assumption is made that the number of additional cells stimulated by increasing the intensity 1 dB is approximately independent of intensity (i.e., that the width of the band due to the interaural intensity difference depends only on the decibel difference). In this case, since the number of cells affected by a fixed interaural delay increases with overall intensity, the amount of delay required to balance a

FIG. 2. Neural structure proposed by van Bergeijk for lateralization. A few cells are shown from corresponding rows in symmetrical nuclei. A cell is excited when a firing from the excitatory fiber arrives before a firing from the inhibitory fiber. The input pathways are assumed to be constructed such that simultaneous acoustic inputs result in simultaneous arrivals of firings at the center cell of the rows in each nucleus, so that in the left nucleus, for example, the cells left of center are inhibited and the cells right of center are excited.

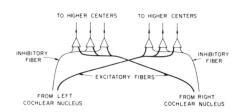

TO HIGHER CENTERS   TO HIGHER CENTERS

INHIBITORY FIBER   INHIBITORY FIBER

EXCITATORY FIBERS

FROM LEFT COCHLEAR NUCLEUS   FROM RIGHT COCHLEAR NUCLEUS

LEFT NUCLEUS   RIGHT NUCLEUS

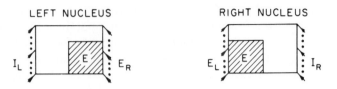

(a) EQUAL AMPLITUDES - NO RELATIVE DELAY - IMAGE CENTERED

(b) LEFT STIMULUS ADVANCED - IMAGE LEFT OF CENTER

(c) LEFT STIMULUS ATTENUATED - IMAGE RIGHT OF CENTER

(d) LEFT STIMULUS ADVANCED AND ATTENUATED - IMAGE CENTERED

FIG. 3. Schematic illustration of excited cells (E) in symmetric nuclei of van Bergeijk's model for impulsive stimuli and various interaural configurations. The blocks for each pair of nuclei are continuous representations of many rows of cells, each row of cells having the structure illustrated in Fig. 2. The input fibers (I_L represents inhibitory fibers from the left and E_R represents excitatory fibers from the right) are arranged such that a larger stimulus amplitude causes firings over a greater vertical extent, i.e., input fibers with higher thresholds are placed higher in the block. The horizontal extent of excited regions is determined, as in Fig. 2, by the interaural time delay. Equal excited areas result in a centered image, and unequal excited areas result in an image that is lateralized on the side with the smaller excited area.

1-dB intensity difference (i.e., the size of the trading ratio) will decrease with overall intensity. It is also clear that this model predicts qualitatively the lateralization of high-frequency tones as well as impulsive stimuli since there are no interaural time effects for such tones and the interaural intensity effects are roughly independent of the stimulus.

A quantitative formulation of this model, as well as application to a larger class of stimuli and experiments, requires additional assumptions about the input firing patterns (including stochastic aspects), inhibitory effects, and the distribution of time delays in the central nuclei. One could make predictions concerning interaural sensitivity by assuming that the difference in the numbers of cells excited in the two nuclei is a decision variable that is used optimally by higher centers. A key feature of this analysis, of course, would have to be the specification of internal noise.

A set of physiological measurements together with calculations based on a model closely related to the preceding models, in which position is determined by the relative number of excited cells in two nuclei and in which the response of a particular cell depends upon the inputs to both ears, was presented by Hall (1965). He measured the electrophysiological responses of cells in cat (the neurons were presumed from indirect evidence to be located in the accessory nuclei of the superior olive) to binaural click stimuli, with average intensity, interaural time delay, and interaural intensity difference as stimulus parameters. Although several types of cells were observed, the study focused on a particular type named "time–intensity trading cells." These cells were excited by contralateral stimulation and inhibited by ipsilateral stimulation, and the degree of inhibition was a function of both the interaural time delay and the interaural intensity difference. Hall demonstrated the compatibility of his physiological data and model with behavioral phenomena by showing that the time–intensity trading ratios computed from his physiological data were comparable to behavioral values. Although Hall's work offers support for a lateralization mechanism that is based upon relative amounts of neural activity and that includes inhibition as a basic component, he did not consider the physiological mechanisms governing the behavior of the time–intensity trading cells. In particular, he did not determine the extent to which the effects of interaural intensity difference were caused by the dependence of latency on intensity at the periphery.

Unlike all the other work on count-comparison models, which focused exclusively on mean responses and ignored response variability, Hall considered the variability observed in his physiological data and the implications of this variability for interaural discrimination. By postulating that both the input patterns and the responses of the time–intensity trading cells are statistically independent from cell to cell and from trial to trial and are memoryless from trial to trial (so that the probability that at least one firing occurs in response to a given click in a given cell—the quantity estimated in the physiological measurements—is constant from trial to trial and is independent of the firings on other trials or in other cells), Hall derived predictions that were found to be roughly consistent with human behavioral data describing the dependence of interaural time and amplitude sensitivity on overall intensity. It is not possible to predict the response of Hall's time–intensity trading cells to stimuli other than clicks since an input–output description of these cells cannot be deduced from available data, especially in the absence of data on multiple firings and latency.

III. INTERAURAL-DIFFERENCE-DETECTOR MODELS

In this section, we discuss models in which it is assumed that the system measures interaural differences in time and, in some cases, amplitude. Most of these models were based upon the early work of Jeffress (1948) on lateralization. Some of these models are directed toward lateralization phenomena and some are applied primarily to detection phenomena; none, however, has satisfactorily described lateralization, interaural discrimination, and detection. In many cases, the internal noise assumptions are not well specified and quantitative predictions are not possible.

Jeffress (1948) outlined a hypothetical neural network that converted interaural time differences in the stimulus into "place information" in the network (i.e., into information that is contained in the average rates of firing of neurons, as opposed to the detailed time patterns of firings). This network is displayed in Fig. 4. Since it is completely symmetric, attention will be confined to the left complex of tertiary fibers. When the stimulus is presented with no interaural differences, the left and right auditory tracts are symmetrically stimulated and, on the average, nerve impulses arrive at X and Y simultaneously, and therefore at the nerve cell of Tertiary Fiber 4 simultaneously. At Cells 3, 2, and 1, the right-tract impulses arrive progressively later than the left-tract impulses, and at Cells 5, 6, and 7, progressively earlier. If we assume that coincident stimulation is more effective in invoking a response from a cell than less coincident stimulation, then Cell 4 responds

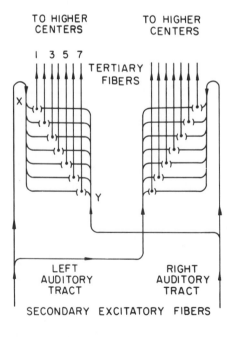

FIG. 4. Neural network proposed by Jeffress for localization of low-frequency tones. The tertiary neurons act as coincidence detectors: a tertiary fiber is more likely to respond when firings from left and right secondary fibers reach the cell body at times that are closer to simultaneity. Interaural time differences in the firings of the input fibers are thus converted to differences in the spatial excitation pattern of the output fibers. The effects of interaural intensity differences are included by assuming that a more intense signal leads to earlier firings in the secondary fibers (the latency hypothesis). [From Jeffress (1948). Copyright 1948 by the American Psychological Association. Reprinted by permission.]

maximally and Cells 3, 2, and 1 and 5, 6, and 7 respond increasingly less when the external interaural time delay is zero. If the left stimulus is presented earlier, coincidence will occur closer to point Y than point X, and the average rate of firing of Cell 4 will be less than the average rate at Cell 5, 6 or 7 (depending upon the delay). Interaural time delay at the input is thus represented by the distribution of the response over cells at different places.

Interaural intensity differences are assumed to change the relative interaural time delays in the primary and secondary fibers (the so-called latency hypothesis) such that a stimulus that is more intense to the left ear, but has no external interaural delay, will generate impulses that arrive earlier at point X than at point Y and therefore affect the neural place information in a way similar to an external delay at the right ear. Thus, Jeffress's network, combined with the latency hypothesis, can be used to interpret the dependence of lateralization on both time and intensity (including time–intensity trading) for any stimulus in which the fibers carry the appropriate timing information.

This model differs in two basic ways from the count-comparison models discussed in the previous section. First, it assumes that the internal representation of the interaural differences consists of a whole distribution of counts over a large number of fibers; in the count-comparison models, this representation is restricted to merely two numbers. Second, it makes use of the latency hypothesis to mediate time–intensity trading; the count-comparison models reject this hypothesis.

A coincidence network essentially equivalent to that of Jeffress was incorporated by Licklider (1959) into his triplex theory for pitch perception. This theory assumes peripheral filters, neural transduction, a cross-coincidence analysis of the signals from opposite ears, an autocoincidence analysis of the outputs of the first coincidence network, and a final analysis by a self-organizing neural network. The cross-coincidence mechanism, the component of the model that is relevant to binaural interaction, "mediates sound localization in phenomenal space" and was added to provide an explanation of Huggins's binaural creation-of-pitch effect (Cramer & Huggins, 1958).

The first interaural-difference-detector models that were applied to masking phenomena were based on Webster's hypothesis that interaural time difference provides the dominant cue for binaural signal detection (Webster, 1951). Webster applied this hypothesis to the detection of narrow-band target signals masked by broad-band random noise. He made use of the critical-band idea that the total stimulus to each ear passes through a narrow bandpass filter centered on the center frequency of the target signal (so that the output can be described as a sinusoidal signal with slowly varying amplitude and phase). He noted that when the interaural relations of the target signal and masking noise are different, the interaural time difference between the outputs of the narrow-band filters depends upon the presence or absence of the target signal. This led Webster to postulate that the advantages achieved in binaural detection (which only occur when the inter-aural differences in the target signal are distinct from those in the masking noise) are the result of detecting the change in interaural time delay when the signal is added. A general block diagram of a detection model based on these ideas is shown in Fig. 5. (The dashed pathways, concerned with interaural amplitude differences, which were not considered by Webster, are discussed on pages 479–480.) The detection, for arbitrary stimulus con-figurations, is assumed to be based on a combination of binaural and mon-aural processing (the latter is required for cases in which the interaural relations of the target signal are identical to those of the masking noise because in these cases the addition of the target signal causes no change in the interaural relations).

Predictions for masked threshold based upon Webster's hypothesis have been compared with results from a wide variety of experiments. Webster (1951) made calculations for narrow-band target signals masked by broad-band random noise assuming that the final processor can detect changes in in-teraural time delay greater than some critical value that is fixed for all condi-tions and frequencies. (This critical value reflects the limited resolution of the binaural system and specifies, indirectly, the effects of internal noise.) In order to simplify the computations, he approximated the band of noise out of the narrow-band filter by a tone with an amplitude equal to the rms value of

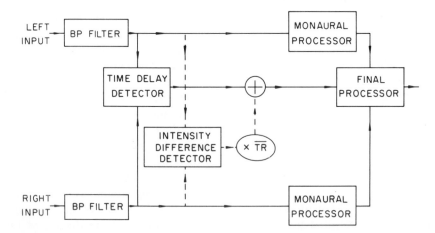

FIG. 5. Block diagram of interaural-difference-detector models. The solid pathways reflect the essential elements of Webster–Jeffress detection models. The dashed pathway shows one way in which interaural intensity differences could be made available in addition to interaural time differences; in this case, the weighting factor $\overline{TR}$ corresponds to the time–intensity trading ratio. The intensity-difference information could also be included by postulating a peripheral time–intensity trade or by postulating interactions in the final processor between the time-delay-detector output and the monaural-processor outputs. Which of these possibilities is most appro-priate depends upon the specific model under consideration (see text).

the noise and a phase that is fixed at a value relative to the phase of the target signal such that the change in the interaural time delay caused by the addition of the target signal is maximized. (Actually, of course, the change in the interaural time delay that occurs in the stimulus when the target signal is added depends on the amplitude and phase of the masking signal relative to the target signal and these vary randomly during the presentation of the target signal at a rate determined by the bandwidth of the peripheral filter.) With these assumptions and approximations, Webster computed the frequency dependence of the detection thresholds of monaural signals and out-of-phase signals in backgrounds of masking noise that is identical in both ears. The application of Webster's hypothesis was then continued, using similar assumptions and approximations, in an important paper by Jeffress, Blodgett, Sandel, and Wood (1956). They considered masking of tones by both tones and noise, and included both monaural and binaural phenomena. The value of the interaural-time-deviation threshold obtained by fitting the data on binaural masked thresholds with this model was found to be of the order of 100 μsec. The decreased sensitivity (i.e., the increase in the minimum achievable threshold) that was observed when the noise image was off the median plane (due to the introduction of interaural differences in the noise) was interpreted in terms of a decrease in the density of cells used to measure interaural time off the median plane.

This interaural-time-detector model has been successful in describing substantial amounts of data on lateralization and binaural masked thresholds. It has numerous inadequacies, however, even though many of them have been ameliorated by later work. Some of these inadequacies are the following. First, it ignores all statistical problems and does not include a description of internal noise or of how the interaural time deviation is used to make decisions. Second, since the interaural-time-deviation threshold is assumed to be independent of level, it does not predict the observed dependence of threshold signal-to-noise ratios on the overall level of the total signals at the two ears or at a single ear. Third, since the same threshold is assumed to be independent of frequency, it predicts arbitrarily low thresholds as frequency decreases, and arbitrarily high thresholds as frequency increases. (This is because a fixed time deviation corresponds to increasingly smaller phase deviations as frequency decreases, and increasingly larger phase deviations as frequency increases, and the interaural phase deviation caused by adding the target signal is independent of frequency.) The value of 100 μsec cited previously for the threshold was obtained for relatively intense levels and for intermediate frequencies (e.g., 200 to 1500 Hz). Fourth, the model is clearly inadequate for describing the lateralization of high-frequency tones since the model does not contain any means for taking into account interaural intensity differences other than the latency hypothesis, whereas it is well known that the auditory system is insensitive to interaural phase for high-frequency tones and that primary auditory-nerve fibers show no synchrony of response to the detailed time structure of such stimuli (i.e., instantaneous rates of firing are approximately constant during a high-frequency continuous-tone stimulus.) Fifth, the model is inadequate for describing the results on sensitivity to interaural time delay obtained in simple discrimination experiments. Among the difficulties in this area are the recently reported results on the influence of interaural amplitude difference on the function describing the dependence of the just-noticeable difference in interaural time on the reference value of interaural time (Domnitz, 1973), and the discrepancy between the value of the interaural-time-deviation threshold obtained from the masking data (roughly 100 μsec) and the value of the just-noticeable difference (jnd) in interaural time obtained from discrimination experiments using comparable stimuli (roughly 10 μsec).

The statistical problems have been approached in a preliminary fashion by Robinson (1966) and Levitt and Lundry (1966a,b) and in an analysis by Henning (1973). Robinson calculated the probability distribution of interaural time delays of the total signals for each of several stimulus configurations containing equally detectable target signals. If these distributions were found to be the same, then any decision rule based on observation of this delay would result in correct predictions. Robinson found that although some of the configurations had a common distribution, others did not. Thus, the model could not be evaluated without a specific decision rule and internal-noise postulates. Levitt and Lundry, who also calculated distributions of delays, postulated that detection of the target occurs if the deviation of the interaural time delay from the noise-alone value exceeds some critical value with a probability p. Using this postulate, they computed the critical value of interaural time deviation required to describe binaural detection data for several frequencies and noise conditions. Their results show that, although the critical value is approximately constant for most conditions with frequencies in the range 500–1000 Hz, a marked decrease in interaural time resolution (i.e., an increase in the critical value) is required for lower frequencies. For frequencies above 1500 Hz, it is necessary to specify another mode of detection. Henning (1973) specified an explicit internal noise for the model; he assumed that half-Gaussian noise was added to the interaural phase shift and he computed the dependence of frequency-discrimination performance on the signal-to-noise ratio for an interaurally phase-inverted sinusoid masked by interaurally identical masking noise. Results of these computations failed to describe the large release from masking obtained in masked frequency-discrimination experiments when the interaural phase of the sinusoid is changed from in-phase to out-of-phase.

The problem associated with the lateralization of high-frequency tones was considered by David et al. (1959) in their important paper on binaural interaction of high-frequency complex stimuli. They suggested that one might explain the effect of interaural amplitude difference on the lateralization of high-frequency tones by incorporating some of Békésy's ideas into

Jeffress's model. They argued that a time comparator excited by neural impulse trains with different average rates could result in an asymmetric (with respect to the midline) distribution of responses in the place dimension. However, since a time comparator (by definition) can operate only on the time structure of the waveforms and since advance and delay are equivalent operations for a homogeneous (time-stationary) input firing pattern, we believe that their argument is incorrect and that no statistical argument will lead to the required asymmetry.

The fact that the use of two ears leads to improved sensitivity for some configurations at high frequencies led Durlach (1964a) to postulate the existence of an interaural-intensity detector in addition to the interaural-time detector. He assumed that the quantity of concern in the binaural masked detection of high-frequency tones is the instantaneous difference in power between the outputs of the two peripheral bandpass filters, and demonstrated quantitatively that this assumption could be used to explain the available high-frequency data. He pointed out, however, that the value of the interaural-intensity-deviation threshold required to fit these data (like the value of the interaural-time-deviation threshold required to fit the lower-frequency masking data) was significantly larger than the corresponding jnd measured in simple discrimination experiments. This extension of the time-detector model can be pictured in terms of Fig. 5 by including the intensity-difference detector and replacing the multiplication by $\overline{TR}$ and the summation (discussed in the next paragraph) by a simple switch to select between the time detector and intensity detector according to the frequency. (If the outputs of the two detectors were combined optimally for all frequencies, the results would be essentially the same.)

Another interaural-difference-detector model, closely related to the previous ones, was proposed by Hafter and Carrier (1970). They continued the line of thought that a change of lateral position or lateral movement is the basic cue used in binaural detection (e.g., Jeffress *et al.*, 1956) and suggested a *lateralization model* in which the decision variable is a linear combination of interaural time difference and interaural intensity difference with relative weights specified by the time–intensity trading ratio $\overline{TR}$. This formulation is supported not only by its consistency with lateralization phenomena (and, in particular, the phenomenon of time–intensity trading), but also by results that show that the distribution of lateralization responses can be used to predict detection performance by applying ideal observer theory to the lateralization data (Hafter, Bourbon, Blocker, & Tucker, 1969; Hafter, Carrier, & Stephan, 1973). The block diagram shown in Fig. 5 (with the dashed lines included) provides one possible visualization of this model. Another visualization can be achieved by omitting the intensity-difference detector pathway and including the influence of intensity difference more peripherally in a manner that is consistent with the latency hypothesis (and Jeffress's original conception).

The lateralization model has been applied to the detection of a tone burst masked by a tone of the same frequency (which is equivalent to the discrimination of simultaneous changes in interaural time delay and interaural amplitude ratio) and to the masking of tone bursts by wide-band noise (Hafter & Carrier, 1970; Hafter, 1971; Yost, 1972). The model was found to be roughly consistent with the tone-on-tone masking data (Hafter & Carrier, 1970; Yost, 1972) using values of $\overline{TR}$ of the order of 10–20 μsec dB^{-1}. However, since the model is based on the notion that interaural time and intensity are completely tradable, its predictions fail to reflect those aspects of the data which contradict this notion. In particular, significant discrepancies between the model and data were noted for cases in which the interaural time and intensity shifts caused by the addition of the target tone were in opposition. Since the data on the detection of narrow-band noise in narrow-band noise generated from the same source (Jeffress & McFadden, 1971; McFadden, Jeffress, & Ermey, 1971; McFadden, Jeffress, & Lakey, 1972) also exhibit incomplete tradability, the model cannot be completely adequate for these data either. Recently, Hafter and Carrier (1972) proposed a "double-image" model in which there are two operative time–intensity trades (with different values of $\overline{TR}$) in order to account for incomplete tradability. Using values of 2.0 μsec dB^{-1} for the smaller ratio and roⁱghly 20 μsec dB^{-1} for the larger, they were able to describe their data on the ability to discriminate between a 500-Hz tone with no interaural differences and a 500-Hz tone with differences that were in opposition. They also presented conjectures about the mechanisms that might underlie the interaction of time and intensity (mechanisms that are less consistent with the block diagram that we have shown in Fig. 5 than with the original latency hypothesis). The application of the single $\overline{TR}$ model to the detection of tones in broad-band noise (Hafter, 1971) was successful in predicting the shape of the dependence of the masked threshold on the interaural amplitude ratio and phase shift of the tone for masking noise that is identical in both ears. However, in order to predict the dependence of the antiphasic threshold on tone frequency, the value of $\overline{TR}$ must be less than a few microseconds per decibels. [The apparent fit obtained with larger trading ratios in Figs. 4 and 5 of Hafter (1971) is invalid and is the result of comparing predictions for thresholds with data for masking-level differences.] Not only is this result inconsistent with the results obtained for $\overline{TR}$ from the tone-on-tone masking data, but with such a small trading ratio, the single-$\overline{TR}$ lateralization model is not significantly different from the pure time-detector model.

Some additional difficulties with interaural-difference-detector models have been pointed out by Henning (1973) in connection with his data describing the effects of interaural signal phase on frequency discrimination and amplitude discrimination of tones in a background of broad-band noise. He showed that the Hafter–Carrier modifications would not significantly reduce the difficulties that were described above for the initial form of the model.

Jeffress (1972) has summarized in broad outline a binaural mechanism that is an extension and refinement of his original proposal. This mechanism again contains a coincidence structure that is spatially distributed in frequency and internal time delay and that becomes less dense away from the median plane. The neural following is assumed to be imperfect and this "neural jitter" is assumed to be an important contributor to the internal noise. This mechanism differs from the one originally proposed in that it rejects the simple latency hypothesis. (This revision is necessitated by the many experimental results which show that time and intensity are not completely tradable.) A model that is consistent with many of Jeffress's ideas, but that differs from all other such models in that it explicitly incorporates a quantitative description of the auditory nerve firing patterns (Colburn, 1969, 1973, 1977a,b), is presented in Section VI.

IV. NOISE-SUPPRESSION MODELS

The approach discussed in this section has been oriented primarily towards the detection of narrow-band signals in backgrounds of broad-band masking noise and describes binaural interaction in terms of operations performed on the two received signals that reduce or eliminate the masking noise. The most prominent and successful example of this approach is the equalization and cancellation (EC) model originally suggested by Kock (1950) and later developed by Durlach and his associates (Colburn & Durlach, 1965; Durlach, 1960, 1962, 1963, 1964b, 1966, 1972; Hershkowitz & Durlach, 1969; Metz, von Bismarck, & Durlach, 1968; Rabiner, Laurence, & Durlach, 1966). A comprehensive and detailed description of most of the work performed on this model prior to 1967 is available in Durlach (1972) (which was actually written in 1967). The basic idea of the EC model is to adjust the received signals so that the masking components are equal in the two channels (equalize) and then to subtract (cancel). If these operations are performed perfectly, and the interaural relations of the target signal are different from those of the masking signal, then the resultant output will contain a component due to the target signal but not the masking signal. In order to exclude arbitrarily good performance, Durlach assumes that the processing is corrupted by random "jitter" in the EC mechanism. Furthermore, he assumes that this jitter can be described in terms of two statistically independent random variables on each channel, a multiplicative amplitude factor $1 - \epsilon$ and a time delay δ. In the preliminary version of the EC model (e.g., see the discussion by Durlach, 1972), it is assumed that the equalizer can effect any operations on the incoming signals, such as interaural time delays, phase shifts, and amplitude adjustments, and that the probability distributions of the random-jitter parameters are independent of the transformation. Although these assumptions are sufficient for a large body of data, they are inadequate for many situations in which the masker is not the same at both ears (i.e., in which an equalization transformation is required). In order to predict the data correctly for these situations, it is necessary to restrict the repertoire of transformations that can be effected by the equalizer and/or to permit the distributions of the jitter parameters to depend on the transformation. (Since no equalization operation is necessary when the masker is the same at both ears, predictions for this case are unaffected by such modifications.)

In the form of the EC model that has been explored most extensively (e.g., Durlach, 1964b, 1972; Rabiner *et al.*, 1966), it is assumed that the distributions of the jitter parameters are fixed, that the permissible transformations are restricted to interaural time delays of limited magnitude, and that, for a given stimulus, the system selects that delay in the repertoire which maximizes the signal-to-noise ratio at the output of the subtractor. This model is outlined in Fig. 6. After passing through the peripheral bandpass filter centered at the target frequency, each incoming signal is multiplied by a random amplitude factor $1 - \epsilon_j$ and delayed by a random delay δ_j. The random variables ϵ_1, ϵ_2, δ_1, and δ_2 are statistically independent, zero-mean, Gaussian random variables with variances σ_ϵ^2 ($= \sigma_{\epsilon_1}^2 = \sigma_{\epsilon_2}^2$) and σ_δ^2 ($= \sigma_{\delta_1}^2 = \sigma_{\delta_2}^2$). The operation of the detector is not specified in detail, but it is assumed that detection is characterized by the signal-to-noise ratio on the channel that has the maximum signal-to-noise ratio. This assumption permits one to predict ratios of threshold signal-to-noise ratios for any two stimulus configurations (including the purely monaural case) without specifying in detail the operation of the detector. The predictions of the model for a specific binaural configuration are calculated in terms of binaural unmasking, that is, the decibel difference between the threshold signal-to-noise ratio for

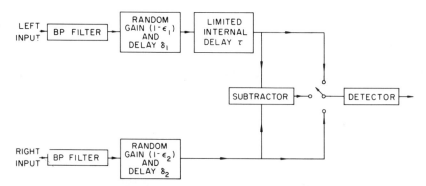

FIG. 6. Block diagram of the equalization–cancellation (EC) model of Durlach. The random parameters ϵ_1, δ_1, ϵ_2, and δ_2 are statistically independent zero-mean Gaussian variables. The variances of ϵ_1 and ϵ_2 are both equal to σ_ϵ^2, and the variances of δ_1 and δ_2 are both equal to σ_δ^2. The performance of the detector is assumed to be determined by the signal-to-noise ratio, and the choices of the internal delay (within the permissible range) and of the three possible inputs to the detector are made to maximize performance.

this binaural configuration and the threshold signal-to-noise ratio for the purely monaural configuration (or, equivalently from an empirical view point, the configuration in which the signal and noise are both interaurally identical). In order to predict the thresholds themselves with this version of the EC model, one must specify a threshold criterion on the signal-to-noise ratio. [In a signal-detection analysis of the EC model, Green (1966) assumed that the energy of the signal at the output of the subtractor is used optimally as the decision variable and, for the few cases studied, obtained essentially the same equations as those obtained with the simple signal-to-noise ratio approach. In this analysis, Green assumed that the frequency of the target signal was sufficiently low to allow him to ignore the effects of the time jitter.] Aside from structural restrictions, the fitting parameters of the model are limited to two fixed numbers, σ_ϵ^2 and σ_δ^2, that are independent of the stimulus parameters and of the transformation chosen by the equalizer.

Under these conditions, several conclusions can be drawn immediately that do not depend upon the repertoire of permitted transformations (so long as the identity transformation is included). First, both amplitude and time jitter are necessary. If there were no amplitude jitter (i.e., $\sigma_\epsilon = 0$), predicted performance would become arbitrarily good as the frequency is decreased (because σ_δ is fixed). If there were no time jitter (i.e., $\sigma_\delta = 0$), predicted performance would fail to decrease as the frequency is increased (because σ_ϵ is fixed). Second, the model fails to predict the observed 3-dB plateau in binaural unmasking that occurs for antiphasic configurations at all frequencies above roughly 1500 Hz. This failure is a direct consequence of the assumption that σ_δ^2 is independent of frequency; at high frequencies, values of δ occur nearly uniformly over a period of the carrier frequency so that the subtraction of the jittered waveforms results in incoherent addition of both target and masker with no net advantage. [This argument depends upon an assumption that has not been discussed here and that is related to the order of averaging the jitter and forming the signal-to-noise ratio (see Durlach, 1972).] Third, and again contrary to the data, predicted binaural unmasking is independent of the overall noise level. This deficiency could be reduced (without violating the constraint that σ_ϵ and σ_δ are fixed) by assuming the existence of an additive internal noise that is constant, i.e., that has a level independent of the external noise level. This assumption, which can be included in almost any model (and is used in some of the models discussed in Section V), was rejected by Durlach (1972) because he found it to be quantitatively inconsistent with the data that were avaliable to him [specifically, the data of Hirsh (1948), which showed that the increase in binaural unmasking with level was essentially linear over a range of more than 50 dB]. Except for the high-frequency problems and the noise-level problem, this version of the EC model, together with the assumption that $\sigma_\epsilon = 0.25$ and $\sigma_\delta = 100$ μsec, describes all available data on the detection of tones masked by broad-band binaurally identical noise. In an initial attempt to predict the values of the jnds in interaural amplitude and time on the basis of these values for σ_ϵ and σ_δ, Durlach (1963) obtained the estimates 1 dB and 150 μsec for these differences. The value of 150 μsec for the interaural time jnd, like the roughly comparable value obtained for the interaural-time-deviation threshold in the interaural-time-detector model (discussed in Section III), is approximately an order of magnitude greater than observed values.

The predictions of the EC model for interaural time delays and phase shifts of the masking noise are directly related to the transformations that are included in the repertoire of the equalizer, and the restriction that the repertoire includes only interaural time delays of limited magnitude was determined largely by the data for these conditions (as well as considerations concerning the transformations that would be required for equalization in natural acoustic environments).

The idea that time delays of at least limited magnitude should be included was suggested by, among other things, the fact that, over a wide variety of conditions, the amount of binaural unmasking obtained when the signal has an interaural delay τ_s and the noise has an interaural delay τ_n is roughly the same as when the signal has a delay $\tau_s - \tau_n$ and the noise has zero delay (the configuration that would result by interaurally delaying the total stimulus of the first configuration interaurally by an amount $-\tau_n$).

The idea that phase shifts should be excluded was suggested by the fact that the amount of binaural unmasking for the configuration signal-in-phase-noise-out-of-phase is generally smaller than for signal-out-of-phase-noise-in-phase. (Compensating for a phase shift in the noise by an internal time delay rather than an internal phase shift reduces the predicted unmasking for the noise-out-of-phase case by an amount that depends on the signal frequency and the bandwidth of the peripheral filter centered on this frequency.)

The idea that the internal interaural delays should be limited in magnitude was motivated by a variety of factors, including the data which show that the function describing the dependence of binaural unmasking on τ_n is a damped periodic function with a period $1/f$ (where f is the signal frequency), a damping factor that corresponds to the correlation time of the filtered noise (determined by the critical bandwidth), and an asymptote for large τ_n (i.e., $\tau_n > 20$ msec) that equals the value obtained for statistically independent noise (Jeffress, Blodgett, & Deatherage, 1952, 1962; Langford & Jeffress, 1964; Rabiner et al., 1966; Robinson & Jeffress, 1963). If the internal delays were unlimited, this function would be strictly periodic for all τ_n. On the other hand, if the magnitudes of the delays are limited to values less than or equal to the half-period $1/2f$ of the target signal, then the system can only compensate for values of τ_n modulo $1/f$ and the results for larger τ_n are degraded by decorrelation in the noise (determined by the bandwidth and the number of "slipped cycles" that occur in the modulo $1/f$ compensation).

Two possible limits were considered for the range of available internal interaural delays (e.g., Durlach, 1972; Rabiner et al., 1966): The half-period $1/2f$ of the tone frequency, and a constant value H of the order .5–1.0 msec (corresponding to the maximum interaural delay naturally experienced and referred to as the "headwidth constraint"). Neither of these constraints, however, was found to be adequate for describing all the binaural unmasking data involving time delays and phase shifts in the noise. In particular, they were both found unsatisfactory for describing the results on τ_n for very low frequencies (i.e., $f \leq 400$ Hz) and τ_n in the interval $H < \tau_n < 1/2f$, where the amount of binaural unmasking for the signal-in-phase case appears to be independent of τ_n (referred to as the "flattening" phenomenon). If H is chosen as the upper limit, then performance for this case is predicted to drop sharply as τ_n increases beyond H. On the other hand, if $1/2f$ is chosen as the upper limit, then performance for this case is predicted to continue increasing as τ_n increases from H to $1/2f$ (just as performance continues to increase with τ_s in this region for the case in which $\tau_n = 0$).

It was also pointed out (Durlach, 1972, p. 434; Rabiner et al., 1966, p. 70) that a contradiction between the model and data exists even if one includes time delays with magnitudes up to $1/2f$ and assumes that σ_δ increases when the magnitude exceeds H. This contradiction was revealed by comparing data for the following four configurations: signal out-of-phase and noise in-phase $[(\pi|0)]$; signal in-phase and noise out-of-phase $[(0|\pi)]$; signal in-phase and noise delayed by a half-period $[(0|1/2f)]$; and signal out-of-phase and noise both out-of-phase and delayed by a half-period $[(\pi|\pi, 1/2f)]$. The last configuration is equivalent to the results that would be obtained for the configuration $(0|\pi)$ at the input to the subtractor if the equilizer applied the interaural delay $1/2f$ to compensate for the interaural phase shift π in the noise (and the target signal is sufficiently narrow band to equate phase shifts and time delays for the target signal). According to the model, the threshold for $(0|\pi)$ is higher than the threshold for $(\pi|0)$ at low frequencies both because of the headwidth effect (i.e., the increase in σ_δ as the magnitude of the internal delay exceeds H) and because of the decorrelation effect (i.e., the degradation that results from compensating for a phase shift with a time delay). The headwidth effect (without contamination by the decorrelation effect) is measured by the extent to which the threshold for the case $(0|1/2f)$ exceeds the threshold for $(\pi|0)$. Similarly, the decorrelation effect (without contamination by the headwidth effect) is measured by the extent to which the threshold for $(\pi|\pi, 1/2f)$ exceeds the threshold for $(\pi|0)$. According to the data, each of these effects by itself is sufficient to explain the observed difference in thresholds between $(\pi|0)$ and $(0|\pi)$; when they are combined, the predicted difference is significantly larger than the observed difference. An analogous argument applies, of course, to a model that assumes that only phase shifts are available. It should be noted, however, that this argument against time delays alone (or phase shifts alone) implicitly assumes that only one time delay is used at any given time. If one assumes alternatively that several time-delay channels can be used simultaneously, then the system can respond to out-of-phase noise equally well with two time delays of the same magnitude ($\pm 1/2f$), each resulting in decorrelation, whereas the system can respond to noise that is time delayed by $1/2f$ without decorrelation by only one time delay ($-1/2f$). A model that makes use of this fact and that adequately describes the data on both time delays and phase shifts in the noise at low frequencies is discussed in Section VI.

It should also be noted that in later work with the EC model, data on phase-shifted noise at low frequencies were very well described by assuming that phase shifts (as well as time delays) are available in the repertoire and that the jitter parameters depend upon the interaural phase and the band width of the noise (Metz et al., 1968). Finally, it should be noted that the model adequately predicts the results on the dependence of binaural unmasking on the correlation of the noise (where the correlation is controlled by varying the amount of noise that is common to both ears relative to the amount that is statistically independent between the ears), but that it fails to predict the dependence on the interaural amplitude ratio of the noise (Durlach, 1964b, 1972).

Although the EC model has been applied primarily to binaural unmasking, it has also been applied (with varying degrees of success) to a variety of other phenomena. Results on Huggins's creation-of-pitch effect (Cramer & Huggins, 1958; Durlach, 1962, 1972) are consistent with available data and include predictions for experiments that have not yet been performed. Also, Bilsen and Goldstein (1974) have shown that the EC model can be used to relate monotic and dichotic repetition pitch by assuming that a single pitch read-out mechanism operates on the monaural spectrum of the monotic repetition-pitch stimulus and on the binaural spectrum of the dichotic repetition-pitch stimulus generated by the EC mechanism. Attempts have also been made to apply the model to interaural jnds in time, amplitude, and correlation (Durlach, 1966, 1972; Hershkowitz & Durlach, 1969). Although preliminary analysis resulted in a common interpretation of all three jnds (for the case in which the reference stimulus is the same in both ears) by assuming that a difference from the reference stimulus in any dimension is just detectable when the energy at the output of the subtractor deviates by a critical amount from the energy that occurs with the reference stimulus, the results have been shown to be inadequate in two respects. First, the value of the critical energy deviation required to fit the jnd data is substantially smaller than the value that would be expected on the basis of binaural unmasking data (Durlach, 1966, 1972). Second, the value of this critical constant was found to be significantly different for interaural time jnds than for interaural amplitude jnds when these jnds were measured on a common set of subjects (Hershkowitz & Durlach, 1969). In addition, the model is totally inadequate for predicting the results on discrimination of simultaneous increments in interaural time and interaural amplitude (tone-on-tone masking). Finally, Henning (1973) has shown that a modified version of the model is consistent with his data on binaural discrimination of amplitude (and, to a lesser extent, frequency) of in-phase and out-of-phase tone bursts in backgrounds of identical noise. In these applications, Henning assumed that the jitter errors occur before the two monaural channels are combined so that they corrupt the signals in the monaural channels as well as in the binaural channel (a revision that has been incorporated in Fig. 6). Also, like Green (1966), he assumed that the binaural processor is capable of addition (which is equivalent to subtraction after an internal phase shift of magnitude π) as well as subtraction, and restricted his work to low frequencies where the effect of the time jitter is negligible.

Although the EC model has generally been found very useful in organizing a large body of data, and many of its implications have been explored in greater quantitative detail than the implications of many of the other models of binaural interaction, the model as presently developed suffers from two major defects. First, it has been addressed exclusively to sensitivity phenomena and has entirely ignored the subjective attributes of the binaural image space that provide the cues that are used to distinguish among stimuli. Although it is conceivable that the model could be extended to include these attributes, it is unlikely that such an extension would be a natural one. Second, it is a completely black-box model and fails to take into account the underlying physiology. Although the postulated processing and the random jitter in this processing could possibly be interpreted in terms that are physiologically reasonable, no effort has been made to construct such an interpretation.

Finally, it should be noted that a somewhat similar approach to the problem of binaural unmasking is evident in the model developed by Schenkel (1967). The structure of this model is based upon addition and subtraction operations followed by unspecified signal-to-noise ratio detectors. No internal noise is explicitly included in this model, but processing imperfections are built into the structure by assuming that the result of the binaural interaction step (addition or subtraction of inputs) is combined with a monaural input before the detector. The amount of unmasking is determined by the relative weighting in the combination. (The result of the binaural interaction step alone would give infinite unmasking and the monaural input alone would give no unmasking.) The weighting coefficient is chosen as a function of frequency to match the frequency dependence of the experimental results. Since the model includes no internal time delay, it cannot describe results as a function of interaural time delay of the noise. Also, the differences between the thresholds for signal-out-of-phase–noise-in-phase and signal-in-phase–noise-out-of-phase that have been repeatedly observed at low frequencies were ignored by Schenkel.

V. CROSS-CORRELATION MODELS

In this section we consider theoretical work in which binaural interaction phenomena are interpreted explicitly and quantitatively in terms of interaural cross correlation. This work includes the modeling of fusion and lateralization by Sayers and his colleagues and of binaural masked detection by Dolan and Robinson, McFadden, Sondhi, Levitt, and Osman. Although the cross-coincidence mechanisms of Jeffress (1948) and Licklider (1959) discussed in Section III are essentially cross-correlation devices, these mechanisms are not sufficiently specified to allow quantitative comparisons with behavioral results and they will not be considered further until the end of the chapter.

The first attempt to describe binaural phenomena quantitatively in terms of interaural correlation was presented by Sayers and Cherry (1957) in their study of binaural fusion and lateralization. Since an acoustic image is generally more fused the more alike the binaural inputs, and since the correlation is a measure of the degree to which waveforms are alike on a point-to-point basis, it is natural to attempt to describe binaural fusion in terms of interaural correlation. Such a description is also consistent with the ability of the auditory system to create an image from complex inputs by selecting the signal components that are common to both ears, and with the observation that the relative influence of a particular common component in a complex stimulus is proportional to the product of the levels of the component at the left and right ears (Sayers & Cherry, 1957). Furthermore, since an interaural time delay in the binaural stimulus shifts the interaural correlation function by an amount equal to this delay (such that, for example, the positions of maxima in the correlation function will be directly related to this delay), the correlation function constitutes a natural means for interpreting the lateralization phenomena associated with interaural time delay.

Perceptual features that are not so natually reflected in the behavior of the correlation function, however, are those concerned with the effects of interaural amplitude difference on lateralization. Specifically, since the lateralization of an image depends upon the direction of an interaural amplitude imbalance, whereas the correlation function depends only on the product of the amplitudes of the two functions being correlated (and is independent of how this product is decomposed into factors), any model for lateralization that is based on interaural correlation must include an additional mechanism for interaural amplitude effects. Sayers and Cherry rejected the latency hypothesis (used by Jeffress, 1948) to account for these effects because their empirical binaural coherence curves, which describe the probability of judging an image to be to the left of center (rather than to the right) as a function of interaural delay, were not consistent with this hypothesis in that an interaural intensity difference was found to displace these curves vertically rather than horizontally. In other words, they took account of the obvious fact that as the intensity in one ear becomes substantially greater than that in the other, the whole function describing the dependence of lateralization on time delay is displaced toward the ear receiving the more intense signal.

The correlation model of Sayers and Cherry (1957) is outlined schematically in Fig. 7. The input signals are first transformed by adding to each a dc term (proportional to signal level) so that the running cross-correlation function of the transformed signals is always positive (and has a dc level proportional to the input signal levels). The running cross-correlation function $R(\tau, t)$ is then computed and weighted by two factors: The first weights the function according to the magnitude of the argument τ so that later processing focuses on values of the function with arguments near zero (and only small internal delays influence the results); the second factor weights values of the function for positive τ arguments by A_R, the level of the right input signal, and values for negative τ arguments by A_L, the level of the left input signal, so that interaural amplitude differences appear distinctly in the weighted function. The weighted, running cross-correlation function is then time-averaged over t (its value for each argument τ is, of course, time-varying) and position judgments are made by comparing the integral of this final function over positive values of τ with the integral over negative values of τ (the integral is denoted by $+$ in the figure). As we shall see, extended

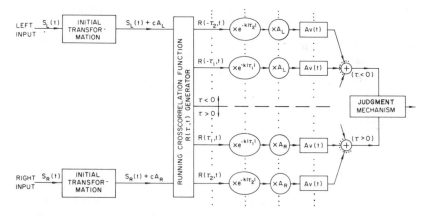

Fig. 7. Block diagram of the model of Sayers and Cherry. The parameters A_L and A_R are the averaged levels (e.g., rms values) of the inputs $S_L(t)$ and $S_R(t)$. The constant c in the initial transformation is postulated to be much greater than unity. The output of the running cross correlator is a continuous function of time t and of internal interaural delay τ, although the output in the τ dimension is represented here as a set of discrete outputs. The time function corresponding to each value of the delay τ is weighted by two factors, one dependent on the magnitude of the delay and the second on the polarity of the delay. The functions are then time averaged and the outputs with common delay polarity are added together. Finally, the resulting two numbers are used by the judgment mechanism to generate responses about the position of the image.

versions of this model preserved the cross-correlation operation, the weighting that serves to limit internal delays, and the weighting that serves to include interaural amplitude differences, but made substantial changes otherwise. Specifically, a multiple output operation was inserted before the cross correlator and each output pair was used as an input pair for a structure like that shown in Fig. 7. In one version, the multiple output operation was a running autocorrelation device (window approximately 1 msec) with outputs corresponding to the autocorrelation delay variable (Cherry & Sayers, 1959; Leaky, Sayers, & Cherry, 1958; Sayers & Cherry, 1957). In a later version only vaguely described, the input signals are spectrum analyzed, the pair of outputs from bandpass filters with the same frequency response are used as the inputs to the cross-correlation device, and the integration over τ and judgment mechanism just described are replaced with a mechanism that relates position to the mean of the peak of the weighted correlation function (Sayers, 1964; Toole & Sayers, 1965). The multiple channel approach (with all channels simultaneously available) was needed to allow a more comprehensive description of monaural and binaural multiple images.

Sayers and his associates have applied the basic model, or variants of it, to a wide variety of fusion and lateralization data. The data described by the model include almost all the coherence-curve data and the results from many lateralization-scaling experiments, including those showing multiple images and the effects of interaural amplitude differences. The basically curve-fit procedure by which the correlation function is weighted by the input signal levels provides an important alternative to other ways of including interaural amplitude information. A discussion of "natural" weighting in a detection-theory context is found in Voelcker (1961).

Finally, in a study directed toward interaural intensity effects with binaural click stimuli, Sayers and Lynn (1968) compare time–intensity trading relations that are derived from physiological experiments on cat and from behavioral centering experiments on man. They demonstrate that, for auditory-nerve fibers, the rates of change with intensity (in microseconds per decibel) of the center of gravity of post stimulus-time histograms are approximately the same as the behavioral trading ratios. This rough equivalence led Sayers and Lynn to speculate that, for transient stimuli, experimental procedures that allow judgment-averaging (such as in a centering task) measure intensity effects that are caused by averaged neural responses, while the experiments tracing single images without judgment-averaging [such as in the lateralization-judgment paradigm introduced by Sayers (1964)] show intensity effects that may be caused by mechanisms in the higher centers of the auditory pathway. This assumption of dual mechanisms was rejected by Békésy on the grounds that there is no reason for the trading ratios to be the same for both mechanisms; we could argue, however, that they should be the same because ultimately they both relate to the position of an object in space and the central mechanism should be calibrated consistently with respect to the peripheral mechanism.

The first explicit consideration of interaural correlation as a general means for organizing binaural unmasking phenomena was made by Jeffress and his associates (Jeffress *et al.*, 1952; Langford & Jeffress, 1964; Robinson & Jeffress, 1963), who examined the extent to which binaural unmasking (the difference between the threshold for a given configuration and the threshold for the purely monaural case) is determined by the correlation coefficient of the masking noise for different types of decorrelation without specifying any underlying binaural-processing mechanism. In particular, they examined binaural masked thresholds for in-phase and out-of-phase 500-Hz tones for two types of noise decorrelation, one achieved by introducing an interaural time delay in the noise and one achieved by adding statistically independent noise at the two ears to a noise signal that is common to both ears. (Negative correlations were achieved by using a phase inversion of the common noise at one ear.) In the latter case, the interaural differences in the noise are statistical rather than deterministic. For the time-delayed noise, the correlation coefficient was computed assuming that the total signals were bandpass filtered at the periphery (with a bandwidth specified by the critical band). Under this assumption, the correlation coefficient is a damped periodic function of time delay with a period equal to the period of the center frequency of the band (i.e., the frequency of the target signal) and a damping factor determined by the bandwidth. A comparison of the data for these two types of decorrelation showed agreement at time delays corresponding to multiples of the half-period of the target tone (the peaks and valleys of the above-mentioned function) and disagreement elsewhere (e.g., at odd multiples of quarter-periods, where the coefficient is zero). These results gave strong support to the notion that the correlation coefficient by itself is an inadequate predictor of the amount of unmasking and that it is necessary to assume the existence of internal interaural delays (i.e., to make use of the correlation *function*). With such delays available, for example, the case in which the target signal is in-phase and the noise is interaurally delayed by a quarter cycle can be reduced to the case in which the target signal is 90° out-of-phase and the noise is interaurally identical. As far as we know, this is the only interpretation that has been used in models of binaural detection to describe these results.

The assumption that binaural unmasking for a fixed target signal is determined by the correlation of the noise was considered further by Dolan and Robinson (1967) and McFadden (1968), who combined this assumption with the assumption of additive internal noise to explain the dependence of binaural unmasking on the overall level and interaural amplitude ratio of the external noise. This internal noise was assumed to be uncorrelated with the external noise and to have a fixed level that is small with respect to the level of the external noise at the high levels used in most masking experiments that are not specifically concerned with the dependence of binaural unmasking on level. Dolan and Robinson (1967) showed that for monaural signal and in-phase noise, the decrease in the amount of unmasking that occurs when the noise in the nonsignal ear is attenuated below the level in the signal ear can be predicted from the decrease in the effective noise correlation caused by the relative increase of the internal noise level at the nonsignal ear. Specifically, they showed that if the detection threshold of a monaurally presented 500-Hz tone is measured both as a function of the external noise level in the nonsignal ear (for perfectly correlated external noise) and as a function of the interaural correlation of the external noise (for equal, high noise levels in the two ears, and using an independent noise source to achieve the decorrelation), then the results of the first experiment can be predicted from the latter by assuming that performance depends only on the effective interaural correlation coefficient. It was necessary to fix the spectrum level of the internal noise at .15% of the reference spectrum level of the external noise (the level that was always used in the signal ear and that was used in both ears for the decorrelation experiment). Since this reference level in these experiments was 45 dB SPL per cycle, the .15% corresponds to a spectral level of the internal noise of 16.8 dB SPL per cycle.

McFadden (1968) showed that the same basic ideas could also be used to describe the dependence of binaural unmasking on noise level for two signal-out-of-phase noise-in-phase cases, one with the noise at the same level in both ears, and one with the noise level reduced in one ear. In the second case, the signal was reduced along with the noise so that the signal-to-noise ratio was always the same in both ears, and the independent variable was the noise level in the ear with a reduced level (the level in the other ear being held fixed at 45 dB SPL per cycle). Unlike the situation for the second case (and unlike the situation considered by Dolan and Robinson), in which the noise level at one ear is always maintained at a level high enough to ignore the fixed-level internal noise in that ear, the situation represented by the first case requires that attention be given to the interaural correlation of the internal noise as well as its level. McFadden estimated the interaural correlation coefficient of the internal noise from his experimental results at very low (or zero) external noise levels [following the work of Diercks and Jeffress (1962) in which absolute binaural thresholds were interpreted in terms of partially correlated internal noise], and chose the level of the internal noise to fit his experimental results at particular (higher) external noise levels. The data of Robinson and Jeffress (1963), which were taken at sufficiently high external noise levels to ensure that the effects of the external noise dominated the effects of the assumed internal noise, were used throughout to describe the dependence of binaural unmasking on decorrelation. The estimates obtained of the interaural correlation and level of the internal noise from the first case were .35 and 4.2 dB SPL per cycle, respectively, and the estimate of the level from the second case was 12.2 dB SPL per cycle. Using these constants, McFadden was able to describe his data with considerable accuracy.

In the approach followed by Dolan and Robinson (1967) and McFadden (1968), it is assumed that the performance of the binaural mechanism responsible for binaural unmasking is determined by the correlation coefficient of the effective masking noise, but there is no specification of how this mechanism operates. Thus, as these investigators point out, the postulate of a fixed-level, partially correlated, additive, internal noise can be adjoined to any model and enable it to predict the dependence of binaural unmasking on the overall level and (in some cases) on the interaural amplitude ratio of the noise, provided only that it (like the interaural-time-detector or EC model) is capable of describing the dependence of binaural unmasking on the decorrelation of the noise. With respect to dependence on the interaural amplitude ratio of the noise, note that this postulate is unable to predict the result (Weston & Miller, 1965) that the detection threshold for monaural signal and in-phase noise increases as the level of the noise in the nonsignal ear is raised above the level in the signal ear.

Binaural detection models that describe the operation of the binaural processing mechanism more specifically and quantitatively and that are based upon the optimum use of a decision variable that includes an internal interaural correlation term have been proposed by Sondhi (1966), Levitt and Lundry (1966b), and Osman (1971). The models of Sondhi and Levitt and Lundry have not been described in detail in the literature. Sondhi's model postulates that detection is based on changes in the correlation coefficient of waveforms generated from the input stimuli by filtering, delaying, inverting, rectifying, and adding internal noise (whose level depends on frequency and the presence or absence of inversion). Levitt and Lundry's model bases decisions on the position and/or amplitude of the main peak in the cross-correlation function of waveforms generated from the input stimuli by filtering, delaying, and adding internal noise (whose level depends on the magnitude of the interaural delay).

Osman (1971) presented a model [outlined schematically in Fig. 8 and called the correlation (ρ) model] that assumes peripheral bandpass filters; an internal interaural delay (and/or phase shift) capability; additive internal noise; and a decision variable D that is a weighted sum of three terms, two monaural energy terms and one interaural correlation term. (The assumptions concerning the system's capability for performing interaural transformations are not clearly stated and it is difficult to tell if they are applied uniformly in Osman's discussion. For example, it is not clear whether the system can perform time shifts alone, phase shifts alone, neither, or both, nor is it clear how large a shift is permitted, $\pi/2$ or π radians. In our block diagram, we have assumed that time delays up to $1/4f_0$ are available, where f_0 is the frequency of the target signal.) The weighting constants A, B, and C used to weight the terms of the decision variable are

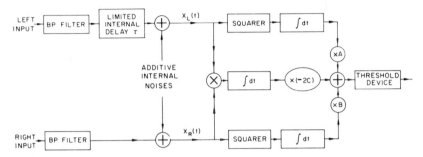

FIG. 8. Block diagram of the correlation (ρ) model of Osman. The additive internal noise is zero-mean, Gaussian noise with interaural correlation coefficient equal to $\rho_I(f)$ and with power spectrum levels equal to $R(f)$ times the external noise spectrum levels. The functions $\rho_I(f)$ and $R(f)$ are chosen to match the frequency dependence of experimental results. The weighting constants A, B, and C are given by $A = 1/(1 - \rho_n^2)$, $B = [1 - \rho_n^2(1 - \eta_{0L}/\eta_{0R})]/(1 - \rho_n^2)$, and $C = \rho_n(\eta_{0L}/\eta_{0R})^{1/2}/(1 - \rho_n^2)$, where ρ_n is the interaural correlation coefficient of the total (internal plus external) noise signals, and η_{0L} and η_{0R} are the power spectrum levels of the total noise signals on the left and right.

specified by the parameters of the internal and external noise. Specifically, they are chosen such that when the internal signals $X_L(t)$ and $X_R(t)$ are linearly transformed to give two waveforms in which the external noise components are uncorrelated point-by-point (i.e., the noise components have a zero interaural correlation coefficient), the decision variable is the total energy in the transformed signals. The internal noise is assumed to be partially correlated between the two ears, and the spectrum level of the internal noise at each ear is assumed to be dependent on (but not necessarily proportional to) the external noise level at that ear. Both the interaural correlation coefficient ρ_I and the ratio R of internal noise level to external noise level are assumed to be functions of frequency, and these two functions are chosen to match the experimental data as functions of frequency. Based on data in which the level of the masking noise is the same in both ears and relatively high, the values obtained for ρ_I range from 0 to .6 (generally decreasing with increasing frequency) and the values of R range from -6 to 9 dB (generally increasing with increasing frequency). With this model, and with values of ρ_I and R within these ranges, Osman (1971, 1973) was able to fit the high-masker-level data on the binaural detection of tones in noise for interaurally identical noise, and for statistically decorrelated noise. He also fit the data for the dependencies on the interaural time delay and phase shifts in the noise, but only for cases in which the tone frequency is not lower than 500 Hz. The correlation model is also able to describe the psychometric functions obtained in binaural detection experiments (Osman, Schacknow, & Tzuo, 1973). As the model currently stands, however, it has no predictions for the results on the overall level of the noise and is completely inadequate for describing the "flattening" phenomenon observed with time delays and phase shifts in the noise at very low frequencies (see Section IV). In addition, it has not been applied to data on the interaural amplitude ratio of the noise or its bandwidth. The only application of the model to experiments other than the detection of tones in noise has been the detection of pulse trains of differing interaural correlation in a background of masking noise (Pohlmann & Sorkin, 1974).

In Osman's model the lack of explicit assumptions about the dependence of the level of the internal noise on the level of the external noise makes it impossible to predict the dependence of thresholds on the level of the masking noise. The two simplest possibilities would be that the level of the internal noise is proportional to the external noise (which would mean that the ratio R in Osman's model would be independent of masker level) or that the level of the internal noise is fixed [as in the work of Dolan and Robinson (1967) and McFadden (1968)]. Clearly, the postulate of additive internal noise, combined with either one of these two assumptions, is, by itself, inadequate. If the first assumption is used, then the model is incapable of predicting the dependence of binaural detection thresholds on masker level. On the other hand, the second assumption is in conflict with Weber's law and with certain results on monaural detection (e.g., Green, 1964; Swets, Shipley, McKey, & Green, 1959). Thus, if the postulate of additive internal noise is to be used, then either a different level assumption must be made, or other types of noise must also be included in the model. With regard to the latter possibility, it is important to recall that in the work of Dolan and Robinson (1967) and McFadden (1968), the additive, fixed-level, internal noise is pictured as only part of the total internal noise that corrupts the processing, because the binaural mechanism that is assumed to be responsible for binaural detection (and the performance of which is assumed to be determined by the effective correlation coefficient) would presumably also include some inherent randomness. If no further loss of information occurred in the processing, the binaural thresholds for high-level, perfectly correlated, external noise would approach zero. This presumption of an additional source of noise in the theoretical work of Dolan, Robinson, and McFadden, but not in the work of Osman, is reflected in the much larger levels of the additive internal noise assumed in the latter work (at 500 Hz and an external noise level of 45 dB SPL, Osman assumes an internal noise level that is 25–35 dB greater than the fixed internal noise levels assumed by the previous investigators).

It should also be noted, as Osman (1971) has pointed out, that the structure of the ρ model is very similar to the structure of the EC model (compare Figs. 6 and 8). Aside from the fact that both models assume peripheral bandpass filters, a limited class of internal interaural time delays, and some internal randomness that affects the signals in both channels before the binaural interaction, the central processing is very similar. In particular, if the EC model detector is based on energy (as is usually assumed, e.g.,

Durlach, 1972; Green, 1966), then the decision variables in both models can be written

$$D = A \int_0^T X_\mathrm{L}^2(t)\, dt + B \int_0^T X_\mathrm{R}^2(t)\, dt - 2C \int_0^T X_\mathrm{L}(t) X_\mathrm{R}(t)\, dt,$$

where $X_\mathrm{R}(t)$ and $X_\mathrm{L}(t)$ are the inputs to the central processor and A, B, and C are weighting factors. In the EC model, the binaural decision variable (i.e., the energy in the output of the subtractor) is obtained by setting $A = B = C$ and the two monaural decision variables are obtained by setting $A = C = 0$ or $B = C = 0$. In the ρ model, the weighting factors are specified as functions of the correlation coefficient ρ_n of $X_\mathrm{L}(t)$ and $X_\mathrm{R}(t)$ (for the case when noise-alone is presented) and of the ratio of the total noise powers (internal noise plus external noise) in the two channels. Clearly, both models are special cases of a general energy-correlation model with a decision variable that is equal to a linear combination of energy terms and a correlation term derived from corrupted external waveforms. With regard to the class of internal interaural transformations that are assumed to be available in the model, both models include the option of choosing a time delay of limited magnitude to optimize performance. Further, it is easy to verify that the problems encountered using the EC model in attempting to interpret the results for time-delayed and phase-shifted noise for very low-frequency target signals also arise with the ρ model, and the discussion of these problems in Section IV carries over to the ρ model with essentially no change.

The principal differences between the EC and ρ models concern the choice of weighting constants, and thereby the extent to which parallel processing is required in the event that a priori information on the stimulus configuration is incomplete, and the postulates for the internal noise.

One difference concerning the choice of weighting constants is that the EC model explicitly assumes that the weighting constants can be chosen such that either monaural channel can be used alone, whereas the ρ model has not been formulated with this assumption. As noted by Osman et al. (1973), however, this assumption may be required to predict the equality of the threshold for the signal-in-phase, noise-in-phase case and the threshold for the signal-monaural, noise-monaural case. There are also differences in the decision variables for some binaural cases. For example, if the level of the external noise is the same in both ears, $A = B = C$ applies to the binaural variable in the EC model and $A = B = C/\rho_\mathrm{n}$ applies to the variable in the ρ model. The relation between the choice of weighting constants and the extent to which a priori information concerning the stimulus configuration is required has been discussed by both Durlach (1972) and Osman (1971). In general, three statements seem clear: Either model can use parallel processing to reduce the need for such information; parallel processing or a priori information about the interaural relations of the masking noise is required in both models for cases in which the noise is time-delayed or phase-shifted by an arbitrary amount; when there are no such time delays or phase shifts (and the system knows it), the ρ model, but not the EC model, can estimate the necessary parameters internally without the use of parallel processing or a priori information (a difference that is associated with the different weighting procedures).

In order to understand the relations between the internal-noise postulates in the two models, it is useful first to observe that the internal noise in the EC model, which has customarily been represented in terms of fixed-variance amplitude and time jitter, can also be represented in terms of additive noise. In order to represent the EC-model noise in this fashion, it is necessary to take the signal that is corrupted by the fixed-variance jitter and subtract from it the signal before it is corrupted, and then identify the additive noise with this difference term. This term has the property (by definition) of producing the corrupted signal when added to the uncorrupted signal, and goes to zero as the jitter variances go to zero. Moreover, it can be shown that its level is proportional to the input level, that the proportionality constant increases with frequency, and that the correlation coefficient between the ears for this term decreases with frequency (properties that are similar to those of the additive noise in the ρ model). Although there are certainly several differences between the internal noises in the two models (e.g., when the EC-model noise is represented in terms of additive noise, the noise is no longer Gaussian), the most important difference concerns the extent to which the properties of the noises are derived from fundamental assumptions as opposed to fitting of data. Whereas in the EC model the frequency dependence of the internal noise follows from the assumption of fixed-variance amplitude and time jitter, in the ρ model it is obtained purely by fitting the behavioral data. (This additional freedom in the ρ model, of course, allows it, unlike the EC model, to fit the binaural detection data at high frequencies.) Although neither model predicts the dependence of binaural detection thresholds on the overall level of the external noise, each model could be expanded by fitting the noise parameters to empirical results. Thus, for example, the EC model could be revised to fit the level data better (without contradicting Weber's law and the results on monaural detection) by permitting the jitter variances to depend on level in the appropriate manner or by including fixed-level additive internal noise in addition to the jitter [as suggested by Dolan and Robinson (1967) and McFadden (1968)]. Similarly, the ρ model could be revised with equivalent results by assuming that the ratio of internal-noise level to external-noise level depends on level in the appropriate manner or by including both a fixed-level, additive internal noise and a fixed-ratio additive internal noise. These revisions would not be a natural consequence of the structures or previous postulates of either model, but would be an expansion in the complexity of the model in an amount comparable to the additional set of data described. Finally, it should be noted that predictions based on the EC model may be more difficult to derive than those based on the ρ model, if the EC predictions are computed by an analysis of the statistics of the decision variable rather than merely by signal-to-noise ratio evaluation. In the decision-variable analyses conducted with the EC model (Green, 1966; Henning, 1973), it has been assumed that the frequency of the target signal is sufficiently low to permit disregarding the time jitter. No one has yet carried out an analysis for target signals that do not satisfy this constraint.

VI. AUDITORY-NERVE-BASED MODEL

In this section, we discuss a model (Colburn, 1969, 1973, 1977a,b) that includes an explicit quantitative description of physiological observations of auditory-nerve firing patterns and in which the black-box modeling is restricted to a central processor that operates on the auditory-nerve patterns as inputs. The performance characteristics are determined by the properties of the peripheral transduction from acoustic waveforms to neural firing patterns, including the probabilistic aspects of this transduction (which constitute the internal noise in this model) and by the structure of the central processor. The model uses the same general approach as that developed by Siebert (1965, 1968, 1970) for analysis of monaural phenomena and the description of auditory-nerve activity is based on the extensive observations of the auditory nerve of cat by Kiang and his associates (Kiang, 1968; Kiang, Watanabe, Thomas, & Clark, 1965).

Included among the general properties that are built into the description of the auditory-nerve firing patterns are the following: restriction of relevant information to the firing times of each fiber, randomness in the transformation from acoustic stimuli to neural firing patterns, frequency selectivity for each fiber, synchrony of firing times to the detailed time structure of the acoustic stimulus, and increase and saturation of the average firing rate and of the degree of synchrony as the stimulus intensity is increased. The activity on the fibers is described in terms of statistically independent, nonhomogeneous, Poisson random processes. This description is consistent with available data that suggest that successive intervals between firings and separate fibers are conditionally statistically independent (given the stimulus) and show that histograms of the lengths of the intervals have approximately exponential envelopes. The description is inconsistent with the relatively small number of very short intervals (refractory behavior). Parametric descriptions that are chosen to be consistent with the physiological data include the following dependencies: frequency selectivity (tuning curve) on the characteristic (most sensitive) frequency of the fiber, degree of synchrony on stimulus frequency, average firing rate and degree of synchrony (including dynamic range) on stimulus intensity, and density of fibers on characteristic frequency. Since a simple systematic dependence of phase on intensity is not seen in the auditory-nerve responses to tones at low and moderate intensities, the phase is assumed to be independent of intensity (i.e., the latency hypothesis is not included in the description). The assumption is made that the phase is independent of level for ongoing signals even though some physiological data, particularly from central nuclei, show changes in response latency with level that are consistent with a latency hypothesis (e.g., Kemp, Coppée, & Robinson, 1937; Thurlow, Gross, Kemp, & Lowy, 1951; Galambos, Rose, Bromiley, & Hughes, 1952).

The initial work on this model (Colburn, 1973) considered the performance that would be obtained with an ideal central processor (i.e., one in which optimum use is made of all the information carried by the auditory-nerve patterns) and demonstrated that some restrictions must be imposed upon the central processor in order to prevent predicted performance from being significantly better than observed performance in interaural time discrimination experiments. It was further demonstrated that performance at least as good as that observed in these experiments could be achieved when the central processor was restricted by two constraints. First, times of firings on a given fiber can be individually compared with times of firings only from a fiber with the same frequency selectivity in the other auditory nerve. Second, for a given pair of fibers, only firings that occur almost simultaneously (within 100 μsec after an internal, interaural delay that is fixed for the pair) can be compared. These restrictions were assumed as a working hypothesis for further development of this model since, although they have not been shown to be necessary, they are reasonable and consistent with a lot of data.

The specific central processor assumed in most of the further work (Colburn, 1977a,b) is outlined in Fig. 9. The model assumes that an "ideal decision maker" uses an overall decision variable that is an optimum combination of three nonoptimum decision variables: a purely monaural variable from each ear and a binaural variable that carries the interaural timing information. The binaural decision variable is generated from an ideal linear combination (i.e., an optimally weighted sum) of outputs from a binaural displayer. The binaural displayer, shown in Fig 9b, is completely specified by the distribution of interaural delays and the properties of the coincidence counters (i.e., the width of the coincidence "windows"). When, in addition, the firing patterns in the auditory nerve fibers are described, the outputs of the display are determined and performance using the binaural decision variable can be computed for any objective experiment on sensitivity.

It is convenient to think of the outputs of the displayer as a display of numbers on a two-dimensional grid, one dimension corresponding to the characteristic frequency f_m of the fiber pair (specifying the frequency response of the fiber pair), and the other dimension corresponding to the relative internal delay τ_m of the fiber pair. The response to any stimulus is a pattern of activity in the (f_m, τ_m) plane, and the task of the binaural analyzer is to make judgments about the stimulus on the basis of this pattern. It is clear from a comparison of Fig. 9b with Fig. 4 that the binaural displayer is

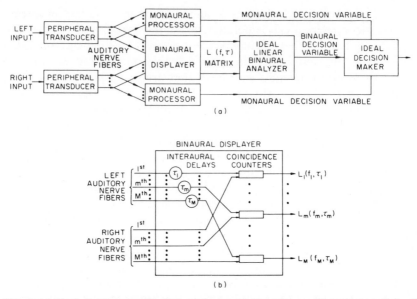

FIG. 9. (a) Block diagram used by Colburn for a model based on auditory-nerve activity. The peripheral transducers relate a random-process description of the auditory-nerve patterns to the acoustic input stimuli. The description is based upon data from single auditory-nerve fibers and includes effects corresponding to the bandpass filters and internal noise generators of other models. A binaural displayer processes the firing patterns on the auditory-nerve fibers to generate a matrix of numbers $L(f,\tau)$ that are the inputs to the ideal linear binaural analyzer. In the analyzer, the outputs of the displayer are multiplied by weighting factors that are optimally chosen for each task, and the weighted outputs are added to form the binaural decision variable. (b) Structure of binaural displayer used in the model. The binaural displayer compares firing patterns from corresponding fibers and limits available information to the number of "coincidences" after an internal, interaural delay that is fixed for each pair and distributed over the set of all pairs independently of other parameters. The density function for the distribution of delays is chosen to match experimental results. [From Colburn (1977a).]

very similar to the mechanism proposed by Jeffress (1948), and that the model discussed in this section can be considered as a quantification and elaboration of some of his ideas. It can also be shown that this model can be considered as a specific mechanism for generating an estimate of the cross-correlation function that has played such a central role in much of the past theoretical work (see Section V). In particular, the coincidence counts L_m, considered as a function of internal delay τ_m for a given characteristic frequency, generate an estimate of the cross-correlation function of the instantaneous firing rates of fiber pairs with this characteristic frequency, and thereby an estimate of the cross-correlation function of bandpass filtered input signals.

This model has been shown to be consistent with nearly all available data on the binaural detection of low-frequency (below 1500 Hz) tones in noise under the assumptions that all the coincidence windows have a width of about 50 μsec and that the distribution of internal interaural delays is given by a fixed specified function. This function is symmetric about zero, decays exponentially after a certain delay is reached, and has an rms width of ~1 msec. [The assumption that this function decays as the delay deviates from zero plays the same role in this model as the assumption that the "cells are less dense away from the median plane" in Jeffress's model, or the assumption in the EC model that the delays are limited or that the jitter factors increase away from the median plane (Metz *et al.*, 1968).] In particular, this model is consistent with the dependence of the binaural masked threshold on the interaural phase shift and amplitude ratio of the tone, the frequency and duration of the tone, the level and bandwidth of the noise, and the interaural correlation, phase shift, time delay, and (in most cases) the amplitude ratio of the noise. [The difficulties encountered by the EC and ρ models in describing the dependence on interaural time or phase shifts in the noise for very low-frequency tones (i.e., below 500 Hz) are avoided in this model by the assumption of multiple pathways with different delays that are simultaneously available together with the assumption that there are fewer pathways with long delays.] The only known inadequacies of this model in describing these data are (*1*) an overall shift of almost 20 dB in predicted signal-to-noise ratios at threshold relative to observations (a shift we believe to be caused by inadequacies in our description of the auditory-nerve firing patterns in response to noise), (*2*) minor discrepancies that arise in certain cases when the binaural masked threshold is nearly as high as the monaural masked threshold (discrepancies caused by inadequate specification of the monaural processing), and (*3*) the failure to predict an increase in the threshold for the case of monaural signal in binaurally identical noise as the level of the noise in the nonsignal ear is raised above the level in the signal ear (Weston & Miller, 1965). We believe that this last difficulty is related to certain difficulties that appear when the model is applied to interaural time discrimination for cases in which the stimuli to be discriminated contain interaural amplitude differences.

Although much of the success of this model in describing these data follows from structural assumptions that are essentially the same as those employed by previous investigators, there are several advantages that result from including an explicit description of the peripheral transformation from stimulus waveforms to auditory-nerve patterns. The incorporation of a quantitative description of the auditory-nerve patterns not only ties the model more closely to physiology while maintaining the ability to make quantitative predictions of behavioral phenomena, but it provides a natural explanation for the dependence of binaural masked thresholds on noise level and frequency. The decrease of the threshold signal-to-noise ratio as the noise level is increased is caused primarily by the increase in the number of fiber pairs that provide relevant information as the level is increased. The frequency dependence of the thresholds results primarily from the frequency dependence of the degree to which the auditory-nerve patterns are phase-locked to the detailed time structure of the stimulus and also from the frequency dependence of the bandwidth of the "tuning curves" of the fibers. (Since the synchrony of the auditory-nerve firings to the detailed time structure is not present at high frequencies, the application of this model to high-frequency detection experiments would have to be based upon synchrony to the envelope of the filtered stimulus or upon a separate mechanism operative at high frequencies.) The main disadvantage of this approach is the increased difficulty in computing predictions. The mathematical problems created by using multidimensional random point processes rather than simple deterministic continuous functions to characterize the inputs to the central processor are substantial and have made it necessary to employ a variety of approximations that are not easily justified. Future work with this model will probably have to make extensive use of computer-simulation techniques.

Finally, it should be noted that although the structure of the central processor in this model was initially motivated by a comparison of the predictions obtained using an ideal central processor with data on the interaural time discrimination of tones (Hershkowitz & Durlach, 1969), the model is not adequate for describing the data that are now available on this topic (e.g., Domnitz, 1973) or the data that are available on detecting simultaneous increments in time and amplitude (such as occur in tone-by-tone masking). This difficulty, of course, is merely another reflection of the fact that any model based on an interaural correlation or coincidence mechanism must include an additional mechanism to account for the effects of interaural amplitude differences in the total signals. (We use the word "total" here in order to distinguish between this case and cases in which the amplitude difference is restricted merely to some components of the total signal, as in many binaural-unmasking configurations.) The inclusion of such a mechanism would have implications not only for the model's predictions for the data just cited, but also for the data on binaural detection in which the configuration consists of a monaural signal and binaural noise and the noise in the nonsignal ear is made more intense than the noise in the signal ear. The most obvious way to include such a mechanism within the context of the present model is to reject the assumption that the constants used to weight the outputs of the binaural displayer (i.e., the coincidence counts from the individual fiber pairs) are chosen optimally by the binaural analyzer, and to assume that they are chosen in such a way as to emphasize the outputs that are associated with the left (right) ear leading whenever the signal to the left (right) ear is more intense. A revision of the model with this sort of weighting (which is similar to that employed by Sayers and his associates) has been explored in a preliminary fashion by Colburn (1969).

The model has not yet been applied to any phenomena other than those concerned with sensitivity. In order to predict properties of subjective attributes, it is necessary to specify a mapping from the binaural display to the perceived-image space.

VII. OVERVIEW

In this section, we present an overview of the various models. Initial discussion is concerned primarily with similarities among the models and, in particular, with the idea that all the models can be considered equivalent in terms of their operations on the acoustic waveforms. The models differ primarily in their internal noise postulates and in the constraints that are imposed on how the internally measured aspects of the waveforms can be combined to generate decision variables. The abilities of the models to describe the various binarual phenomena are then outlined with emphasis on these differences.

A. Similarities among the Models

Figure 10 shows a block diagram of a general model that includes elements that are common to almost all the models that we have considered. The two acoustic signals shown coming in on the left side of the figure are first bandpass filtered and then corrupted by noisy transformations. The noisy transformation can be as simple as a device that adds an internal noise to the signal or as elaborate as a device that transforms the filtered signal to a point-event process like a neural firing pattern. The transformed corrupted

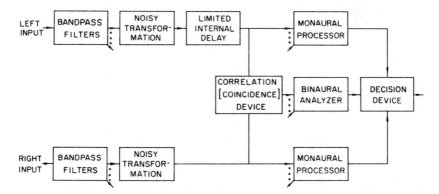

FIG. 10. Block diagram of a general model summarizing the elements that are common to almost all models of binaural interaction. The assumption of simultaneously available, multiple pathways in some of the models is represented by the multiple outputs of the bandpass filters. Each output pair is processed in the manner shown, and the multiple pathways are recombined in the binaural analyzer and in the monaural processors. The binaural analyzer and the decision device are not easily separated in some of the models, and the distinction between them is not important for the discussion in this section.

signals undergo a relative interaural time delay of limited magnitude. Each channel then splits and leads to an interaural cross-correlation device and to a monaural processor. The cross-correlation device can be represented as a cross-coincidence mechanism when its inputs (the outputs of the noisy transformation) are point-event signals. For simplicity in the following discussion, the monaural processors can be thought of as energy computers or the equivalent. The output of the binaural analyzer (which "reads" the output of the correlation device) and of the two monaural processors are combined in the final decision device to form a decision variable that is compared with some criteria to make a decision. For some models, it is necessary to include multiple channels between the bandpass filters and the binaural analyzer and the monaural processors, each pair of channels following the same structure as that indicated in the figure for a single pair of channels. This possibility is indicated in Fig. 10 by the multiple outputs of the bandpass filters and the multiple inputs to the binaural analyzer and monaural processors.

The most direct comparisons of this structure with published models can be made with the equalization–cancellation (EC) model of Durlach and with the correlation (ρ) model of Osman. We have already argued (in Section V) that these models are closely related special cases of a more general energy-correlation model. This more general model is itself a special case of the model that is described by Fig. 10. [The fact that the internal delay precedes the noisy transformation in the ρ model (Fig. 8) is not an essential difference; this ordering was chosen merely to simplify calculations.]

The structure of the general model can also be easily compared with several correlation or coincidence models through a consideration of the model based on auditory-nerve data developed by Colburn. A block diagram of this model is shown in Fig. 9a. The first stage of the model relates the stimulus waveforms to activity on auditory-nerve fibers and includes a bandpass filter and a noisy transformation for each fiber. The binaural processor consists of a binaural displayer and an ideal linear analyser that sums the outputs of the displayer with optimum weights. The binaural displayer, shown in detail in Fig. 9b, includes the internal delays and a coincidence mechanism that generates an output for each fiber pair. The monaural-processor inputs separate off before the internal delays merely for convenience, and the decision device is represented as an "ideal decision maker" that has inputs from the monaural processors and a binaural processor. This model is clearly a special case of the general model with multiple channels.

As we have pointed out in Section VI, the binaural displayer in Colburn's model is very similar to Jeffress's original lateralization model and Colburn's model can be interpreted as a quantification and elaboration of Jeffress's without the latency hypothesis (even though Colburn's displayer grew out of an optimum-processing analysis of auditory-nerve firing patterns). Thus, Jeffress's model can also be regarded as a special case of the general model, provided the latency hypothesis is dropped or included in the noisy transformation or in the internal delay by specifying a dependence on the interaural amplitude ratio. Furthermore, since a coincidence network with internal delays can be used to measure changes in delay resulting from the addition of a signal to a background of noise, the interaural-time-detector model of Webster and of Jeffress, Blodgett, Sandel, and Wood for binaural detection can also be regarded as a special case of the general model. Finally, the lateralization model of Hafter and Carrier can be included in the general model by regarding it as a version of Jeffress's model in which latency depends linearly on stimulus amplitude, or by assuming that the decision device estimates the amplitude ratio from the monaural signals and combines this estimate with the estimate of delay from the binaural analyzer. Including interaural amplitude comparisons in the decision device would also enable the general model to include the interaural-intensity-detector model discussed by Durlach for binaural unmasking at high frequencies.

As discussed in Section VI, if the outputs L_m of the binaural displayer in Colburn's model are grouped according to characteristic frequencies (best frequencies of the bandpass filters), then the outputs in any group considered as a function of the internal delays constitute an estimate of the cross-correlation function of the bandpass-filtered input. The Colburn model can therefore also be viewed as a physiologically reasonable realization of the cross-correlation model of Sayers and his associates, provided the weights in the binaural analyzer are chosen in the appropriate, nonoptimum way. (Note, however, that a strict realization of the Sayers model in terms of the general model would require either that the binaural analyzer be influenced by the outputs of the monaural processors or that the binaural analyzer have two outputs leading to the decision device, one for positive and one for negative internal delays). Similar arguments apply to the work of Sondhi and Levitt.

The models that are most difficult to fit into the basic structure of the general model outlined in Fig. 10 are the count-comparison models discussed in Section II. However, models that are equivalent to these models with respect to the information that is derived from the stimuli and used to make decisions can be fit into the general structure by assuming additional constraints on how time and amplitude information are combined in the decision device of the general model. Although a slightly different argument is required for each specific model, the essential points are the same for all of them and we consider only that of van Bergeijk (illustrated by Figs. 2 and 3). In the displays shown in Fig. 3, cells are arranged in rows such that the relative intensities of the stimuli determine whether the cells in each row are all excited, all inhibited, or divided into these two categories by a boundary. The horizontal dimension in each row corresponds to internal interaural delay and the position of the boundary for a given binaural stimulus is the point at which the excitatory input from one side and the inhibitory input from the other side arrive simultaneously. The position of the boundary and the relative intensities determine the number of excited cells in each population, and thereby, the lateralization. In the general model, the relative intensities are specified by the outputs of the monaural processors. Also, the position of the boundary in the van Bergeijk model can be identified in the general model with the output of the binaural analyzer. Finally, the constraint that only the numbers of excited cells influence the lateralization perception can be incorporated in the general model by assuming that the decision device in the general model is constrained to compute these numbers (deduced from the monaural information and the information presented by the binaural analyzer) as the first step in the decision procedure.

Although the elements of the general binaural model outlined in Fig. 10 may not be uniquely determined by available data, it is easy to justify the reasonableness of each element by reference to these data. The peripheral elements in the model, namely, the bandpass filters and the noisy transformation, are suggested by a wide variety of perceptual phenomena, both binaural and monaural, and by extensive physiological data. Included among the binaural phenomena that require the bandpass filters are the ability of the binaural system to independently lateralize stimulus components that occupy different spectral regions, and the quasi-periodic form of the function describing the dependence of the binaural detection threshold of a tone on the interaural time delay of the masking noise. The location of at least part of the internal noise near the periphery is needed for all explanations of binaural phenomena that assume at least partially uncorrelated noise between the two ears. The cross-correlation device constitutes a simple, mathematically tractable mechanism that is well matched to the ability of the auditory system to form a fused image from signal components that are common to both ears while rejecting other components, to the dependence of binaural detection on the interaural parameters of the target signal for interaurally identical noise, and to the dependence of binaural detection on the interaural correlation of the noise (where the correlation is controlled by the use of independent sources). In addition, it provides adequate information for the observed ability to discriminate interaural time delay. Given a device that computes the correlation coefficient, it is easy to justify the need for a limited internal delay (i.e., a limited-delay version of the correlation function) on the basis of the data describing the dependence of lateralization and fusion on interaural delay and the dependence of binaural detection on the interaural delay of the masking noise. Finally, given that binaural processing is based on correlation or coincidences, monaural pathways are needed to interpret lateralization and interaural discrimination data for cases in which the amplitudes at the two ears are unequal, since some of these cases definitely cannot be interpreted in terms of the latency hypothesis and since the correlation operation is symmetric with respect to input amplitude imbalances. In addition, the monaural channels are required in connection with binaural detection in order to provide an independent measure of the masking noise so that the effects of the variability due to the statistical nature of the masking noise can be effectively eliminated from the decision variable used for detection. (In considering the monaural channels in Fig. 10, it should be noted that, at the level of generality of this discussion, it makes no difference whether they are combined with the binaural channel in the decision device, as pictured, or in the binaural analyzer.) These informal intuitive arguments clearly do not prove that the elements in the general model are necessary, but they do provide indications of why these elements are so prevalent in the specific models that have been proposed.

B. Abilities of the Different Models to Describe Different Types of Data

Although all the binaural interaction models can be described, at least roughly, in terms of the basic elements we have discussed, it is evident that there are important differences in the assumptions characterizing these elements. These differences have significant consequences for the ability of each model to describe available data. The most important differences seem to be in the assumed constraints on how interaural time information and interaural amplitude information are combined, and in the postulates defining the internal noise. These differences will be explored briefly in connection with a summary of the abilities of the various models to describe the various types of experimental data. The data considered here are separated into descriptions of lateralization phenomena, binaural detection of tones masked by noise, and discrimination of interaural parameters. We omit consideration of other types of data (such as those relating to binaurally created pitch or binaural loudness summation) since so few of the models have been applied to these other data.

1. LATERALIZATION

In order for a model to describe lateralization phenomena, the model must contain or generate an internal variable that corresponds to the subjective attribute of lateralization. For those models that do have such a variable, the fundamental differences in the models concern the mechanism for combining the effects of interaural time delay and interaural amplitude ratio, and, more specifically, how peripherally this mechanism is located.

In the Jeffress model (and presumably in the latency-version of the Hafter–Carrier lateralization model), the internal variable that corresponds to lateralization for low frequencies is the place of maximum coincidence along the internal delay dimension. Changes in amplitude are assumed to cause changes in the latency of the nerve-pattern inputs to the coincidence devices; the mechanism thus corresponds to time–intensity trading at the periphery (even if two trades create two separate images). In the count-comparison models, the internal variable is the difference in the counts in the two cell populations at which the monaurally determined patterns first come together. Interaural time and intensity differences have distinct effects in the cell populations; the mechanism thus corresponds to time–intensity interaction after the coincidence device in the general model. In the model of Sayers and Cherry, the internal variable is an integrated, weighted, cross-correlation function (the sum of weighted coincidence outputs). The amplitude effects are mediated by weighting factors, and the time–intensity interaction again occurs after the correlation–coincidence operation. The fact that the interaction occurs before the coincidence device in the first case, but after the coincidence device in the second and third cases, is reflected in the different predictions for the effect of amplitude difference on the function describing how lateralization depends on delay. Whereas in the first case an amplitude difference is predicted (incorrectly) to offset the independent variable (delay), in the second and third cases, an amplitude difference is predicted (correctly) to offset the dependent variable (lateralization). In the other models that we have discussed, no internal variables have been identified with lateralization, and therefore no predictions can be made for these data. It appears obvious, however, that many of these models could be extended to describe at least certain of the lateralization phenomena by incorporating some additional constraints.

It is uncertain whether any of the models that we have discussed are capable of describing both the vertical shift and the diffused or split images that have been reported when there is an amplitude difference. Although the two-trading-ratio model of Hafter and Carrier could be used to predict some changes in the form of the lateralization curve with variations in amplitude difference by assuming that the single lateralization response required in most lateralization experiments is constructed by averaging the lateralizations of the two images, it does not appear that this model could predict a vertical shift since neither curve by itself exhibits such a shift.

2. BINAURAL DETECTION OF TONES IN NOISE

Predictions of binaural detection performance (like predictions of any type of sensitivity, but unlike predictions of mean lateralization responses) depend on the internal-noise postulates. Presumably, these predictions should also depend on the assumptions concerning the interaction of time and intensity. The fact that these assumptions have generally not been very important in this area is probably nothing more than a reflection of the fact that relatively little attention has been given to cases in which the level of the masking noise is unequal in the two ears. Although the results for some of these cases, such as those studied by Dolan and Robinson (1967) and McFadden (1968), can be explained without considering these assumptions, we expect that other cases cannot. Included among these other cases are the case in which the target signal is presented monaurally and the masking noise in the nonsignal ear is raised above the level in the signal ear, and the case in which the masking noise involves both an interaural amplitude difference and an interaural time delay.

Almost all models of binaural detection appear to be capable of describing the data on how the detection threshold varies with the interaural parameters of the target signal for the case of interaurally identical noise. In other words, the predictions for this body of data appear to be relatively insensitive to the detailed assumptions of the model. Although the basic reason for this lack of sensitivity is not entirely clear, recent work has shown that under the assumption of small signal-to-noise ratio (which is applicable to most binaural masked detection data), there are a wide variety of operations that can be performed on the received signals and a wide variety of internal-noise postulates that lead to the same results (Domnitz & Colburn, 1976). Specifically, it has been shown that the predicted results for ratios of thresholds involving stimulus configurations in which the target signal is not interaurally identical are independent of whether the decision variable is identified with the interaural correlation coefficient, the ratio of complex amplitudes of the signals at the two ears, or the magnitude or phase of this ratio. When the masking noise is constrained to be interaurally identical, the only ratios for which the internal noise influences the results are those that involve an interaurally identical target signal. As long as the internal noise is chosen to fit the amount of binaural unmasking for one nontrivial configuration, the model will automatically fit the other configurations.

Predictions that reflect the internal noise postulates in the models much more directly and in greater detail are those that are concerned with the dependence of the threshold signal-to-noise ratio on the overall level of the masking noise and the frequency of the target signal. Internal noise postulates that lead to the false prediction that the threshold signal-to-noise ratio is independent of the noise level include (1) internal noise that is added to the signals before the binaural interaction takes place and that has a level that is proportional to the external noise level, (2) multiplicative internal noise that is inserted before the binaural interaction (with or without time jitter) and that has a variance which is independent of the external noise level (Durlach's EC model), and (3) fixed-variance internal noise that is added to the output of a binaural-interaction mechanism which measures interaural time difference and/or interaural amplitude ratio (a postulate that is equivalent to the postulate of a fixed-deviation threshold that is used in the interaural-time-detector model of Webster and of Jeffress, Blodgett, Sandel, and Wood and in the lateralization model of Hafter and Carrier). As discussed previously, models with these postulates could be revised to better fit the dependence on noise level, without contradicting other data, by including additional fixed-level internal noise that is added before the binaural interaction (Dolan & Robinson, 1967; McFadden, 1968). A more natural fit to the level dependence, however, has been obtained with Colburn's model in which the internal noise postulates are derived from a statistical description of the auditory-nerve firing patterns. In this description, the patterns are described by Poisson processes with rate functions that saturate and that are nonzero when the stimulus is zero. Thus, the internal noise in this model is neither independent of the external level nor proportional to the external level; it exhibits features that are characteristic of both assumptions.

Predictions of the frequency dependence of binaural detection have been derived for a variety of models. However, the method used to generate these predictions, as well as the frequency region over which the predictions are adequate, varies considerably among the models. In Osman's correlation model, the frequency dependence is described merely by allowing the internal noise to vary with frequency in a manner that produces a good fit. In the EC and interaural-time-detector models, a good fit to the intermediate frequency region 500–1500 Hz is obtained by assuming a fixed-variance temporal noise (or its equivalent). The decrease in binaural performance with increasing frequency then results from the effect of frequency on the relation between time and phase (higher frequencies leading to increased phase noise). The EC model, but not the interaural-time-detector model, also provides a reasonable fit to the frequency dependence at lower frequencies, where the fixed-variance amplitude jitter in the EC model limits performance. Neither model, however, is capable of predicting the results at higher frequencies, where the fixed-variance temporal noise becomes large with respect to the period of the tone. In order to describe the data in this region, it is necessary either to allow the characteristics of the internal noise to depend on frequency, or to assume that different operations are performed on the received signals (as in Durlach's power-difference model or, possibly, in Hafter and Carrier's lateralization model). The frequency dependence predicted by the auditory-nerve-based model, which is consistent with data at both intermediate and low frequencies, is derived in part from the dependence on frequency of the synchrony in the neural firing patterns. This synchrony is constant at very low frequencies and decreases as frequency increases. At frequencies above roughly 800 Hz, the assumption of a decrease in the synchrony parameter of approximately 6 dB octave^{-1} appears to be sufficient to describe both the limited amount of available auditory-nerve data on this function and the behavioral detection data. This decrease, moreover, is precisely the decrease that one would predict from a fixed time jitter, as assumed explicitly in the EC model and implicitly in the interaural-time-detector model. In order to fit the data at high frequencies, the auditory-nerve-based model must rely on synchrony with the envelope of the filtered input waveform.

Predictions concerning the dependence of binaural detection on the interaural differences in the noise are generally more sensitive to the structure of the model and to the internal noise postulates than predictions of the dependence on interaural differences in the target signal. The only apparent exception to this statement concerns the case in which the noise is decorrelated through the use of independent noise sources. Practically all models that are sufficiently developed to permit quantitative predictions of these data are able to fit these data with reasonable accuracy. The empirical results that provide the strongest constraints on the models are those describing the dependence of binaural detection on the interaural time delay, phase shift, or amplitude ratio of the noise. The time-delay and phase-shift data not only require the assumption of some limited internal-delay or phase-shift capability in the model, but as indicated previously, the flattening phenomenon that occurs in these data at low frequencies suggests that this capability must be structured in a rather special way. At present, the only model that adequately describes all these time-delay and phase-shift data is the model based on auditory-nerve firing patterns. The ability of this model to fit these data results from the assumption that there are fewer fiber pairs with long delays than short ones (which implies that the effective internal noise increases with internal delay, since there are fewer pairs over which the coincidence information can be averaged), and from the assumption that a variety of delays are available simultaneously. Presumably, other models could also be made to fit these data by the use of equivalent assumptions, but this work has not been carried out. An initial step in this direction is evident in the work by Metz, von Bismarck, and Durlach on the EC model. Also, it is clear that the same basic ideas, although not worked out quantitatively, are contained in the original lateralization model of Jeffress.

Since many of the effects of interaural amplitude differences in the noise are closely related to the dependence on overall noise level, only those models that can describe this dependence (e.g., the models of Dolan and Robinson, McFadden, and Colburn) can possibly describe all these effects. As pointed out previously, however, an adequate description of all these effects probably requires an appropriate assumption concerning the interaction of time and intensity. No model has yet provided a satisfactory explanation of the observed increase in threshold that occurs when the signal is monaural and the noise in the nonsignal ear is raised above its level in the signal ear.

3. INTERAURAL DISCRIMINATION

Predictions concerning the ability to discriminate interaural parameters are sensitive to both the internal noise postulates and the constraints imposed on the interaction of time and intensity. Compared to the work on the detection of tones in noise, and despite the close relationship between binaural unmasking and interaural discrimination, surprisingly little effort has been made to apply quantitative models of binaural interaction to data on interaural discrimination. Moreover, in most cases where an effort has been made, only a limited class of data has been considered and/or the success achieved has been limited. Of all the possible experiments on interaural discrimination that might be considered, the ones that have proved most interesting for models of binaural interaction are those involving incremental changes in interaural time delay, either with or without simultaneous changes in interaural amplitude ratio. (Coherent masking, such as tone-on-tone masking, is included as a special case of simultaneous changes in time delay and amplitude ratio.)

Predictions of the jnd in interaural time delay for the case in which the reference stimulus is interaurally identical have been derived explicitly from Durlach's EC model, Colburn's auditory-nerve-based model, and Hall's count-comparison model. The predictions based on the EC model are consistent with the data (as are predictions of the jnds in interaural amplitude and correlation) when all the parameters of the model are chosen separately for each set of data. There are difficulties, however, when one set of parameters is used to describe all the data. For example, if all the parameters of the model are chosen to fit the binaural unmasking data, the predicted interaural time jnd is too large. Similarly, the model based on auditory-nerve data correctly predicts the interaural time jnd, but the thresholds of detection for binaural unmasking are predicted to be about 20 dB lower than observed. This deviation is in the same direction as that predicted by the EC model when the parameters of the EC model are chosen to fit the discrimination data. Hall's model correctly predicts the interaural time jnd for a click stimulus. However, since this model cannot be applied to other stimuli (including those used in masked detection experiments) without additional physiological data, we do not know whether the same difficulties in fitting both discrimination and detection data would be encountered by this model with a single set of parameters. Although no explicit quantitative predictions for the interaural time jnd have been stated for the interaural-time-detector model (Webster; Jeffress, Blodget, Sandel, and Wood), the lateralization model (Hafter and Carrier), or the ρ model (Osman), it appears that these models would encounter essentially the same problem as that encountered by the EC model and the model based on auditory-nerve data.

Predictions for the dependence of the interaural time jnd on interaural time delay and interaural amplitude ratio depend upon the assumed interaction of time and amplitude, as well as the internal noise postulates. The available data on this dependence reflect an interaction that is totally inconsistent with a simple, peripheral time–intensity trade (as specified, for example, by the latency hypothesis). According to these data, the ability to detect a small increment in interaural time delay is better when the stimulus in which the increment is inserted has an internal time delay and an internal amplitude ratio that are collateral than when they are antilateral. None of the models that we have discussed appear to be capable of describing these data satisfactorily.

Further predictions that reflect the assumed constraint on the interaction of time and intensity are those describing the ability to detect simultaneous changes in interaural time delay and interaural amplitude ratio. The observation that simultaneous antilateral increments in time delay and amplitude ratio are more difficult to detect than the corresponding time increments alone or than the corresponding simultaneous collateral increments indicates that the increment in delay cannot be measured independently of the increment in amplitude ratio, and that only a combined effect of the two increments is available to the final decision device. On the other hand, the data on the discrimination of simultaneous increments show that time and intensity are only partially tradable. Thus, whatever constraint is required on how the individual effects are combined, it cannot be described merely as a simple time–intensity trade. To date, no model has shown itself to be capable of predicting all these data in quantitative detail. Models that do not explicitly postulate some form of time–intensity interaction (such as the EC model, the ρ model, the internal-time-detector model without the latency hypothesis, and the auditory-nerve-based model) appear to be totally inadequate for describing these data. Of those models that do incorporate such a postulate, only the lateralization model of Hafter and Carrier has been applied quantitatively to these data. Although the single-image (single-trading-ratio) version of this model is inadequate for describing the details of all these data, the multiple-image (multiple-trading-ratio) version may not be inadequate. No attempt has been made to apply the ideas concerning time–intensity interaction that are used in the count-comparison models or the correlation model of Sayers and Cherry to these data.

Finally, it should be noted that discrimination experiments in which no time increment is involved have played a relatively small role in the development of models of binaural interaction. The fact that discrimination of pure amplitude increments has been relatively unimportant is not surprising since the available psychophysical results of such studies can be explained (appropriately or not with respect to the underlying physiological mechansims) solely on the basis of information in the monaural channels (e.g., Colburn, 1973). Similarly, discrimination of frequency differences has been relatively uninteresting because, for low- and intermediate-frequency tones, a small interaural difference in frequency can be represented, and is percieved, as a slowly varying interaural time delay. If the duration of the stimuli is sufficiently great, the only limitation on performance in this case would appear to arise from imperfect memory.

In contrast to amplitude and frequency, however, we see no logical reason for the fact that discrimination of interaural correlation of noise signals (where the correlation is controlled by independent sources) has played such a small role. The ability to discriminate along this dimension, both with equal and with unequal noise levels at the two ears, would appear to be an important ability to consider in developing an adequate model of binaural interaction. This ability [which has been measured for certain cases by Pollack and Trittipoe (1959a,b)], has been considered only in connection with the EC model, and then only briefly.

C. Concluding Remarks

In considering the material presented in this section, two points should be immediately apparent.

First, in order to provide an adequate overview of the models, a great deal of further work is required. Not only is our discussion in this section both crude and incomplete, but it contains some statements that are based more on speculation than on fact. For example, in some cases we have attempted to evaluate a model's capabilities for describing certain data, even though the detailed analysis required to support such an evaluation has not yet been carried out. It is possible that some of our evaluations will prove to be incorrect. Similar remarks apply to our attempts to identify the underlying assumptions that are responsible for particular characteristics of a model's predictions. Despite these limitations, we decided to include this section because we believe that the development of an adequate overview is vital to further progress in this field.

Second, despite all the work that has been performed on models of binaural interaction, there is no model now available that is satisfactory. Aside from the general fact that none of the existing models is capable of predicting more than a small portion of all the existing data on binaural interaction, they are all deficient in at least one (and often all) of the following areas:

1. Providing a complete quantitative description of how the stimulus waveforms are processed and of how this processing is corrupted by internal noise.
2. Deriving all the predictions that follow from the assumptions of the model and comparing these predictions to all the relevant data.
3. Having a sufficiently small number of free parameters in the model to prevent the model from becoming merely a transformation of coordinates or an elaborate curve-fit.
4. Relating the assumptions and parameters of the model in a serious manner to known physiological results.
5. Taking account of general perceptual principles in modeling the higher-level, more central portions of the system for which there are no adequate systematic physiological results available.

The explicit inclusion of a quantitative description of the peripheral transformation from acoustic waveforms to neural firing patterns in the auditory nerve would appear to be a reasonable step toward achieving a satisfactory model (and certainly constitutes a natural means for generating at least a portion of the internal noise that is required in any such model). However, neither the auditory-nerve-based model nor any of the other existing models has been shown capable of solving the outstanding problem that has faced theorists in this area for many years, namely, the problem of specifying a mechanism that leads to an adequate description of all the data on time–intensity interaction. Perhaps the outline of a solution to this problem will only become clear when improved experimental techniques are developed for specifying the complex spatial properties of the in-head binaural image.

Note. This chapter reviews research conducted prior to 1974 (the year the chapter was written). Reports of more recent research can be found in the journals cited in the reference list (particularly the *Journal of the Acoustical Society of America*).

Acknowledgments

This work was supported by Public Health Service Grants NIGMS-5-PO1-GM14940 and NINCDS-5-RO1-NS10916. Many helpful comments on an earlier draft of this chapter were received from our colleagues, especially E. Osman and D. McFadden.

References

Békésy, G. von. Zur Theorie des Hörens. *Physikalische Zeitschrift*, 1930, **31**, 857–868. [Translation in Chapter 8 of *Experiments in hearing*, G. V. Békésy (E. G. Wever, Ed. and Trans.). New York: McGraw-Hill, 1960.]

Bilsen, F. A., & Goldstein, J. L. Pitch of dichotically delayed noise and its possible spectral basis. *Journal of the Acoustical Society of America*, 1974, **55**, 292–296.

Cherry, E. C., & Sayers, B. McA. On the mechansim of binaural fusion. *Journal of the Acoustical Society of America*, 1959, **31**, 535.

Colburn, H. S. Some physiological limitations on binaural performance. Unpublished dissertation, Ph.D., Elec. Eng. Dept., M.I.T., 1969.

Colburn, H. S. Theory of binaural interaction based on auditory-nerve data. I. General strategy and preliminary results on interaural discrimination. *Journal of the Acoustical Society of America*, 1973, **54**, 1458–1470.

Colburn, H. S. Theory of binaural interaction based on auditory-nerve data. II. Detection of tones in noise. *Journal of the Acoustical Society of America*, 1977, **61**, 525–533. (a)

Colburn, H. S. "Theory of Binaural Interaction Based on Auditory-Nerve Data. II. Detection of Tones in Noise. Supplementary Material," Am. Inst. Physics, Physics Auxiliary Publication Service document No. PAPS, JASMA-61-525-98, 1977; also appears in *Current Physics Microfilm*, 1977. (b)

Colburn, H. S., & Durlach, N. I. Time-intensity relations in binaural unmasking. *Journal of the Acoustical Society of America*, 1965, **38**, 93–103.

Cramer, E. M., & Huggins, W. H. Creation of pitch through binaural interaction. *Journal of the Acoustical Society of America*, 1958, **30**, 413–417.

David, E. E., Jr., Guttman, N., & van Bergeijk, W. A. Binaural interaction of high-frequency complex stimuli. *Journal of the Acoustical Society of America*, 1959, **31**, 774–782.

Diercks, K. J., & Jeffress, L. A. Interaural phase and the absolute threshold for tone. *Journal of the Acoustical Society of America*, 1962, **34**, 981–984.

Dolan, T. R., & Robinson, D. E. Explanation of masking-level differences that result from interaural intensive disparities of noise. *Journal of the Acoustical Society of America*, 1967, **42**, 977–981.

Domnitz, R. The interaural time jnd as a simultaneous function of interaural time and interaural amplitude. *Journal of the Acoustical Society of America*, 1973, **53**, 1549–1552.

Domnitz, R., & Colburn, H. S. Analysis of binaural detection models for dependence on interaural target parameters. *Journal of the Acoustical Society of America*, 1976, **59**, 598–601.

Durlach, N. I. Note on the equalization and cancellation theory of binaural masking-level differences. *Journal of the Acoustical Society of America*, 1960, **32**, 1075–1076.

Durlach, N. I. Note on the creation of pitch through binaural interaction. *Journal of the Acoustical Society of America*, 1962, **34**, 1096–1099.

Durlach, N. I. Equalization and cancellation theory of binaural masking-level differences. *Journal of the Acoustical Society of America*, 1963, **35**, 1206–1218.

Durlach, N. I. Note on binaural masking-level differences at high frequencies. *Journal of the Acoustical Society of America*, 1964, **36**, 576–581. (a)

Durlach, N. I. Note on binaural masking-level differences as a function of the interaural correlation of the masking noise. *Journal of the Acoustical Society of America*, 1964, **36**, 1613–1617. (b)

Durlach, N. I. On the application of the EC model to interaural jnd's. *Journal of the Acoustical Society of America*, 1966, **40**, 1392–1397.

Durlach, N. I. Binaural signal detection: Equalization and cancellation theory. In J. V. Tobias (Ed.), *Foundations of modern auditory theory*. New York: Academic Press, 1972.

Erulkar, S. D. Comparative aspects of spatial localization of sound. *Physiological Review*, 1972, **52**, 237–360.

Galambos, R., Rose, J. E., Bromiley, R. B., & Hughes, J. R. Microelectrode studies on medial geniculate body of cat. II. Response to clicks. *Journal of Neurophysiology*, 1952, **15**, 359–380.

Green, D. M. Consistency of auditory detection judgments. *Psychological Review*, 1964, **71**, 392–407.

Green, D. M. Signal detection analysis of EC model. *Journal of the Acoustical Society of America*, 1966, **40**, 833–838.

Hafter, E. R. Quantitative evaluation of a lateralization model of masking-level differences. *Journal of the Acoustical Society of America*, 1971, **50**, 1116–1122.

Hafter, E. R., Bourbon, W. T., Blocker, A. S., & Tucker, A. A direct comparison between lateralization and detection under conditions of antiphasic masking. *Journal of the Acoustical Society of America*, 1969, **46**, 1452–1457.

Hafter, E. R., & Carrier, S. C. Masking level differences obtained with pulsed tonal maskers. *Journal of the Acoustical Society of America*, 1970, **47**, 1041–1047.

Hafter, E. R., & Carrier, S. C. Binaural interaction in low-frequency stimuli: The inability to trade time and intensity completely. *Journal of the Acoustical Society of America*, 1972, **51**, 1852–1862.

Hafter, E. R., Carrier, S. C., & Stephan, F. K. Direct comparison of lateralization and the MLD for monaural signals in gated noise. *Journal of the Acoustical Society of America*, 1973, **53**, 1553–1559.

Hall, J. L., II. Binaural interaction in the accessory superior-olivary nucleus of the cat. *Journal of the Acoustical Society of America*, 1965, **37**, 814–823.

Henning, G. B. Effect of interaural phase on frequency and amplitude discrimination *Journal of the Acoustical Society of America*, 1973, **54**, 1160–1178.

Henning, G. B. Lateralization and the binaural masking-level difference. *Journal of the Acoustical Society of America*, 1974, **55**, 1259–1262.

Hershkowitz, R. M., & Durlach, N. I. Interaural time and amplitude jnds for a 500-Hz tone. *Journal of the Acoustical Society of America*, 1969, **46**, 1464–1467.

Hirsh, I. J. The influence of interaural phase on interaural summation and inhibition. *Journal of the Acoustical Society of America*, 1948, **20**, 536–544.

Jeffress, L. A. A place theory of sound localization. *Journal of Comparative and Physiological Psychology*, 1948, **41**, 35–39.

Jeffress, L. A. Binaural signal detection: Vector theory. In J. V. Tobias (Ed.), *Foundations of modern auditory theory*. New York: Academic Press, 1972.

Jeffress, L. A., Blodgett, H. C., & Deatherage, B. H. The masking of tones by white noise as a function of the interaural phases of both components. I. 500 cycles. *Journal of the Acoustical Society of America*, 1952, **24**, 523–527.

Jeffress, L. A., Blodgett, H. C., & Deatherage, B. H. Masking and interaural phase. II. 167 cycles. *Journal of the Acoustical Society of America*, 1962, **34**, 1124–1126.

Jeffress, L. A., Blodgett, H. C., Sandel, T. T., & Wood, C. L., III. Masking of tonal signals. *Journal of the Acoustical Society of America*, 1956, **28**, 416–426.

Jeffress, L. A., & McFadden, D. Differences of interaural phase and level in detection and lateralization. *Journal of the Acoustical Society of America*, 1971, **49**, 1169–1179.

Kemp, E. H., Coppée, G. E., & Robinson, E. H. Electric responses of the brain stem to unilateral auditory stimulation. *American Journal of Physiology*, 1937, **120**, 304–315.

Kiang, N. Y. S. A survey of recent developments in the study of auditory physiology. *Annals of Otology, Rhinology, and Laryngology*, 1968, **77**, 656–675.

Kiang, N. Y. S., Watanabe, T., Thomas, E. C., & Clark, L. F. *Discharge patterns of single fibers in the cat's auditory nerve*. Research Monograph 35, Cambridge, Massachusetts: M.I.T. Press, 1965.

Kock, W. E. Binaural localization and masking. *Journal of the Acoustical Society of America*, 1950, **22**, 801–804.

Langford, T. L., & Jeffress, L. A. Effect of noise cross-correlation on binaural signal detection. *Journal of the Acoustical Society of America*, 1964, **36**, 1455–1458.

Leakey, D. M., Sayers, B. McA., & Cherry, E. C. Binaural fusion of low- and high-frequency sounds. *Journal of the Acoustical Society of America*, 1958, **30**, 222–223.

Levitt, H., & Lundry, E. A. Some properties of the vector model for binaural hearing. *Journal of the Acoustical Society of America*, 1966, **39**, 1232. (a)

Levitt, H., & Lundry, E. A. Binaural vector model: Relative interaural time differences. *Journal of the Acoustical Society of America*, 1966, **40**, 1251. (b)

Licklider, J. C. R. Three auditory theories. In E. S. Koch (Ed.), *Psychology: A study of a science*. Study 1, Vol. 1. New York: McGraw-Hill, 1959.

Matzker, J. Versuch einer Erklärung des Richtungshörens auf Grund feinster Zeitunterschieds-registrierungen. *Acta Oto-Laryngologica*, 1958, **49**, 483–494.

McFadden, D. Masking-level differences determined with and without interaural disparities in masker intensity. *Journal of the Acoustical Society of America*, 1968, **44**, 212–223.

McFadden, D., Jeffress, L. A., & Ermey, H. L. Differences of interaural phase and level in detection and lateralization: 250 Hz. *Journal of the Acoustical Society of America*, 1971, **50**, 1484–1493.

McFadden, D., Jeffress, L. A., & Lakey, J. R. Differences of interaural phase and level in detection and lateralization: 1000 Hz and 2000 Hz. *Journal of the Acoustical Society of America*, 1972, **52**, 1197–1206.

Metz, P. J., Bismarck, G. von, & Durlach, N. I. Further results on binaural unmasking and the EC model. II. Noise bandwidth and interaural phase. *Journal of the Acoustical Society of America*, 1968, **43**, 1085–1091.

Osman, E. A correlation model of binaural masking level differences. *Journal of the Acoustical Society of America*, 1971, **50**, 1494–1511.

Osman, E. Correlation model of binaural detection: Interaural amplitude ratio and phase variation for signal. *Journal of the Acoustical Society of America*, 1973, **54**, 386–389.

Osman, E., Schacknow, P. N., & Tzuo, P. L. Psychometric functions and a correlation model of binaural detection. *Perception and Psychophysics*, 1973, **14**, 371–374.

Pohlman, L. D., & Sorkin, R. D. Binaural masking level differences for pulse train signals of differing interaural correlation. *Journal of the Acoustical Society of America*, 1974, **55**, 1293–1298.

Pollack, I., & Trittipoe, W. J. Binaural listening and interaural noise crosscorrelation. *Journal of the Acoustical Society of America*, 1959, **31**, 1250–1252. (a)

Pollack, I., & Trittipoe, W. J. Interaural noise correlations: Examination of variables. *Journal of the Acoustical Society of America*, 1959, **31**, 1616–1618. (b)

Rabiner, L. R., Laurence, C. L., & Durlach, N. I. Further results on binaural unmasking and the EC model. *Journal of the Acoustical Society of America*, 1966, **40**, 62–70.

Robinson, D. E. Some computations relevant to the Webster-Jeffress model for binaural signal detection. *Journal of the Acoustical Society of America*, 1966, **39**, 1232.

Robinson, D. E., & Jeffress, L. A. Effect of varying the interaural noise correlation on the detectability of tonal signals. *Journal of the Acoustical Society of America*, 1963, **35**, 1947–1952.

Sayers, B. McA. Acoustic-image lateralization judgments with binaural tones. *Journal of the Acoustical Society of America*, 1964, **36**, 923–926.

Sayers, B. McA., & Cherry, E. C. Mechanism of binaural fusion in the hearing of speech. *Journal of the Acoustical Society of America*, 1957, **29**, 973–987.

Sayers, B. McA., & Lynn, P. A. Interaural amplitude effects in binaural hearing. *Journal of the Acoustical Society of America*, 1968, **44**, 973–978.

Schenkel, K. D. Accumulation theory of binaural-masked thresholds. *Journal of the Acoustical Society of America*, 1967, **41**, 20–31.

Siebert, W. M. Some implications of the stochastic behavior of primary auditory neurons. *Kybernetic*, 1965, **2**, 206–215.

Siebert, W. M. Stimulus transformations in the peripheral auditory system. In P. A. Kolers & M. Eden (Eds.), *Recognizing patterns*. Cambridge, Massachusetts: M.I.T. Press, 1968.

Siebert, W. M. Frequency discrimination in the auditory system: Place or periodicity mechanisms? *Proceedings of the IEEE*, 1970, **58**, 723–730.

Sondhi, M. M. Crosscorrelation model for binaural unmasking. *Journal of the Acoustical Society of America*, 1966, **39**, 1232.

Swets, J. A., Shipley, E. F., McKey, M. J., & Green, D. M. Multiple observations of signals in noise. *Journal of the Acoustical Society of America*, 1959, **31**, 514–521.

Thurlow, W. R., Gross, N. R., Kemp, E. H., & Lowy, K. Microelectrode studies of neural auditory activity of cat. I. Inferior colliculus. *Journal of Neurophysiology*, 1951, **14**, 289–304.

Toole, F. E., & Sayers, B. McA. Inferences of neural activity associated with binaural acoustic images. *Journal of the Acoustical Society of America*, 1965, **38**, 769–779.

van Bergeijk, W. A. Variation on a theme of von Békésy: A model of binaural interaction. *Journal of the Acoustical Society of America*, 1962, **34**, 1431–1437.

Voelcker, H. B. A decision-theory approach to sound lateralization. In C. Cherry (Ed.), *Information theory*. London: Butterworth, 1961.

Webster, F. A. The influence of interaural phase on masked thresholds. I. The role of interaural time-deviation. *Journal of the Acoustical Society of America*, 1951, **23**, 452–462.

Weston, P. B., & Miller, J. D. Use of noise to eliminate one ear from masking experiments. *Journal of the Acoustical Society of America*, 1965, **37**, 638–646.

Yost, W. A. Tone-on-tone masking for three binaural listening conditions. *Journal of the Acoustical Society of America*, 1972, **52**, 1234–1237.

Part V

Psychology of Music

Chapter 12

MUSICAL ACOUSTICS

JEAN-CLAUDE RISSET

I. INTRODUCTION

Musical acoustics faces the challenge of dealing scientifically with music, an aesthetic activity that raises philosophical questions and involves a Weltanschauung (Lesche, cited in Music and Technology, 1971, pp. 39–55). Science is not a normative activity like aesthetics; however, it can clarify some musical issues and show that they are burdened with many myths. There is an urge for a better understanding of musical behavior: It would be valuable to gain insight on such a human experience, deeply involving perceptual and motor abilities, and capable of rousing strong motivations. Moreover, such understanding is needed to make good musical use of the technological progress and of the new and powerful tools it can provide.

An acoustic signal becomes music only when it is perceived as such, through ear and brain. So hearing and auditory perception are central to musical acoustics. However, hearing has been studied mostly in terms of reactions to simple stimuli (see Part III, this volume, Chapters 6–9). This is

HANDBOOK OF PERCEPTION, VOL. IV

understandable, but musical sounds are not simple stimuli, so psychoacoustic results have to be qualified. More important, the stimulus and response situation of many sensory experiments is remote from the experience of music. To obtain significant results on music, we must take in account very complex situations. Must we agree with Eddington that a science with more than seven variables is an art, and conclude that musical acoustics is either irrelevant or unscientific?

There are some specific research subjects that are relevant to music and can legitimately be isolated from the intricate context involved in music. Moreover, powerful new tools and new methods are available to study more and more complex situations and to isolate what is musically relevant in this complexity. Thanks to recording, evanescent sounds become objects that can be scrutinized at leisure. New devices, especially the general purpose digital computer, permit us to analyze complex data—psychological judgments as well as sounds—or to formulate elaborate models of perception, musical sounds, and musical composition. Recent progress in musical acoustics is encouraging, although it is slowed down by lack of support. (Important results often come as by-products of research in other fields.) So a number of questions asked 30 years ago (Young, 1944) are still unanswered (Small & Martin, 1957).

This chapter reviews some important topics in musical acoustics, but it merely scratches the surface. The reader looking for a more complete treatment is directed to a number of varied references.

II. MUSIC, HEARING, AND PERCEPTION

A. Parameters of Musical Sounds

Perception implies generalization and discrimination. The discriminating power of hearing determines the smallest differences that can be used significantly in music. For instance, the steps of a musical scale should not be smaller than the just noticeable pitch difference. Hence the psychoacoustic study of the listener's response to separate parameters of sound is of interest; however, it provides only a bounding of the area of musical perception, rather than determining what happens in that area (Poland, 1963). There is evidence that limens, measured in laboratory conditions, are smaller than the differences that can be detected in complex listening tasks (Plomp, 1966, p. 19) like attending to music (Jacobs & Wittman, 1964). Perception also implies construction and abstraction. Interaction between separate parameters is important in musical perception, which takes place in a complex context (Francès, 1958) (see Section II,F).

In works on musical acoustics, we generally consider four parameters—or attributes—of auditory events: pitch, duration (related to rhythm), loudness, and timbre. Pitch and duration are marked carefully in conventional occidental music notation, which resembles a system of cartesian coordinates (pitch versus time); loudness is marked more crudely, and timbre is determined by the musical instruments for which the music is written (e.g., violin) and the way they are played (e.g., pizzicato). In some manuscripts by Bach, the instruments are not even specified and no dynamic marking is provided. Duration and especially pitch are regarded as the most important musical parameters. A review entitled Musical Perception (Ward, 1970) deals almost exclusively with pitch perception. Yet other parameters are also important, especially in certain types of music: Some nonwestern notational systems contain information related to timbre and intensity.

We might question the choice of the parameters of sound just mentioned. As Seashore (1938, p. 16) clearly states, this choice stems from the assumption that the hearing of tones is an imperfect copy of the physical characteristics of the sound. Periodic sound waves can be described in terms of frequency, amplitude, duration, and form; hence, the auditory correlates should be the four characteristics of musical tones. This assumption is disputable: It is now clear that periodic sound is not synonymous of musical tone (see Section II,D); also, pitch and timbre are correlated (see Section II,B,6). However the description of musical sounds in terms of pitch, duration, loudness, and timbre remains widespread and most useful, but we must remind ourselves that these parameters are seldom treated independently in music.

B. Musical Pitch

1. HEARING AND MUSICAL PITCH

Music calls for appreciation of pitch intervals. Musicians consistently judge that a constant musical interval between two pitches corresponds over a wide range to a constant ratio between the two corresponding frequencies. This seems to be at variance with psychophysical experiments of pitch scaling (Stevens & Volkmann, 1940); however, pitch scaling involves a very special task for subjects. As Ward (1970) strongly states, "it is nonsense to give musical pitch a cavalier dismissal simply because an octave interval has a different size in mels depending on the frequency range."

Precise appreciation of pitch intervals is not possible throughout the entire frequency range of audible sounds. According to Watt (1917, p. 63), the *musical range* of pitch may be defined as the range within which the octave is perceived. Using this definition, Guttman and Pruzansky (1962) find that the lower limit of musical pitch is around 60 Hz (the frequency of the lowest note of the piano is about 27 Hz); similarly there is a breakdown in the precision and the consistency of intervallic judgments above 4000 Hz, which corresponds roughly to the highest note of the piano. This does not mean that frequencies below 60 Hz or above 4000 Hz are never used in music (Attneave & Olson, 1971). In the range of musical pitch, the octave relationship is very strong—and will be discussed in Section I,B,6.

The pitch of a sinewave depends upon the intensity (Stevens & Davis, 1952); this effect varies with listeners, it is usually quite small (Cohen, 1961), and it is weaker for complex tones or for modulated sine tones than for unmodulated sine tones (Seashore, 1938, p. 64). Thus, the effect of intensity on pitch is, fortunately, of little significance in music.

Presbycusis—that is, the normal hearing loss at high frequencies occurring with age—does not interfere too much with musical pitch discrimination, although it influences judgments on the tone quality of the sounds.

2. MUSICAL SCALES

Most music uses scales (Sachs, 1943). A *musical scale* is a set of tone steps (or notes) selected from the continuum of frequencies and bearing a definite interval relation to each other. There exists a considerable amount of literature on the frequency ratios corresponding to the scales used in music (Barbour, 1953; Billeter, 1970; Ellis, 1954; Lloyd & Boyle, 1963; Partch, 1949).

The brief discussion that follows is restricted to occidental music. Pythagoras is credited for the design of a scale in which the frequencies of the tone steps are deduced in turn from the frequency of one of them by multiplications by $\frac{3}{2}$—corresponding to an interval of a *perfect fifth* (and divisions by 2, to bring back the notes in the proper octave). Aristoxenus is sometimes credited for a slightly different scale (also called just intonation or Zarlino scale) with simple frequency ratios; the notes of the scale are the tones obtained on a string instrument by dividing the string into 2, 3, 4, etc. equal sections, and bringing them back in the proper octave. Early occidental music used so-called diatonic scales comprising 7 (unequal) intervals per octave, which were slightly different in the Pythagoras and Aristoxenus designs. However, these scales were unpractical for *modulation,* that is, change of *tonality,* tonality meaning here the note chosen as the origin of the successive intervals of the scale. A keyboard instrument would have required many dozens of keys per octave to give the proper intervals in several tonalities. With the increasing use of modulation between the sixteenth and eighteenth centuries, compromises had to be adopted for the tuning of fixed pitch instruments (especially keyboard instruments). *Equal temperament* is the best known: The octave is divided into 12 equal intervals, named semitones, forming a so-called chromatic scale (a semitone thus corresponds to a frequency ratio of $2^{1/12}$). From the tones of the chromatic scales, one can select 12 major and 12 minor tempered scales corresponding to different tonalities. Expressed in number of semitones, the succession of intervals of the major scales is (2,2,1,2,2,2,1) (Backus, 1969, p. 127; Barbour, 1953). Bach's "well-tempered clavier" illustrates the use of all tonalities: however the question whether this *well-tempered clavier* really used the *equally tempered* tuning is not settled (Billeter, 1970). Equal temperament was widely used in classical, romantic, and contemporary occidental music: Schoenberg's 12-tone technique uses the notes of the chromatic scale. Yet several twentieth century composers, specially Varèse, were not satisfied with what they considered a somewhat arbitrary and aurally unsatisfactory pitch system (Ouelette, 1968). Special instruments were designed for other scales (van Esbroeck & Montfort, 1946; Partch, 1949). The development of electronic sources of sound (see Section V) makes it easier for the musician to escape equal temperament and to freely choose his own scales.

Despite considerable speculation about the justification of the frequency ratios used in various scales (see Section II,B,3), there are few data about tuning, intonation, and intervals used in actual musical practice or preferred by listeners. The tuning of pianos is usually *stretched,* that is, the high tones are higher and the lower notes are lower than what would correspond to the tempered scale. This can be ascribed partly to the inharmonicity of piano strings (Schuck & Young, 1943), yet stretched tuning seems to take place also in the gongs of the Indonesian Gamelans (Hood, 1974), so it may relate to universal perceptual characteristics such as the stretching of the subjective octave (Sundberg & Lindqvist, 1973). Stretched tuning is preferred over unstretched by listeners (Ward & Martin, 1961). Violinists have been said to follow a Pythagorean scale (van Esbroeck & Montfort, 1948; Greene, 1937), which may result from practice on an instrument tuned by fifths. However, the departure from equal temperament is not very significant except that notes other than the tonic (in tonal music) tend to be played sharp. Also, contextual effects in tonal music have a significant influence on intonation, for example, the interval C to F sharp (an augmented fourth) is played larger than the interval C to G flat (a diminished fifth), although these intervals are identical in equal temperament (Small, 1936; Sackford, 1961, 1962). Extensive listening tests, performed with the help of a specially designed organ, failed to give clear trends about the preferences of listeners for a given type of tuning (van Esbroeck & Montfort, 1948). Well-tempered intervals tend to be preferred in melodies, which may be due to familiarity with the piano, whereas results are unclear in chords (Ward & Martin, 1961). Listeners tend to prefer intonations in which the notes are sharp as compared with a tempered scale (Boomsliter & Creel, 1963). In the performance of solo music, wind instruments are played with a stretched frequency scale, which agrees with the fact that the subjective musical octave systematically exceeds a 2:1 frequency ratio (Sundberg & Lindqvist, 1973; Fransson *et al.,* 1970; Music, Room, and Acoustics, 1977).

Nonoccidental music uses other scales: Indian music, for instance, has a larger variety of scales than western music (Ellis, 1954). Many of these scales have five or seven steps per octave, and this has been linked to "the magical number seven plus or minus two" which, according to Miller (1969), measures in *items* (digits, letters, notes) the span of immediate memory. The intervals of octave, fifth and fourth, seem to be present in many exotic scales (Sachs, 1943).

3. CONSONANCE AND DISSONANCE

A *consonance* is a combination of two or more simultaneous tones that is judged pleasing to listen.

Pythagoras noticed that consonant intervals like the octave, the fifth, and the fourth, correspond to simple frequency ratios like $\frac{2}{1}$, $\frac{3}{2}$, $\frac{4}{3}$ (actually Pythagoras measured ratios of string *length* on a string instrument, the monochord). Aristoxenus held a more relativist view on consonance. Later, numerological explanations were advocated by Leibniz [who asserted that unconscious counting by the brain was the basis for the feeling of consonance or dissonance (cf. Revesz, 1954, p. 50, Euler, Schopenhauer; Meyer, 1899: "the brain dislikes large numbers")]. Some authors still claim that the ear appreciates the numerical complexity of an interval, either melodic—notes played in succession—or harmonic—simultaneous notes (Boomsliter & Creel, 1963; cf. Cazden, 1959). There have been attempts (e.g., R. Tanner) to attribute to a given frequency ratio a multiple-valued complexity, in order to explain that the same frequency ratio can be heard as two different intervals (Canac, 1959, pp. 83–102; also Tanner, 1972). (For example, on a piano keyboard, F sharp and G flat correspond to the same note, yet one can mentally switch and hear the interval this note forms with the C below either as diminished –C–G flat—or as augmented –C–F sharp— implying different harmonic resolutions.)

Numerological theories of consonance suffer difficulties. Because of the ear's tolerance, intervals corresponding to 3 : 2 (a simple ratio) and 300,001: 200,000 (a complex ratio) are not discriminated. Also psychophysiological evidence indicates that numerical ratios should not be taken for granted. The subjective octave corresponds to a frequency ratio a little larger than 2, and reliably different for different individuals (Sundberg & Lindqvist, 1973; Ward, 1954); this effect is increased by sleep deprivation (Elfner, 1964).

There are also physical theories of consonance. Helmholtz (1954) links the degree of dissonance to the audibility of beats between the partials of the tones. (Intervals judged consonants like the octave, fifth, fourth, usually evoke no beat, although the fifth corresponding to frequencies of 32 and 48 Hz does evoke an audible beat.) This theory is hardly tenable, because the pattern of beats, for a given interval, depends very much on the placement of the interval within the audible frequency range. Some observations (Plomp, 1966) suggest an improved physical explanation of consonance. Listeners find that the dissonance of a pair of pure tones is maximum when the tones are about a quarter of a critical bandwidth apart; the tones are judged consonant when they are more than one critical bandwidth apart. Based on this premise, Pierce (1966) (cf. von Foerster & Beauchamp, 1969, pp. 129–132)

has used tones made up of nonharmonic partials, so that the ratios of fundamentals leading to consonance are not the conventional ones. Kameoka and
Kuriyagawa (1969a,b) have developed an involved method to calculate the
magnitude of dissonance by taking into account the contribution of separate
frequency components.

Although the explanation put forth by Plomp can be useful to evaluate the
consonance, smoothness, or *roughness* of a combination of tones, it is certainly insufficient to account for musical consonance. In a laboratory study,
van de Geer *et al.* (1962) found that intervals judged the most consonant by
laymen do not correspond to the ones usually termed consonant. This result
is elaborated by work by Fyda (1975). The term consonance seems ambigu-
ous, since at the same time it refers to an elemental level, where smoothness
and roughness are evaluated, and to a higher aesthetic level, where consonance can be functional in a given style. The two levels are related in a
culture-bound fashion. In music, we do not judge only the consonance of
isolated tones. As Cazden (1945) states, "context is the determining factor. . . . The resolution of intervals does not have a natural basis; it is a
common response acquired by all individuals within a culture ᴖrea" (see also
Lundin, 1947). Musical consonance is relative to a musical style (Guernesey,
1928), so ninth chords, dissonant in Mozart's music, are treated as consonant
by Debussy (Cazden, 1962, 1968, 1972; Chailley, 1951). The cultural and
contextual aspects of musical consonance are so important that, despite
nativists' claims to the contrary, purely mathematical or physical explanations
can only be part of the story (Costère, 1962).

4. RELATIVE PITCH AND MELODY

Relative pitch, akin to intervallic sense (Revesz, 1954), is a basic ingredient of musical aptitude (Lundin, 1967). Given a pitch reference (e.g.,
the A of a tuning fork or a pitchpipe), an individual with good relative pitch
will be able to sing or identify any note of the scale. As Ward (1970) puts it,
the Western musician "apparently has an internal scale of relative pitch, a
movable conceptual grid or template so to speak, that specifies the pitch
relations among the notes of our Western scale."

Relative pitch is an acquired ability. Apparently the child first appreciates
the general contour of melodies—only in a latter stage of development can he
appreciate the intervals accurately, granted sufficient exposure to music
(Brehmer, 1925; Francès, 1958; Zenatti, 1969). Intervallic sense is not immediate but abstracted from familiarity with melodies (Teplov, 1966). Experiments (Dowling & Fujitani, 1971) confirm that subjects have good long-term
memory for exact interval sizes in the context of familiar tunes and establish
(Dowling, 1971) that interval size and melodic contour are handled differently by the listener. An experiment by Bever and Chiarello (1974) indicates
that the perceptual processing of melodies can switch from the right to the
left hemisphere of the brain while children are learning music, which con-

firms the acquisition of a more analytic ability. A melody is not perceived as a sequence of isolated tones, but as a pattern of grouped sounds; perception involves grouping of tones in streams and segregation of different streams. For example, a simple melodic instrument, rapidly alternating high and low tones, can be heard as playing two melodies (Bregman & Campbell, 1971; cf. van Norden, 1975; Pikler, 1966a; Warren et al., 1969). Similar processes, as well as interaction between pitch and localization, probably intervene in Deutsch's striking musical illusions, obtained by presenting certain sequences of tones to both ears (Deutsch, 1975a). For example, when a sequence consisting of a high tone (800 Hz) alternating with a low tone (400 Hz) is presented so that when one ear receives the high tone, the other ear receives the low tone, and vice versa, most right-handed subjects hear a high tone in the right ear alternating with a low tone in the left ear; the effect is not changed by reversing the earphones.

Active processes play a part in melodic perception. As Creel et al. (1970) say, "the singer sings a note flat–flatter than what?—than our internal pattern of expectations" (see also Boomsliter & Creel, 1963). The constructive aspect of perception has been stressed in other fields (Neisser, 1967). According to Licklider (1967), "one is proposing and testing hypotheses, actually hearing, not the sensory data, but the winning hypothesis." Genetic and cultural factors favor the supply of certain types of hypotheses (Francès, 1958; Risset, 1968, p. 102). This fact can explain the reference grid or template, constituted by familiarity with a cultural pitch system. Such a grid makes pitch perception more consistent, systematic, and easier to remember, but also particularized and biased. Large frequency deviations in artistic singing are not perceived as such, but the pitches heard correspond to the conventional scale (Seashore, 1938, pp. 256–272). Different musical civilizations use different scales, but intervals are naturalized (Francès, 1958, pp. 47–49). Thus, a Western musician will interpret intervals of an Eastern scale in terms of the Western scale template. For instance, listening to two different steps, he may assimilate, incorporate the steps to his template, and say, this is a low F, this is a sharp F. This categorization into scale steps is analogous to phoneme perception. Apparently it is possible only for children to accommodate efficiently (Piaget & Inhelder, 1969) the template to different scales. There is some evidence that the development of pitch sense can be inhibited at an early age by culture-bound conditions (Tanner & Rivette, 1964). Clearly, relative pitch perception is not naive; it involves unconscious abstraction, influenced by the cultural history of the listener (Allen, 1967; Francès, 1958).

5. Standard of Pitch

A scale, defined as a succession of intervals, must be anchored on a note of fixed frequency, called *standard of pitch*, or *diapason*. It is customary to take the frequency of A above middle C as the standard of reference (Backus, 1969).

As can be inferred from the tuning of organs, three centuries ago the frequency of A above middle C varied between some 375 and 500 Hz (Ellis, 1954). Later the latitude was reduced, and an official standard pitch was adopted first at A = 435 Hz and then at A = 440 Hz. However, there are many complaints that the standard of pitch actually used in rising, which imposes difficulties to musicians—especially singers—and to instrument-makers. Responsibility for this rise often is ascribed to instrumentalists and instrument-makers who want a more brilliant sound, but other reasons inter-vene. The pitch given by a pipe depends upon the temperature, and coun-teradjustments in pipe length affect the pitches given by the holes of the instrument. A wind instrument player can compensate this only to a small extent, at the expense of ease of playing and quality of intonation. Hence, the standard of pitch should be prescribed at a specified temperature (Young & Webster, 1958). Yet the intonation of different instruments does not de-pend the same way of temperature. Measurements performed at the Opera of Paris (Leipp, 1971, pp. 132, 328–329) indicate that many factors affect the orchestral pitch, including the tempo and the excitement of the performance.

6. THE RIDDLE OF PERFECT PITCH

Good musicians possess good relative pitch. But an aura of mystery sur-rounds *perfect pitch,* a rare ability even among musicians. The choir leader gifted with perfect pitch does not need a pitchpipe or a tuning fork to give the reference tone A to his chorus: Somehow he has an internal reference of standard pitch. The term perfect pitch is favored by musicians. Many scien-tists prefer the term *absolute pitch* (AP), since it refers to identification of tones on an absolute basis.

There has been much controversy over AP: Is it a specific ability? Is it an inborn, hereditary faculty, or can it be learned?

Neu (1947) claims that AP is nothing more than a fine degree of accuracy of pitch discrimination. This view seems untenable. Oakes (1955) has shown that pitch-naming ability and differential pitch sensitivity are independent. Also, the absolute note recognition seems to involve a different process: Subjects with AP have much faster response (Baird, 1917; Gough, 1922). According to Revesz (1954) or Bachem (1950), there is a clear-cut difference between subjects with AP and those with *regional pitch,* which simply nar-rows the interval of errors. Other experimenters (Oakes, 1955) contend there is a continuous distribution of subjects in AP test performance (cf. Ward, 1963).

Seashore (1938), Revesz (1954), and Bachem (1950) contend that AP is hereditary, whereas Neu (1947) holds that it is a product of environment. Pitch discrimination can indeed improve with practice (Lundin, 1967). Yet attempts by adults to acquire AP by training have been poor. Although their performance is improved, it is far from that of a recognized possessor of AP (Brady, 1970; Cuddy, 1970; Lundin & Allen, 1962; Meyer, 1899, 1956). Ac-cording to Copp (1916), pitch-naming is easy to develop in children—early years are critical. This suggests that AP can be acquired at some critical stage of development, a process similar to imprinting (Jeffress, 1962). The nature–nurture argument is hard to settle. Possessors of AP tend to cluster in families, but this does not prove that AP is hereditary, since it is in these families that AP is more likely to be recognized, valued, and fostered by musical exposure. Clearly, a child can learn to name notes only if he is told their names, which will not occur in just any environment. In a most commendable review on AP, Ward (1963) advocates a viewpoint put forth by Watt (1917): AP is perhaps an inborn ability in all of us, which may be "trained out of us in early life" (Ward, 1970). This ability is normally reinforced, but it is rather inhibited by the generalization involved in tasks such as recognition of transposed melodies. There is some indication that AP is related to a special ability for memory retrieval rather than storage.

Although AP is exceptional, absolute identification of vowels, using timbre cues, is commonplace. It has been suggested that AP was mediated by a proficient use of timbre clues. The performance of subjects on AP tests often depends highly on the musical instrument on which the pitches are produced (Baird, 1917). On the other hand, Brentano (1907), Revesz (1954), and Bachem (1950) claim that AP involves recognition of a certain quality, called *tone chroma* or *tonality,* which endows all Cs with a certain C-ness, all Ds with a certain D-ness, regardless of the octave placement and timbre (hence octave errors are not surprising). This implies that pitch is a compound attribute. Other authors have supported a two-component theory of pitch (Köhler, 1915; Meyer, 1904; Stumpf, 1890; cf. Teplov, 1966); all theories are not identical. According to Revesz (1954) the pitch continuum can be represented as a helix drawn on a cylinder (cf. Pikler, 1966b). The vertical coordinate, along the axis, corresponds to an attribute named *tone height,* which varies monotonically with the frequency. When the frequency is increased, the other attribute, the *chroma,* represented by the position around a circular section, varies cyclically. A rise of an octave corresponds to one turn around the circle. Such a view was often not taken seriously, until Shepard (1964) succeeded in demonstrating circularity of relative pitch, using a specially contrived computer, synthesized sounds comprising only octave components. Shepard synthesized 12 tones, forming a chromatic scale which seems to go up endlessly when the 12 tones are repeated.

We can go further in contriving the stimuli to divorce chroma and tone height. Sounds have been generated that go down the scale while becoming shriller and different listeners can make different pitch judgments about such stimuli, depending whether they weigh more one aspect or another. For example, stimuli made with stretched octaves are heard by most listeners to go down in pitch when their frequencies are doubled, because chroma cues dominate the conflicting tone height cue (Risset, 1971). Moreover tone chroma (like speech) appears to be processed by the left brain hemisphere, whereas tone height is processed by the right hemisphere (Charbonneau and

Risset, 1975). The basis for chroma is the strength of the octave relation. Octave similarity is perceived by all subjects, although more strongly by trained musicians (Allen, 1967), and there are striking indications that tonal pitch memory is organized in a way that allows disruptions to generalize across octaves (Deutsch, 1972). The aforementioned demonstrations involved artificial stimuli with only octave components, which creates special situations. Certainly the octave is not always "the Alpha and the Omega of . . . the musical ear [Revesz, 1954, p. 61]." Tune recognition is very much disturbed by playing the different notes at different octaves (Deutsch, 1972; see also Bregman & Campbell, 1971). Yet pitch perception certainly seems to involve both a focalized aspect (associated with the periodicity of the waveform) and a distributed aspect (associated with the spectral distribution and closely related to timbre (Licklider, 1956; Watt, 1917). The focalized aspects only lends itself to precise pitch-matching (Köhler, 1915). Although the two aspects are not normally divorced, in some cases the clues for the two aspects are contradictory. It is then clear that subjects rely mostly on one or the other (Risset, 1971). For instance many nontrained subjects do not immediately perceive the low pitch of the residue (Plomp, 1966), but rather a high *formant pitch* (Meyer-Eppler, in Die Reihe, 1958, p. 60). To some extent, we can learn to improve pitch-naming from clues of the distributed aspect (Gough, 1922; Köhler, 1915), but in addition to intervallic sense, characteristic cases of AP seem to involve a special ability to deal with the focalized aspect, regardless of timbre cues (Bachem, 1950).

Absolute pitch can help the intonation of singers, especially in atonal music; it is also useful to the conductor. However, it can have drawbacks. Possessors of AP can be annoyed by changes in the pitch standard. Apparently a number of great composers did not have AP, among them Schumann and Wagner, although such data are hard to check (Teplov, 1966, p. 194). Many points on AP are not settled; cross-cultural data might be enlightening. Passion pervades the issues of AP (Ward, 1963) and this shows even in the expression *perfect pitch*.

C. Duration and Rhythm

The music listener does not, in most cases, attend to durations of isolated events. The rhythmic organization of music often involves a metric grid somewhat similar to the pitch scale, which helps judging duration relationships in a precise and consistent way. Subjects that have much difficulty in halving a duration can solve complex rhythmic problems in the context of music (Teplov, 1966, pp. 358–376). Listeners have an amazing inability to detect temporal order—except in the highly structured patterns of speech and music (Warren *et al.,* 1969; Bregman & Campbell, 1971). As in pitch, there are intended deviations from a mathematically accurate division of time. Rhythmic organization and "chunking" of the musical flux seem critical to its memorization (Dowling, 1973). For more information on rhythm, meter, and duration, see Cooper and Meyer (1960), Farnsworth (1934), Fraisse (1956), Jacques-Dalcroze (1921), Ruckmick (1918), Sachs (1953), Stetson (1905), Teplov (1966), Bengtsson and Gabrielson (in Music, Room, and Acoustics, 1977, pp. 19–59), Fraisse *et al.* (1953), Simon (1972), Restle (1970), and Jones (1976). To do justice to musical rhythm, we should keep in mind its relation to the other aspects of the music (for instance, the harmonic aspect for tonal Western music).

D. Timbre

Timbre, the attribute of the tone that can distinguish it from other tones of the same pitch and loudness, is also called *tone color* or *tone quality*. For periodic tones, timbre has been ascribed to the form of the wave, and subsequently to the harmonic spectrum, assuming that the ear is insensitive to phase relations between harmonics (Helmholtz, 1954; Olson, 1967, p. 206; Backus, 1969, pp. 94–100). Actually phase changes can alter the timbre in certain conditions, yet their aural effect on periodic tones is very weak, especially in a normally reverberant room where phase relations are smeared (Cabot *et al.,* 1976; Schroeder, 1975; Wightman & Green, 1974).

Even a sinewave changes quality from the low to the high end of the musical range (Köhler, 1915; Stumpf, 1890). In order to keep the timbre of a periodic tone approximately invariant when the frequency is changed, should the spectrum be transposed so as to keep the same amplitude ratios between the harmonics, or should the spectral envelop be kept invariant? This question raised a debate between Helmholtz and Hermann (see Winckel, 1967, p. 13). In speech, a vowel corresponds approximately to a specific formant structure (a formant is a peak of the spectral envelope, often associated with a resonance in the sound-producing system). We may say that a fixed formant structure gives a timbre that varies less with frequency than a fixed spectrum (Slawson, 1968). To some extent, one can correlate a particular spectrum and the resulting timbre (Schaeffer, 1952; Stumpf, 1890). The concept of critical bandwidth, linked to the spectral resolution of the ear (Plomp, 1966), may permit a better understanding of this correlation. In particular, if many high order harmonics lie close together, the sound becomes very harsh. Hence, for instance, antiresonances in the frequency response of the string instruments play an important part to ensure acceptable timbres.

So for periodic tones, the timbre depends upon the spectrum. It has long been thought that musical tones were periodic (see Section III,B). However, manipulations of sound, including simple tape reversal (Schaeffer, 1952; Stumpf, 1926), electronic and computer sound synthesis (Chowning, 1973; Risset & Mathews, 1969) indicate that strictly periodic tones are dull and that timbre is very sensitive to temporal factors. It is not surprising that hearing does not rely only on the exact structure of the spectrum to evaluate timbre and identify the origin of the sound, since this structure is severely distorted during the propagation of the sound (Wente, 1935; Young, 1957). Timbre perception involves a pattern recognition process, which resorts to factors resistant to distorsion. Specific variations of parameters throughout the sound often are not perceived as such, but rather as characteristic tone qualities (see Section III,B). This is especially true for rapid variations during the attack (Stumpf, 1926), and also for the slow frequency modulation known as *vibrato,* whose rate is around 6 or 7 Hz (Seashore, 1938, p. 256). Departures from regular periodicity can make the sound livelier (Booms-liter & Creel, 1970). Many musical sounds are inharmonic, which means that the partials' frequencies are not exact multiples of the fundamental frequencies. This contributes to subjective warmth (Fletcher *et al.,* 1962). The presence of many simultaneous players or singers affects the tone quality as well as the intensity. This so-called chorus effect leads to the widening of spectral lines; in fact, there is no clear-cut barrier between musical tones and noise (Winckel, 1967). The acoustics of the listening room can have an important influence on the tone quality (see Chapter 11; see also Schroeder, 1966). As for pitch, timbre perception depends upon the internal timbre references of the listener, which are related to the sounds (e.g., to the musical instruments) he is accustomed to hearing and identifying. Abilities in musical instrument recognition vary widely among individuals.

A single spectrum is thus inadequate to characterize the timbre of an arbitrary sound. Useful representations of sounds are provided by the sound spectrograph (Potter *et al.,* 1947), which displays the temporal evolution of the spectrum in a crude but often meaningful way (Leipp, 1971; Fig. 1). Other modalities for analysis—especially for a running analysis—are helpful for the investigation of timbre (Moorer, 1977). An inspection of analysis results reveals physical features that may affect timbre; however, this enumeration of features remains speculative until their aural significance has been ascertained by synthesis (Risset & Mathews, 1969).

Multidimensional scaling promises to clarify the concept of timbre by providing geometrical models of subjective timbral space, which reveal the principal dimensions of timbre differentiation (Grey, 1977; Miller & Carterette, 1975; Wessel, 1973). The initial results tend to support the hypothesis (Huggins, 1952) that in order to identify the source of a sound, hearing attempts to separate the temporal properties in the sound, attributable to the excitation, and the structural properties, unchanged with time and related to a response in the sound source.

Further details will be given in Sections III,B and V,C. An understanding of the physical correlates of timbre is of great relevance to the production of better instruments and better synthetic sounds; timbral maps may help explore and organize new sound material (Ehresman & Wessel, 1978; Wessel, 1978).

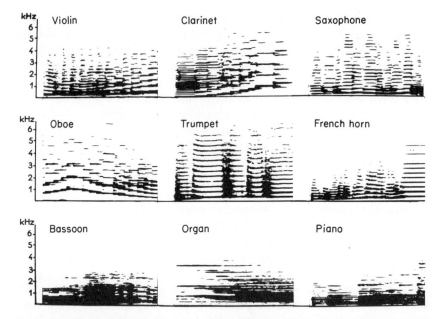

FIG. 1. Sound spectrograms (frequency versus time) of tones played by various instruments. The duration of sound is 1 sec for each instrument. [From Leipp (1971), *Acoustique et musique*. Copyright 1971 by Masson. Reprinted by permission.]

E. Criteria for Musical Aptitude Tests

Tests have been developed to evaluate musical aptitude. Such tests embody the conceptions of their authors on the measurement of musical aptitude and the factors of musical talent, and these conceptions are hard to evaluate objectively. But the tests can be appraised in terms of reliability—reproducibility of the results—and validity: Does the test measure what it claims to? It is straightforward, although tedious, to determine the reliability? The validity can be evaluated by comparing the results with other appraisals of subjects' musical aptitude, by matching the results with those of an assumed valid test, or by careful study of the test's procedures. Other criteria can be of importance: ease of administration; objectivity (the person scoring the test should not influence the results); economy (in terms of time and money); and standardization.

We can find an appraisal of some tests in Lundin (1967) and Lehman (1968). In general, musical tests leave much to be desired in reliability and relevance. Their indications may help to make a better than random evaluation, but the appraisals they warrant should not be taken for granted. Tests reflect the conceptions of their authors, and they should not be regarded absolute, especially tests of appreciation. The factors measured may not be the important ones in all conditions. There is still much research to be done on the relevance of the testing procedures.

F. Music Perception and Musical Preference

1. THE PERCEPTION OF MUSIC

We can already infer from the previous sections that the perception of music involves a wealth of natural and cultural factors, and that it depends in an intricate way on the context and on the listener's *set* (Francès, 1958; Poland, 1963). Several volumes could not exhaust this topic. This section only gives some leads that may help explore the tangle of subjective musical preference.

Strong hopes have been placed in *information theory* (Cherry, 1961; Pierce, 1962; Shannon, 1948) as a framework suitable to study musical perception. Information theory provides a quantitative definition of *information*, related to the complexity and the unpredictability of the message. The theory has been successful in determining the maximum information that could be conveyed on communication channels, and also in predicting that proper *redundancy* (related to internal structure lowering the information rate) made it possible to code messages so as to protect them against the detrimental effects of noisy channels. The language of information theory helps to clarify some concepts relevant to musical communication (Berlyne, 1971; Cohen, 1962; Hiller & Isaacson, 1959, pp. 22–35; Le Caine, 1956; Meyer, 1967; Meyer-Eppler, 1952, 1965; Moles, 1966) especially message intelligibility. A message with a very low information rate arouses no interest in the listener: It is too predictible and banal (like the endless repetition of a note or a pattern). But if the information rate is too high, the message is not intelligible: It is too original and unpredictible (like white noise). Compositional redundancy reduces the information rate—provided the listener possesses the *code*, that is, has a knowledge of the rules of the game, of the constraints of the compositional style.

As listeners learn a style through familiarity with the music, the redundancy becomes clear to them, and the music gets banal—especially for musicians who overlearn the style. Hence, historically, music tends to get more complex (Meyer, 1967, p. 117). From the time of Ars Nova (fourteenth century) to the present, new music has often been termed *noise*. It was too original for the listeners until they had become familiar with the new style. But contemporary music is in an unprecedented situation in that respect. Most music listeners are heavily exposed to music—classical, background, pop and jazz heard on radio, television, in shopping centers, and in factories (Soibelman, 1948)—that has a tonal syntax. Listeners overlearn this syntax, which prepares them for appreciating seventeenth to nineteenth century music, but not early occidental music, music of other civilizations, or contemporary music. [This does not mean that tonal and nontonal music can be perceived in the same way (see Francès, 1958).]

However, the previous theses are only qualitative, and they could have been formulated without the help of information theory. Few data are available on the correlation between information rate and perceived complexity. Pitts and de Charms (1963) indicate that this correlation can be strong, but that unexpected factors intervene. For example, an intricate piece of music can be judged simple because it is written in waltz tempo. Pitts and de Charms also gathered some evidence supporting a model proposed by McClelland *et al.* (1953) and whose application to music resembles the preceding information theory considerations. According to this model, positive affective arousal results from small deviations in perceived complexity from the level to which the listener is adapted. Similarly, Berlyne (1971) claims that complexity and novelty interact to determine listeners' preference for stimuli. This is supported by experiments on the relation between auditory complexity and preference (Duke & Gullickson, 1970; Vitz, 1964). However, the measurement of information, designed to deal with independent or statistically related events, is inadequate for organized signals (Green & Courtis, 1966) like music, and it cannot thoroughly take into account the effect of context and of previous musical experiences. Yet information theory has been an incentive for computer statistical analysis of musical styles (Bowles, 1966; Fucks, 1962; Hiller & Bean, 1966; Lefkoff, 1967; Lincoln, 1970; cf. Cohen, 1962) and for proposing models of musical composition that can be implemented with computers (see Section V,C).

Different aspects come into play in the perception of music. Lee (1932) surveyed about 200 musicians from England, France, and Germany on the meaning of music. About half of them said that the meaning resided in music itself; the other half said music implied for them an extramusical message. There have been heated debates between the *absolutists,* who insist that musical meaning lies in the perception of musical form (e.g., Hanslick, 1891; Schoen, 1940; Stravinsky, 1947), and the *referentialists,* who contend that music conveys extramusical feelings, concepts, and meaning (e.g., Teplov, 1966; cf. Meyer, 1956). According to absolutists, extramusical associations are not natural and universal. Referentialists, however, can retort that musical symbolism is present in all musical civilizations, and quite precise in the Orient (Sachs, 1943). These opposing viewpoints coexist rather than being mutually exclusive (Francès, 1958; Meyer, 1956). In them we can distinguish 2 aspects in the perception of music: a formal, syntactic, cognitive aspect, and a referential, emotional, affective aspect (Tischler, 1956). These aspects are linked to *definite* and *indefinite* listening (Vernon, 1934; Moles, 1966; cf. Poland, 1963). Definite listening implies active attention to perceive relations; indefinite listening is more passive and vague. Different aspects of pitch (see Section II,B,6) or consonance (see Section II,B,3) relate to either definite or indefinite listening.

The viewpoint of Meyer (1956, 1967) bridges the gap between the formalist and the referentialist aspects of music. According to this viewpoint, perception of music involves anticipation. Continuous fulfillment of expectations would cause boredom. Music arouses tendencies of affect when an expectation is inhibited or blocked (expectations are, of course, relevant to the particular style of a composer). This view is akin to McClelland's model cited previously. Meyer believes that these cerebral operations evoke all responses to music, and that it is the listener with his cultural history who brings to musical experience a disposition that leads to intellectual, emotional, or referential response.

The preceding observations do not consider much the materialization of music into sound. Varèse complained that "the corporealization" of musical intelligence (also significant to Stravinsky) was neglected in occidental music (see Schwartz & Childs, 1967, p. 198). This condition has changed somewhat, and contemporary composers are often interested in controlling sound structure in music (Erickson, 1975). In primitive civilizations, some practices (e.g., pounding of drums) probably contributed to the magic and therapeutic effects of music (Schullian & Schoen, 1948). Much of the organ's impact comes from low frequencies, some of them felt by the body although inaudible. A number of rock groups now achieve an almost intoxicating effect on listeners by using very high sound intensities; they can even be detrimental to hearing (Chadwick, 1973). Despite the existence of this sensual aspect, experiments on the *pleasantness* of isolated sounds, chords, or sequences (Butler & Daston, 1968) are probably of little relevance to musical preference (Langer, 1951, p. 171).

According to Osmond-Smith (1971), the response to music can be studied from the viewpoint of two disciplines: experimental psychology (Francès, 1958; Lundin, 1967), and semiotics. Although linguistic concepts and methods should not be applied to music without caution, some musical phenomena are clearly of a semiological nature (Harweg, 1968; Nattiez, 1972; Ruwet, 1972; Springer, 1956). Musical semiotics is still in infancy. The bridge between the viewpoint of experimental psychology and semiotics is perhaps to be found in an approach focusing on the cognitive processes involved in the perception of music (Harwood, 1972).

2. MUSICAL PREFERENCE

At the time of Gregorian chant, the question of musical preference did not often arise; sacred music was meant for rituals, not for comparisons. Now a great variety of music is available through recordings. Record companies take their own view of musical preference into account to make marketing evaluations influencing availability and advertisement of records, which in turn prejudice the buyers' preferences. The relevance of *musical taste* depends upon the function of music. This relevance is probably maximum in our occidental civilization where music has lost most of its magic, therapeutic, or ritual significance (Schullian & Schoen, 1948).

It is not easy to evaluate musical preferences. Record sales as a measure of preference is clearly biased, and it does not permit us to analyze the effect of factors such as listeners' origin or personality. Analyses of concerts or radio music programs (Moles, 1966) do not either. An urge for objectivity has led some to measure physiological responses to music (Phares, 1934); however, these responses are not clearly and reliably related to music appreciation (Eaton, 1971; Podolsky, 1954; cf. Schoen, 1927). Most investigators revert to recordings and comparisons of the listeners' verbalized reactions. [It might be interesting, although perhaps misleading, to study the effect of music on faces and behavior (see Lundin, 1967).]

If we crudely compare the music of various civilizations, it appears that most classical Western music favors stable rhythmic pulses, very elaborate harmony, involving attractions, and resolutions, correlated with rhythmic accents, and developed at the expense of tuning subtlety and of melodic richness. Africans use complicated rhythmic patterns, the organization of which is often not perceived by Occidentals, and a large variety of instruments, often with indefinite pitch. Oriental music, in addition to elaborate rhythmic systems, often calls for varied tuning systems and significant pitch deviations around the notes (Leipp, 1971; Sachs, 1943). Efforts are now made to preserve musical traditions and to protect them against a rapid contamination (Farnsworth, 1950, 1958) by Western tonal music. Contemporary occidental music often tries to incorporate features of other musical civilizations.

More specific data about the effect of various factors on music preference in Western culture are reported by Lundin (1967). Preference is clearly a complex function of the musical *stimulus,* but also of the listener, of his history of contacts with this kind of music, and of his concept of the function of music (background music? dance music? *pure* music?). Sometimes a particular type of music becomes a token of a subculture (e.g., pop music, free jazz, folk songs). This is a factor in its acceptance or refusal; in this case, superficial characteristics (in instrumentation, rhythm or melody, for example) may suffice for many listeners. There are also definite cases of specific associations; for instance, some listeners claim to be oppressed by sirenlike glissandi sometimes used in contemporary music (Xenakis, 1971) because they evoke war memories.

Despite such specific effects, a wide survey performed over half a century ago and analyzing 20,000 verbal reports indicated that affective reactions to musical compositions are strikingly similar for a large majority of listeners regardless of training, age, or experience (Schoen, 1927). The conformity of concert programs (Mueller & Hevner, 1942) and the uniformity of radio (and now television) exposure can be partly responsible for that. Also, the effect of reverence for highly regarded cultural values should not be underestimated. Farnsworth (1950) finds a strong agreement between musicologists, students, and high school students, on composers judged eminent, even though their many responses may be based on little personal listening experiences.

This is not of course the only effect of education. Early musical training strongly develops musical perception abilities (Copp, 1916; Teplov, 1966). In teenagers, musical sophistication is related to socioeconomic status (Bauman, 1960). The effects of variations in the structure of the music on the affective response and the significations elicited have been studied (Mueller & Hevner, 1942). The association of the minor mode with sadness is frequent (although not constant) but for Western listeners only, and it seems to be learned (Heinlein, 1928). With repetitions, classical selections gain more in enjoyment than popular selections—the latter often lose (Schoen, 1927; see also Getz, 1966). Popular tunes get quickly "worn out"; satiety is hastened with the new media. This can be understood in terms of the conceptions of McClelland or Meyer (see Section II,F,1). In an experiment on the preference of harmonic sequences (Lundin, 1967), it was found that musically sophisticated subjects reject the sequences that are too predictable, whereas unsophisticated subjects rejected the too unpredictable ones. The aesthetic response depends upon attention and attitude. Some listeners prefer a familiar, reassuring music; others have a strong curiosity for novelty and can impose a form on a random pattern. Mikol (1960) reported that in an appreciation study, the more receptive and less dogmatic students showed improved taste for modern music over repeated hearings (see also Mull, 1957).

III. MUSICAL INSTRUMENTS

The acoustical study of musical instruments has progressed along two main lines: understanding their physical behavior and determining the cues used to identify and evaluate them. Both approaches can be useful in order to improve instrument making. The former correlates variations in instrument design and building with variations in the physical parameters of the sounds produced. The latter indicates which configurations of physical parameters should be achieved in the sound.

A. Physical Behavior of Musical Instruments

Musical instruments are very complex mechanical systems and are far from being thoroughly understood (see Backus, 1969; Benade, 1976; for data on instrument tone spectra and instrument directivity, cf. Culver, 1947; Meyer, 1966; Meyer & Buchmann, 1931; Miller, 1926; Olson, 1967). Instrument design has evolved mostly empirically, yet in many cases remarkable skill is shown in the way instrument making takes into account properties of sound, characteristics of hearing, and necessities of music (Leipp, 1971; Benade, 1976).

This is well exemplified by string instruments such as the violin, considered to have been brought to a high level of perfection by the Italian masters at a time when its physical behavior was not well understood. The bow catches the string and pulls it to one side until the string separates from the bow and flies back. The string is then caught again, and so on. This behavior takes place because friction between bow and string is higher at slow speeds; this is relatively well known from the work of Helmholtz (1954), Raman (1918), and a number of others (e.g., Hutchins, 1962a,b; Leipp, 1971). Bowed string vibrations have been filmed, picked up magnetically (Kohut & Mathews, 1971), and simulated by computer from the differential equations of motion (Hiller & Ruiz, 1971). The waveform is approximately triangular, and the flyback time depends upon the position along the string. The plucked string's behavior is simpler. In both cases the period of the vibration is determined by the time it takes a perturbation to travel two string lengths (this time depends on string length, tension, and material). The violin body is necessary to convey efficiently vibratory motion from the string to the air, that is, to match impedances. It is not a *resonator* (if it were, the instrument would emphasize too much the resonant frequency). In fact the response curve of a violin body has many peaks and valleys (Hutchins, 1962a,b; Meinel, 1957), and it can be approximated by a number of resonances at different frequencies (Mathews & Kohut, 1971). Fine variations in the structure of the violin body and the elastic properties of the wood affect the tone and its evenness. It is of utmost importance to control adequately the lowest air and wood resonances, which good violin-makers do. We are close to being able to make better (or less expensive) instruments thanks to acoustical progress (Agren & Stetson, 1972; Hutchins, 1962a,b, 1975, 1976; Jansson, 1973).

The piano could be considered a percussion instrument, since its strings are struck by hammers. The hammers are set into motion by the keys. The action (i.e., the mechanical transmission between keyboard and hammers) is quite elaborate. The hammer must escape the string after striking, the inertia must be small, and a damper must stop the vibration when the key is released. Each hammer strikes one (in the low range) to three strings (in the medium and high range). The string vibrations are transmitted to the soundboard, which radiates into the air. The strings exert a considerable tension on the frame (up to 30 tons), so piano frames are made of iron (Blackham, 1965). The area hit by the hammer affects the spectral pattern of the string vibration, which also depends upon the action, the hammer's speed, and its surface (soft or hard). Due to the stiffness of the piano string, the vibration is inharmonic; that is, partials are not quite harmonic (see Section II,B,2) (Schuck & Young, 1943). Thus piano sounds are not quite periodic. The string vibrations decay because of friction and radiation; the higher the pitch, the faster the decay. The initial rate of decay is faster than the decay rate of the latter part of the sound (Martin, 1947). When a pianist plays an isolated note, he can only control the velocity of the hammer and subsequently the damping (Hart *et al.*, 1934). This leaves, however, considerable room for differences between different pianists' *touch* (levels of individual notes, overall level, staccato–legato and pedals skill) (Ortmann, 1962).

In wind instruments, a resonant air column is coupled to a valve mechanism (a *reed*) that modulates a steady air stream at audiofrequencies. Complex interactions between the valve mechanism and the air column determine the frequency and waveform of the sound (Benade, 1960; Nederveen, 1969).

In the case of the so-called woodwind instruments, the air column *dominates* the reed to determine the frequency, and holes in the tube allow variation in the vibration wavelength, hence the frequency. Woodwinds use tubes that have an almost cylindrical (flute, clarinet) or conical (oboe, bassoon) bore. This permits the use of the same holes in two registers (Benade, 1960). Switching to a high register, that is, to a higher resonance mode of the air column, is done by overblowing; it can be helped by a special *register* hole. The material of woodwind instruments has very little influence on the tone (Backus, 1969, p. 208). Thus flutes, formerly made of wood, are now made of metal. In the flute or the recorder, the air column is excited by a stream of air striking against a sharp edge at the embouchure. The valve operates by air deflection in and out of the embouchure hole under the influence of the vibrating air column. The flute was greatly improved more than a century ago by Boehm (Benade, 1960; Boehm, 1964; cf. Coltman, 1966). In the clarinet or the saxophone, a single vibrating reed modulates the flow of air from the lungs. The reed's behavior partly explains the fact that the clarinet tone does not contain only odd-numbered partials, as a simplistic theory would state; it also explains that the playing frequencies of the clarinet are lower than the resonance frequencies of the tube (Backus, 1969, pp. 193, 200). The oboe and the bassoon use a double reed. The intonation of woodwinds still raises many problems (Young & Webster, 1958): The physical situation is very complex (Bouasse, 1929), and despite ingenious compromises the player has to adjust the pitch by a delicate control of the lips. According to Backus (1969, p. 202), the bassoon "badly needs an acoustical working-over."

In the brass instruments, the reed is formed by the player's lips, which are heavy in comparison with wood reeds. The lip action is influenced, although not dominated, by the air column (Benade, 1970). The player produces different frequencies by adjusting the tension of the lips. The instruments take advantage of the resonance peaks of the air column, which helps intonation. The length of the tube can be modified by using valves (e.g., in the trumpet) or a sliding piece of tubing (e.g., in the trombone). To position the peaks close to musically useful frequencies, the tube departs from a cylindrical shape. The adjustment is done empirically, but it is now possible to calculate the impedance corresponding to various horn shapes with the help of a computer (Young, 1960). The sound radiates from a large area at the flaring end (the bell). This increases the output level and accounts for the marked directivity of the instrument at high frequencies (Martin, 1942). The oscillations within the horn comprise amounts of nth harmonic growing as the nth power of the first component pressure (Worman, 1971). Mutes can be inserted into the bell to soften or modify the tone.

The organ is a special kind of wind instrument. Organ pipes are excited by vibrating reeds or by edge tones. Sets of pipes are grouped in various ways to form so-called stops. The organ console comprises stop knobs and a variable number of keyboards. This complex organ action has evolved—there are organs with mechanical, pneumatic, and electric actions. The action can affect the tone transients (Richardson, 1954) as well as the ease of playing. The revival of interest in ancient organs has resulted in a better knowledge of the various styles of organ-making (Lottermoser, 1957), an art involving considerable expertise. The reverberant environment of the organ is of utmost importance.

The human voice is perhaps the oldest musical instrument. It can be considered a wind instrument for the glottis (the vocal chords) acts somewhat like lip reeds. However, unlike brass instruments, the coupling is very weak between the vocal chords and the vocal tract. Hence the fundamental frequency is determined by control of the vocal chords, while the vocal tract resonances determine formants, responsible for the vocalic quality (Flanagan, 1972). A fixed formant near 3000 Hz, regardless of the vowel being sung, has been evidenced in operatic singing (Vennard, 1967). This had been ascribed to a special glottis behavior, but recent investigations suggest that it is due to special vocal tract configurations adopted in singing, and that it helps the singer to resist being masked by the accompanying orchestra (Sundberg, 1974, 1977; Music, Room, and Acoustics, 1977). Vibrato (see Section II,D) has a considerable importance in operatic singing (Seashore, 1938, pp. 42, 256); it seems to imply a control loop (Deutsch & Clarkson, 1959).

There is a large variety of percussion instruments, so called because the sound is produced by hitting them with sticks, soft or hard mallets, or with various other tools including the hands. Most of them involve vibrations of membranes, bars, or plates. Such vibrations are complex; the partials are not harmonic (Olson, 1967, pp. 75–83). So it may be difficult to ascribe a pitch to the sound. When one partial or a group of closely or equally spaced partials is dominant, a definite pitch can be identified. Among percussion instruments with definite pitch, the timpani (or kettledrums) use a membrane stretched over a hemispherical bowl. The xylophone consists of tuned wooden bars coupled to an air resonant column. The vibraphone is similar, but uses metal bars, and the columns can be closed periodically to yield a characteristic amplitude modulation; the bells are empirically shaped so that the frequencies of the first partials are tuned according to euphonious intervals (van Heuven, 1949). Among instruments with indefinite pitch, the snare drum consists of a short cylinder onto which a membrane is stretched at both ends. Metallic snares can be set along the bottom membrane to add a rattle quality to the sound. Gongs and cymbals are circular plates that have many closely spaced resonances.

There are many more instruments (see Baines, 1969). Interest is growing in nonoccidental instruments. Despite an understandable inertia in the composition of the Western orchestra, acoustical progress leads to modification of existing instruments and to design of new acoustical instruments. This is evidenced by inspection of numerous patents (each issue of the *Journal of the Acoustical Society of America* reviews new patents). However, electronic or hybrid musical instruments (see Section V) seem to develop at a faster rate, and they now promise to provide interesting musical possibilities (Mathews & Kohut, 1973).

B. Correlates of Timbre of Musical Instruments

It has long been believed that musical tones were periodic, and that the tone quality was associated solely with the waveform or with the relative amounts of the various harmonics present in the frequency spectrum (see Section II,D). Many analyses of musical instrument tones have been performed (Culver, 1947; Miller, 1926; Olson, 1967). However, most of these analyses did not adequately characterize the instrument timbre. A successful analysis should yield a physical description of the sound from which we could synthesize a sound that, to a listener, is nearly indistinguishable from the original. In many cases the previously mentioned descriptions of musical instrument tones fail the foolproof synthesis test (Risset & Mathews, 1969).

Only recently has it been possible to analyze transient rapidly evolving phenomena. Older instruments gave steady-state analyses, yielding either the frequency spectrum averaged over some duration or the spectrum of a particular pitch period (assumed to be repeated throughout the note). Helmholtz (1954) was aware that "certain characteristic particularities of the tones of several instruments depend on the mode in which they begin and end," yet he studied only "the peculiarities of the musical tones which continue uniformly," considering that they determined the "musical quality of the tone." The temporal characteristics of the instruments were averaged out by the analyses—yet different instruments had different average spectra, so it was thought that this difference in average spectrum was solely responsible for timbre differences. Helmholtz followers do not appear to have felt the importance of temporal changes for tone quality; there were a few exceptions, such as Seashore (1938, p. 102) and Stumpf (1926). The latter had found that removing the initial segment of notes played by various instruments impaired the recognition of these instruments. This motivated analyses of the attack transients of instrument tones (Backhaus, 1932; Meyer & Buchmann, 1931; Richardson, 1954). However, transients are complex and they are not quite reproducible from one tone to another, even for tones that sound very similar (Schaeffer, 1966). Most analyses have been restricted to a limited set of tones, and their authors have tended to generalize conclusions that may well be valid only for that set of tones. These shortcomings have produced many discrepancies in the literature and cast an aura of doubt on the entire body of acoustic data.

Thus it is necessary to isolate, from complex physical structures, those significant features that are both regular and relevant to timbre. There are now various ways to control the psychoacoustical and musical relevance of the features extracted from the analysis. The most elegant one is the synthesis approach. These extracted features are used to synthesize tones. Listeners judge how similar the synthetic and real tones sound, with results that indicate whether the physical description is sufficient. If it is not, additional analysis work has to be performed to find the proper parameters. Then systematic variations in the parameters (one at a time) enable listeners to evaluate the aural relevance of each of these parameters. The irrelevant parameters can then be discarded to simplify the description (Beauchamp, 1967; Fletcher *et al.*, 1962; Freedman, 1967; Grey & Moorer, 1977; Risset, 1969; Risset & Mathews, 1969; Strong & Clark, 1967a; Sundberg, cited in Music, Room, and Acoustics, 1977, pp. 57–81). Methods starting from actual instrument tones and studying the effect of various alterations of these tones on listeners' recognition have also provided insight. Thus it has been shown that the attack of the tone is an important recognition clue for a number of instruments (Berger, 1964; Saldanha & Corso, 1964; Schaeffer, 1966). The analysis of confusions between speeded-up instrument tones suggests there is a perceptual basis for grouping the instruments into families such as the string or the brass family (Clark *et al.*, 1964).

Temporal changes can be essential: A fast attack followed by a slow decay gives a plucked quality to any waveform. Schaeffer (1966) distinguishes between the sound *material* (matière), corresponding to a spectral cross section, and the sound *shape* (forme), corresponding to the evolution in time [similar concepts had been introduced under the names timbre and sonance by Seashore (1938, p. 103)]. By appropriate modifications of material and/or shape (that is, of spectrum and/or temporal envelop), it is possible to transmute, for example, a piano tone into a guitarlike tone, or an oboelike tone into a harpsichordlike tone (Risset, 1969; Schaeffer, 1966).

In most cases, one cannot isolate a single physical invariant characteristic of the timbre of a musical instrument. Throughout the pitch and loudness range, the physical parameters of the sound of a given instrument vary considerably, to the extent that the perceptual invariance, the unity of timbre of an instrument such as the clarinet seems to be a learned concept. However, a property, a law of variation, rather than an invariant, often appears to play an important part in the characterization of an instrument (or a class of similar instruments). In the piano, from treble to bass, the attack gets less abrupt while the spectrum gets richer (Schaeffer, 1966). Throughout part of the range, the sound of the clarinet can be grossly imitated by a symetrical nonlinear scheme giving a sinewave at low amplitude and odd partials at higher intensity, provided the temporal envelope is smooth enough (Beauchamp, 1975; Risset, 1969). The violin's quality is ascribed to a triangular source waveform modified by a steady and complex spectral response with many peaks and valleys (Mathews & Kohut, 1973). This scheme explains the richness of the vibrato, which modulates the spectrum in a complex way; the presence of vibrato makes violin recognition easier (Fletcher & Sanders, 1967; Saldanha & Corso, 1964). The brassy quality seems to be associated primarily to spectral variation with loudness, since increasing loudness causes a strong increase in the intensity of higher partials (Risset & Mathews, 1969). Within the brass family, different instruments present different spectral patterns and different temporal envelopes (Luce & Clark, 1967). That these features indeed characterize to a large extent stringed and brassy timbres can be demonstrated with Mathews' electronic violin (Mathews & Kohut, 1973). This instrument, played with a bow, can sound like an ordinary violin, but also like a trumpet if it is given the spectral characteristic of the brass.

Very often idiosyncrasies of sound production result in tone particularities that are strong cues for instrument recognition. Examples are frequency glides between notes in the trombone, because of the slide; intonation errors (cracked notes) in the horn because of the difficulty in hitting the right mode; initial, noisy impulsive vibration in string instruments when the string is first set into motion by the bow; and the burst of tonguing noise at the onset of a recorder note. Such particularities help make imitative synthesis very realistic (Morrill, 1977).

Some instruments can be grossly characterized by the combination of a few factors. A smooth temporal envelope, a spectrum with a predominant fundamental, a proper amplitude modulation with a regular and an irregular component yield a flutelike sound. A rapid attack followed by a fast decay, imposed on a low-frequency inharmonic spectrum plus a high-frequency noise band, resembles a snare drum. On the other hand, the naturalness and tone of a bell-like sound are critically dependent on the harmonic composition and on the decay characteristics (Risset, 1969). To characterize economically the tones of various wind instruments has been attempted—the respective importance of the temporal and the spectral envelopes for one instrument has been assessed by exchanging these envelopes between instruments (Strong & Clark, 1967).

The importance of a given cue can depend on context. For instance, details of the attack of trumpetlike tones (especially the rate at which various partials rise with time) are more significant for timbre in long sustained tones than in brief or evolving tones (Risset & Mathews, 1969). In the case of a very short rise time (as in the piano), the subjective feeling for the attack is actually correlated with the shape of the beginning of the amplitude decay (Schaeffer, 1966). The influence of the room acoustics is quite important and complex (Benade, 1976; Schroeder, 1966). Details of a fast decay can be masked in a reverberant environment like that of the organ. For percussion instruments with low damping (like bells, gongs, or low piano tones), the instrument's decay usually dominates the room's reverberation. In such cases, the details of the decay have a strong bearing on the timbre. If the partials decayed synchronously, the sound would be unnatural, *electronic* (Risset, 1969). Generally, the lower the component's frequency, the longer its decay time. Liveliness and warmth of the sound are increased by a complex pattern of beats between the components of the sound—warmth has been ascribed to inharmonicity in the piano tones (Fletcher *et al.*, 1962).

Although much remains to be done, the recent work on analysis and synthesis of musical instrument tones has brought substantial insight to the correlates of musical instrument timbre (Grey & Moorer, 1977) to the extent that it is now possible to simulate a number of instruments using simplified descriptions, for example, descriptions in terms of Chowning's (1973) powerful frequency modulation technique for sound synthesis (Morrill, 1977; Schottstaedt, 1977).

IV. MUSICAL REPRODUCTION

Most music heard nowadays comes from loudspeakers. Electroacoustic transducers—the microphone and the loudspeaker—have made it possible to use electronic amplification and modification of signals, and to achieve high standards of quality in sound recording and reproduction.

Present reproduction systems can be divided conceptually into four parts (some of which may or may not be assembled in one piece of equipment): the signal sources (phonograph, radio tuner, or tape deck), which supply electrical signals corresponding to audio-information; the preamplifier (or control amplifier), which modifies the electrical signals, performing amplification and equalization (that is, restoring of a proper spectral balance); the power amplifier, which boosts the power of the signals to a level adequate for driving the loudspeakers; and the loudspeakers, which convert the electrical signals into sound.

The main defects of a reproduction system are linear and nonlinear distortions. Linear distortion is nonuniform response to various frequencies in the reproduced band (it can be evaluated from the frequency response of the separate components, which should be as smooth and as flat as possible). Nonlinear distortion creates additional harmonics and very objectionable intermodulation distortion heard as noise (hiss or hum). Irregular rotation of a turntable results in flutter and wow, also very objectionable. Various other imperfections can affect the recording, such as microphone placement and balance, recording room acoustics, an imperfect rendering of the spatial distribution of sound, the acoustics of the listening room, or an inappropriate listening level [because of the hearing characteristics as shown by Fletcher and Munson curves (Stevens & Davis, 1952), high and low frequencies are quite weakened by low-level listening].

In the present state of the art (Crowhurst, 1971; Olson, 1967; cf. Villchur,

1965), power amplifiers and even preamplifiers can be made near perfect (although cheap ones can be of very poor quality). The weak points are the storage medium (disk records, tape) and the transducers (phonograph pickup, loudspeaker). Disk records cannot accommodate the full range of dynamics of orchestral music (about 80 dB between the softest and the loudest passages), although this has been improved by intensity compression before recording and compensating expansion at playback. The curvature of the groove introduces distortion, especially near the center of the disk. Records wear very much. Tape storage is much better in that respect, yet it is prone to deterioration with time. Tape also suffers from noise and there is a trade-off between noise (at low recording levels) and distortion (at high levels), which can be improved by compression and expansion (Blackmer, 1972; Dolby, 1967). Although still in its infancy and expensive, digital recording promises to offer higher quality and durability: Digital encoding affords substantial protection against the deficiencies and fragility of the recording medium. (David *et al.*, 1959; Kriz, 1975; Stockham, 1941).

The components of a musical reproduction system should be properly matched in quality. It is often the speaker that limits the quality of the set. The electrodynamic speaker is still the most widely accepted. Multiple speakers are generally used, small ones (tweeters) for high frequencies and large ones (woofers) for low frequencies, with the signal divided into low and high frequency parts by a crossover network before feeding the speakers. Speaker enclosures are necessary, and their design and realization have a strong effect upon the sound. The art of making loudspeakers is still evolving. The principle of motional feedback can be applied advantageously. Also, the desirable spatial distribution of the loudspeaker sounds still needs careful study.

Some of the spatial quality of music is rendered through the use of stereophony, which needs two recording channels and two speakers to create the illusion of auditory perspective. The next step is quadriphony (use of four channels). It has been shown that powerful control of the position and movement of the virtual sound source in the horizontal plane could be achieved with four channels (Chowning, 1971). However this may not be necessary for the rendering of classical music. Some quadriphony systems only use two recording channels, which are properly delayed in time and reverberated before being fed to the additional speakers, in an attempt to approximate the auditory environment of a concert hall in a listening room.

Hi-fi is an art of illusion. Faithful objective reproduction is impossible. Music reproduction must take advantage of the limitations of hearing and maintain the defects and distortion of the system at a low enough level to satisfy the listener (Jacobs & Wittman, 1964). Relevant to this problem are tests performed by Olson (1967, p. 388), which indicate that listeners are much more tolerant of distortions if the high-frequency cutoff is lower (they also show that speech is less impaired by distortion than music). Chinn and

Eisenberg (1945) tested the frequency range preference for reproduced speech and music. Surprisingly, they found that a majority of subjects preferred a narrow band system to a medium and a wide band system. Olson (1967, p. 393) objected that the amount of distortion may have been significant, so that in fact Chinn and Eisenberg may have measured the effect of bandwidth on distortion tolerance. Olson tested the preferred frequency range of live music, using acoustical filters, and found that subjects preferred the full-frequency range. Kirk (1956) proved that the judgment of subjects was biased by their expectations and that unfamiliarity with wide-range reproduction systems could explain Chinn and Eisenberg's results. Repeated listenings of the wide or narrow band system shifted subjects' preference toward the wide or narrow band system. Indeed AM radio and television teach many listeners to expect a narrow frequency range in music reproduction. There are also instances of hi-fi fans disappointed by listening to live music.

Music reproduction is not always used in a neutral way. Balance can be intentionally changed, some instruments can be emphasized, special effects can be used, and many pop music recordings have necessitated much sound processing. So far, music reproduction equipment has been designed for signals having the frequency distribution of instrumental music (Bauer, 1970). Inferior quality equipment has specifications chosen to minimize aural impairment for this type of music, and it can be quite detrimental to synthetic music with much energy in the low or high frequency range.

V. SYNTHETIC AND ELECTRONIC MUSIC

A. The Forerunners

Musical automata already existed at the end of the Middle Ages. In the seventeenth century, Kircher (1650) built music machines using pneumatic action. The score was recorded on punched tape (Kircher also built devices that automatically implemented certain rules of musical composition). There appeared a wealth of pianos, organs, wind, and percussion instruments, activated by a clock or a pneumatic mechanism. There were even automated *orchestras,* like the Panharmonicon of Maelzel (the inventor of the metronome), for which Beethoven specially composed *La Bataille de Vittoria* in 1813.

Recording and electrical transmission of sound appeared at the end of the nineteenth century. The techniques involved also have been used for the creation of new instruments and new music. In 1897, Cahill built an enormous "electrical factory of sounds," the telharmonium (see Russcol, 1972). A few composers were calling for new instruments, specially Varèse, who wrote in 1917, "Music . . . needs new means of expression, and science alone can infuse it with youthful sap'' (see Ouelette, 1968). Varèse wanted to escape the scale limitations and timbre restrictions imposed by the conventional instruments. Between the two World Wars, he tried in vain to originate research towards "the liberation of sound." A number of electronic instruments were built at that time, but most of them were designed or used with a traditional turn of mind, e.g., the electronic organ (Dorf, 1963; cf. Douglas, 1957, 1962). Among the most novel electronic instruments were Mager's Sphaerophon, Termen's Theremin, Trautwein's Trautonium, and the Ondes Martenot (Crowhurst, 1971; Dorf, 1963). Such instruments were used by composers such as Strauss, Hindemith, Honneger, Messiaen, and Jolivet. The performer used a keyboard or other device (e.g., the displacement of a ribbon, or the capacitance effect of the hand) to modify the adjustments of electronic circuits, producing electrical waves that were sent to a loudspeaker.

During that time period, several composers, including Milhaud, Hindemith, and Varèse, experimented with phonograph manipulations. Varèse proposed the generalization of music to organized sound. Stokowski foresaw the direct creation into tone, not paper. Cage predicted "the synthetic production of music . . . through the aid of electrical instruments which will make available for musical purposes any and all sounds that can be heard" (see Russcol, 1972, p. 72) and realized this in the 1939 *Imaginary Landscape No. I,* a piece using recorded sound produced by instruments and oscillators. It can be considered the first piece of electronic music—at any rate, the first musical work to exist only as a recording.

B. Electronic Music

After World War II, the progress of electronics and recording techniques fostered new and important developments (Beranek, 1970; Music and Technology, 1971).

Thanks to recording on magnetic tape, sounds could be dealt with as material objects. In 1948 Schaeffer (1952, 1966) started at the French Radio systematic experiments on modifications of sounds. He made recordings, performed so as to achieve special effects rather than fidelity, and used loops, tape reversal, tape splicing, mixing, filtering, etc. (see Olson, 1967; Ussachevsky, 1958). These experiments led to production of *musique concrète,* using processed recorded sounds of natural origin, including those of musical instruments. The name musique concrète refers to the process of building the music directly by sound manipulation instead of using an abstract medium—the score—between the conception and the realization of the music. The Schaeffer group attempted to uncover empirically some criteria helpful in musically assembling diversified and complex sounds. It was found essential to dissimulate the nature of the sound source by proper transformations. A priori any sound-producing object is adequate for musique concrète, be it a piano, played in any conceivable way, or a garbage lid; however, the identification of the piano or the garbage lid would hinder listening to the sounds for themselves.

Electronic music appeared a couple of years later, first in Germany, then in Italy, Holland, and Japan. The promotors, Meyer-Eppler and Eimert, were joined by composers like Stockhausen, Pousseur, and Koenig (Die Reihe, 1958; Russcol, 1972) who adopted a formalist approach quite different from the empirical approach of musique concrète. Instead of relying on aural control to assemble complex sounds, the emphasis was on the precise building and organization of compositions calling for sounds of well-known physical parameters; often a precise graphic score was produced before the composition was realized into sound. Initially the sounds were mostly combinations of sinusoidal tones and band-limited noises, produced by a battery of electronic equipment.

Tape music, started at Columbia University in 1952 by Ussachevsky and Luening, used freely electronic or natural sounds; in 1953 a work for orchestra and magnetic tape was presented. The theoretical and technical gap between the original electronic music and musique concrète has gradually been bridged. The term electronic music now refers to essentially any process using electronic equipment for the production of sound. Varèse used both electronic and natural sounds in *Déserts* (1954) and in *Poème Électronique* (1957). For this latter work, a number of loudspeakers were used so that the sound could travel in space. Cage and Stockhausen later used real-time electronic processing of musical instrument sounds.

Many studios devoted to the production of electronic music were built for universities, radio stations (Le Caine, 1956), and even private composers (see Mumma, 1964). Five thousand electronic music compositions are listed in a catalog compiled several years ago (Davies, 1968; see also Cross, 1967). Originally, electronic music studios used recording equipment plus electronic equipment, such as wave generators or filters, not specifically designed for music. Later, music synthesizers appeared. The R.C.A. synthesizer designed in 1955 by Olson (1967, pp. 415–426) is an enormous but powerful machine comprising many electronic circuits for the production of sound, controlled by instructions recorded on punched paper tape. Voltage control of oscillators and amplifiers was first applied to the design of electronic music equipment around 1964. Instead of requiring manual adjustment of a knob, parameters like frequency can thus be set by an input voltage (Moog, 1967). The equipment can be controlled by electrical signals, produced by a keyboard, a knob, or possibly other sources such as biological sensors (Eaton, 1971) or computers (see Section V,C; Mathews & Moore, 1970). Voltage-controlled oscillators, amplifiers, modulators, and filters now are often assembled in compact and convenient music synthesizers that can be used as performing instruments as well as part of electronic music studios (Appleton & Perera, 1975; Electronic Music Review, 1967–1968; Strange,

1972). For this reason they had an immediate appeal, especially in the field of pop music, and they helped live electronic music come of age, after pioneer realizations such as those of the Barrons (Barron & Barron, 1959). However, one may object to the rather mechanical sound that synthesizers often produce.

Electronic music has produced striking effects and powerful pieces of music. There is, however, some dissatisfaction with electronic music among many composers who feel that they cannot exert subtle enough control upon the elaboration of the sound structure. The lack of variety and richness is a strong limitation of purely electronic sounds, which are not complex enough (see Section II,D) unless they are manipulated in complex ways; however, the user then loses control of the parameters. Natural recorded sounds are varied and often rich, but one cannot easily exercise fine compositional control over them, since there is a disparity between the rich sounds and the rudimentary means of transforming them.

C. Computer Music

1. COMPOSITION WITH COMPUTERS

The digital computer can be used to relieve the composer from mechanical tasks, like transposing or inversing a melody (Smith, 1972); it can even be given a demanding duty—that of composing the music. If musical composition is regarded as the assembling of elements of a symbolic repertoire in some structured way (Moles, 1966), it can be performed automatically, provided the rules for selecting and assembling the elements are embodied in a computer program. Rules of counterpoint, as well as other rules, have thus been programmed (Barbaud, 1966; Hiller & Isaacson, 1959; Koenig, 1970). Statistical constraints, based on statistical analyses of existing music, permit us to grossly imitate a style or a composer (Olson, 1967, p. 430). Also, the composition of stochastic music, where compositional control is only statistical, can be carried out by computer (Tenney, 1969; Xenakis, 1971). It is easy to produce automatically random compositions with structure imposed as a sequential dependency, but this does not yield readily perceivable long range structures (Denes & Mathews, 1968). Indeed Markov processes, used to generate music in which the probabilities of successive notes depend on the preceding ones, are inadequate to generate certain musical structures, such as self-imbedded structures. Processes similar to Chomsky's generative grammars were proposed by Schenker half a century ago as models of tonal composition (see Kassler, 1964). Automatic musical composition faces problems as difficult as those of artificial intelligence in general. It is hard to express all the criteria of compositional choice in a computer program, but the very deficiencies of automatic composition bring insight to the creative process. Moreover the computer, instead of taking composition completely in charge, can efficiently help the composer in specific compositional tasks or in testing compositional rules.

2. Sound Synthesis with Computers

A computer is much more versatile than ordinary electronic equipment. Computer synthesis of sound can offer varied and precisely controllable sounds. The computer also permits us to complete complex mathematical or logical operations, including automatic musical composition.

Direct digital synthesis was introduced in 1958 and developed by Mathews (1963, 1969). The computer directly calculates the sound waveform—it computes samples of the waveform, e.g., values of the acoustical pressure at equally spaced time intervals. The numbers are then put out and converted into electrical pulses by a digital-to-analog converter. The pulses are smoothed by an appropriate low-pass filter to produce a continuously varying voltage that drives a loudspeaker. The sampling theorem (Shannon, 1948) states that, provided the sampling rate is high enough (e.g., 40,000 Hz), we can thus produce any bandlimited waveform (e.g., up to 20,000 Hz). In essence, the computer directly controls the motion of the loudspeaker. Direct digital synthesis is the most general sound synthesis process available.

To use digital synthesis efficiently, however, two problems must be solved. First, one needs a convenient program to control the computer. Programs like MUSIC V enable the user to produce a wide variety of sounds, even very complex ones, provided their physical structure is thoroughly specified (Mathews, 1969). Second, the user—the composer—must be able to provide very thorough descriptions of sound. It was soon realized after the first experiments (Foerster & Beauchamp, 1969; Mathews, 1963) that a body of psychoacoustical knowledge, relating the physical parameters of musical sounds and their subjective effect, was needed and lacking. Fortunately, computer sound synthesis is invaluable for progress in this field as well as for psychoacoustics and speech synthesis research. Every result of interest can be retained and pooled between the users, through examples of synthetic sounds comprising a listing of the synthesis data, which provide a complete and precise description of the sounds, and a recording of the sounds, which users can listen to in order to subjectively evaluate the timbres (Chowning, 1973; Morrill, 1977; Risset, 1969). So psychoacoustic expertise can accumulate cooperatively to increase the gamut of musically useful sounds available by computer synthesis and even by other processes of electronic synthesis.

Digital synthesis has helped us understand the physical correlates of the timbre of traditional instruments. Consequently it can generate sounds reminiscent of those instruments (see Section III,B). It has also already permitted us to achieve unprecedented control over various aspects of the sound, for example, controlling independently and/or precisely various cues for pitch (Risset, 1971) or space (Chowning, 1971), or interpolating between instrumental timbres (Grey, 1977), thus yielding novel musical possibilities. Among the most promising areas that can be explored through computer synthesis is the use of tones built up from arbitrarily chosen inharmonic frequency components, which may favor new melodic and harmonic relationships between the tones, as indicated by Pierce (1966). The computer thus affords sonic resources of unprecedented diversity and ductility. The musician can now envision working in a refined way with the continuum of sound.

However direct digital synthesis is difficult. A lot of computing is involved, so the computer cannot work in real time; a complete sound description must be specified in advance. This does not permit the user to react and modify the sound while listening. However, this possibility, whereby the composer can introduce performance nuance in real time, is provided by hybrid systems that interpose a computer between the composer–performer and an electronic sound synthesizer. As a result, the computer is freed from the computation of all the temporal details of the waveform; it only has to provide control signals for the synthesizer. Thus real-time operation is possible, and the user can control the sound in elaborate ways with various devices attached to the computer, like *programmed* knobs or keyboards. Thus we can program the performance of electronic music without tape recorders. The computer storage and editing facilities considerably extend the possibilities that would be available with the synthesizer alone. New situations can be set up where the user of the system can conduct, perform, and improvise. The performance can be perfected with the help of the computer (e.g., the intonation can be corrected, or the voice played may be harmonized). This may contribute to revive musical practice in nonexpert amateurs (Mathews & Moore, 1970; Mathews *et al.*, 1974; Music and Technology, 1971). Of course, the sounds produced by hydrid systems are inherently limited by the possibilities of the synthesizer attached to the computer. However, it is now possible to build digital synthesizers that are stable, accurate, and powerful (Alonso *et al.*, 1975; Alles & Di Giugno, 1977; Moorer, 1977), so that we will be able to take advantage of real-time operation while benefiting from the rich sonic possibilities of direct digital synthesis.

Electronic music has grown rapidly as a new medium of expression. From an economic standpoint, computer prices now compare with the prices of the analog equipment in a traditional electronic music studio. It seems that we are at the beginning of a new era for the development of electronic music, due to the considerable progress of digital microelectronics and digital sound processing techniques. Electronic music will probably use more and more computers (or microprocessors) in conjunction with a battery of digital circuits acting as powerful special-purpose sound processing computers (Moorer, 1977; Music and Technology, 1971, p. 129). However, progress in psychoacoustical expertise and music theory as well as ingenuity in musical system design are required, if such systems are to be musically efficient.

Acknowledgments

The author is indebted to E. C. Carterette, J. Grey, D. Harwood, M. V. Mathews, and D. Wessel for helpful comments and criticism.

References

Agren, C. H., & Stetson, K. A. Measuring the resonances of treble viol plates by hologram interferometry and designing an improved instrument. *Journal of the Acoustical Society of America,* 1972, **51,** 1971–1983.

Allen, D. Octave discriminability of musical and non-musical subjects. *Psychonomic Science,* 1967, **7,** 421–422.

Alles, H. G., & Di Giugno, P. A one-card 64-channel digital synthesizer. *Computer Music Journal,* 1977, **1,** 7–9.

Alonso, S., Appleton, J. H., & Jones, C. A special purpose digital system for the instruction, composition and performance of music. Proc. of the 1975 Conference on Computers in the undergraduate Curricula 6, 17–22.

Appleton, J. H., & Perera, R. C. (Eds.) *The development and practice of electronic music.* Englewood Cliffs, New Jersey: Prentice Hall, 1975.

Arfib, D. Digital synthesis of complex spectra by means of multiplication of nonlinear distorted sine waves (Preprint No. 1319). Hamburg: 59th Convention of the Audio Engineering Society, 1978.

Attneave, F., & Olson, R. K. Pitch as a medium: a new approach to psychophysical scaling. *American Journal of Psychology,* 1971, **84,** 147–165.

Babbitt, M. Contemporary music composition and music theory as contemporary intellectual history. In *Perspectives in musicology.* New York: W. W. Norton, 1972. Pp. 151–184.

Bachem, A. Tone height and tone chroma as two different pitch qualities. *Acta psychologica* 1950, **7,** 80–88.

Backhaus, W. Die Ausgleichvorgänge in der Akustik. *Zeitschrift für Technische Physik,* 1932, **13,** 31.

Backus, J. Small vibration theory of the clarinet. *Journal of the Acoustical Society of America,* 1963, **35,** 305–313.

Backus, J. *The acoustical foundations of music.* New York: W. W. Norton, 1969.

Baines, A. (Ed.) *Musical instruments through the ages.* Middlesex, England: Penguin Books, 1969.

Baird, J. W. Memory for absolute pitch. In *Studies in psychology.* Titchener commemorative volume Worcester: L. N. Wilson, 1917. Pp. 43–78.

Barbaud, P. *Initiation à la composition musicale automatique.* Paris: Dunod, 1966.

Barbour, J. M. *Tuning and temperament.* (2nd ed.) East Lansing, Michigan: Michigan State College Press, 1953.

Barron, L., & Barron, B. Electronic non-music: Problems of an orphan art. Audio Engineering Society, N.Y., 1959.

Bauer, B. B. Octave-band spectral distribution of recorded music. *Journal of the Audio Engineering Society,* 1970, **18,** 165–172.

Bauman, V. H. Teen-age music preferences. *Journal of Research in Music Education,* 1960, **8,** 75–84.

Beauchamp, J. W. A computer system for time-variant harmonic analysis and synthesis of musical tones. Technical Report no. 15, Experimental Music Studio, University of Illinois, 1967.

Beauchamp, J. W. Analysis and synthesis of cornet tones using non linear interharmonic relationships. *Journal of the Audio Engineering Society,* 1975, **23,** 778–795.

Benade, A. H. *Horns, strings and harmony*. Garden City, New York: Doubleday Anchor Books, 1960.

Benade, A. H. *Fundamentals of musical acoustics*. New York: Oxford University Press, 1976.

Beranek, L. L. *Music, acoustics and architecture*. New York: J. Wiley, 1962.

Beranek, L. L. Digital synthesis of speech and music. *I.E.E.E. Trans. on Audio Electroacoustics*, 1970, AU 18 no. **4**, 426–433 (record attached).

Berger, K. W. Some factors in the recognition of timbre. *Journal of the Acoustical Society of America*, 1964, **36**, 1888–1891.

Berlyne, D. E. *Aesthetics and psychobiology*. New York: Appleton, 1971.

Bever, T., & Chiarello, R. J. Cerebral dominance in musicians and nonmusicians. *Science*, 1974, **185**, 537–539.

Billeter, B. Die Silbermann-Stimmungen. *Archiv für Musikwissenchaft*, April 1970.

Blackham, E. D. Physics of the piano. *Scientific American*, 1965, **213**, 88–99.

Blackmer, D. E. A wide dynamic range noise reduction system. *DB, The Sound Engineering Magazine*, 1972, **6**, 23–26.

Boehm, T. *The flute and flute playing*. Translated by D. C. Miller. New York: Dover, 1964.

Boomsliter, P. C., & Creel, W. The long pattern hypothesis in harmony and hearing. *Journal of Music Theory*, 1961, **5**, 2–30.

Boomsliter, P. C., & Creel, W. Extended reference: An unrecognized dynamic in melody. *Journal of Music Theory*, 1963, **7**, 2–22.

Boomsliter, P. C., & Creel, W. Hearing with ears instead of instruments. *Journal of the Audio Engineering Society*, 1970, **18**, 407–412.

Bouasse, H. *Les instruments à vent*. Paris: Delagrave, 1929.

Bouhuys, A. Physiology and musical instruments. *Nature*, 1969, **221**, 1199–1204.

Boulez, P. *Notes of an apprenticeship*. New York: Knopf, 1968.

Bowles, E. A. *Computers and research in the humanities*. Englewood Cliffs, New Jersey: Prentice Hall, 1966.

Brady, P. T. Fixed-scale mechanism of absolute pitch. *Journal of the Acoustical Society of America*, 1970, **48**, 883–887.

Bregman, A. S., & Campbell, J. Primary auditory stream segregation and perception of order in rapid sequences of tones. *Journal of Experimental Psychology*, 1971, **89**, 244–249.

Brehmer, F. *Melodieauffassung u. melodische Begabung des kindes*. Leipzig, 1925 (cited in Teplov, 1966).

Brentano, F. *Untersuchungen zur sinnespsychologie*. Leipzig, 1907 (cited in Teplov, 1966).

Butler, J. W., & Daston, P. G. Musical consonance as musical preference: a cross cultural study. *Journal of General Psychology*, 1968, **79**, 129–142.

Cabot, R. C., Mino, M. G., Dorans, D. A., Tackel, I. S., & Breed, H. E. Detection of phase shifts in harmonically related tones. *Journal of the Audio Engineering Society*, 1976, **24**, 568–571.

Canac, F. (Ed). Acoustique musicale. Ed. du C.N.R.S., Paris 7°, 1959.

Cazden, N. Musical consonance and dissonance—a cultural criterion. *Journal of Aesthetics and Art Criticism*, 1945, **IV**, 3–11.

Cazden, N. Musical intervals of simple number ratios. *J. Res. Music. Educ.*, 1959, **20**, 301–319.

Cazden, N. Sensory theories of musical consonance. *Journal of Aesthetic and Art Criticism*, 1962, **20**, 301–319.

Cazden, N. The harmonic evolution of Jacques Chailley. *Journal of Music Theory*, 1968, **12**, 119–159.

Cazden, N. The systemic reference of musical consonance response. *International Review of the Aesthetics and Sociology of Music*, 1972, **12**, 217–243.

Chadwick, D. L. Music and hearing. *Proceedings of the Royal Society of Medicine*, 1973, **66**, 1078–1082.

Chailley, J. *Traité historique d'analyse musicale*. Paris: A. Leduc, 1951.

Charbonneau, G., & Risset, J. C. Différences entre oreille droite et oreille gauche pour la perception de la hauteur des sons. *C.R. Acad. Sci. Paris,* 1975, Série D, **281,** 163–166.

Cherry, C. *On human communication.* New York: Science editions, 1961.

Chinn, H. A., & Eisenberg, P. Frequency range preference for reproduced speech and music. PIRE, 1945, **33,** n° 9, 571.

Chowning, J. The simulation of moving sound sources. *Journal of the Audio Engineering Society,* 1971, **19,** 2–6.

Chowning, J. The synthesis of complex audio spectra by means of frequency modulation. *Journal of the Audio Engineering Society,* 1973, **21,** 526–534.

Clark, M., Jr., Robertson, P., & Luce, D. A preliminary experiment on the perceptual basis for musical instrument families. *Journal of the Audio Engineering Society,* 1964, **12,** 199–203.

Cohen, A. Further investigation of the effects of intensity upon the pitch of pure tones. *Journal of the Acoustical Society of America,* 1961, **33,** 1363–1376.

Cohen, J. E. Information theory and music. *Behavioral Science,* 1962, 7,137–163.

Coltman, J. W. Resonance and sounding frequencies of the flute. *Journal of the Acoustical Society of America,* 1966, **40,** 99–107.

Computer Music Journal (from 1977). Box E, Menlo Park, Ca. 94025.

Cooper, G., & Meyer, L. B. *The rhythmic structure of music.* Chicago: The University of Chicago Press, 1960.

Copp, E. F. Musical ability. *Journal of Heredity,* 1916, **7,** 297–305.

Costère, E. *Mort ou transfigurations de l'harmonie.* Paris: Presses Universitaires de France, 1962.

Creel, W., Boomsliter, P. C., & Powers, S. R.. Jr. Sensations of tone as perceptual forms. *Psychological Review,* 1970, **77,** 534–545.

Cross, M. L. (Ed.) *A bibliography of electronic music.* Toronto, Canada: University of Toronto Press, 1967.

Crowhurst, N. H. *Audio systems handbook.* Blue Ridge, Pennsylvania: TAB Books, 1969.

Crowhurst, N. H. *Electronic musical instruments.* Blue Ridge, Pennsylvania: TAB Books, 1971.

Cuddy, L. L. Training the absolute identification of pitch. *Perception and Psychophysics,* 1970, **8,** 265–269.

Culver, C. A. *Musical Acoustics.* Philadelphia: Blakiston, 1947.

David, E. E., Jr., Mathews, M. V., & McDonald, H. S. A high-speed data translator for computer simulation of speech and television devices. Proceedings of the I.R.E. Western Joint Computer Conference, 1959, 354–357.

Davies, H. (Ed.) International electronic music catalog. Cambridge, Massachusetts: The MIT Press, 1968.

DeGeorge, D., & Cook, G. E. Statistical music analysis: An objection to Fuck's curtosis curve. *IEEE Transactions on Information Theory,* 1968, **14,** 152–153.

Denes, P. B., & Mathews, M. V. Computer models for speech and music appreciation. Fall Joint Computer Conference, 1968, 319–327.

Deutsch, D. Octave generalization and tune recognition. *Perception and Psychophysics,* 1972, **11,** 411–412.

Deutsch, D. Musical illusions. *Scientific American,* 1975, **233,** 92–104. (a)

Deutsch, D. The organization of short-term memory for a single acoustic attribute. In *Short-term memory.* New York: Academic Press, 1975. Pp. 107–151. (b)

Deutsch, J. A., & Clarkson, J. K. Nature of the vibrato and the control loop in singing. *Nature,* 1959, **183,** 167–168.

Die Reihe *Electronic music.* Bryn Mawr, Pennsylvania: Th. Presser, 1958.

Dolby, R. M. An audio noise reduction system. *Journal of the Audio Engineering Society,* 1967, **15,** 383–388.

Dorf, R. H. *Electronic musical instruments.* Mineola, New York: Radiofile, 1963.

Douglas, A. *The electrical production of music.* New York: Philosophical Library, 1957.

Douglas, A. *The electronic musical instrument manual*. New York: Pittman, 1962.

Dowling, W. J. Recognition of inversions of melodies and melodic contours. *Perception and Psychophysics*, 1971, **9**, 348–349.

Dowling, W. J. Rhythmic groups and subjective chunks in memory for melody. *Perception and Psychophysics*, 1973, **14**, 37–40.

Dowling, W. J., & Fujitani, D. S. Contour, interval and pitch recognition in memory for melodies. *Journal of the Acoustical Society of America*, 1971, **49**, 524–531.

Duke, A. W., & Gullickson, G. R. Children's stimulus selection as a function of auditory stimulus complexity. *Psychonomic Science*, 1970, **19**, 119–120.

Eaton, M. L. *Bio-music*. Kansas City: Orcus, 1971.

Ehresman, D. L., & Wessel, D. L. *Perception of timbral analogies*. Paris: IRCAM Report No. 13, 1978.

Electronic Music Reports. The Institute of Sonology at Utrecht State University, Holland, 1969.

Electronic Music Review. Vol. 1–6. Trumansburg, New York: R. A. Moog Co., 1967–1968.

Elfner, L. Systematic shifts in the judgment of octaves of high frequencies. *Journal of the Acoustical Society of America*, 1964, **36**, 270–276.

Ellis, A. J. *Additions to the translation of the book On the sensations of tone by Helmholtz 1855*. New York: Dover, 1954.

Erickson, R. *Sound structure in music*. Berkeley/Los Angeles: University of California Press, 1975.

Esbroeck, J. van, & Montfort, F. *Qu'est-ce que jouer juste?* Bruxelles: Ed. Lumière, 1946.

Farnsworth, P. R. Studies in the psychology of tone and music. *Genetic Psychology Monographs*, 1934, no. **1**.

Farnsworth, P. R. *Musical taste: Its measurement and cultural nature*. Stanford: Stanford University Press, 1950.

Farnsworth, P. R. *The social psychology of music*. New York: The Dryden Press, 1958.

Flanagan, J. L. *Speech analysis, synthesis and perception*. New York: Academic Press, 1972.

Fletcher, H., Blackham, E. D., & Stratton, R. Quality of piano tones. *Journal of the Acoustical Society of America*, 1962, **34**, 749–761.

Fletcher, H., & Sanders, L. C. Quality of violin vibrato tones. *Journal of the Acoustical Society of America*, 1967, **41**, 1534–1544.

Foerster, H. V., & Beauchamp, J. W. *Music by computers*. New York: J. Wiley, 1969.

Fraisse, P. *Les structures rythmiques*. Paris: Erasme, 1956.

Fraisse, P., Oleron, G., & Paillard, J. Les effets dynamogéniques de la musique, étude expérimentale. *Année psychologique*, 1953, **53**, 1–34.

Francès, R. *La perception de la musique*. Paris: Vrin, 1958.

Fransson, F., Sundberg, J., & Tjerlund, P. Statistical computer measurements of the tone scale in played music (Rep. STL-QPSR 2–3). Stockholm: Speech Transmission Lab, 1970. Pp. 41–45.

Freedman, M. D. Analysis of musical instrument tones. *Journal of the Acoustical Society of America*, 1967, **41**, 793–806.

Fucks, W. Mathematical analysis of formal structure in music. *IRE Trans. on Inf. Th.*, 1962, **8**, 225–228.

Fyda, M. C. Perception and internal representation of musical intervals. M. A. thesis, Michigan State University, East Lansing, 1975.

Geer, J. P. van de, Levelt, W. J. M., & Plomp, R. The connotation of musical intervals. *Acta Psychologica*, 1962, **20**, 308–319.

Getz, R. P. The effects of repetition on listening response. *Journal of Research in Music Education*, 1966, **14**, 178–192.

Gordon, H. W. Hemispheric asymmetry and musical performance. *Science*, 1975, **189**, 68–69.

Gough, R. The effects of practice on judgments of absolute pitch. *Arch. Psychol.*, 1922, **7**, 47.

Gravesaner Blätter, *Gravesano Review*. Switzerland, 1956–1966, Mainz, Germany: Schott.

Green, R. T., & Courtis, M. C. Information theory and figure perception. The metaphor that failed. *Acta Psychologica*, 1966, **25**, 12–35.

Greene, P. C. Violin intonation. *Journal of the Acoustical Society of America*, 1937, **9**, 43–44.

Grey, J. M. Multidimensional perceptual scaling of musical timbres. *Journal of the Acoustical Society of America*, 1977, **61**, 1270–1277.

Grey, J. M., & Moorer, J. A. (1977). Perceptual evaluation of synthesized musical instrument tones. *Journal of the Acoustical Society of America*, 1977, **62**, 454–466.

Guernesey, M. The role of consonance and dissonance in music. *American Journal of Psychology*, 1928, **XL**, 173–204.

Guttman, N., & Pruzansky, S. Lower limits of pitch and musical pitch. *Journal of Speech and Hearing Research*, 1962, **5**, 207–214.

Hanslick, E. *The beautiful in music*. Translated by G. Cohen. Novello, London: Ewer, 1891.

Hart, H. C., Fuller, M. W., & Lusby, W. S. Precision study of piano touch and tone. *Journal of the Acoustical Society of America*, 1934, **6**, 80–94.

Harweg, R. Language and music: An immanent and sign theoretic approach. *Foundations of language*, 1968, **4**, 270–281.

Harwood, D. L. Towards a cognitive psychology of music. Unpublished thesis, Dept. of Psychology, University of California, Los Angeles, 1972.

Heinlein, C. P. The affective characters of the major and minor modes in music. *Journal of Comparative Psychology*, 1928, **8**, 101–142.

Helmholtz, H. *Sensations of tone, 1877*. English translation with notes and appendix by E. J. Ellis. New York: Dover, 1954.

Heuven, E. W. van *Acoustical measurements on church-bells and carillons*. The Hague: Van Cleef, 1949.

Hiller, L. A., & Bean, C. Information theory analysis of four sonata expositions. *Journal of Music Theory*, 1966, **10**, 96–138.

Hiller, L. A., Jr., & Isaacson, L. M. *Experimental music*. New York: McGraw Hill, 1959.

Hiller, L., & Ruiz, P. Synthesizing musical sounds by solving the wave equation for vibrating objects. Pt 1. *Journal of the Audio Engineering Society*, 1971, **19**, 463–470.

Hood, M. Indonesian music. In H. Kähler (Ed.), *Handbuch der Orientalistik*, 3rd ed., Vol. 6. Leiden, Netherlands: E. J. Brill, 1974.

Hornbostel, E. von Musikalische Tonsysteme. *Handbuch der Physik*, 1927, **VIII**.

Huggins, W. H. A phase principle for complex-frequency analysis and its implication in auditory theory. *Journal of the Acoustical Society of America*, 1952, **24**, 582–589.

Hutchins, C. M. The physics of violins. *Scientific American*, 1962, **289**, 79–93. (a)

Hutchins, C. M. Founding a family of fiddles. *Physics Today*, 1962, **20**, 23–37. (b)

Hutchins, C. M. (Ed.) *Musical acoustics: Benchmark papers on acoustics* (Pt. I, *Violin family components*, 1975; Pt. II, *Violin family functions*, 1976). Stroudsburg, Pennsylvania: Dowden, Hutchinson & Ross, 1975/1976.

Imberty, M. Intégration formelle et pouvoir impressif de l'oeuvre musicale. *Sciences de l'Art—Scientific Aesthetics*, 1974, **9**, 15–32.

Jacobs, J. E., & Wittman, P. Psychoacoustics, the determining factor in stereo disc recording. *Journal of the Audio Engineering Society*, 1964, **12**, 115–123.

Jansson, E. An investigation of a violin by laser speckle interferometry and acoustical measurements. *Acustica*, 1973, **29**, 21–28.

Jansson, E., & Sundberg, J. Long-term average spectra applied to analysis of music. *Acustica*, 1975/1976, **34**, 15–19 and 269–274.

Jacques-Dalcroze, E. *Rhythm, music and education*. New York: Putman, 1921.

Jeans, Sir James. *Science and music*. London: Cambridge University Press, 1937.

Jeffress, L. A. Absolute pitch. *Journal of the Acoustical Society of America*, 1962, **34**, 987.

Jones, M. R. Time, our lost dimension: Toward a new theory of perception, attention, and memory. *Psychological Review*, 1976, **83**, 323–355.

Kameoka, A., & Kuriyagawa, M. Consonance theory. Part I. Consonance of Dyads. *Journal of the Acoustical Society of America*, 1969, **45**, 1451–1459. (a)

Kameoka, A., & Kuriyagawa, M. Part II. Consonance of complex tones and its calculation method. *Journal of the Acoustical Society of America*, 1969, **45**, 1460–1469. (b)

Kassler, M. A report of work directed toward explication of Schenker's theory of tonality. Princeton University, 1964.

Kircher, A. *Musurgia universalis*. Rome, 1650.

Kirk, R. E. Learning, a major factor influencing preference for high fidelity reproducing systems. *Journal of the Acoustical Society of America*, 1956, **28**, 1113–1116.

Koenig, G. M. A program for musical composition. Electronic Music Reports, 1970, **2**, 32–44.

Köhler, W. Akustische Untersuchungen. *Zeitschrift für Psychologie*, 1915, **72**, 159.

Kohut, J., & Mathews, M. V. Study of motion of a bowed string. *Journal of the Acoustical Society of America*, 1971, **49**, 532–537.

Kriz, J. S. A 16 bit A.D.A. conversion system for high fidelity audio research. *IE.E.E. Trans. on Acoustics, Speech and Signal Processing ASSP*, 1975, **23**, 146–149.

Langer, S. K. *Philosophy in a new key*. Cambridge, Massachusetts: Harvard Univ. Press, 1951.

Le Caine, H. Electronic music. *Proceedings of the Institute of Radio Engineers*, 1956, **44**, 457.

Lee, V. *Music and its lovers*. London: Allen and Unwin, 1932.

Lefkoff, G. (Ed.) *Computer applications in music*. Morgantown: West Virginia University Library, 1967.

Lehman, P. R. *Tests and measurements in music*. Englewood Cliffs, New Jersey: Prentice Hall, 1968.

Leipp, E. *Acoustique et musique*. Paris: Masson, 1971.

Licht, S. *Music in medicine*. Boston: New England Conservatory of Music, 1946.

Licklider, J. C. R. Auditory frequency analysis. In C. Cherry, (Ed.), *Information Theory*. New York: Academic Press, 1956.

Licklider, J. C. R. Phenomena of localization. In A. B. Graham, (Ed.), *Sensorineural hearing processes and disorders*. Boston: Little Brown, 1967.

Lieberman, L. R., & Walters, Jr., W. M. Effects of repeated listening on connotative meaning of serious music. *Perceptual and Motor Skills*, 1968, **26**, 891–895.

Lincoln, H. B. *The computer and music*. Ithaca, New York: Cornell University Press, 1970.

Lloyd, L. S., & Boyle, H. *Intervals, scales and temperaments*. New York: St. Martin's Press, 1963.

Lomax, A. *Folksong style and culture*. Washington, D.C.: American Association for the Advancement of Science, 1968.

Lottermoser, W. Acoustical design of modern German organs. *Journal of the Acoustical Society of America*, 1957, **29**, 682–689.

Lottermoser, W., & Meyer, J. Orgelakustik in Einzeldarstellung. Frankfurt: Ed. Das Musikinstrument, 1966.

Luce, D., & Clark, Jr., M. Physical correlates of brass-instrument tones. *Journal of the Acoustical Society of America*, 1967, **42**, 1232–1243.

Lundin, R. W. Toward a cultural theory of consonance. *Journal of Psychology*, 1947, **23**, 45–49.

Lundin, R. W. *An objective psychology of music*. New York: Ronald Press, 1967.

Lundin, R. W., & Allen, J. D. A technique for training perfect pitch. *The Psychological Record*, 1962, **12**, 139–146.

Martin, D. W. Directivity and acoustic spectra of brass wind instruments. *Journal of the Acoustical Society of America*, 1942, **13**, 309–313.

Martin, D. W. Decay rates of piano tones. *Journal of the Acoustical Society of America*, 1947, **19**, 535–541.

Martin, D. W., & Ward, W. D. Subjective evaluation of musical scale temperament in pianos. *Journal of the Acoustical Society of America*, 1961, **33**, 582–588.

Mathews, M. V. The digital computer as a musical instrument. *Science*, 1963, **142**, 553–557.

Mathews, M. V. *The technology of computer music*. Cambridge, Massachusetts: MIT Press, 1969.

Mathews, M. V. Violin resonances studied by electrical simulation. *Journal of the Acoustical Society of America*, 1971, **50**, 128.

Mathews, M. V., & Kohut, J. Electronic simulation of violin resonances. *Journal of the Acoustical Society of America*, 1973, **53**, 1620–1626.

Mathews, M. V., & Moore, F. R. Groove—a program to compose, store and edit functions of time. *Communic. of the ACM*, 1970, **13**, 715–721.

Mathews, M. V., Moore, F. R., & Risset, J. C. Technology and future music. *Science*, 1974, **183**, 263–268.

McClelland, D. C., Atkinson, J. W., Clark, R. A., & Lowell, E. L. *The achievement motive*. New York: Appleton, 1953.

Meinel, H. Regarding the sound quality of violins and a scientific basis for violin construction. *Journal of the Acoustical Society of America*, 1957, **29**, 817–822.

Mendel, A., Sachs, C., & Pratt, C. C. *Some aspects of musicology*. New York: Liberal Arts Press, 1957.

Meyer, E., & Buchmann, G. *Die Klangspektren der Musikinstrumente*. Berlin: Akademie der Wissenschaften, 1931.

Meyer, J. *Akustik der Holzblasinstrumente in Einzeldarstellung*. Frankfurt: Ed. Das Musikinstrument, 1966.

Meyer, J. *Acoustics and the performance of music*. Translated by J. Bowsher and S. Westphal. Frankfurt: Das Musikinstrument, Verlag Erwin Bochinsky, 1977.

Meyer, L. B. *Emotion and meaning in music*. Chicago: University of Chicago Press, 1956.

Meyer, L. B. *Music, the arts and ideas*. Chicago: University of Chicago Press, 1967.

Meyer, M. Is the memory of absolute pitch capable of development by training? *Psychological Review*, 1899, **6**, 514–516.

Meyer, M. On the attribute of the sensations. *Psychological Review*, 1904, **11**.

Meyer, M. On memorizing absolute pitch. *Journal of the Acoustical Society of America*, 1956, **28**, 718–719 (L).

Meyer-Eppler, W. Informationsthoerie. *Naturwissenschaften*, 1952, **39**, 341.

Meyer-Eppler, W. Musical communication as a problem of information theory. *Graves. Blätter*, 1965, **26**, 98–102.

Mikol, B. The enjoyment of new musical systems. In M. Rokeach (Ed.), *The open and closed mind*. New York: Basic Books, 1960.

Miller, D. C. *Science of musical sounds*. New York: MacMillan, 1926.

Miller, G. A. *The psychology of communication*. Baltimore: Penguin Books, 1969.

Miller, J. R., & Carterette, E. C. Perceptual space for musical structures. *Journal of the Acoustical Society of America*, 1975, **58**, 711–720.

Moles, A. *Information theory and esthetic perception*. Urbana: University of Illinois Press, 1966.

Moog, R. A. Electronic music—its composition and performance. *Electronics World*, 1967.

Moorer, J. A. The synthesis of complex audio spectra by means of discrete summation formulas. *Journal of the Audio Engineering Society*, 1976, **24**, 717–727.

Moorer, J. A. Signal processing, aspects of computer music: A survey. *Proc. of the I.E.E.E.*, 1977, **65**, 1108–1137.

Morrill, D. Trumpet algorithms for computer composition. *Computer Music Journal*, 1977, **1**, 46–52.

Mueller, J. H., & Hevner, K. Trends in musical taste. *Indiana University Publ.*, Humanity Series, 1942, no. 8.

Mull, H. K. The effect of repetition upon the enjoyment of modern music. *Journal of Psychology*, 1957, **43**, 155–162.

Mumma, G. An electronic music studio for the independent composer. *Journal of the Audio Engineering Society*, 1964, **12**, 240–244.

Mursell, J. L. *The psychology of music.* New York: W. W. Norton, 1937.

Music, Room, and Acoustics. Stockholm, Sweden: Royal Swedish Academy, 1977 (record attached).

Music and Technology. *La Revue Musicale,* Paris. Proceedings of the Stockholm Meeting June 8–12, 1970 organized by UNESCO, 1971.

Nattiez, J. J. Is a descriptible semiotics of music possible? *Language Sciences,* 1972, **23**, 1–7.

Nederveen, C. J. *Acoustical aspects of wind instruments.* Amsterdam: Knuf, 1969.

Neisser, U. *Cognitive psychology.* New York: Appleton, 1967.

Neu, D. M. A critical review of the literature on "absolute pitch." *Psychological Bulletin,* 1947, **44**, 249–266.

Oakes, W. F. An experimental study of pitch naming and pitch discrimination reactions. *Journal of Genetic Psychology,* 1955, **86**, 237–259.

Olson, H. F. *Music, physics and engineering.* New York: Dover, 1967.

Ortmann, O. *The physiological mechanics of piano technique.* New York: Dutton, 1962. (first published 1929).

Osmond-Smith, D. Music as communication: Semiology or morphology? *International Review of the Aesthetics and Sociology of Music,* 1971, **II**, 108–111.

Ouelette, F. *Edgard Varèse.* New York: Orion Press, 1968.

Partch, H. *Genesis of a new music.* Madison: Univ. of Wisconsin Press, 1949.

Patterson, B. Musical dynamics. *Scientific American,* 1974, **231**, 78–95.

Phares, M. L. Analysis of music appreciation by means of the psychogalvanic response technique. *Journal of Experimental Psychology,* 1934, **17**, 119–140.

Piaget, J., & Inhelder, B. *The psychology of the child.* Translated by Helen Weaver. New York: Basic Books, 1969.

Pierce, J. R. *Symbols, signals and noise.* London: Hutchinson, 1962.

Pierce, J. R. Attaining consonance in arbitrary scales. *Journal of the Acoustical Society of America,* 1966, **40**, 249.

Pikler, A. G. History of experiments on the musical interval sense. *Journal of Music Theory,* 1966a, Spring, 54–95.

Pikler, A. G. Logarithmic frequency systems. *Journal of the Acoustical Society of America,* 1966b, **39**, 1102–1110.

Pitts, C. E., & De Charms, R. Affective arousal to music as a function of deviations in perceived complexity from an adaptation level. Washington Univ., St. Louis, Technical Report no. 19, AD–413 361, June, 1963.

Plomp, R. Experiments on tone perception. Institute for Perception. RVO-TNO, Soesterberg, The Netherlands, 1966.

Podolsky, E. (Ed.) *Music therapy.* New York: Philosophical Library, 1954.

Poland, W. Theories of music and musical behavior. *Journal of Music Theory,* 1963, **7**, 150–173.

Potter, R. K., Kopp, G. A., & Green, H. C. *Visible speech.* New York: Van Nostrand, 1947.

Rabson, G. R. The influence of age, intelligence and training on reactions to classic and modern music. *Journal of Genetic Psychology,* 1940, **22**, 413–429.

Raman, C. V. On the mechanical theory of the vibrations of bowed strings and of musical instruments of the violin family, with experimental verification of the results. New Delhi: The Indian Association for the Cultivation of Science, Bulletin No. 15, 1918.

Restle, F. Theory of serial pattern learning: Structural tree. *Psychological Review,* 1970, **7**, 481–495.

Revesz, G. *Introduction to the psychology of music*. Norman: University of Oklahoma Press, 1954.

Richardson, E. G. The transient tones of wind instruments. *Journal of the Acoustical Society of America*, 1954, **26**, 960–962.

Risset, J. C. Sur certains aspects fonctinnels de l'audition. *Annales des Télécomm.*, 1968, **23**, 91–120.

Risset, J. C. An introductory catalog of computer-synthesized sounds. Bell Telephone Laboratories, 1969 (record attached).

Risset, J. C. Paradoxes de hauteur: Le concept de hauteur sonore n'est pas le même pour tout le monde. *Proceedings of the Seventh International Congress on Acoustics, Budapest*, 1971, paper 20S10.

Risset, J. C., & Mathews, M. V. Analysis of musical instrument tones. *Physics Today*, 1969, **22**, 23–30.

Roederer, J. *Introduction to the physics and psychophysics of music*. New York: Springer-Verlag, 1972.

Rossing, T. D. Resource letter MA.1: Musical acoustics. *American Journal of Physics*, 1975, **43**, 944–953.

Ruckmick, C. A. A bibliography of rhythm. *American Journal of Psychology*, 1918, **29**, 214–218.

Russcol, H. *The liberation of sound: An introduction to electronic music*. Englewood Cliffs, New Jersey: Prentice Hall, 1972.

Ruwet, N. *Langage, musique, poésie*. Paris: Ed. du Seuil, 1972.

Sachs, C. *The history of musical instruments*. New York: Norton, 1940.

Sachs, C. *The rise of music in the ancient world, east and west*. New York: Norton, 1943.

Sachs, C. *Rhythm and tempo*. New York: Norton, 1953.

Sackford, C. Some aspects of perception. *Journal of Music Theory*, 1961, **5**, 162–202 (I).

Sackford, C. Some aspects of perception. *Journal of Music Theory*, 1962, **6**, 66–90 (II).

Saldanha, E. L., & Corso, J. F. Timbre cues and the identification of musical instruments. *Journal of the Acoustical Society of America*, 1964, **39**. 2021–2026.

Schaeffer, P. *A la recherche d'une musique concrète*. Paris: Ed. du Seuil, 1952.

Schaeffer, P. *Traité des objets musicaux*. Paris: Ed. du Seuil, 1966.

Schoen, M. (Ed.) *The effects of music*. New York: Harcourt, 1927.

Schoen, M. *The psychology of music*. New York: Ronald Press, 1940.

Schottstaedt, B. The simulation of natural instrument tones using frequency modulation with a complex modulating wave. *Computer Music Journal*, 1977, **1**, 46–50.

Schroeder, M. R. Architectural acoustics. *Science*, 1966, **151**, 1355–1359.

Schroeder, M. R. Models of hearing. *Proceedings of the Institute of Electrical and Electronics Engineers*, 1975, **63**, 1332–1350.

Schuck, O. H., & Young, R. W. Observations on the vibrations of piano strings. *Journal of the Acoustical Society of America*, 1943, **15**, 1–11.

Schullian, D., & Schoen, M. (Eds.), *Music and medicine*. New York: Aberland Schuman, 1948.

Schwartz, E. *Electronic music, a listener's guide*. New York: Praeger, 1973.

Schwartz, E., & Childs, B. *Contemporary composers on contemporary music*. New York: Holt, Rinehart and Winston, 1967.

Seashore, C. E. *Psychology of music*. New York: McGraw-Hill, 1938.

Shannon, C. E. A mathematical theory of communication. *Bell Systems Technical Journal*, 1948, **27**, 379–423.

Shepard, R. N. Circularity in judgments of relative pitch. *Journal of the Acoustical Society of America*, 1964, **36**, 2346–2353.

Simon, H. A. Complexity and the representation of patterned sequences of symbols. *Psychological Review*, 1972, **79**, 369–382.

Slawson, A. W. Vowel quality and musical timbre as functions of spectrum envelope and fundamental frequency. *Journal of the Acoustical Society of America*, 1968, **43**, 87–101.

Small, A. M. An objective analysis of violin performance. *Univ. of Iowa Studies in the Psychology of Music*, 1936, **4**, 172–231.

Small, A. M., & Martin, D. W. Musical acoustics: Aims, problems, progress and forecast. *Proceedings of the Second International Congress of Acoustics, American Institute of Physics*, 1957, 68–75.

Smith, L. Score: A musical approach to computer music. *Journal of the Audio Engineering Society*, 1972, **20**, 7–14.

Soibelman, D. *Therapeutic and industrial uses of music*. New York: Columbia Univ. Press, 1948.

Springer, G. P. Language and music: Parallel and divergencies. In M. Halle, H. Lunt, and H. McClean (Eds.), *For Roman Jakobson*. La Hague: Mouton, 1956. Pp. 504–613.

Stetson, R. B. A motor theory of rhythm and discrete succession. *Psychological Review*, 1905, **XII**, 250–270 and 293–350.

Stevens, S. S. (Ed.), *Handbook of experimental psychology*. New York: J. Wiley, 1951.

Stevens, S. S., & Davis, H. *Hearing*. New York: J. Wiley, 1952.

Stevens, S. S., & Volkmann, J. The relation of pitch to frequency: A revised scale. *American Journal of Psychology*, 1940, **53**, 329–353.

Stockham, T. G. A-D and D-A converters: Their effect on digital audio fidelity. Preprint no. 834, 41st Meeting of the Audio Engineering Society, 1941, New York, N.Y.

Strange, A. *Electronic music: Systems, techniques and controls*. Dubuque, Iowa: W. C. Brown, 1972.

Stravinsky, I. *Poetics of music*. Cambridge, Massachusetts: Harvard Univ. Press, 1947.

Strong, W., & Clark, M., Jr. Synthesis of wind-instrument tones. *Journal of the Acoustical Society of America*, 1967, **40**, 39–52. (a)

Strong, W., & Clark, M., Jr. Perturbations of synthetic orchestral wind-instrument tones. *Journal of the Acoustical Society of America*, 1967, **41**, 277–285. (b)

Stumpf, C. *Ton psychologie*. Leipzig: Hirzel, 1883 and 1890.

Stumpf, C. *Die Sprachlaute*. Berlin: Springer-Verlag, 1926.

Sundberg, J. Voice source properties of bass singers. *Proceedings of the Seventh International Congress on Acoustics, Budapest*, 1971 paper 20S 5.

Sundberg, J. Articulatory interpretation of the "singing formant." *Journal of the Acoustical Society of America*, 1974, **55**, 838–844.

Sundberg, J. The acoustics of the singing voice. *Scientific American*, 1977, **236**, 82–91.

Sundberg, J. E. F., & Lindqvist, J. Musical octaves and pitch. *Journal of the Acoustical Society of America*, 1973, **54**, 922–929.

Tanner, R. La différenciation qualitative des psycharithmes et des intervalles musicaux. *La revue musicale*, 1972, **825**.

Tanner, W. P., & Rivette, C. L. Experimental study of "tone deafness." *Journal of the Acoustical Society of America*, 1964, **36**, 1465–1467.

Taylor, C. A. *The physics of musical sounds*. New York: Elsevier, 1965.

Tenney, J. C. Computer music experiments. *Electronic Music Reports* (Utrecht State Univ.), 1969, **1**, 23–60.

Teplov, B. M. *Psychologie des aptitudes musicales*. (Translated from Russian into French.) Paris: Presses Universitaires de France, 1966.

Terhardt, E. Pitch, consonance and harmony. *Journal of the Acoustical Society of America*, 1974, **55**, 1061–1069.

Tischler, H. The aesthetic experience. *Music Review*, 1956, **17**, 189.

Ussachevsky, V. A. The processes of experimental music. *Journal of the Audio Engineering Society*, 1958, **6**, 202–208.

van Esbroeck, G., & Montfort, G. *Qu'est-ce que jouer juste?* Brussels: Lumière, 1948.

van Norden, L. P. A. S. Temporal coherence in the perception of tone sequences. Eindhoven, Holland: Institute for Perception Research, thesis, 1975 (record attached).

Vennard, W. *Singing: The mechanism and the technique.* New York: Fischer, 1967.

Vernon, P. E. (1934). Auditory perception: I. The Gestalt approach. II. The evolutionary approach. *British Journal of Psychology,* 1934, **25,** 123–139 and 265–283.

Villchur, E. M. *Reproduction of sound.* New York: Dover Public, 1965.

Vitz, P. C. Preferences for rates of information presented by sequences of tones. *Journal of Experimental Psychology,* 1964, **68,** 176–183.

Ward, W. D. Subjective musical pitch. *Journal of the Acoustical Society of America,* 1954, **26,** 369–380.

Ward, W. D. Absolute pitch. Pt I *Sound,* 1963, 2(3), 14–21, Pt II *Sound,* 1963, 2(4), 33–41.

Ward, W. D. Musical perception. In J. V. Tobias (Ed.), *Foundations of modern auditory theory.* Vol. 1. New York: Academic Press, 1970. Chapter II, 407–447.

Ward, W. D., & Martin, D. W. Psychophysical comparison of just tuning and equal temperament in sequences of individual tones. *Journal of the Acoustical Society of America,* 1961, **33,** 586–588.

Warren, R. M., Obusek, C. J., Farmer, R. M., & Warren, R. P. Auditory sequence: Confusion of patterns other than music. *Science,* 1969, **164,** 586–587.

Watt, H. J. *The psychology of sound.* Cambridge, England: University Press, 1917.

Wente, E. C. Characteristics of sound transmission in rooms. *Journal of the Acoustical Society of America,* 1935, **7,** 123.

Wessel, D. L. Psychoacoustics and music: A report from Michigan State University. *Page: Bulletin of the Computer Arts Society,* 1973, **30,** 1.

Wessel, D. L. Low dimensional control of musical timbre (Preprint No. 1337). Hamburg: 59th Convention of the Audio Engineering Society, 1978.

Wightman, F. L., & Green, D. M. The perception of pitch. *American Scientist,* 1974, **62,** 208.

Winckel, F. *Music, sound and sensation.* New York: Dover, 1967.

Worman, W. Unpublished doctoral thesis. Case Western Reserve Univ., Cleveland, Ohio, 1971.

Wright, D. F. Musical meaning and its social determinants. *Sociology,* 1975, **9,** 419–435.

Xenakis, I. *Formalized music.* Bloomington: Indiana Univ. Press, 1971.

Young, F. J. The natural frequencies of musical horns. *Acustica,* 1960, **10,** 91–97.

Young, R. W. Some problems for postwar musical acoustics. *Journal of the Acoustical Society of America,* 1944, **16,** 103–107.

Young, R. W. Sound absorption in air in rooms. *Journal of the Acoustical Society of America,* 1957, **29,** 311.

Young, R. W. A decade of musical acoustics. *Proceedings of the Fourth International Congress on Acoustics,* 1962, **II,** 231–250.

Young, R. W., & Webster, J. C. Tuning of musical instruments: The clarinet. *Graves. Blätter,* 1958, **4,** 182–186.

Zenatti, A. Le développement génétique de la perception musicale (Monographies françaises de Psychologie, No. 17). Paris: Centre National de la Recherche Scientifique, 1969.

Part VI

Stress, Trauma, and Pathology

Chapter 13

EFFECTS OF HEARING IMPAIRMENT ON THE AUDITORY SYSTEM

DONALD D. DIRKS

I. HISTORICAL PERSPECTIVE

The impact of severe hearing loss or complete deafness on social communication has been appreciated at least since Biblical times. So-called "deaf-mutism" was described in the Bible and by early Greek and Latin writers. The concept that deafness and muteness depended on a common abnormality was one of many false notions that have characterized the history of the problem. Early laws and regulations reflected such misunderstandings, and the deaf were often denied legal rights and, in some instances, considered mentally incompetent. The realization that a person with a severe hearing loss could acquire speech evolved slowly, and the various oral and manual methods of training the deaf did not appear until the Renaissance period.

HANDBOOK OF PERCEPTION, VOL. IV

Fundamental to the rehabilitation or training of persons with hearing impairment is the development of suitable diagnostic procedures to assess the magnitude of hearing loss and the specific functional problems associated with the various types of hearing impairment. Such diagnostic methods have been slow in development, awaiting, first, solid concepts regarding auditory physiology and, second, technological advances in acoustic instrumentation. In addition, the practical need for precise diagnosis was motivated by the development of innovative middle-ear surgical techniques, which occurred around 1935–1945 and the recognized necessity for aural rehabilitative services for the large number of World War II veterans with hearing loss.

The need to determine the magnitude of residual hearing a deaf or hard-of-hearing child possessed was emphasized by Urbantschitsch, a Viennese otologist, toward the end of the nineteenth century. He stressed the possibility of exercising such residual hearing to make the deaf child aware of sounds and his own voice. However, the most sophisticated methods of measuring human hearing during the nineteenth century employed tuning forks and live voice.

Following World War I, advances in electronics provided the necessary technology for improving hearing tests (electronic audiometers) and for the more adequate use of residual hearing (electrical amplification). As mentioned previously, the need for precise diagnosis of auditory disorders gained impetus during the period from 1935 to 1945 with the successful development of surgical procedures to alleviate hearing loss due to impairments of the middle ear. During World War II, the establishment of aural rehabilitation centers focused further attention on the problems of impaired hearing. Responsibilities in these centers included development of tests of hearing function and selection of hearing aids as well as the development of rehabilitation techniques. The rapid progress in technology during this period provided the necessary instrumentation to precisely generate and manipulate auditory signals. This greater technical precision facilitated investigations that have led to a steady increase in our understanding of the functional handicaps that occur with different types of auditory lesions. Thus, modern clinical auditory measurements are a result of the need to establish techniques that delineate the distinguishing characteristics among a variety of auditory disorders and permit detailed diagnosis of hearing impairment.

The purpose of this chapter is to review some of the effects of lesions occurring at specific sites in the auditory system, especially as these effects provide for the differential diagnosis of hearing disorders. In doing so, the diagnostic test procedures that have been found especially useful will be described and, from such results, a profile of symptoms that characterize the various hearing disorders will be developed. In addition, several factors that must be considered in determining the magnitude of the handicap imposed by hearing impairment are discussed.

II. BASIC CONSIDERATIONS

A. Types of Hearing Impairment

Auditory impairments usually produce two major types of receptive disorders: (1) a loss of auditory sensitivity and (2) dysacusis. A loss of sensitivity is characterized by a reduction in or absence of response to sounds that would normally be heard, whereas dysacusis refers to impairments of hearing that are not primarily losses of auditory sensitivity. Dysacusis often accompanies a sensitivity loss, but each may occur independently. Loss of sensitivity is no doubt the most common finding in hearing disorders and usually is a result of impairment in the peripheral auditory system, including the external ear, the middle ear, the cochlea, and the first-order neuron of the VIIIth cranial nerve. Sensitivity loss is not a common characteristic associated with lesions of the central auditory nervous system; that is, of the brainstem pathway and the primary auditory projection area of the temporal lobe (Bocca & Calearo, 1963; Jerger, 1973a).

In practice, dysacusis is usually associated with disorders of the sensorineural system. Various types of dysacusis have been described, but the most common is a reduction in speech discrimination performance even though the stimulus is delivered at sound pressure levels (SPLs) well above the individual's threshold for hearing. Other common forms of dysacusis are diplacusis (tones presented to an impaired ear have a different pitch than in the normal ear), recruitment (a rapid increase in subjective loudness as a function of sound pressure), and auditory agnosia or central auditory imperception. It may be apparent from these examples that, unlike sensitivity losses, dysacusis is not totally alleviated by simple amplification, via hearing aids.

B. Basic Audiometric Assessment

The most common symptom of an auditory disorder, especially in the peripheral auditory system, is a loss of sensitivity. Thus, an estimate of the magnitude of the sensitivity loss forms the nucleus of most auditory examinations and descriptions of hearing impairment. In practice, the magnitude of the loss is usually determined from the threshold of hearing for pure tones at selected frequencies within the major useful range of human hearing ($\sim$125–8000 Hz).

In delineating a loss of sensitivity, the crucial question is whether or not the patient deviates in sensitivity from a normal group of listeners, that is, from "audiometric zero." The establishment of a standard for normal air-conduction threshold is thus of paramount importance.

In the early days of electronic audiometers, there were no accepted standards for specifying the sound stimulus levels for the normal air-conduction

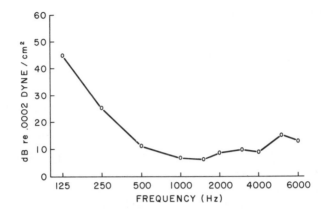

Fig. 1. Normal threshold levels re .0002 dyne cm⁻² for air conduction via a TDH-39 earphone fitted with a MX-41/AR cushion. [Reproduced with permission from American National Standard 53.6-1969, copyright 1969 by the American National Standards Institute, copies of which may be purchased from the American National Standards Institute at 1430 Broadway, New York, New York 10018.]

threshold of hearing. Likewise, no guidelines existed regarding the acceptable signal parameters for the test procedures. In the United States, the National Bureau of Standards and other regulatory groups have established standards for audiometer calibration. Prior to 1951, audiometers were calibrated from physical reference values based on thresholds obtained from the U.S. Public Health Survey of 1935–1936 (Bulletin 1–7, 1938). SPLs close to those obtained in the Public Health Survey were used later by the American Standard Association to establish a standard on audiometers (ASA Z24.5–1951). However, threshold levels averaging ~10 dB lower than those suggested in the ASA 1951 standard were occasionally reported in laboratory and field surveys. The International Organization for Standardization investigated the problems involved in such discrepancies and recommended new, threshold levels in 1964 (ISO R389-1964). The differences in recommended threshold levels are no doubt the result of differences in choice of normal populations, improvements in physical, environmental, and procedural controls, and advancements in calibration procedures that have occurred during the period since the U.S. Public Health Survey. Threshold levels close to those recommended in the ISO 1964 recommendation were adopted in the United States by the American National Standards Institute in the current standard on audiometers, ANSI S3.6-1969.

Figure 1 shows the decibel levels* for normal threshold as suggested in

*The decibel is often used to quantitatively describe the sound pressure level of various auditory signals. The reference pressure for the decibel scale in this instance is 2×10^{-4} μbar, a physical reference. Two decibel levels, *hearing level* and *sensation level*, are commonly used in describing hearing loss. Hearing level (HL) is used to designate a quantitative deviation of the hearing threshold from a prescribed standard, or the number of decibels that an individual threshold is above the standard "zero" of the audiometer at a particular frequency. The term sensation level (SL) is used to describe the pressure level of a sound in decibels above its threshold of audibility for an individual observer or group of individuals.

ANSI S3.6-1969. The output SPLs for normal hearing are specified in terms of the acoustic calibration of earphones. The sound SPLs from the earphone are measured in couplers or so-called "artificial ears," which have been developed to simulate impedance characteristics of the ear. The standard also specifies other requirements such as the minimum desirable frequency and intensity ranges for testing, switching rates, and allowable distortions.

The basic procedures used in clinical pure tone audiometry were established more than 30 years ago (Hughson & Westlake, 1944) and subsequently have achieved widespread clinical acceptance. The general principles have remained essentially unchanged, although variations in technique have appeared (Carhart & Jerger, 1959). The development of an automatic audiometer by Békésy (1947) presents one of the most notable additions to the original pure-tone testing procedures. In this self-recording audiometer, both the frequency and the signal intensity are motor operated, while the patient (via a manual switch) records his thresholds by controlling the direction of the intensity change. Although originally not designed for diagnostic purposes, the introduction of semiautomatic audiometers has provided a valuable tool for screening and industrial audiometric programs and, under certain conditions, for the differential diagnosis of auditory disorders. The latter use of automatic audiometry will be described later.

Figure 2 contains examples of two pure-tone audiograms obtained from a 5-year-old child (Fig. 2A) with serous otitis media (fluid in the middle ear) and from a 70-year-old male (Fig. 2B) with presbycusis (hearing loss due to aging). The audiogram in Fig. 2A indicates a mild hearing impairment with the loss greatest in the low frequencies (125–500 Hz). The audiometric configuration of Fig. 2B shows a moderate hearing loss, with the magnitude of the loss increasing with frequency. Such audiograms are commonly observed among populations of patients seen in hearing clinics. However, the audiometric configurations of pure-tone loss vary greatly among patients and

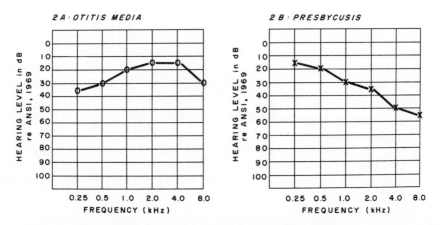

FIG. 2. Typical examples of clinical pure-tone audiograms.

in themselves contain only information concerning the magnitude of the sensitivity deficit.

Pure-tone audiometry has tended to dominate audiometric diagnosis for at least two major reasons. First, pure-tone signals can be closely controlled in calibration and appear to be relatively simple to administer. Second, pure-tone audiometric results provide a very useful description of the magnitude of the hearing loss throughout the major audible frequency range. With few exceptions, however, little differential diagnostic information can be obtained merely from air-conducted pure-tone audiometry, since hearing disorders at various anatomical sites of the ear may result in similar patterns of sensitivity loss. As a consequence, numerous more sophisticated hearing tests have been developed with the specific purpose of distinguishing among the types of auditory disorders.

III. DIFFERENTIAL DIAGNOSIS OF AUDITORY DISORDERS

A. Diagnostic Strategy

The results of auditory test procedures specifically designed for differential diagnosis most commonly permit classification of auditory impairments on the basis of the anatomical site of the lesion underlying the hearing disorder. The findings from these auditory tests can be of great assistance when establishing a medical diagnosis of the hearing problem. Differential diagnostic auditory measurements, however, are not used in and of themselves to determine the disease process. From the results of auditory tests together with information provided by the case history and other medical diagnostic procedures, the disease process must be inferred.

For many years, hearing losses were divided into two anatomical–physiologic classifications: middle-ear or *conductive loss* and inner-ear or *neural loss*. Conductive loss applied to any hearing loss resulting from disorders of the external and/or middle ear. The terms *nerve loss* and *perceptive loss* have often been applied to hearing disorders involving the cochlea and VIIIth nerve. This classification is clearly an oversimplification. Individuals with hearing impairment due to lesions in this part of the auditory system are somewhat more appropriately classified as sensorineural disorders. *Sensori* refers to lesions principally involving the receptors (hair cells) within the cochlea and *neural* to lesions of the VIIIth nerve. This division has become functionally useful since patients with cochlear disorders respond to some auditory tests in a markedly different manner from patients with known VIIIth nerve disorders.

The results of modern diagnostic test procedures are currently helpful in differentiating between disorders located in the peripheral and central auditory system. The three major locations of impairments in the peripheral system are (*1*) the external and/or middle ear, (*2*) the cochlea, and (*3*) the VIIIth nerve. The two principal sites of an auditory disorder in the central nervous system are (*1*) the brainstem, from the second-order neurons of the afferent auditory nerve in the cochlear nucleus up to the cortex, and (2) the primary auditory projection area located in the superior convolution of the temporal lobe. The rationale for this general method of classifying the results of the various differential diagnostic tests was discussed by Jerger (1973b). A distinction between peripheral and central loci becomes necessary because peripheral disorders appear to modify the systems response to auditory signals in a manner that is fundamentally different from central disorders. Accordingly, the specific diagnostic procedures used may differ, depending on the supposed anatomical site of the lesion. It should be understood that although the division of auditory impairments into specific anatomical sites has been found quite useful for diagnostic purposes, in practice, diseases and injuries may often cause more generalized damage than merely to one specific anatomical location. Thus, the auditory changes described in this chapter are those most commonly associated with a specific site of damage. For individual patients, however, the test results and the location of the lesion may not always be so definitive.

B. External- and Middle-Ear Disorders

External- and middle-ear disorders occur from a wide variety of causes (Goodhill *et al.*, 1971). The impairment may range in seriousness from a simple accumulation of cerumen (wax) to a potentially dangerous middle-ear otitis secondary to an infectious disease, such as scarlet fever. Regardless of the etiology, the conditions that lead to the impariment always produce changes in the mechanics of the external- or middle-ear system and usually result in a reduction of sound transmission or conduction to the cochlea.

Several major mechanical changes are most often associated with external- and middle-ear impairments:

(*1*) Blocking of external meatus by foreign bodies or accumulation of cerumen.

(*2*) Loading of the tympanic membrane from an accumulation of fluid in the middle ear, due commonly to respiratory infections and allergic reactions or failure of pressure equalization when the eustachian tube remains closed.

(*3*) Perforation of the tympanic membrane from penetrating objects or resulting from severe middle-ear infection.

(*4*) Myringo–malleal fixations, from immobilization by tympanosclerosis, or by bony or fibrous fixating lesions.

(*5*) Incudostapedial fixations, such as observed with otosclerosis a disease of the otic capsule, which causes stapes or ossicular fixations.

(6) Incudostapedial discontinuities from necrosis, atrophy, or trauma resulting in a gap or discontinuity at the incudo-stapedial joint.

The major dysfunction observed in conductive disorders is a loss in sensitivity. The magnitude of the loss varies greatly due to the severity and type of physical change imposed on the mechanical system of the middle ear. For example, small perforations of the tympanic membrane often result in only minor sensitivity losses. However, complete fixations of the ossicular chain due to far advanced otosclerosis result in conductive losses that may be as large as 60–70 dB, owing to the additional stiffness of the ossicular system from the disease.

For several decades, the classical diagnostic procedure used to ascertain the presence or absence of an external or middle-ear lesion and estimate the integrity of the sensorineural system has been the difference between thresholds for air-conducted and bone-conducted tones. Stimulation by bone conduction is accomplished by placing a vibrator in direct contact with the skull. The diagnostic utility of the difference between air- and bone-conduction thresholds (air–bone gap) is based primarily on two assumptions: first, that the air-conduction threshold reflects the function of the total hearing system, both conductive and sensorineural, and second, that the threshold for bone-conduction is a measure of the integrity of the sensorineural auditory system and thus essentially not influenced by the status of the external and middle ear. As a consequence, the discrepancy between the air- and bone-conduction thresholds should indicate the magnitude of the conductive component of the hearing loss. Theoretically, in a purely conductive loss the bone-conduction thresholds should be completely normal. However, it has been demonstrated conclusively (Békésy, 1932; Barany, 1938; Tonndorf, 1966) that both the external and middle ear contribute to the bone-conduction threshold. As a result, elevated bone-conduction thresholds may partially result from middle-ear abnormalities and not necessarily from sensorineural impairment. Despite this limitation, the difference between air- and bone-conduction thresholds has considerable clinical utility. Some restraint, however, must be exercised in the complete acceptance of a bone-conduction threshold as a pure measure of sensorineural integrity or so-called "cochlear reserve."

Clinical measurements of bone conduction are generally carried out with small hearing-aid type bone vibrators coupled to the mastoid process or the frontal bone via a headband. Carhart (1950) was among the first investigators to lay a solid foundation for the quantitative use of bone-conduction measurements clinically. But bone-conduction audiometry has been continually beset with several problems: *(1)* the lack of a reliable method of physically calibrating bone vibrators; *(2)* the necessity of masking the nontest ear because skull vibration cannot be isolated to the area under the stimulating vibrator; and *(3)* the influence of middle-ear pathology on the total bone-conduction response. The first of these problems is reaching solution with the development of reliable artificial mastoids (Weiss, 1960; Whittle & Robinson, 1967) that simulate the mechanical impedance characteristics of human heads (Dadson, Robinson, & Grieg, 1954; Corliss & Koidan, 1955). A standard for the physical specification of artificial mastoids (ANSI S3.13-1972) has been established and values for the normal threshold of hearing by bone conduction have been reported (Lybarger, 1966; Dirks & Kamm, 1975). The difficulties of clinical masking essentially involve the risk that masking delivered via a headphone may cross the head by bone conduction (Zwislocki, 1953) and influence the test ear. Some increase in transcranial attenuation may be achieved by insert receivers (Zwislocki, 1953; Studebaker, 1962) instead of the customary over-the-ear type earphones. Also, the use of narrow-band noise instead of wide-band noise reduces the effects of "crossover" since narrow bands are more efficient maskers (Hood, 1957; Studebaker, 1964, 1967). The influence of the external and middle ear on bone-conduction thresholds has already been mentioned. Perhaps the most well-known, but not exclusive, examples are patients with stapes fixations, who often show a loss in bone conduction in the frequency region around 2000 Hz. Figure 3 illustrates the air- and bone-conduction thresholds observed in such a patient with surgically confirmed stapes fixation due to otosclerosis. The hearing loss had progressed gradually over a period of 10 years starting at 30 years of age. Thus, the fixation process was far advanced at the time of testing and accounts for the moderate-to-severe

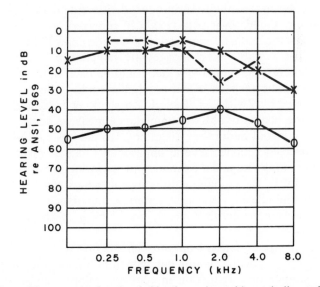

FIG. 3. Air- and bone-conduction thresholds of a patient with surgically confirmed stapes fixation due to otosclerosis. Pre-op AC: O—O; post-op AC: ×—×; pre-op BC: ⟨--⟨.

air-conduction loss. Notice, however, that the bone-conduction thresholds are essentially normal except for a notch-shaped reduction centered at 2000 Hz. This notch effect was originally described by Carhart (1950) and now bears his name. It is due to mechanical changes in the middle ear that reduce the middle-ear contribution to the bone-conduction threshold. The place of maximal loss along the frequency scale is determined by the resonance of the middle ear, which, in humans, is near 2000 Hz (Tonndorf, 1966). The additional audiometric curve ($\times$——$\times$) in the figure represents the postoperative air-conduction thresholds following stapes mobilization surgery, which successfully restored the hearing to near normal levels, including the frequency region of the notch.

Diagnostic evaluation of middle-ear disorders has been significantly expanded with the successful development of measurements of acoustic impedance at the tympanic membrane. Such measurements have been a serious subject of investigation for several decades. However, the vast clinical applications of impedance measurements have developed more recently and are rapidly becoming part of standard diagnostic procedures. The clinical value of impedance measurements evolves from the fact that various disease processes modify the transmission characteristics of the middle ear in markedly different and predictable ways; thus, differential diagnostic information concerning the status of the middle ear is possible from these measurements.

Schuster (1934) made an early systematic attempt to adapt the theory of acoustic impedance to a practical method of evaluating the function of the human ear. But it was Metz (1946) who initially demonstrated that various disease processes in the middle ear produced different changes in impedance at the eardrum. Later, Zwislocki (1957a,b) reported more comprehensive results on the static acoustic impedance of normal ears. These results led to development of a stable mechanoacoustic impedance bridge (Zwislocki, 1963; Zwislocki & Feldman, 1963) that could be used in the clinic.

Both the acoustic resistance and reactance could be measured with the bridge developed by Zwislocki. Table I (Zwislocki & Feldman, 1970, p. 36) summarizes the results of absolute impedance measurements that might be observed for selected middle-ear disorders. On the basis of absolute impedance measurements alone, several impairments can be distinguished: ossicular discontinuity, stapedial fixation, and sensorineural disorders (normal impedance results). Other malfunctions such as adhesions, retracted drums, and fluid in the middle ear also cause abnormal impedance results but are not distinguishable from each other merely on the basis of absolute impedance measurements.

Specifically, stapes fixation from otosclerosis produces an increase in the mechanical stiffness of the middle ear, which is reflected as an increase in acoustic reactance or a reduction in acoustic compliance as suggested in Table I. The fixation process may cause the normal mechanical impedance of the cochlea to increase. This characteristic is observed as a higher than

TABLE I

ACOUSTIC IMPEDANCE SYMPTOMATOLOGY ASSOCIATED WITH SELECTED MIDDLE-EAR PATHOLOGIES SHOWN BY X[a]

Pathology	Compliance				Resistance		
	Very low	Low	Normal	High	Low	Normal	High
Ossicular separation							
Distal to stapedius				X	X		
Proximal to stapedius				X	X		
Stapes ankylosis							
Complete		X				X	(X)
Partial		X				X	
Massive adhesions	X						X
Retracted adhesions	X						X
Middle-ear fluid	X	(X)				(X)	X
Sensorineural hearing loss			X			X	

[a] The (X) indicates symptoms that occasionally may be present. From Zwislocki and Feldman [1970, *Acoustic Impedance of Pathological Ears* (ASHA Monograph No. 15, Table 2, p. 36). Copyright 1970 by the American Speech and Hearing Association].

normal acoustic resistance, but depends on the probe frequency used (Feldman & Zwislocki, 1965). An ossicular discontinuity, on the other hand, reduces both the stiffness (increases the compliance) and the resistance components. The middle-ear system becomes very compliant and the resistance component, which has its origin in the cochlea, can be substantially reduced by the interruption. The presence of fluid in the ear reduces the compliance even more than in stapes fixation, whereas the resistance may be normal or slightly high.

Changes in acoustic impedance at the eardrum can be measured by increasing or decreasing air pressure in the external auditory meatus (Terkildsen & Thomsen, 1959) and during contraction of the tympanic muscles (Metz, 1946; Klockhoff, 1961). Two widely used clinical measurements have evolved from these observations: (1) tympanometry, or the measurement of certain acoustic properties of the middle ear as a function of variations in external canal air pressure, and (2) measurements of the middle-ear muscle reflex, most often from stapedius muscle contraction induced by acoustic stimulation.

Tympanometry and middle-ear reflex measurements have become important diagnostic procedures for identifying the presence of a middle-ear disorder, and, as will be developed later, for differentiating between cochlear and retrocochlear impairments. Most clinical impedance measurements are car-

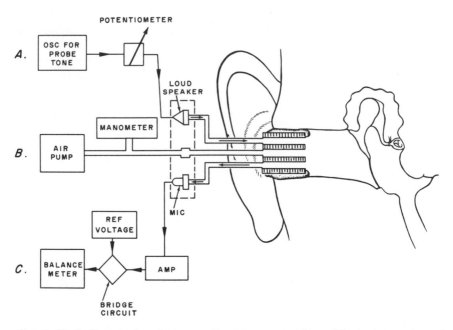

Fig. 4. Block diagram of an electroacoustic system commonly used for tympanometry and middle-ear reflex measurements.

ried out with one of several types of electroacoustic instruments. These devices are balanced electrically and measure either the impedance or admittance* at the eardrum.

Figure 4 is an example of one electroacoustic system used to perform tympanometry and the measurement of middle-ear muscle contraction. Other impedance and admittance measuring systems are available for clinical use, but most have certain features in common with the example illustrated in Fig. 4. A probe tone is fed to a loudspeaker or receiver (A in Fig. 4) via an attenuator that allows adjustment of the output level. In some instruments, the output may be fixed at a predetermined level. The probe tone output of the receiver is introduced into the external canal through a flexible tube in the probe unit which is placed firmly in the ear canal with an airtight seal. Through a second tube (C in Fig. 4), the SPL of the signal developed in the ear canal can be monitored by a microphone. The microphone output is usually amplified, filtered, rectified, and led to one side of a zero-indicating device whereas the other side of the instrument is balanced with a constant voltage. If the probe-tone level is kept constant, the SPL in the ear canal will be a function of the impedance of the ear canal,

*Admittance is the reciprocal of a complex impedance. The complex admittance $Y = G + jB$ has a real part G, called *conductance*, and an imaginary part B, called *susceptance*.

eardrum, and middle ear. The probe tone can be adjusted until the instrument is "in balance" for a specific ear. Changes in impedance are measured from a variation in this balance point which corresponds in time to middle-ear muscle contraction or induced external-ear canal pressure changes.

The impedance-measuring instrument also includes an air pump (B in Fig. 4) connected to the third tube in the ear canal. This system is used to vary the air pressure within the external ear canal. The pressure is determined from readings on a manometer. In practice, tympanometry is usually performed by initially inducing a positive air pressure equivalent to 200 mm H_2O (98.1 N m^{-2}) in the external canal. It is assumed that with a pressure equivalent to 200 mm H_2O or greater, the tympanic membrane and middle ear become effectively rigid. Thus the impedance measured should essentially represent the volume enclosed in the canal itself. As the air pressure in a normal ear is reduced, a point is reached where the middle-ear pressure and the pressure in the external canal are equal. At this point, maximum transmission of sound to the middle ear has been reached and the air pressure of the middle ear can be inferred. As the external canal pressure is reduced further with negative pressures, the SPL developed in the canal is again reduced.

Figure 5 shows a representative tympanogram (Lilly, 1970) from a normal ear obtained with an instrument as described in Fig. 4. Notice the point of maximum transmission was reached at an air pressure value of 0 mm H_2O. The static impedance can be calculated by subtracting the volume of the external canal (result at +200 mm H_2O) from the equivalent volume of the external canal and middle-ear system combined (the latter corresponding to the point where maximum sound transmission is found). In the example, the impedance was calculated at 1062 ohms on the first test and 1082 ohms on a retest. Tympanometry thus provides quantitative information concerning middle-ear air pressure, changes in impedance at the tympanic membrane as a function of air pressure, and, through calculation (from results obtained at maximum compliance and ±200 mm pressure), an estimate of static impedance.

Figure 6 shows an example of an abnormal tympanogram observed on an impedance system identical to that described in Fig. 4. The results are from the left and right ears of a 6-year-old male with bilateral serous otitis media, more severe in the right ear. Note that in the left ear, the middle-ear air pressure (estimated from the maximum transmission point) is −300 mm H_2O and the impedance is high (4889 ohms). The right ear has a much higher impedance than the left and the impedance remains essentially constant as the external air pressure changes.

As mentioned previously, the admittance of the tympanic membrane can be measured clinically with at least one commercially available instrument (Grason-Stadler Otoadmittance Meter 1720). This unit is an electroacoustic

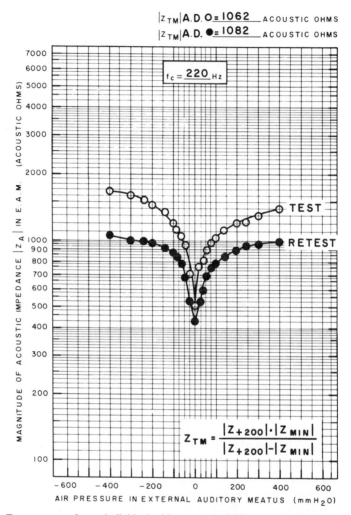

FIG. 5. Tympanogram for an individual with a normal middle-ear system. Results are shown for an initial test and a retest. [From Lilly (1970), *A Comparison of Acoustic Impedance Data Obtained with Madsen and Zwislocki Instruments.* Paper presented to the American Speech and Hearing Association, New York, 1970.]

device, but unlike the instrument in Fig. 4, the phase angle of the impedance can be measured. Tympanograms can also be obtained at two probe frequencies (220 and 660 Hz) and separately for acoustic susceptance (B_A) and for acoustic conductance (G_A). Static values for B_A and G_A can then be converted to both complex acoustic admittance (Y_A) and its reciprocal acoustic impedance (Z_A). Thus the effects of middle-ear disorders on each component of the admittance can be distinguished.

Figures 7 and 8 show susceptance and conductance results at the two probe frequencies for two patients, one with a normal ear (Fig. 7) and the other with an ossicular discontinuity (Fig. 8). Even from these few examples, it is obvious that considerable detailed information concerning the status of the middle ear can be gained with multiple probe tones and analysis of susceptance and conductance components. The effect of ossicular interruption is more evident in the tympanograms at 660 Hz than at 220 Hz. Notice the double peaks in both the B_A and G_A tympanograms with the 660-Hz probe tone. Because of the discontinuity the system is mass-controlled and the effect is more dramatic at the higher probe frequency, nearer the resonance point of the middle ear. There is some controversy among inves-

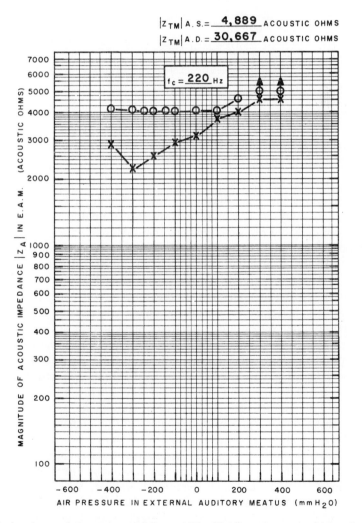

FIG. 6. An abnormal tympanogram from a child with bilateral serous otitis media. [From Lilly (1970), *A Comparison of Acoustic Impedance Data Obtained with Madsen and Zwislocki Instruments*. Paper presented to the American Speech and Hearing Association, New York, 1970.]

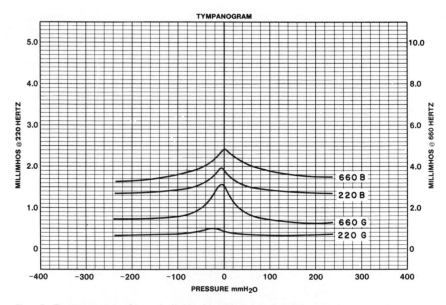

FIG. 7. Tympanograms for an individual with a normal middle ear, for the probe-tone frequencies 220 and 660 Hz and for conductance G, and susceptance B.

tigators concerning the exact diagnostic value of multiple probe frequencies and component analysis. The final decision awaits a better understanding of the rather complicated physical changes that occur in various pathologies.

The middle-ear reflex is most often elicited by a loud sound (approximately 80 dB above behavioral threshold for tones) delivered to the ear contralateral to the one containing the probe tone. Since the reflex is activated bilaterally, this arrangement (probe tone in one ear and stimulating tone in the other) is practically useful and effectively isolates the probe from the stimulating tone. When both stimuli are presented in the same ear, considerable care must be exercised to eliminate or reduce acoustic interaction in the external-ear canal. In patients with middle-ear disorders, changes in impedance from stapedial contraction to loud sounds will generally not be observed because of the malfunction that impairs the ossicular chain or results in very high impedance (Jepsen, 1963; Klockhoff, 1961). The absence of a reflex in such cases provides another useful diagnostic tool for distinguishing between middle-ear and cochlear disorders.

The information gained from the impedance measurements establishes whether or not the middle ear is functioning normally. These measurements have the important advantage of objectivity, because they require no subjective response on the part of the patient. Their use in testing of infants, children, and uncooperative adults is of great importance. The interested reader will find that Lilly (1973) has provided a comprehensive review of basic concepts of impedance along with a significant reference list of investigations on the clinical use of impedance measurements.

Fortunately, a majority of auditory disorders due to external- and middle-ear impairment can be completely or partially improved by surgical or medical treatment. Among those individuals in whom hearing cannot be satisfactorily restored, hearing-aid amplification can be used to eliminate or reduce the effects of the sensitivity loss. Once the sensitivity loss is overcome, either by surgery or amplification, speech and other auditory signals are usually transmitted effectively to the cochlea. Thus, relatively good success

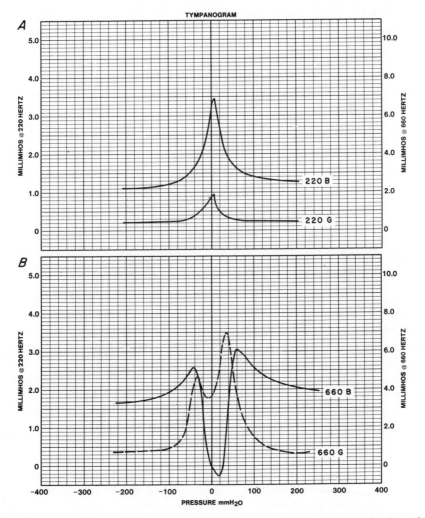

FIG. 8. Abnormal tympanograms for a patient with an ossicular discontinuity, for the probe-tone frequencies 220 (A) and 660 (B) Hz and for conductance G, and susceptance B.

in understanding amplified speech is achieved by patients with conductive loss so long as the disorder is isolated to impairment of the middle-ear system and is not compounded by a concomitant sensorineural hearing loss.

C. Cochlear Disorders

In clinical practice, a significant number of sensorineural lesions involve degeneration or atrophy of the sensory cells (hair cells) along the basilar membrane, although conductive impairments within the cochlea itself have also been reported (Schuknecht, 1975). Hearing losses due to cochlear dysfunction may be hereditary (Goodhill *et al.*, 1971) or acquired. Among the major causes of acquired cochlear hearing loss are presbycusis, noise exposure, ototoxic drugs, various infections (Rubella, mumps), and disease processes (Ménière's disease).

Sensitivity loss is almost always observed in cochlear disorders and the magnitude of the loss ranges from mild to profound. Although the magnitude of the hearing loss is often greatest at frequencies above 2000 Hz, exceptions to this rule are frequent. For example, one notable exception is the greater low-tone-frequency loss often observed in the early stages of Ménière's disease (Williams, 1952).

During the past 30 years, several symptoms typically associated with cochlear hearing loss have been described. The development of differential diagnosis in this area was originally enhanced by the observations of E. P. Fowler, Sr. (1928, 1936). He was able to differentiate between two types of lesions on the basis of the perception of the growth of loudness above threshold. In one type of patient with unilateral hearing loss (conductive loss), given changes in intensity were observed to elicit identical increments in loudness growth in both the normal and pathological ear. In another set of patients (sensorineural loss), loudness growth above threshold was found to be greater in the pathological than in the comparison normal ear. This phenomenon, called *recruitment*, was further localized by Dix, Hallpike, and Hood (1948) to disorders of the cochlea. These investigators demonstrated that, regardless of the severity of the hearing loss, a judgment of equality in loudness between a normal ear and one with cochlear loss may be produced at equal SPLs slightly above the threshold in the impaired ear. Thus, at suprathreshold intensity levels, the judgment of loudness for an auditory signal in the ear with a cochlear disorder becomes equivalent to the perceived loudness of the same signal in the comparative normal ear.

Figure 9 describes the results of the alternate binaural loudness balance test for recruitment in an individual with a unilateral loss due to Ménière's disease. Loudness balancing was accomplished at the two pure-tone frequencies of 1000 and 4000 Hz where the hearing loss was 40 and 60 dB, respectively. At both frequencies, the loudness in the pathological ear became equivalent to that of the normal ear at levels approximately 20 dB

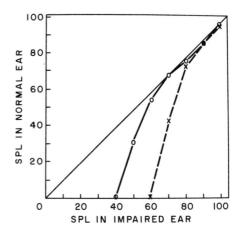

FIG. 9. Results from the alternate binaural loudness balance test demonstrating the presence of loudness recruitment in a patient with unilateral Ménière's disease. 1000 Hz: O—O; 4000 Hz: ×--×.

above the impaired thresholds. Thereafter, the loudness growth remained essentially the same for both ears.

Another characteristic often observed in cochlear-impaired ears is *hypersensitivity* to intensity change. Numerous attempts at the clinical measurement of the difference limen (DL) for intensity (Hirsh, Palva, & Goodman, 1954; Jerger, 1952, 1953; Lüscher & Zwislocki, 1951) have been reported. The effectiveness and reliability of these results, however, were often influenced by procedural variables. Such considerations led to the development of the Short Increment Sensitivity Index (SISI Test; Jerger, Shedd, & Harford, 1959). This procedure was based on the quantal psychophysical method and, because of the ease of administration and repeatability, has often been used as a clinical measure of intensity discrimination during the past two decades. Generally, the patient is asked to identify the presence of 1-dB intensity increments superimposed on a steady state tonal stimulus. The stimulus is conventionally presented at a SPL of 20 dB above the threshold of the impaired ear. Detection of 1 dB changes in sound intensity usually cannot be recognized at sensation levels (SL) of 20 dB among persons with normal hearing, or for patients with hearing loss due to middle-ear or auditory-nerve pathology. However, increments of 1 dB are routinely heard by patients with cochlear impairments.

Several investigators (Martin, 1970; Swisher, 1966; Thompson, 1963; Young & Harbert, 1967) have explored the response of normal ears to the SISI stimulus at high intensity levels. As with the DL for intensity, the ability to detect small changes increases as a function of intensity. Such results suggest that the hypersensitivity for intensity change attributed to the cochlear-impaired ear may only be observed when the test is conducted at equal SLs above the normal and impaired ear thresholds but not at equivalent SPLs.

Adaptation to continuous tonal stimulation at or near threshold has also been studied extensively among individuals with cochlear and other auditory impairments. Excessive threshold adaptation (which will be described later) is associated with retrocochlear rather than cochlear disorders. Clinical investigators have measured threshold "adaptation" principally with so-called "threshold tone-decay procedures" (Carhart, 1957; Hood, 1955) or Békésy audiometry (Békésy, 1947; Jerger, 1960a; Lierle & Reger, 1955). Basically, either procedure is carried out by determining the threshold level or the minimum suprathreshold level necessary for a patient to hear a continuous tone over a period of 60 sec. With conventional tone-decay procedures, the patient is asked to respond as long as he hears the stimuli. When he fails to respond, the intensity of the signal is increased manually in predetermined steps. The duration of the response and the intensity increments needed to maintain the stimulus for 60 sec are recorded.

When the automatic audiometer of Békésy (1947) is used to measure adaptation, comparative changes in auditory threshold for interrupted and continuous stimulation are automatically recorded depending on the patients reception of each stimulus over several minutes. For a patient with normal hearing or a middle-ear disorder, sustained tones are traced at SPLs identical to tones that are interrupted (200 msec on/200 msec off). Similar results are sometimes observed for patients with cochlear disorders; however, in many instances, the threshold for a sustained tone at higher frequencies is traced at levels 10–15 dB below the threshold for the interrupted tones. Figure 10 shows a Békésy audiogram from a patient with Ménière's disease (Hughes, 1972). The top portion of Fig. 10 contains results for sweep-frequency Békésy audiometry whereas the bottom part of the figure illustrates selected fixed-frequency data for the same patient. Note that the thresholds for continuous tones are traced at SPLs 10 to 20 dB greater than for the interrupted tones. This characteristic is typical of hearing loss of cochlear origin and indicates the presence of mild threshold adaptation, usually in the high frequencies.

Small threshold changes to continuous pure-tone stimulation are often observed on conventional manually controlled tone-decay tests for individuals with cochlear hearing loss. In order to reduce certain experimental artifacts associated with threshold tone-decay procedures, Olsen and Noffsinger (1973) recently suggested performing the tone decay tests at a SPL 20 dB above the impaired threshold. They observed that persons with cochlear loss were able to hear a continuous tone stimulus for at least one minute at this SL. Laboratory evidence (Dirks, Morgan, & Bray, 1974; Margolis & Wiley, 1976; Wiley, Lilly, & Small, 1976) has also indicated that young adults with cochlear loss due to noise exposure show no appreciable suprathreshold loudness adaptation. The general picture of cochlear impairment that emerges from results obtained by the threshold decay, Békésy audiometry, and suprathreshold loudness adaptation procedures is one of minimal threshold decay and little or no suprathreshold loudness adaptation.

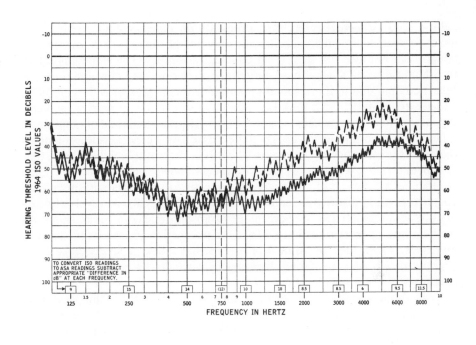

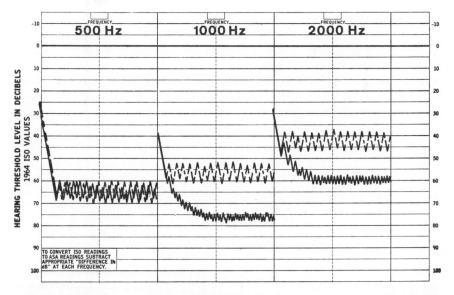

FIG. 10. Sweep-frequency Békésy audiogram (upper) for a patient with cochlear disorder displaying thresholds for interrupted (broken line) and continuous tones (unbroken line), and fixed-frequency Békésy tracings (lower) at three test frequencies. [From Hughes (1972), Békésy audiometry. In J. Katz (Ed.), *Handbook of Clinical Audiology,* Chapter 12. Copyright 1972 by Williams & Wilkins.]

Intra-aural stapedial reflex measurements on patients with hearing loss have become increasingly useful not only in the diagnosis of middle-ear impairment but also for identifying cochlear disorders. The stapedius reflex threshold for tones among these patients is often observed at sound pressure levels comparable to those found in normal listeners (Jerger & Jerger, 1972; Liden, 1970; Metz, 1952; Terkildsen & Thomsen, 1959). However, as hearing loss increases, especially above ~60 dB HL, the likelihood of obtaining a reflex at near normal levels begins to decrease. As a general rule, so long as the cochlear loss does not exceed ~60 dB HL, there is a high likelihood that a stapedial reflex will be observed. Figure 11 shows the incidence of reflex absence as a function of the degree of loss for 515 patients with presumed cochlear hearing disorders (Jerger & Jerger, 1972, p. 520). At levels of hearing loss less than 60 dB, the percentage of absent reflexes is quite small. As the hearing loss increases above 60 dB, the proportion of absent reflexes also increases. Thus, the appearance of a stapedial reflex at levels close to or slightly higher than for normal listeners can usually be considered another manifestation of a cochlear lesion.

Even though the measurement of speech discrimination among clinical patients has become a standard audiometric procedure, the diagnostic significance of the performance score has not been highly efficient in distinguishing disorders at the various locations in the sensorineural auditory system. One limitation has been that speech discrimination tests are often administered at only one SL. Generally, the SL chosen is well above threshold, at a level where maximal discrimination performance is usually observed. The maximum speech discrimination score for cochlear hearing loss patients is often found to be reduced from those observed in normal listeners, although it is generally not as poor as those reported for VIIIth nerve problems (Schuknecht & Woellner, 1955). Unfortunately, there are also patients with a medical diagnosis of cochlear hearing loss for whom the speech discrimina-

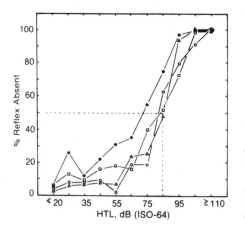

FIG. 11. Incidence of reflex absence and degree of hearing loss in 515 patients with sensorineural loss. △ 500 Hz; ○ 1000 Hz; □ 2000 Hz; ● 4000 Hz. [From Jerger and Jerger (1972), Studies in impedance audiometry. I. Normal and sensorineural ears. *Archives of Otolaryngology*, **96**, 513–523.]

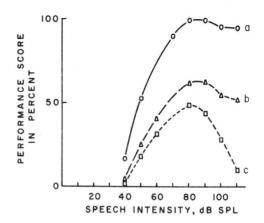

FIG. 12. Comparative performance-intensity functions for phonetically balanced word lists for patients with (a) a middle-ear disorder, O—O, (b) a cochlear lesion, Δ--Δ, and (c) an VIIIth nerve lesion, □---□.

tion scores may be quite low. Thus, a typical performance range of difficulty on a speech discrimination test cannot be identified for persons with cochlear disorders. Observations by Jerger and Jerger (1971) suggest, however, that cochlear losses can be differentiated from retrocochlear disorders on the basis of a change in speech discrimination performance as the intensity of the speech signal is raised to quite high intensity levels (100 dB HL or more). Their results indicate that once a maximum discrimination score is reached for a cochlear hearing loss, further increases in speech stimulus levels do not result in significant reductions in speech discrimination. In contrast, patients with retrocochlear disorders exhibit a so-called "rollover" function; that is, as speech level is increased to very high intensities, speech discrimination tends to decrease significantly.

Comparative examples of speech discrimination functions for three individuals with 40 dB hearing losses are shown in Fig. 12. Once the sensitivity loss is exceeded, the intelligibility function for the patient with conductive loss is similar to that observed in normal listeners (Fig. 12a). The maximum score remains high as the intensity of the speech is progressively raised. For the patient with cochlear loss, the maximum discrimination score (70%) never reaches normal as the intensity of the speech stimulus is increased to high SPLs, however, the intelligibility score remains constant and then decreases slightly (Fig. 12b). For the patient with an VIIIth nerve disorder, increases in speech level result in significant decreases in intelligibility after maximum performance is reached (Fig. 12c). Palva (1952) and Liden (1954) have also reported little or no rollover among individuals with cochlear loss. Further confirmation of these results is necessary, however, since Huizing and Reyntjes (1952) and Schultz and Streepy (1967) observed rollover effects in some individuals with presumed cochlear hearing loss, although the degree of rollover generally was not as severe as that reported by Jerger and Jerger (1971) for VIIIth nerve impairments.

Numerous other test procedures have also been developed to diagnose and describe cochlear disorders. In general, procedures other than those described have not been as thoroughly studied, or extensively used. However, several procedures deserve mention. Early reports by Miskolczy-Fodor (1953, 1956) suggested that it may be possible to differentiate cochlear loss from other sites of hearing impairment on the basis of response to pure tones of brief duration (e.g., 10–500 msec). Evidence has been presented (Wright, 1968) indicating that individuals with cochlear involvement require less change in intensity than normal listeners to maintain threshold response to short duration stimuli. Apparently there are still questions, however, concerning the application of this result to all types of cochlear lesions (Martin & Wofford, 1970; Sanders & Honig, 1967). The most recent comparative brief-tone audiometry results among normal listeners, cochlear impaired, and VIIIth nerve disorder patients (Olsen, Rose, & Noffsinger, 1974) suggested different integration slopes across these groups. But the overlap between the various groups was large and the cochlear loss patients did not form a distinctive diagnostic group. These investigators pointed out the need for greater precision in defining the site and function of the lesion with the brief-tone test procedure.

Several experiments concerned with masking and distortion effects have led to the conclusion that listeners with sensorineural loss show greater aural distortion than normal listeners. For example, results from masking experiments have suggested that greater upward spread of masking is found in patients with sensorineural loss than in normals (Jerger, Tillman, & Peterson, 1959). Lower thresholds of aural overload have been reported for sensorineural-loss ears than normal ears (Lawrence & Yantis, 1956; Opheim & Flottorp, 1955), and results of mistuned-octave masking experiments have indicated lower thresholds of octave masking (Clack & Bess, 1969) for sensorineural-loss patients than for normal listeners. In contrast, results from other masking experiments (Rittmanic, 1962) have not demonstrated significant upward spread of masking among sensorineural-loss ears, and de Boer and Bouwmeester (1975) report that masking extends over an abnormally wide range of frequencies for some but not all patients with sensorineural loss. Nelson and Bilger (1974a,b) reported pure-tone octave masking evidence, which suggested that the sensorineural-loss group studied did not perform differently from normal ears. The conclusion that cochlear impaired ears produce greater aural distortion than normal ears at equivalent SPLs is not clearly established. The Nelson and Bilger results would suggest the opposite, that ears with cochlear loss do not exhibit abnormal distortion.

In summary, cochlear impairment commonly results in (*1*) a sensitivity loss that may range from mild to severe, (*2*) the presence of loudness recruitment, (*3*) minimal or no loudness adaptation at threshold or suprathreshold levels, (*4*) "hypersensitivity" to suprathreshold intensity change, and (*5*) moderate-to-severe reductions in speech discrimination ability.

D. VIIIth Nerve Disorders

The investigation of the effects of peripheral VIIIth nerve disorders on the auditory system has been primarily carried out on surgically confirmed cases of VIIIth nerve tumors. These patients are of great research and clinical interest. Acoustic tumors constitute one of the few auditory neural disorders in which the presence and specific location of the lesion can be confirmed from surgery. Diagnostically, the early detection of an acoustic tumor is of great importance, since these intracranial tumors are capable of producing a variety of undesirable symptoms besides hearing loss.

Although auditory investigation of patients with confirmed acoustic tumors form a major source of subjects with VIIIth nerve disorders, secondary nerve degeneration is also associated with hearing loss due to presbycusis (Schuknecht, 1975). Further reports indicate that vascular problems and viral infections can attack the VIIIth nerve, although the clinical diagnosis in these instances is usually on more tenuous grounds and not verified surgically.

Most of the test procedures that have been previously described for use in diagnosing cochlear disorders are also employed when there is a suspicion of VIIIth nerve impairment. In many instances, response to these tests is markedly different for individuals with VIIIth nerve involvement than for those with cochlear disorders. For example, loudness recruitment tends to be present in cochlear disorders but absent in VIIIth nerve loss. Abnormal and rapid loudness adaptation is one of the more dramatic features often associated with VIIIth nerve impairment (Reger & Kos, 1952; Jerger, 1960). The adaptation can be measured with threshold tone decay procedures or by Békésy audiometry. Figure 13 illustrates preoperative sweep-frequency (upper part) and fixed-frequency (lower part) Békésy tracings for an individual with an acoustic neurinoma. Notice that the sensitivity loss for interrupted tones is relatively mild, but the adaptation to continuous tonal stimulation is extremely rapid and appears even at the lowest test frequencies. The magnitude and time course of the rapid adaptation are found to differ greatly among patients with VIIIth nerve disorders and in some instances, especially where small tumors are present, abnormal adaptation may not be observed.

Results of intensity discrimination tasks, such as the SISI test (Jerger, Shedd, & Harford, 1959), have also been reported for patients with VIIIth nerve impairment. Whereas, in the cochlear hearing loss, an apparent hypersensitivity to intensity change is observed at levels slightly above the impaired threshold, the opposite is found among VIIIth nerve disorders. Even at extremely high SPLs, the patient is often unable to identify even large changes (5 dB) in the intensity of a continuous tone. As with the results of adaptation tests, patients with VIIIth nerve disorders who have acoustic tumors vary widely in their ability to detect changes in intensity. Note,

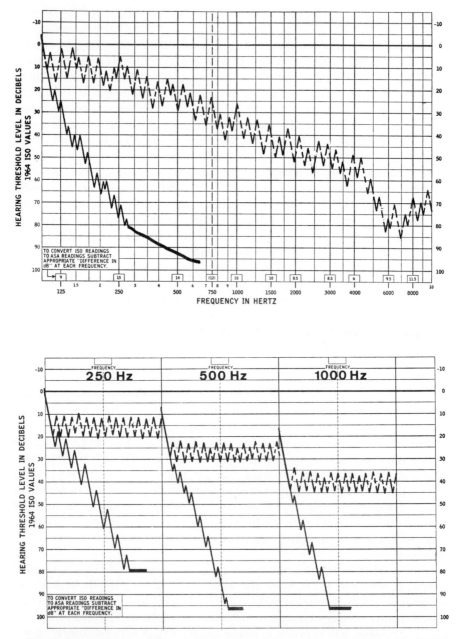

FIG. 13. Sweep-frequency Békésy audiogram (upper) for a patient with VIIIth nerve disorder displaying thresholds for interrupted (broken line) and continuous tones (unbroken line), and fixed-frequency Békésy tracings (lower) at three test frequencies. [From Hughes (1972), Békésy audiometry. In J. Katz (Ed.), *Handbook of Clinical Audiology*, Chapter 12. Copyright 1972 by Williams & Wilkins.]

however, that these patients are studied at different stages of VIIIth nerve impairment and there is often a progression of auditory symptoms as the acoustic tumor develops (Jerger & Jerger, 1968).

As reviewed previously, a reduction in speech discrimination among VIIIth nerve losses in and of itself cannot necessarily be considered pathognomonic. However, the presence of a substantial rollover effect (see Fig. 12c), observed in cases with VIIIth nerve disorder indicates that speech discrimination ability may be severely impaired and often decreases as the speech intensity level increases.

In summary, peripheral VIIIth nerve problems are often readily distinguishable from other types of auditory disorders. They characteristically show the following symptoms: (1) a mild sensitivity loss, although again the range of hearing loss is large; (2) the absence of loudness recruitment; (3) the presence of abnormal adaptation to continuous stimulation; (4) poor intensity discrimination, even at high intensity levels; and (5) poor speech discrimination, sometimes decreasing from a maximum as the sound intensity of the speech signal is raised.

E. Central Auditory Nervous System Disorders

Until the early 1950s, attempts to determine the effect of central nervous system disorders on the auditory system met with little success. In contrast to the peripheral auditory system, where injuries are easily revealed, the central auditory nervous system appeared highly immune to sensitivity loss even when the damage was massive. Some investigators and clinicians did refer to "central deafness" (inferring a threshold acuity deficit due to a central nervous system disorder), but there was general recognition that unilateral lesions did not produce a loss in sensitivity at either ear. However, some diagnosticians felt that rare bilateral lesions might cause a sensitivity loss or even total deafness. Subsequently, it has been demonstrated (Bocca, 1955; Bocca & Calearo, 1963; Goldstein, Goodman, & King, 1956; Jerger, 1960b, 1964; Korsan-Bengtsen, 1973) that hearing loss for pure tones and highly redundant speech is conspicuously absent in patients with unilateral temporal lobe disorders involving the primary auditory areas. Jerger, Weikers, Sharbrough, and Jerger (1969) did describe one patient who sustained two separate cerebral infractions with considerable damage to both temporal lobes. A pronounced hearing loss was initially observed but recovered quickly to near-normal hearing. Except perhaps for several reports of lesions involving the pathways in the lower brainstem, the central auditory nervous system is highly resistive to hearing loss for pure tones and ordinary speech messages.

Undistorted speech, with its high redundancy, presents more information to the listener than is required for normal reception. The complicated anatomy of the central auditory nervous system with both cochleas represented bilaterally in each auditory cortex and numerous junctions at different levels in the pathways appears to guarantee efficient speech reception. Because of this extrinsic (highly redundant speech) and intrinsic (complex anatomy of the system) redundancy, routine undistorted speech discrimination tests have generally failed to reveal lesions of the auditory cortex and the central auditory pathways in the brainstem.

The first significant breakthrough in devising tests that demonstrated deficits due to central auditory system damage was achieved by Bocca and his colleagues in 1955. Following the lead of Bocca, the diagnosis of central auditory impairment has been enhanced by the use of speech materials that have been physically modified or distorted to reduce the redundancy of the message. The early investigation by Bocca showed that patients with unilateral temporal lobe tumors had considerable difficulty in understanding frequency-distorted speech presented to the ear contralateral to the side of lesion. Since that time, various methods of modifying speech for diagnosis of central auditory disorders have been devised. These include time compression, frequency distortion, interruptions, acceleration, and masking with a competing message. Much of the pertinent literature on this topic has been reviewed by Bocca and Calearo (1963) and by Korsan-Bengtsen (1973). There is a growing body of literature indicating that the clinical response to certain auditory tests differs for patients with lesions in the central pathways of the brainstem as opposed to lesions of the auditory cortex. Accordingly, this review will describe results from patients with brainstem and cortical lesions separately.

Anywhere along their course through the brainstem and up to the outer layers of the temporal lobe, the central auditory pathways can be affected by brain tumors, cerebral hemorrhage, cerebral emoblisms or thrombosis, multiple sclerosis, arteriosclerosis, syphilis, or brain abscesses. In addition, birth injuries, gunshot wounds, and skull fractures are not uncommon problems causing damage or scarring to the auditory cortex.

Figures 14 and 15 (from Jerger & Jerger, 1974) present representative auditory results on two patients with intra-axial brainstem lesions due to pontine gliomas. They were selected to illustrate two patterns of results that characterize lesions in the auditory pathways of the lower brainstem. In Fig. 14 the glioma is primarily located on the left side of the brainstem. There is no hearing loss and the Békésy audiograms are Type I (Jerger, 1960b), indicating no abnormal adaptation to sustained pure-tone stimulation. The rollover effect (decreased performance as speech intensity level is raised), described in Section III,C, is observed when the right ear (contralateral to side of lesion) is stimulated. Likewise, a deficit in identification of sentence materials (SSI; Speaks & Jerger, 1965) is found when the sentences are presented to the right ear with background competition (ICM, ipsilateral competing message). The main results are a reduction in speech discrimination either for very intense speech or speech degraded by background competition. However, with

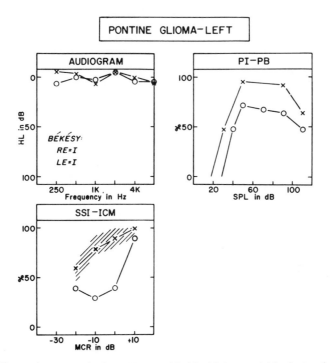

FIG. 14. Diagnostic test results for a 17-year-old girl with intra-axial brainstem lesion on the left side. Hatched area represents normal range for SSI-ICM. [From Jerger and Jerger (1974), *Archives of Otolaryngology*, **99**, 342–350. Copyright 1974, American Medical Association.]

either speech test, the reduction in performance is observed in the ear contralateral to the affected side of the brainstem.

Figure 15 shows results of another patient with a pontine glioma eccentric to the right side. There is a mild bilateral loss with abnormal adaptation (Békésy IV) in the right ear. The performance-intensity function for phonetically balanced word lists (PI–PB function) shows severely reduced performance on both ears but slightly greater on the left. The sentence identification in competition test (SSI–ICM) shows a deficit in both ears, but somewhat larger in the left. In this case, the distinction between a brainstem disorder is complicated by the Type IV Békésy audiogram on the right side. The glioma has produced bilateral effects, although the speech test results are poorer on the left ear (contralateral to the location of a major portion of the glioma). Similar bilateral effects, even occasionally with mild bilateral hearing loss, have also been reported by Calearo and Antonelli (1968), Dix and Hood (1973), and Korsan-Bengtsen (1973) for patients with intra-axial brainstem lesions. These reports demonstrate that brainstem lesions may result in either bilateral or monolateral (in ear contralateral to side of lesion) problems. As will be described, documented lesions in the temporal lobe almost always have resulted in monolateral deficits. Calearo and Antonelli

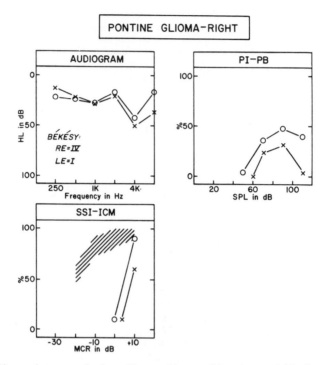

FIG. 15. Diagnostic test results for a 35-year-old man with an intra-axial brainstem lesion on the right side. Hatched area represents normal range for SSI-ICM. [From Jerger and Jerger (1974), *Archives of Otolaryngology,* **99,** 342–350. Copyright 1974, American Medical Association.]

(1968) have remarked on this division of results between brainstem and cortical problems. In explanation, they suggest the following considerations. In the brainstem, the auditory pathways from both sides are concentrated in an extremely limited space, in contrast to the cortex, where the primary auditory areas are separated in two hemispheres. Thus, equally extended lesions would yield a higher incidence of severe and bilateral problems when located in the brainstem than in the cortex. These investigators observed, as did Jerger and Jerger (1974), that when speech discrimination deficits occur, it is often in the ear contralateral to the side of the lesion, whereas, when pure-tone threshold loss is found, the ear affected is always homolateral. These results probably depend upon the level of the lesion, so that the condition (i.e., affected ear) changes whether the involved auditory pathways are before (at the cochlear nuclei) or after crossing in the lower brainstem.

Lesions in the auditory cortex ordinarily present symptoms found in the ear opposite the affected hemisphere. Figure 16 shows the results of a patient following right temporal lobectomy due to the presence of a tumor. No hearing loss is observed, and speech discrimination is normal for undistorted speech materials. The only deficit is for distorted speech words presented to the left ear, that is, the side contralateral to the lesion. In the example, words for the sensitized speech tests have undergone frequency distortion.

It is important to consider several limitations of the distorted-speech-test procedures. First, patients with cochlear hearing loss show impairment in discrimination when sensitized speech (Korsan-Bengtsen, 1973) is used. This means that the results of sensitized-speech tests are difficult to evaluate in patients who have concomitant sensitivity losses due to lesions in other parts of the auditory system. Second, because of large individual variations in response to sensitized-speech tests, many researchers have restricted investigations to patients with unilateral central nervous system lesions. The response due to stimulation of the auditory system on the normal side can then be used as an internal control or reference. A weakness in this approach is that the task must be adjusted in difficulty to meet the needs of the individual patients and has not as yet lent itself to standardization.

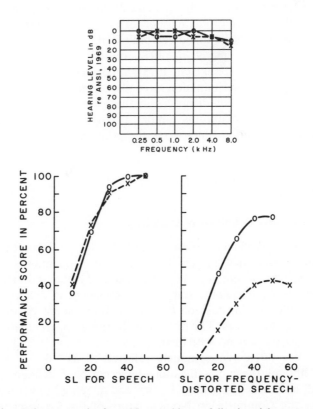

FIG. 16. Diagnostic test results for a 35-year-old man following right temporal lobectomy. Right ear: ○; left ear: ×.

In summary, the results of lesions of the central auditory nervous system suggest the following observations:

1. Patients with lesions involving the auditory cortex characteristically exhibit no sensitivity loss but rather, a significant difference in discrimination is found when distorted speech stimuli are presented contralateral to the affected side. The greater functional significance of the auditory-nerve fibers that cross in the brainstem to the side opposite the stimulated ear may be inferred from such speech-intelligibility performance.
2. Patients with temporal lobe lesions not involving primary or secondary auditory cortex show no difference in interaural discrimination. Thus, for cortical lesions, the reduction in discrimination is related directly to lesions that affect the auditory cortex itself.
3. Interaural differences in response to speech tests are also observed in patients with brainstem lesions. In contrast to those with temporal lobe lesions, these patients may show a greater deficit on the ipsilateral side. Depending on the site and size of the brainstem impairment, however, bilateral symptoms may occur (Jerger & Jerger, 1974).
4. For some patients with lower brainstem disorders, such as multiple sclerosis (Noffsinger et al., 1972) or infiltrating tumors in the pons (Liden & Korsan-Bengtsen, 1973), abnormal loudness adaptation, and poor intensity discrimination have also been reported. This last observation suggests that disorders in the lower brainstem may manifest some auditory symptoms similar to those found in the peripheral VIIIth nerve and at times mask the primary site of disorder.

IV. HANDICAPPING INFLUENCE OF HEARING LOSS

A. Classification and Definition of Handicap

The handicapping influence of an auditory disorder is difficult to establish, since hearing impairment affects the economic, educational, emotional, and social aspects of life and is complicated by the individual's interactions with his environment. Even the assessment of the effects of the magnitude of the hearing loss on communication cannot be isolated from other interacting influences. The difficulties become apparent when attempts are made to classify persons with hearing loss. For example, individuals with hearing loss are often synonymously referred to as "deaf" or "hard of hearing." Although these classifications have not been defined to the satisfaction of all authorities, a widely known and accepted definition has been proposed by the Committe on Nomenclature of the Conference of Executives of American Schools for the Deaf in 1937 (as reported by Silverman,

1971, pp. 401–402). In that proposal, the committee recognized the importance of the magnitude of the loss and the time of onset of the hearing disorder in defining severity of the handicap. Deaf individuals were defined as

> Those in whom the sense of hearing is nonfunctional for the ordinary purposes of life. This general group is made up of two distinct classes based entirely on time of the loss of hearing. (a) The congenitally deaf: those who are born deaf. (b) The adventitiously deaf: those who were born with normal hearing but in whom the sense of hearing becomes nonfunctional later through illness or accident.

The hard of hearing included "those in whom the sense of hearing, although defective, is functional with or without a hearing aid."

In order to establish some distinctions between the concepts of "no handicap" to "extreme handicap," Davis (1965) and others for the American Academy of Ophthalmology and Otolaryngology (AAOO) attempted to categorize the degree of handicap associated with hearing loss. The overall hearing handicap was estimated by this group in terms of the ability to hear everyday speech well enough to understand it. Since the average pure-tone threshold level for the frequencies of 500, 1000, and 2000 Hz corresponds closely to the hearing level for speech reception, Davis defined the degree of handicap in terms of pure-tone audiometric measurements (average pure-tone loss at frequencies of 500, 1000, and 2000 Hz). Table II shows the classes of hearing handicap using this procedure. The classification system provides general reference information for determining the usual handicap of an average individual under the varying circumstances of everyday life. Note that this classification system is not by definition related to medical diagnosis of the hearing disorder. Also, certain other considerations may sometimes supersede the handicap estimated from the table. For example, the time of onset of the hearing loss may affect the educational development patterns and may preclude the appropriate use of this classification system. Even among hearing-impaired adults with the same magnitude of loss, some will understand speech more easily and accurately than suggested by the table. Conversely, some individuals with demanding communicative vocational settings will realize a greater handicap due to a mild hearing loss than is suggested by the AAOO classification system. However, the classification of hearing handicap as shown Table II offers a reasonable reference for estimating the practical handicap resulting from the magnitude of hearing loss in the frequency range necessary for understanding speech.

Several systematic attempts have also been made to predict the level of everyday efficiency in hearing. The Social Adequacy Index (SAI) (Davis, 1948; Silverman et al., 1948) utilized speech reception threshold and speech discrimination results using phonetically balanced word lists to predict the speech handling capacity of hearing-impaired individuals. These word lists

TABLE II
CLASSES OF HEARING HANDICAP[a]
ISO—1964

| | | | Average hearing threshold level for 500, 1000, and 2000 in the better ear[b] | | |
dB	Class	Degree of handicap	More than	Not more than	Ability to understand speech
25	A	Not significant		25 dB (ISO)	No significant difficulty with faint speech
40	B	Slight handicap	25 dB (ISO)	40 dB	Difficulty only with faint speech
55	C	Mild handicap	40 dB	55 dB	Frequent difficulty with normal speech
70	D	Marked handicap	55 dB	70 dB	Frequent difficulty with loud speech
90	E	Severe handicap	70 dB	90 dB	Can understand only shouted or amplified speech
	F	Extreme handicap	90 dB		Usually cannot understand even amplified speech

[a] From Davis (1965, p. 741).

[b] Whenever the average for the poorer ear is 25 dB or more greater than that of the better ear in this frequency range, 5 dB are added to the average for the better ear. This adjusted average determines the degree and class of handicap. For example, if a person's average hearing threshold level for 500, 1000, and 2000 Hz is 37 dB in one ear and 62 dB or more in the other, his adjusted average hearing threshold level is 42 dB and his handicap is Class C instead of Class B.

have subsequently undergone several modifications and changes. Since estimates of social adequacy predicted from results with the original word lists do not apply to more current speech lists with varying degrees of difficulty, the use of the SAI has not been pursued. More recent questionnaires (Dirks & Carhart, 1962; High, Fairbanks, & Glorig, 1964) have also been devised to relate subjective impressions of hearing difficulty in everyday listening situations to severity of hearing loss. However, at present, none of these procedures is used extensively.

B. Other Considerations

Other important factors that must be considered in determining the handicapping influence of a hearing loss include the age of onset of loss, the effect of the anatomical site of the disorder on auditory function, the capacity of the hearing-impaired person to understand speech, and the use of amplification to compensate for the hearing loss. The initial factor, the age of onset of the hearing loss, has been referred to in the discussion on the congenitally versus the adventitiously deaf and the effects of the anatomical site of the lesion have been adequately considered in previous sections of this chapter.

1. Speech Discrimination

Since hearing is the primary communication sense, most evaluations of hearing problems include the evaluation of speech reception as well as puretone audiometry. Despite many difficulties, such as choosing the appropriate type of speech stimulus (nonsense syllables, words, and sentences) and physically specifying a fluctuating and complicated speech signal, speech audiometry has become an indispensable clinical tool in determining receptive communication efficiency.

It was mentioned earlier that speech intelligibility was often normal or near normal in patients with pure middle-ear impairment but could be mildly or severely affected by cochlear or neural disorders. Figure 17 shows examples of speech discrimination functions for standardized monosyllabic word lists as a function of speech intensity level. Curve A is a typical speech discrimination function for a normal listener. Curve B shows the function for a patient with a middle-ear disorders of 30 dB. The function is merely displaced from normal by 30 dB. Curves C and D illustrate two types of speech discrimination functions often observed for individuals with sensorineural hearing losses. The patient in Curve C has a 50-dB loss and a maximum discrimination score of 70%. Even though the speech stimulus is raised to

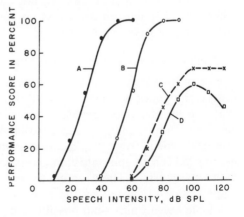

Fig. 17. Performance-intensity functions for phonetically balanced word lists for a normal listener and selected patients with hearing loss. A: normal ear; B: conductive loss; C: sensorineural loss; D: sensorineural loss.

levels above this maximum, the performance score remains the same. Curve D shows a 50-dB loss with a maximum score of 69%. However, for this patient, increases in speech level above maximum discrimination actually cause moderate reductions in performance.

There are a number of poorly understood factors that influence the speech-reception performance of patients with sensorineural hearing loss. The changes in the speech discrimination functions commonly observed in persons with sensorineural impairment are attributed to alterations in the loudness function above the threshold (effects of recruitment) and the often observed greater hearing loss for the high frequencies (filter effect). If speech is presented to persons with sensorineural impairments, it is likely that the weak sounds (consonants) will be inaudible or heard at abnormally low levels and thus not easily understood. If the speech level is raised, as, for example, by amplification devices, these same sounds may be presented at optimal levels but the louder sounds may now be abnormally loud and mask (Martin & Pickett, 1970) the weaker consonants. In addition, many individuals with sensorineural losses are handicapped by a greater hearing loss for the high frequencies. Consonants rich in high-frequency energy are thus particularly vulnerable under these conditions. Amplification systems with frequency selective characteristics are available to compensate partially for this problem.

Everyday listening situations where background noise or competition is present may provide an additional problem for the person with sensorineural loss. At speech-to-competition ratios that result in only a small reduction in intelligibility for a normal listener, individuals with sensorineural loss may have severe problems (Carhart, 1967a,b; Olsen & Carhart, 1967; Olsen & Tillman, 1968; Tillman *et al.*, 1970). These results suggest that, at certain signal-to-competition ratios, the speech level may need to be raised by as much as 14 dB for persons with sensorineural hearing loss than individuals with normal hearing in order to obtain equal intelligibility. Although the explanations for such results are not clear at this time, the handicapping influences of a sensorineural loss on speech discrimination can be severe and are not always appreciated.

2. Amplification by Hearing Aids

Except for surgical and medical therapy for patients with middle-ear disorders, the greatest assistance in alleviating the handicap of hearing loss is provided by means of amplification via hearing aids. Within limitations, it has been established that a majority of individuals with sensorineural hearing loss can benefit from amplification systems. Unfortunately, however, no hearing aid can compensate completely for a hearing loss, especially in cases with dysacusis. There are many practical limits to hearing-aid amplification—imposed by the size, weight, electronics, expense, etc., of available hearing aids—but possibly the greatest limitation is imposed by the sensorineural hearing loss itself. If the hair cells in the cochlea or the nerve fibers have degenerated, no hearing aid can force these cells to transmit sound.

Practical considerations regarding hearing-aid specification, selection, and use have been topics of clinical concern since the development of the electric hearing aids in the early part of the twentieth century (Berger, 1970). Several areas of investigation include (1) physical specification of electroacoustic characteristics of hearing aids, (2) effects of modifications of ear-molds (used to couple the hearing aid to the ear) on the amplified signals, (3) procedures for selection of hearing aids for individuals with various auditory impairments, and (4) techniques of counseling and orientation for the new hearing aid user. A substantial body of literature has accumulated on each of these topics. Detailed discussion of these issues is beyond the scope of this chapter. However, several pertinent references related to hearing aid research can be found in the Suggested Readings on Hearing Aid Amplification at the end of this chapter.

V. CONCLUDING REMARKS

The primary purpose of this chapter has been to review the present status of knowledge concerning the effects of auditory impairments on hearing. Special emphasis was placed on well-established characteristics of auditory impairments that can be attributed to specific anatomical sites of lesions. In addition, several aspects of the handicapping influence of a hearing loss on an individual were considered. The results from electrophysiologic procedures such as evoked potential audiometry and electrocochleography are notable by their absence. Although important information has been gathered about the potentials generated in the auditory system, much of this literature deals with the normal auditory system.

It should be apparent that hearing impairments can impose a variety of complex and, as yet, poorly understood changes on auditory function. Diagnostic procedures have typically been employed to determine the anatomical site of the lesion, contributing to the final medical diagnosis and describing some characteristics of hearing loss. This general strategy, however, must be improved and directed toward obtaining more detailed information about auditory processing in both the normal and impaired listener. The complete understanding of the effects of impairment on auditory processing should lead to improved techniques for preventing and alleviating hearing impairment. The task is indeed monumental, but so are the consequences.

References

American National Standards Institute. American standard for audiometer for general diagnostic purposes. ASA Z24.5-1951. New York, 1951.

American National Standards Institute. Specification for audiometers. ANSI S3.6-1969. New York, 1970.

American National Standards Institute. Specification for an artificial headbone. ANSI S3.13-1972. New York, 1972.

Barany, E. A contribution to the physiology of bone conduction. *Acta Oto-Laryngologica*, 1938, Suppl. 26.

Békésy, G. von. Zur Theorie des Horens bei der Schallaufnahme durch Knochenleitung. *Annelender Physik*, 1932, **13**, 111–136.

Békésy, G. von. A new audiometer. *Acta Oto-Laryngologica*, 1947, **35**, 411–422.

Berger, K. The first electric hearing aids. *Hearing Dealer*, 1970, **21**, 23–28.

Bocca, E. Binaural hearing: Another approach. *Laryngoscope*, 1955, **65**, 1164–1171.

Bocca, E., & Calearo, C. Central hearing processes. In J. Jerger (Ed.), *Modern Developments in Audiology*. New York: Academic Press, 1963. Pp. 337–370.

Calearo, C., & Antonelli, A. Audiometric findings in brain stem lesions. *Acta Oto-Laryngologica*, 1968, **66**, 305–319.

Carhart, R. The clinical application of bone-conduction audiometry. *Archives of Otolaryngology*, 1950, **51**, 798–807.

Carhart, R. Clinical determination of abnormal auditory adaptation. *Archives of Otolaryngology*, 1957, **65**, 32–39.

Carhart, R. Discussion on the first round table international audiology conference. Mexico City, 1967. *International Audiology*, 1967, **6**, 285–289. (a)

Carhart, R. The advantages and limitations of a hearing aid. *Minnesota Medicine*, 1967, **50**, 823–826. (b)

Carhart, R., & Jerger, J. Preferred method for clinical determination of pure tone thresholds. *Journal of Speech and Hearing Disorders*, 1959, **24**, 330–345.

Clack, T., & Bess, F. Aural harmonics: the tone-on-tone masking versus the best-beat method in normal and abnormal listeners. *Acta Oto-Laryngologica*, 1969, **67**, 399–412.

Corliss, E. L. R., & Koidan, W. Mechanical impedance of the forehead and mastoid. *Journal of the Acoustical Society of America*, 1955, **27**, 1164–1172.

Dadson, R. S., Robinson, D. W. & Greig, R. G. P. The mechanical impedance of the human mastoid process. *British Journal of Applied Physics*, 1954, **5**, 435–442.

Davis, H. The articulation area and the social adequacy index for hearing. *Laryngoscope*, 1948, **58**, 761–778.

Davis, H. Guide for the classification and evaluation of hearing handicap in relation to the international audiometric zero. *Transactions of the American Academy of Ophtholmology and Otolaryngology*, 1965, **69**, 740–751.

de Boer, E. J., & Bouwmeester, J. Clinical psychophysics illustrated by the problem of auditory overload. *Audiology*, 1975, **14**, 274–299.

Dirks, D., & Carhart, R. A survey of reactions from users of binaural and monaural hearing aids. *Journal of Speech and Hearing Disorders*, 1962, **27**, 311–322.

Dirks, D., & Kamm, C. Bone vibrator measurements: Physical characteristics and behavioral thresholds. *Journal of Speech and Hearing Research*, 1975, **18**, 242–260.

Dirks, D., Morgan, D., & Bray, D. Perstimulatory loudness adaptation in selected cochlear impaired and masked normal listeners. *Journal of the Acoustical Society of America*, 1974, **56**, 554–561.

Dix, M. R., Hallpike, C. S., & Hood, J. D. Observations upon the loudness recruitment phenomenon with especial reference to the differential diagnosis of disorders of the internal ear and eighth nerve. *Proceedings of the Royal Society of Medicine*, 1948, **41**, 516–526.

Dix, M., & Hood, J. D. Symmetrical hearing loss in brain stem lesions. *Acta Oto-Laryngologica*, 1973, **75**, 165–177.

Feldman, A. S., & Zwislocki, J. Effect of the acoustic reflex on the impedance at the eardrum. *Journal of Speech and Hearing Research*, 1965, **8**, 213–222.

Fowler, E. P. Marked deafened areas in normal ears. *Archives of Otolaryngology,* 1928, **8,** 151–155.

Fowler, E. P. A new method for the early detection of otosclerosis. *Archives of Otolaryngology,* 1936, **24,** 731–741.

Goldstein, R., Goodman, A., & King, R. Hearing and speech in infantile hemiplegia before and after left hemispherectomy. *Neurology,* 1956, **6,** 869–872.

Goodhill, V., Guggenheim, P., Hoversten, G., & MacKay, D. Pathology, diagnosis and therapy of deafness. In L. Travis (Ed.), *Handbook of speech pathology and audiology.* New York: Appleton, 1971. Pp. 279–346.

High, W., Fairbanks, G., & Glorig, A. Scale for self-assessment of hearing handicap. *Journal of Speech and Hearing Disorders,* 1964, **29,** 215–230.

Hirsh, I., Palva, T., & Goodman, A. Difference limen and recruitment. *Archives of Otolaryngology,* 1954, **60,** 525–540.

Hood, J. D. Auditory fatigue and adaptation in the differential diagnosis of end-organ disease. *Annals of Otology Rhinology and Laryngology,* 1955, **64,** 507–518.

Hood, J. D. The principles and practice of bone conduction audiometry. A review of the present position. *Proceedings of the Royal Society of Medicine,* 1957, **50,** 689–697. Reprinted in *Laryngoscope,* 1960, **70,** 1211–1228.

Hughes, R. L. Békésy audiometry. In J. Katz (Ed.), *Handbook of clinical audiology.* Baltimore: Williams & Wilkins, 1972, Chapter 12.

Hughson, W., & Westlake, H. Manual for program outline for rehabilitation of aural casualties both military and civilian. *Transactions of the American Academy of Ophthalmology and Otolaryngology,* 1944 **Suppl. 48,** 1–15.

Huizing, H., & Reyntjes, J. Recruitment and speech discrimination loss. *Laryngoscope,* 1952, **62,** 521–527.

International Standards Organization. A standard reference zero for the calibration of pure-tone audiometers. *ISO Record,* 1964.

Jepsen, O. Middle-ear muscle reflexes in man. In J. Jerger (Ed.), *Modern developments in audiology.* New York: Academic Press, 1963. Pp. 193–239.

Jerger, J. A difference limen recruitment test and its diagnostic significance. *Laryngoscope,* 1952, **62,** 1316–1332.

Jerger, J. DL difference test. *Archives of Otolaryngology,* 1953, **57,** 490–500.

Jerger, J. Békésy audiometry in analysis of auditory disorders. *Journal of Speech and Hearing Research,* 1960, **3,** 275–287. (a)

Jerger, J. Observations in auditory behavior in lesions of the central auditory pathways. *Archives of Otolaryngology,* 1960, **71,** 797–806. (b)

Jerger, J. (Ed.). *Modern developments in audiology.* New York: Academic Press, 1963.

Jerger, J. Auditory tests for disorders of the central auditory mechanism. In W. Fields (Ed.), *Neurological aspects of auditory and vestibular disorders.* Springfield, Illinois: Thomas, 1964. Pp. 1–17.

Jerger, J. (Ed.). *Modern developments in audiology* (2nd ed.). New York: Academic Press, 1973. (a)

Jerger, J. Diagnostic audiometry. In J. Jerger (Ed.), *Modern developments in audiology.* New York: Academic Press, 1973. Pp. 75–115. (b)

Jerger, J., & Jerger, S. Progression of auditory symptoms in a patient with acoustic neurinoma. *Annals of Otology, Rhinology and Laryngology,* 1968, **77,** 230–242.

Jerger, J., & Jerger, S. Diagnostic significance of PB word functions. *Archives of Otolaryngology,* 1971, **93,** 573–580.

Jerger, J., & Jerger, S. Studies in impedance audiometry. I. Normal and sensorineural ears. *Archives of Otolaryngology,* 1972, **96,** 513–523.

Jerger, J., & Jerger, S. Auditory findings in brain stem disorders. *Archives of Otolaryngology,* 1974, **99,** 342–350.

Jerger, J., Shedd, J., & Harford, E. On the detection of extremely small changes in sound intensity. *Archives of Otolaryngology,* 1959, **69,** 200–211.

Jerger, J., Tillman, T., and Peterson, J. Masking by octave bands of noise in normal and impaired ears. *Journal of the Acoustical Society of America,* 1959, **32,** 385–390.

Jerger, J., Weikers, N., Sharbrough, F., & Jerger, S. Bilateral lesions of the temporal lobe: A case study. *Acta Oto-Laryngologica,* 1969, **Suppl. 258.**

Klockhoff, I. Middle ear muscle reflexes in man. *Acta Oto-Laryngologica,* 1961, **Suppl. 164.**

Korsan-Bengtsen, M. Distorted speech audiometry. *Acta Oto-Laryngologica,* 1973, **Suppl. 310.**

Lawrence, M., & Yantis, P. Thresholds of overload in normal and pathological ears. *Archives of Otolaryngology,* 1956, **63,** 67–77.

Liden, G. Speech audiometry: An experimental and clinical study with Swedish language material. *Acta Oto-Laryngologica,* 1954, **Suppl. 114.**

Liden, G. The stapedius muscle reflex used as an objective recruitment test. In G. Wolstenholme & I. Knight (Eds.), *Ciba Foundation Symposium on Sensorineural Hearing Loss.* London: Churchill, 1970. Pp. 295–308.

Liden, G. & Korsan-Bengtsen, M. Audiometric manifestation of retrocochlear lesions. *Oto-Rhino-Laryngology,* 1973, **20,** 271–287.

Lierle, D. M., & Reger, S. N. Experimentally induced temporary threshold shifts in ears with impaired hearing. *Annals of Otology, Rhinology and Laryngology,* 1955, **64,** 263–272.

Lilly, D. A comparison of acoustic impedance data obtained with Madsen and Zwislocki instruments. Paper presented to the American Speech and Hearing Association, New York, 1970.

Lilly, D. Measurement of acoustic impedance at the tympanic membrane. In J. Jerger (Ed.), *Modern Developments in Audiology* (2nd ed.). New York: Academic Press, 1973. Pp. 345–406.

Lüscher, E., & Zwislocki, J. Comparison of the various methods employed in determination of the recruitment phenomenon. *Journal of Laryngology,* 1951, **65,** 187–195.

Lybarger, S. Special report: Interim bone conduction thresholds for audiometry. *Journal of Speech and Hearing Research,* 1966, **9,** 483–487.

Margolis, R., & Wiley, T. Monaural loudness adaptation at low sensation levels in normal and impaired ears. *Journal of the Acoustical Society of America,* 1976, **59,** 222–224.

Martin, E. S., & Pickett, J. M. Sensorineural hearing loss and upward spread of masking. *Journal of Speech and Hearing Research,* 1970, **13,** 426–437.

Martin, F. N. Subjective loudness and the SISI test. Paper read before the Tenth International Congress of Audiology, Dallas, Texas, 1970.

Martin, F. N., & Wofford, M. Temporal summation of brief tones in normal and cochlear impaired ears. *Journal of Auditory Research,* 1970, **10,** 82–86.

Metz, O. The acoustic impedance measured on normal and pathological ears. *Acta Oto-Laryngologica,* 1946, **Suppl. 63.**

Metz, O. Threshold of reflex contractions of muscles of middle ear and recruitment of loudness. *Archives of Otolaryngology,* 1952, **55,** 536–543.

Miskolczy-Fodor, F. Monaural loudness-balance test and determination of recruitment degree with short sound impulses. *Acta Oto-Laryngologica,* 1953, **43,** 573–595.

Miskolczy-Fodor, F. The relation between hearing loss and recruitment and its practical employment in the determination of receptive hearing loss. *Acta Oto-Laryngologica,* 1956, **46,** 409–415.

Nelson, D. A., & Bilger, R. C. Pure-tone octave masking in normal-hearing listeners. *Journal of Speech and Hearing Research,* 1974, **17,** 223–233. (a)

Nelson, D. A., & Bilger, R. C. Pure-tone octave masking in listeners with sensorineural hearing loss. *Journal of Speech and Hearing Research,* 1974, **17,** 234–251. (b)

Noffsinger, D., Olsen, W., Carhart, R., Hart, C., & Sahgal, V. Auditory and vestibular aberrations in multiple sclerosis. *Acta Oto-Laryngologica,* 1972, **Suppl. 303.**

Olsen, W., & Carhart, R. Development of test procedures for evaluation of binaural hearing aids. *Bulletin of Prosthetic Research*, 1967, **10–7**, 22–49.

Olsen, W., & Noffsinger, D. Comparison of one new and three old tests of auditory adaptation. *Archives of Otolaryngology*, 1974, **99**, 94–99.

Olsen, W. A., Rose, D. E., & Noffsinger, D. Brief-tone audiometry with normal, cochlear, and eighth nerve tumor patients. *Archives of Otolaryngology*, 1974, **99**, 185–189.

Olsen, W., & Tillman, T. Hearing aids and sensorineural hearing loss. *Annals of Otology, Rhinology, and Laryngology*, 1968, **77**, 717–726.

Opheim, O., & Flottorp, G. The aural harmonics in normal and pathological hearing. *Acta Oto-Laryngologica*, 1955, **45**, 513–531.

Palva, T. Finnish speech audiometry. *Acta Oto-Laryngologica*, 1952, **Suppl. 101**.

Reger, S., & Kos, C. Clinical measurements and implication of recruitment. *Annals of Otology, Rhinology, and Laryngology*, 1952, **61**, 810–820.

Rittmanic, P. A. Pure tone masking by narrow noise bands in normal and impaired ears. *Journal of Auditory Research*, 1962, **2**, 287–304.

Sanders, J. W., & Honig, E. A. Brief tone audiometry results in normal and impaired ears. *Archives of Otolaryngology*, 1967, **85**, 640–647.

Sanders, J., & Rintelmann W. Masking in audiometry. *Archives of Otolaryngology*, 1964, **80**, 541–556.

Schuknecht, H. F. *Pathology of the ear*. Cambridge, Massachusetts: Harvard University Press, 1975. Pp. 398–403.

Schuknecht, H., & Woellner, R. An experimental and clinical study of deafness from lesions of the cochlear nerve. *Journal of Laryngology*, 1955, **69**, 75–97.

Schultz, M., & Streepy, C. The speech discrimination function in loudness recruiting ears. *Laryngoscope*, 1967, **77**, 2114–2127.

Schuster, K. Eine Methode zum Vergleich akusticher Impedanzer. *Physik Zelforschs* 1934, **35**, 408–409.

Silverman, S. R. The education of deaf children. In L. Travis (Ed.), *Handbook of speech pathology and audiology*. New York: Appleton, 1971. Pp. 399–430.

Silverman, S., Thurlow, W., Walsh, T., & Davis, H. Improvement in the social adequacy index of hearing following the fenestration operation. *Laryngoscope*, 1948, **58**, 607–631.

Speaks, C., & Jerger, J. Method of measurement of speech identification. *Journal of Speech and Hearing Research*, 1965, **8**, 185–194.

Studebaker, G. A. On masking in bone conduction testing. *Journal of Speech and Hearing Research*, 1962, **5**, 215–227.

Studebaker, G. A. Clinical masking of air- and bone-conduction stimuli. *Journal of Speech and Hearing Disorders*, 1964, **29**, 23–25.

Studebaker, G. A. Clinical masking of the non-test ear. *Journal of Speech and Hearing Disorders*, 1967, **32**, 360–371.

Swisher, L. P. Response to intensity change in cochlear pathology. *Laryngoscope*, 1966, **76**, 1706–1713.

Terkildsen, K., & Thomsen, K. A. The influence of pressure variations on the impedance of the human ear drum. *Journal of Laryngology and Otology*, 1959, **73**, 409–418.

Thompson, G. A modified SISI technique for selected cases with suspected acoustic neurinoma. *Journal of Speech and Hearing Disorders*, 1963, **28**, 299–302.

Tillman, T., Carhart, R., & Olsen, W. Hearing aid efficiency in a competing speech situation. *Journal of Speech and Hearing Research*, 1970, **13**, 789–811.

Tonndorf, J. Bone conduction: Studies in experimental animals. *Acta Oto-Laryngologica*, 1966, **Suppl. 213**.

U.S. Public Health Service. National Health Survey (1935–1936): Preliminary Reports, Hearing Study Series. Bulletins 1–7. U.S. Public Health Service, Washington, D.C., 1938

Weiss, E. An air-damped artificial mastoid. *Journal of the Acoustical Society of America*, 1960, **32**, 1582–1588.

Whittle, L. S., & Robinson, D. W. An artificial mastoid for the calibration of bone vibrators. *Acustica*, 1967, **19**, 80–86.

Wiley, T., Lilly, D., & Small, A. Loudness adaptation in listeners with noise induced hearing loss. *Journal of the Acoustical Society of America*, 1976, **59**, 225–227.

Williams, H. L. *Menière's disease*. Springfield, Illinois: Thomas, 1952.

Wright, H. N. Clinical measurement of temporal auditory summation. *Journal of Speech and Hearing Research*, 1968, **11**, 109–127.

Young, I. M., & Harbert, F. Significance of the SISI test. *Journal of Auditory Research*, 1967, **7**, 303–311.

Zwislocki, J. Eine verbesserte Vertäubungsmethode für die Audiometrie. *Acta Oto-Laryngologica*, 1951, **39**, 339–356.

Zwislocki, J. Acoustic attenuation between the ears. *Journal of the Acoustical Society of America*, 1953, **25**, 752–759.

Zwislocki, J. Some measurements of the impedance at the eardrum. *Journal of the Acoustical Society of America*, 1957, **29**, 349–356. (a)

Zwislocki, J. Some impedance measurements on normal and pathological ears. *Journal of the Acoustical Society of America*, 1957, **29**, 1312–1317. (b)

Zwislocki, J. An acoustic method for clinical examination of the ear. *Journal of Speech and Hearing Research*, 1963, **6**, 303–314.

Zwislocki, J., & Feldman, A. Post-mortem acoustic impedance of human ears. *Journal of the Acoustical Society of America*, 1963, **35**, 104–107.

Zwislocki, J., & Feldman, A. *Acoustic impedance of pathological ears*. ASHA Monograph No. 15, American Speech and Hearing Assoc., Washington, D.C., 1970.

Suggested Readings in Hearing Aid Amplification

Berger, K. W. *The hearing aid: Its operation and development* (2nd ed.). Livonia, Michigan: National hearing Aid Society, 1974.

Davis, H., & Silverman, S. R. *Hearing and deafness*. New York: Holt, 1960. Pp. 265–329.

Katz, J. *Handbook of clinical audiology*. Baltimore, Maryland: Williams and Wilkins, 1972. Pp. 564–656.

Pollack, M. C. *Amplification for the hearing impaired*. New York: Grune and Stratton, 1975.

Chapter 14

EFFECTS OF NOISE ON PEOPLE*

J. D. MILLER

I. INTRODUCTION

An old riddle asked, "What comes with a carriage and goes with a carriage, is of no use to the carriage and yet the carriage cannot move without it?" The answer: "A noise." And yet (sound) is of great use to us and to all animals. Many events of nature, whether the meeting of two objects or the turbulent flow of air, radiate a tiny part of their energy as pressure waves in the air. A small fraction of the energy that is scattered enters our ears, and we hear it and thus we know of the event. Hearing is a late development in evolution but it has become the sentinel of our senses, always on the alert. But hearing does more. The ear and the brain analyze these sound waves and their patterns in time, and thus we know that it was a carriage, not footsteps that we heard. What is more, we can locate the position of the carriage, and tell the direction in which it is moving. . . . Many birds and animals have also learned to signal one another by their voices, both for warning and for recognition. But we humans, with good ears and also mobile tongues and throats, and above all, our large complex brains, have learned to talk. We attach arbitrary and abstract meanings to sounds, and we have language. We communicate our experiences of the past and also our ideas and plans for future action. For human beings, then, the loss of hearing brings special problems and a special tragedy. . . . Human society creates a special problem even for those with perfect hearing—the problem of unwanted sound, of noise, which is as much a hazard of our environment as disease germs or air pollution. . . . All of (these subjects) are important. Sounds may be small and weak, but civilization could not have grown without them. [Introduction to *Sound and Hearing,* Life Nature Library, by Hallowell Davis, M. D., published by Time–Life Books, Inc., 1965.]

The role of sound and hearing in man's life can be best understood in evolutionary terms. The ear, the auditory nervous system, and their relations with the remainder of man's bodily and behavioral functions developed to meet the demands of adaptation to the environment. But the pace of genetic change is slow compared to the rapid environmental change brought

* Chapters 14, 15, and 16 originally appeared in the *Journal of the Acoustical Society of America,* Vol. 56, No. 3, September 1974, pp. 729–764. © 1974 Acoustical Society of America. Reprinted by permission of the Acoustical Society of America.

on by technology. Our genes prepare us for the environment of the past, and it will be knowledge of that preparation that will allow us to specify a compatible environment. Each of the adverse effects on people of excess or unwanted sounds can be linked either to positive, adaptive effects of sound or to the absence of protective mechanisms that were not previously required.

Hearing evolved to play a role in both individual and social adaptation to the environment. For individual efforts at survival, hearing is indeed the "sentinel of our senses, always on the alert." By hearing, man can detect a sound-making object or event, day or night. Often man can localize the direction of an object or event and sometimes identify it by its sound alone. To increase the chances of identifying objects or events and to insure appropriate preparation for response, evolution has closely tied hearing to man's activating and arousal systems. These systems energize us. In addition, specific auditory–muscular reflexes cause one to orient his head and eyes in an appropriate direction to aid recognition and identification of the sound-making object or event.

Hearing is also involved in social mechanisms of adaptation to the environment. With our voices and ears we can "communicate our experiences of the past and also our ideas and plans for future action." In addition, language, dialect, and manner of speech are important determiners of the actions and cohesiveness of social groups.

The close ties of hearing to arousal, muscular actions, and social relations provide the biological foundations for the mood-influencing and esthetic properties of auditory experience. For hearing not only serves as an ever-vigilant warning system and as the avenue of speech reception, but also acts to influence man's moods, feelings of well-being, and esthetic sensibilities. Many of these responses to sound are culturally determined and represent learned attitudes, but surely there are biological bases for development of music with its associated emotional responses along with the muscular responses of rhythmic movement and dance. Some of these biological bases stem from adaptive interrelations between the auditory system and the arousal and muscular systems. Others may be simply accidents of the evolution of the auditory system.

Thus, sound is of great value to man. It warns him of danger and appropriately arouses and activates him. It allows him the immeasurable advantage of speech and language. It can be beautiful. It can calm, excite, and it can elicit joy or sorrow. The recent discovery that 5-day-old infants will work to produce a variety of sounds (Butterfield & Siperstein, 1970) only reinforces the everyday observation that man enjoys hearing and making sounds.

Unfortunately, excess sound generated by sources irrelevant to the individual can arouse him too often or with no adaptive advantage or can simply be ugly. Also, excess sound can interfere with the perception of important, relevant auditory signals. Furthermore, one imagines that the evolving auditory system did not need to develop mechanisms to protect it from intense sustained sounds. To be sure, the ear had to be able to withstand the intense but brief sounds of thunder and the moderately intense sounds of windstorms and rain; but these rarely lasted more than a few hours. In general, the evolving ear did not have to cope with either frequent, very intense sounds or even moderately intense sounds that were maintained day after day. Only near some beaches, waterfalls, or areas with sustained winds would moderately intense sound levels have continued for prolonged periods of time. It is interesting in this regard that ancient travelers noted that villagers who lived near the cataracts of the Nile appeared to have hearing loss (Ward, 1970a). It should not surprise us then to learn that overexposure of the ear can cause it to temporarily and sometimes permanently suffer a loss of function.

Thus, irrelevant or excessive sound is undesirable. Such unwanted sound is noise. The definition of noise includes a value judgment, and for a society to brand some sounds as noises requires an agreement among the members of that society. Sometimes such agreements can be achieved readily. Other times considerable analysis and debate is required before agreement can be reached.

For example, while machines are useful and valuable, they often produce as a by-product too much sound—noise. On the other hand, since machines can be dangerous, undoubtedly they should make enough sound to warn us of their approach or of the danger from their rapidly moving, powerful parts. But how much and what kinds of sound? Also, sounds that are valuable in one location may travel to places where they may interfere with and disrupt useful and desirable activities. Some sounds seem to serve no useful purpose, anywhere or anytime to anyone. These sounds are unwanted and they clearly are noises. Other sounds are noises only at certain times, in certain places, to certain people. It is these complexities that require considerable analysis and thought to enable us to reach agreement about what is noise and what is not. Scientists and citizens have engaged in such analysis and thought and some of the results of their efforts are described in this paper.

II. AUDITORY EFFECTS

The auditory system is exquisitely sensitive to sound. The acoustical power at the eardrum associated with a sound so loud as to produce discomfort (120 dB) is only about 1/10,000 of a watt. The sound power of the same sound impinging over the entire surface of the body is of the order of 1 W. Furthermore, the boundary between the skin of the body and the surrounding air is such that little of the acoustical power of audible sound is actually transmitted into the body. Even for very loud sounds only a small amount of acoustical power actually reaches the body. Therefore, it is not surprising that noise has its most obvious effects on the ear and hearing, since these are especially adapted to be sensitive to sound.

One set of auditory effects is noticeable after a noise has passed; these are temporary hearing loss, permanent hearing loss, and permanent injury to the inner ear. Another set of auditory effects is noticeable while a noise is present; these are masking and interference with speech communication. Both of these sets of adverse auditory effects are discussed below.

A. Ear Damage and Hearing Loss

Exposure to noise of sufficient intensity for long enough periods of time can produce detrimental changes in the inner ear and seriously decrease the ability to hear. Some of these changes are *temporary* and last for minutes, hours, or days after the termination of the noise. After recovery from the temporary effects, there may be residual *permanent* effects on the ear and hearing that persist throughout the remainder of life. Frequent exposures to noise of sufficient intensity and duration can produce temporary changes that are *chronic,* though recoverable when the series of exposures finally ceases. Sometimes, however, these chronically maintained changes in hearing lose their temporary quality and become permanent.

The changes in hearing that follow sufficiently strong exposure to noise are complicated. They include distortions of the clarity and quality of auditory experience as well as losses in the ability to detect sound. These changes can range from only slight impairment to nearly total deafness.

1. EAR DAMAGE

a. HOW EAR DAMAGE FROM NOISE IS STUDIED. Conclusive evidence of the damaging effects of intense noise on the auditory system has been obtained from anatomical methods applied to animals. One group of animals is exposed to noise and a comparable control group is not. After a wait of a few months, both groups of animals are sacrificed and their inner ears are prepared for microscopic evaluation. The primary site of injury is found to be in the receptor organ of the inner ear. Modern quantitative methods allow an almost exact count of the numbers of missing sensory cells in the inner ears of noise-exposed animals. These can be compared to the numbers of missing cells in the inner ears of control animals. Other signs of injury such as changes in the accessory structures of the inner ear can also be observed.

These anatomical methods are limited for two reasons. The integrity of crucial structures, such as the connections between the hairs of the hair cells and the tectorial membrane, cannot be evaluated, and also the functional properties of cells that are present cannot be assessed. That is, when a cell is present, the anatomist can only guess at its functional state. The absent cell is clearly identifiable and the interpretation of its function is obvious.

The inner ears of human beings have also been examined. Some patients with terminal illness have volunteered their inner ears to temporal bone banks. Such specimens are collected at the time of a postmortem examination. The anatomist tries to relate the condition of the human ear to the patient's case history after making allowances for postmortem changes in the inner ear and possible premortem changes associated with the terminal illness or its treatment. In spite of these difficulties, observations of human cochleas are extremely important and in combination with animal experiments provide a fairly clear description of the damaging effects of noise on the inner ear.

Because of the limitations of anatomical methods and the lack of complete knowledge of the relations between hearing abilities and the anatomy of the auditory system, it is not possible to predict completely the hearing changes from the anatomical changes. However, physiological observations that include measurement of changes in biochemical state and electrical responses of the cochlea and auditory nerve help to reveal the functional changes produced by exposure to noise.

b. KINDS OF EAR DAMAGE AND MAJOR FINDINGS. The outer ear, eardrum, and middle ear are almost never damaged by exposure to intense noise. The eardrum, however, can be ruptured by extremely intense noise and blasts (von Gierke, 1965). The primary site of auditory injury from excessive exposure to noise is the receptor organ of the inner ear. This has been known for many years, and excellent illustrations of such damage were published near the turn of the century (Yoshii, 1909).

The receptor organ of the inner ear is the organ of Corti, and its normal structure is illustrated in cross section in Panel a of Fig. 1. Here one can identify the auditory sensory cells (hair cells) and the auditory nerve fibers attached to them, as well as some of the accessory structures of the receptor organ. A brief account of the function of the organ of Corti is as follows. Through a complicated chain of events, sound at the eardrum results in an up-and-down movement of the basilar membrane. The hair cells are rigidly fixed in the reticular lamina of the organ of Corti which in turn is fixed to the basilar membrane. As the basilar membrane is driven up and down by sound, a shearing movement is generated between the tectorial membrane and the top of the organ of Corti. This movement bends the hairs at the top of the hair cells. This bending, in turn, causes the hair cells to stimulate the auditory nerve fibers. As a result, nerve impulses arise in the nerve fibers and travel to the brainstem. From the brainstem, the nerve impulses are relayed to various parts of the brain and in some unknown way give rise to auditory sensations. The point to be made is that the integrity of the sensory cells and the organ of Corti is important for normal hearing.

Excessive exposure to noise can result in the destruction of hair cells and collapse or total destruction of sections of the organ of Corti. In addition, auditory neurons may degenerate. Figure 1 illustrates these injuries. The

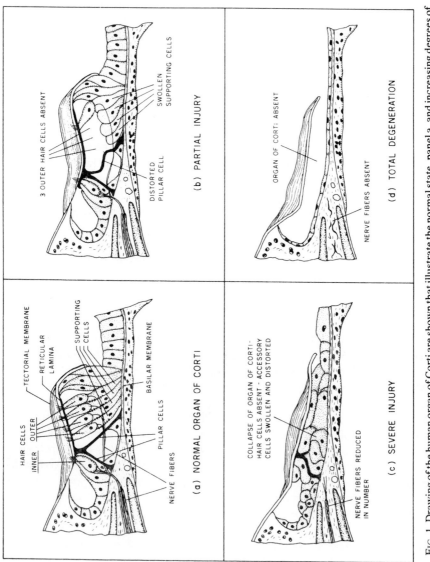

Fig. 1. Drawing of the human organ of Corti are shown that illustrate the normal state, panel a, and increasing degrees of noise-induced permanent injury, panels b, c, and d.

injury illustrated in Panel b includes absence of three outer hair cells, distortion of a pillar cell, and swelling of the supporting cells. In Panel c, there is a complete collapse of the organ of Corti with the absence of hair cells, distortion of the accessory structures, and a reduction in the number of nerve fibers. This section of the organ of Corti is almost certainly without auditory function. The injury shown in Panel d is obvious; there is complete degeneration of the organ of Corti.

Figure 2 shows photomicrographs of cross sections of the organ of Corti from postmortem human specimens. These photographs were provided by Dr. Harold F. Schuknecht of the Massachusetts Eye and Ear Infirmary of Boston, Massachusetts. The organ of Corti in Panel a of Fig. 2 is essentially normal and can be compared with the drawing in Panel a of Fig. 1. Shown in Panel b of Fig. 2 is a cross section of the organ of Corti from a man who worked for a few years in small compartments of boilers where for prolonged periods of time he was exposed to the noise of riveting machines. In this cross section the inner hair cell is present, but only one outer hair cell can be seen where one would normally expect to see four. The example in Panel c is from a man who worked in the noisy environment of a steel factory. There is collapse of the organ of Corti with complete absence of normal receptor cells.

The injuries of Figs. 1 and 2 are from selected locations within the ear. For proper perspective it is important to know that the human organ of Corti is about 34 mm in length with about 395 outer hair cells and 100 inner hair cells per mm (Bredberg, 1968). These total about 17,000. Thus, the five hair cells shown in a single location represent but a small fraction of the receptor organ. The magnitude of injury to the inner ear and the associated hearing loss depend not only on the severity of the injury at any one location but also on the spread of the injury along the length of the organ of Corti.

The loss of hearing abilities depends, in a complicated way, on the extent of the injury along the organ of Corti. Total destruction of the organ of Corti for 1 or 2 mm of the total 34 mm may or may not lead to measurable changes in hearing. Recent evidence from human cases and animal experiments suggests that the loss of sensory cells must be quite extensive in the upper part of the cochlea (that part which is important for the perception of low-frequency sounds) before this damage is reflected as a change in threshold. In the lower part of the cochlea (that part which is important for the perception of high-frequency sounds) losses of sensory cells over a few millimeters are sometimes reflected in changes in hearing (Bredberg, 1968).

The mechanism by which overexposure to noise damages the auditory receptor is not well understood. Very intense noise can mechanically damage the organ of Corti. Thus, loud impulses such as those associated with explosions and firing of weapons can result in vibrations of the organ of Corti that are so severe that some of it is simply torn apart. Other very severe exposures to noise may cause structural damage that leads to rapid "break-

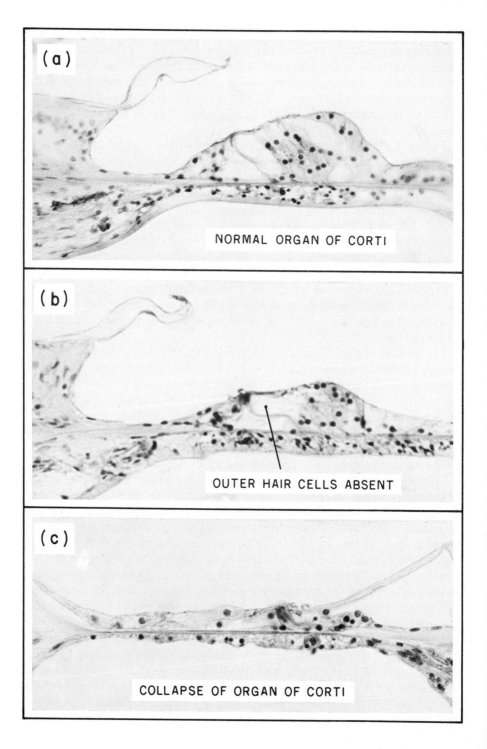

(a) NORMAL ORGAN OF CORTI

(b) OUTER HAIR CELLS ABSENT

(c) COLLAPSE OF ORGAN OF CORTI

down'' of the processes necessary to maintain the life of the cells of the organ of Corti. Such an injury is an *acoustic trauma*.

Overexposure to noise of lower levels for prolonged periods of time also results in the degeneration of the hair cells and accessory structures of the organ of Corti. Such injuries are called *noise-induced cochlear injuries*. Many theories have been proposed to explain noise-induced cochlear injuries. One notion is that constant overexposure forces the cells to work at too high a metabolic rate for too long a period of time. As a result the metabolic processes essential for cellular life become exhausted or poisoned, and this leads to the death of the cells. In a sense, the receptor cells can die from overwork.

No matter what theory is eventually found to be correct, certain facts are established beyond doubt. Excessive exposure to noise leads to the destruction of the primary auditory receptor cells, the hair cells. There can be other injuries to the organ of Corti that can range from mild distortion of its structure to collapse or complete degeneration. The auditory neurons may also degenerate. All of these cells are highly specialized. Once these cells are destroyed, they *do not regenerate* and *cannot* be stimulated to regenerate; they are lost forever.

2. HEARING LOSS

a. HOW HEARING LOSS DUE TO NOISE IS STUDIED. Experiments on hearing loss are sometimes done with animals because one would not deliberately deafen a human subject. For these experiments it is necessary to train the animal subjects so that their ability to detect faint tones can be measured. The measure of this ability is the intensity level of the faintest tone that can be detected. This is called the hearing threshold level. The greater the hearing threshold level, the poorer the ability to hear. The hearing thresholds of trained animals are measured by methods similar to those used with human patients. After the animal's normal thresholds have been measured, it is exposed to noise under controlled laboratory conditions. After the cessation of the noise, changes in the animal's thresholds are measured. Subsequently, its ears are evaluated by physiological and anatomical methods.

Experiments with human subjects are limited to exposures to sound that produce only temporary changes in the hearing mechanism. In such experiments, measures of some auditory capability are made prior to exposure and also at various specified times after its termination. One of the advantages of laboratory studies is the fact that precise measures of hearing are made before and after exposures to a noise whose properties are exactly known.

FIG. 2. Photomicrographs of cross sections of the human organ of Corti are shown: panel a, normal; panels b and c, injuries most probably produced by exposure to noise. Similar injuries have frequently been seen in experimental animals after exposure to noise. [These photographs were provided by Dr. Harold F. Schuknecht of the Massachusetts Eye and Ear Infirmary of Boston, Massachusetts.]

Measurements of the effects of noise on human hearing are also collected in field and clinical case studies. These data are subject to considerable error, but several well-done field studies have been completed or are now in progress. Threshold measurements are made on persons who are regularly exposed to noise. These exposures usually occur in an occupational setting. Noise levels are measured and the progress of hearing thresholds is followed. While it is true that the actual occupational exposures vary from day to day and moment to moment within a day, some rather clear trends emerge when a sufficient number of persons are carefully studied. For comparison, similar measurements are made on persons whose life patterns include very little exposure to noise.

Well-done studies of individual patients in the clinic have suggested hypotheses and have also been an important source of data.

b. TEMPORARY, COMPOUND, AND PERMANENT THRESHOLD SHIFTS— SINGLE EXPOSURES. The primary measure of hearing loss is the hearing threshold level. The hearing threshold level is the level of a tone that can just be detected. The greater the hearing threshold level, the greater the degree of hearing loss or partial deafness. An increase in a hearing threshold level that results from exposure to noise is called a *threshold shift*.

Some threshold shifts are temporary and they diminish as the ear recovers after the termination of the noise. Frequently repeated exposures can produce temporary threshold shifts that are chronic, though recoverable when the exposures cease. When a threshold shift is a mixture of temporary and permanent components, it is a compound threshold shift. When the temporary components of a compound threshold shift have disappeared (that is, when the ear has recovered as much as it ever will), the remaining threshold shift is permanent. Permanent threshold shifts persist throughout the remainder of life.

Temporary threshold shifts can vary in magnitude from a change in hearing sensitivity of a few decibels restricted to a narrow region of frequencies to shifts of such extent and magnitude that the ear is temporarily, for all practical purposes, deaf. After cessation of an exposure, the time for hearing sensitivity to return to near-normal values can vary from a few hours to 2 or 3 weeks. In spite of efforts in many laboratories, the laws of temporary threshold shifts have not yet been completely determined. There are large numbers of variables that need to be explored. Also, there are probably several different underlying processes which need explication before the laws of noise-induced temporary threshold shifts will be completely understood.

Nonetheless, certain generalizations seem to be correct (Ward, 1963). Noises with energy concentrations between about 2000 and 6000 Hz probably produce greater temporary threshold shifts than noises concentrated elsewhere in the audible range. In general, A-weighted sound levels must exceed 60–80 dB before a typical person will experience temporary threshold shifts even for exposures that last as long as 8–24 hours. All other things being equal, the greater the intensity level above 60–80 dB and the longer the time in noise, the greater the temporary threshold shift. However, exposure durations beyond 8–24 hours may not produce further increase in the magnitude of the shift (Mills *et al.*, 1970; Mosko *et al.*, 1970). Another interesting property of temporary threshold shifts is that such shifts are usually greatest for test tones .5–1 octave above the frequency region in which the noise that produces the shift has its greatest concentration of energy. It should also be noted that under certain conditions, contractions of the muscles of the middle ear can offer significant protection from exposure to intense sound. Finally, there is less temporary shift when an exposure has frequent interruptions than when an exposure is continuous.

People differ in their susceptibility to temporary threshold shifts. Unfortunately, these differences in susceptibility are not uniform across the audible range of frequencies. Indeed, one person may be especially susceptible to noises of low pitch, another to noises of medium pitch, and another to noises of high pitch. In general, women appear to be less susceptible to temporary threshold shifts from low-frequency noises than are men, and this relation is reversed for high-frequency noises (Ward, 1966, 1968a).

An impression of the quantitative facts of temporary threshold shifts can be obtained from Figs. 3 and 4. All of the dashed lines indicate extrapolations based on current research. While it is likely that the general trends shown on these figures will be verified by additional research, the exact values cannot be expected to be accurate. For short durations of exposures to high intensities there may even be some changes in the rank ordering of the initial segments of curves. Nonetheless, these graphs provide an adequate summary of reasonable extrapolations of available data.

Consider Fig. 3. The time in noise is plotted along the horizontal axis, while the amount of threshold shift measured in decibels at 2 min after the cessation of the exposure is plotted on the vertical axis. These curves represent probably the worst possible situation in that the noise is in the region, 2400–4800 Hz, to which the ear is most susceptible, and the test tone is at 4000 Hz where threshold shifts are often large. Certain facts are obvious from the graph. The more intense the noise, the more rapidly threshold shifts accumulate as the time in noise is extended. When the noise is only 60 dB, a typical person has to be exposed for several hours before any significant threshold shift can be detected. However, when the noise is very intense, say 120 dB, a typical person exposed for only 5 min reaches dangerous levels of threshold shift. Notice that the combinations of intensity level and duration that produce threshold shifts greater than about 40 dB are said to be in the *region of possible acoustic trauma*. In this region, for some people, the normal processes of the ear may "break down" and permanent threshold shifts—hearing loss—may result from even a single exposure to noise. Remember, however, that these relations are for the worst possible situation

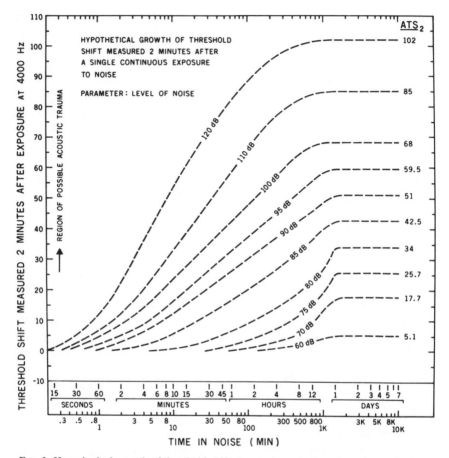

FIG. 3. Hypothetical growth of threshold shift after various single and continuous exposures to noise. These curves represent predictions for an average, normal-hearing young adult exposed to a band of noise or pure tone centered near 4000 Hz. These are "worst-case" conditions as the ear is most susceptible to noise in this region. These hypothetical curves were drawn to be consistent with current facts and theory. They are for an average ear; wide differences among individuals can be expected. In many cases extrapolations had to be made from appropriately corrected data from animals (cats and chinchillas). Other relevant data can be found in papers by Botsford (1971), Carder and Miller (1972), Davis *et al.* (1950), Miller *et al.* (1963, 1971), Mills *et al.* (1970), Mosko *et al.* (1970), and Ward (1960, 1970b).

where the noise is concentrated in the region from 2400 to 4800 Hz. While exposures to other noises lead to qualitatively similar changes in hearing thresholds and to similar risks, the *quantitative* relations (even when the noise is measured in *A*-weighted sound level) may be different.

Recovery from threshold shifts after the cessation of an exposure to noise depends on a variety of factors and is not completely understood. Sometimes recovery from a threshold shift is complete in 200–1000 min. Such rapid recovery from a threshold shift has been observed when the threshold shift is small, less than 40 dB, and the duration of the exposure is short, less than 8 hours (Ward *et al.*, 1959a). Less rapid recovery from threshold shifts is illustrated in Fig. 4. The straight dotted line indicates the course of recovery from a threshold shift that has often been assumed (Ward *et al.*, 1959a,b; Kryter *et al.*, 1966). The data points (filled circles) represent the decline of threshold shift after an exposure at 95 dB for 102 min as actually measured for human listeners. The accuracy of the extrapolation of the dotted line beyond the data points is unknown. Clearly, however, recovery from the exposure of 95 dB for 102 min (dotted line) is more rapid than recovery from the exposure for 3 days (dashed lines).

The slow recovery from noise-induced threshold shifts illustrated in Fig. 4 by the dashed lines probably holds whenever the exposure is severe either in terms of the total duration or in terms of the amount of threshold shift

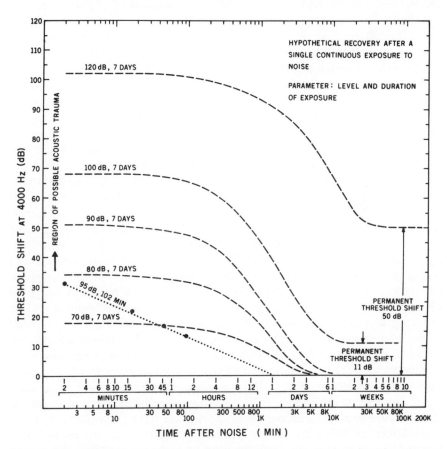

FIG. 4. Hypothetical recovery from threshold shift after various single and continuous exposures to noise. See legend of Fig. 3 for additional explanation.

present a few minutes after the termination of the noise. Recovery from temporary threshold shift appears to be very slow when the initial threshold shift exceeds 35–45 dB (Ward, 1960), when the exposure lasts as long as about 12 hours (Mills *et al.*, 1970; Mosko *et al.*, 1970), or after some long but intermittent exposures to noise (Ward, 1970b). For example, it has been shown that exposure to a noise with an *A*-weighted sound level of about 80 dB for 2 days results in small temporary threshold shifts that do not completely disappear for several days (Mills *et al.*, 1970).

Very severe exposures to noise can produce compound threshold shifts from which complete recovery is impossible. After recovery from the temporary component of a compound threshold shift, there remains a permanent threshold shift. Some examples are shown in Fig. 4. The ear's recovery from compound threshold shifts is often quite slow, and this recovery probably represents a "healing" process. There can be no additional recovery (healing) beyond 2 to 12 weeks after an exposure (Miller *et al.*, 1963).

c. NOISE-INDUCED PERMANENT THRESHOLD SHIFTS—REPEATED EXPOSURES. Sometimes people encounter single exposures to steady noises that produce permanent threshold shifts. This only happens rarely as people usually will not tolerate such severe exposures (see Figs. 3 and 4).

More commonly, noise-induced permanent threshold shifts accumulate as exposures are repeated on a near-daily basis over a period of many years. The best examples of such cases are from field studies of occupational deafness.

An unusually thorough study was done of jute weavers (Taylor *et al.*, 1965). These weavers were all women with little exposure to noise other than that received on the job. The noise exposures had been nearly constant in the mills for almost 52 years, and employees who had worked in the mills for 1–52 years were available for testing. All audiometry (measurement of hearing thresholds) was done with a properly calibrated instrument by a trained physician. Hearing thresholds were measured after a weekend away from the noise. This means that about $2\frac{1}{2}$ days of recovery were allowed and probably only a small recoverable component remained in the measured threshold shift (see Fig. 4). Since the noise in the mill had an *A*-weighted sound level of about 98 dB, a working-day exposure of 8 hours would be expected to produce 35–65 dB of temporary threshold shift in a typical, young adult female for a test tone of 4000 Hz. In $2\frac{1}{2}$ days, this threshold shift would be expected to decay to within about 5 dB of normal (see Figs. 3 and 4). Of course, wide variations can be expected. What happens when such an exposure is repeated about 5 days a week, 50 weeks a year, year after year? The results are shown in Fig. 5. These thresholds are typical for the jute weavers and the expected changes with age have been subtracted.

Evidently, as the exposures are repeated year after year, the ear becomes less and less able to recover from the temporary threshold shift present at the end of each day. It also seems likely that as the exposures are repeated, the

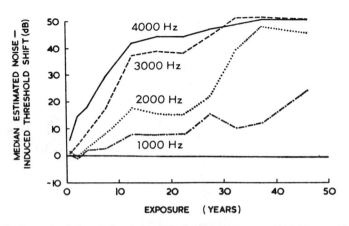

Fig. 5. Median noise-induced threshold shifts for jute weavers with 1 to over 40 years of occupational exposure to noise with an A-weighted sound level of about 98 dB. These threshold shifts have been corrected for the expected changes in thresholds with age in persons who are not exposed to noise. [Reprinted from Taylor *et al.* (1965), by permission of the Acoustical Society of America.]

amount of threshold shift present at the end of each day's work might creep upward toward the asymptote appropriate to the level of the noise as indicated on Fig. 3.

In any case, as the exposures are repeated, the noise-induced temporary threshold shifts become permanent or nearly so. It is also significant that on weekdays there are only 16 hours of recovery between work exposures. Therefore, from the *first day* of *employment,* most of these weavers will be living with a chronic threshold shift of 25–55 dB at 4000 Hz (see Figs. 3 and 4). Only on Saturday and Sunday will their hearing be near normal even during the first year of employment. As the years roll by, these jute weavers become partially deaf even on the weekends.

Similar data have been gathered on male workers in noisy industries in the United States (Nixon & Glorig, 1961). Age-corrected threshold shifts at 4000 Hz are shown for these workers in Fig. 6. The average A-weighted noise levels for the workers environments A, B, and C were about 83, 92, and 97 dB, respectively. Presumably, most of the threshold shifts were measured $2\frac{1}{2}$ days after the last workday and probably contain temporary components of less than 7–10 dB.

The important points to notice on Fig. 6 are *(a)* there is an orderly relation between the median amount of noise-induced threshold shift and the intensity level of the noise, and *(b)* the amount of threshold shift at 4000 Hz from these occupational exposures shows no further increase after about 10 years of exposure, although the threshold shifts for lower frequencies (not shown) continue to increase.

The results shown on Figs. 5 and 6 are medians. These orderly trends do

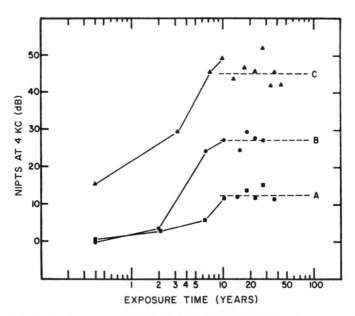

FIG. 6. Noise-induced permanent threshold shifts (NIPTS) plotted against years of occupational exposure to noise for workers in three levels of noise. These threshold shifts have been corrected for the changes with age found in persons without occupational exposure to noise. The graphs are for a test tone of 4000 Hz and the data points are medians. The average A-weighted sound levels were 83 dB for group A, 92 dB for group B, and 97 dB for group C. [Reprinted from Nixon and Glorig (1961), by permission of the Acoustical Society of America.]

not reflect the large differences among individual ears in susceptibility to noise-induced hearing loss. In fact, within a group of similarly exposed people some will exhibit very large threshold shifts while others will exhibit only small threshold shifts. The extent of these differences for jute weavers is shown on Fig. 7. Some of the differences between similarly exposed people are due to differences in susceptibility to noise, and some are due to actual differences in the noise levels encountered. In an industrial situation, the measurement of noise is an average over space and time, and, therefore, all workers do not necessarily receive exactly the same exposure.

d. THRESHOLD SHIFTS FROM IMPULSIVE NOISE. Intense impulsive noise can be particularly hazardous to hearing. The reason is that in addition to the processes involved in noise-induced threshold shifts there is the added risk of a "breakdown" in the inner ear. Permanent threshold shift due to acoustic trauma may result. For example, a single impulse because of its high amplitude might rip or tear a crucial tissue barrier (say the reticular lamina which protects the hair cells and nerves from the fluids of scala media) and a considerable degeneration of the organ of Corti may result.

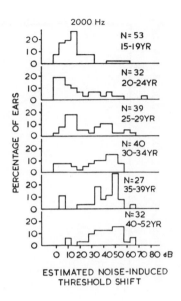

FIG. 7. The distribution of noise-induced threshold shifts of jute weavers exposed for various numbers of years (parameter). The test frequency is 2000 Hz. Notice the large difference among people with regard to the effects of noise on the magnitude of the threshold shift. [Reprinted from Taylor *et al.* (1965), by permission of the Acoustical Society of America.]

When a gun is fired or a hammer strikes metal, very large peak sound pressures may be generated at the eardrum. Idealized waveforms of two types of impulse noises are shown in Fig. 8. In Fig. 9 are shown the combinations of peak sound pressure and duration that can be allowed if as many as 100 impulses were delivered to the ear over a period of four minutes to several hours each day. It is presumed that only 5% of the persons receiving a criterion exposure would have temporary threshold shifts that exceed 10

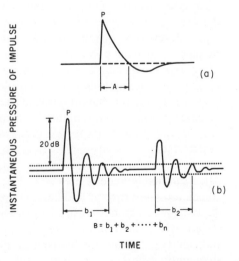

FIG. 8. Idealized pressure waveforms of impulse sounds. On line (a) is shown a single, well-damped impulse. Its duration is taken as the time period indicated by the letter A. On line (b) is shown an impulse that has several oscillations. Also shown is a single reflection. Its duration is taken as the time period $B = b_1 + \cdots + b_n$. The amplitudes of both types of impulse noises are taken as the peak value P expressed in decibels. For more details see Ward (1968b).

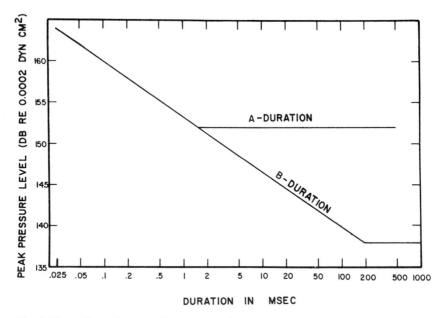

FIG. 9. Upper limits of acceptable exposure to impulse noise as defined by Working Group 57 of the NAS–NRC Committee on Hearing, Bioacoustics, and Biomechanics (Ward, 1968b). The A and B durations are measured as indicated in Fig. 8.

dB at 1000 Hz or below, 15 dB at 2000 Hz, or 20 dB at 3000 Hz or above. Details of these criteria and their derivation can be found elsewhere (Ward, 1968b).

Samples of permanent threshold shifts produced by a single firecracker explosion or the repeated firing of guns are shown in Figs. 10 and 11.

The description of impulse noise and its relation to hearing loss and ear damage is far from complete. The criteria summarized in Figs. 8 and 9 are only provisional and are limited to those acoustic impulses that are similar to gunfire. Another approach to the problem is to describe impulses in terms of their spectra rather than in terms of the instantaneous waveforms. One then assumes that energy in separate frequency bands can be integrated in characteristic ways to account for ear damage and hearing loss in a manner similar to that used for steady noises (Kryter, 1970). This last approach has merit and deserves further experimental and theoretical exploration. However, when the instantaneous pressure of any noise within the audible range becomes too high, the ear and hearing are threatened by acoustic trauma even though a much longer noise of equal energy may be less noxious. Otherwise stated, when the amplitude of vibration of the basilar membrane becomes sufficiently great, the mechanisms of injury to the inner ear probably become sufficiently different to require a different model for the process.

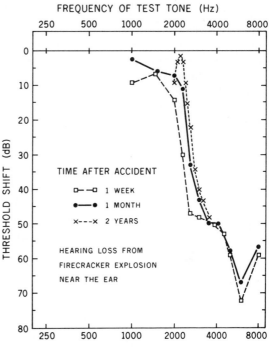

FIG. 10. Permanent threshold shifts produced by a single exposure to a firecracker explosion. The change in hearing is shown by the difference between the thresholds taken before and after the accident. The firecracker was an ordinary flashlight cracker about 2 in. in length and $\frac{3}{16}$ in. in diameter. It was about 15 in. from the patient's right ear when it exploded. [After Ward and Glorig (1961), by permission of *Laryngoscope.*]

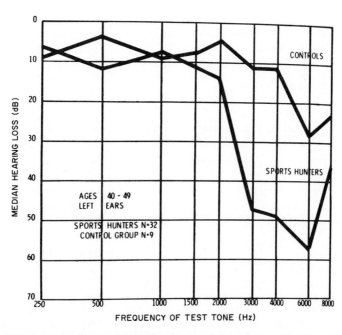

FIG. 11. Median hearing loss in habitual sports shooters and age-matched controls. [From Taylor and Williams (1966), by permission of *Laryngoscope.*]

3. IMPLICATIONS OF EAR DAMAGE AND HEARING LOSS

a. INTERPRETATION OF NOISE-INDUCED HEARING LOSS. There has been and continues to be considerable debate about the implications and significance of small amounts of ear damage and hearing loss. The most recent statement of the Committee on Hearing of the American Academy of Ophthalmology and Otolaryngology on Hearing Handicap is given in Fig. 12. Prior to 1965, this group had used the terms hearing impairment, hearing handicap, and hearing disability almost synonymously and in accordance with the categories displayed in Fig. 12.

In 1965, this committee offered these definitions of terms related to hearing loss. *Hearing Impairment:* a deviation or change for the worse in either structure or function, usually outside the normal range. *Hearing Handicap:* The disadvantage imposed by an impairment sufficient to affect one's efficiency in the situation of everyday living. *Hearing Disability:* Actual or presumed inability to remain employed at full wages.

By these definitions, any injury to the ear or any change in a hearing threshold level that places it outside of the normal range constitutes a *hearing impairment*. Whether a particular impairment constitutes a *hearing handicap*

CLASS	DEGREE OF HANDICAP	AVERAGE HEARING THRESHOLD LEVEL FOR 500, 1000, AND 2000 IN THE BETTER EAR		ABILITY TO UNDERSTAND SPEECH
		MORE THAN	NOT MORE THAN	
A	Not significant		25 dB	No significant difficulty with faint speech
B	Slight Handicap	25 dB	40 dB	Difficulty only with faint speech
C	Mild Handicap	40 dB	55 dB	Frequent difficulty with normal speech
D	Marked Handicap	55 dB	70 dB	Frequent difficulty with loud speech
E	Severe Handicap	70 dB	90 dB	Can understand only shouted or amplified speech
F	Extreme Handicap	90 dB		Usually cannot understand even amplified speech

FIG. 12. Guideline for the relations between the average hearing threshold level for 500, 1000, and 2000 Hz and degree of handicap as defined by the Committee on Hearing of the American Academy of Ophthalmology and Otolaryngology. [From Davis (1965), by permission of *Transactions of the American Academy of Ophthalmology and Otolaryngology*.]

or a *hearing disability* can only be judged in relation to an individual's life pattern or occupation.

The guideline for the evaluation of hearing handicap shown in Fig. 12 uses only thresholds for tones in the region most important for the reception of speech (500, 1000, and 2000 Hz), and judgments of handicap are based on the associated ability to understand connected speech in quiet surroundings. While most authorities agree that a person in Category B or worse has a hearing handicap, there is debate over whether handicap exists when a person in Category A also has large hearing threshold levels above 2000 Hz.

Examples of audiograms that would fall into Category A and also exhibit large hearing threshold levels above 2000 Hz are shown in Figs. 10 and 11. Notice that the guideline of Fig. 12 indicates that such audiograms do not represent a significant handicap. Those who question the guideline of Fig. 12 rally certain facts. For example, some individuals with sizable hearing threshold levels above 2000 Hz may experience considerable difficulty in understanding speech in moderate levels of background noise even though their average hearing threshold levels at 500, 1000, and 2000 Hz do *not* exceed 25 dB (Niemeyer, 1967). Also, persons with hearing loss primarily above 2000 Hz may not be able to distinguish the sounds of certain consonants. Sometimes hearing loss above 2000 Hz may be especially important to a person; for example, piccolo players or specialists concerned with bird song may experience handicap whereas many others might not.

More generally, individuals will react differently to a hearing loss. One may be particularly upset by his inability to understand his children; another may feel handicapped by his inability to participate in rapid verbal patter; and others may miss the sounds of music or those of nature.

There is little room for controversy over the question of handicap when losses become as severe as those of Category C of Fig. 12. Persons with losses this severe or worse are aware that they have lost part or all of a precious gift.

b. HEARING AIDS AND NOISE-INDUCED HEARING LOSS. People with partial deafness from exposure to noise do not live in an auditory world that is simply "muffled." Even those sounds that are heard may be distorted in loudness, pitch, apparent location, or clarity. While a hearing aid sometimes can be useful to a person with noise-induced hearing loss, the result is not always satisfactory. The modern hearing aid can amplify sound and make it audible, but it cannot correct for the distortions that often accompany injury to the organ of Corti.

c. PRESBYCUSIS AND ENVIRONMENTAL NOISE. With age, people almost uniformly experience increasing difficulty in understanding speech. Undoubtedly, some of this loss is due to the degeneration of neurons in the brain which generally accompanies advancing age. Some of this loss is due to changes in middle or inner ears. Some of the changes in the inner ear are due to normal aging processes; some are undoubtedly due to toxic drugs; some, to disease processes; and some, to incidental, recreational, and occupational exposures to noise. Clear evidence is available that noises with A-weighted sound levels above 80 dB can contribute to inner ear damage and eventual hearing handicap if such noises are frequently and regularly encountered. Beyond this, the evidence does not warrant stronger statements about the role of noise in progressive hearing loss with age. Theoretical grounds do suggest that *frequent* exposures of *sufficient duration* to noises with A-weighted sound levels greater than 70–80 dB could contribute to the "normal loss of hearing with age."

At least some aspects of hearing loss with age seem to add to hearing loss from noise exposure (Glorig & Davis, 1961). This means that a small loss of hearing from exposure to noise may be insignificant when one is middle-aged, but might, when combined with other losses due to age, become significant as one reaches an advanced age.

4. PREVENTION OF EAR DAMAGE AND HEARING LOSS FROM NOISE

Hearing loss and ear damage due to noise can be eliminated if exposures to noise are *(1)* held to sufficiently low levels, *(2)* held to sufficiently short durations, or *(3)* allowed to occur only rarely.

The regulation of the acoustic environment in such a way that hearing loss and ear damage from noise are eliminated poses several problems. For example, the chances that a person will develop a hearing impairment due to noise depends on the pattern of exposure from all sources of noise that he happens to encounter. Some of these exposures from particular sources may be innocuous in isolation. But these same noises, which are innocuous by themselves, may combine with noises from other sources to form a total sequence of noises sufficient to produce hearing impairment (Cohen *et al.,* 1970). While it may be possible to control the total exposure in an occupational setting during a day's work, it is nearly impossible to control an individual's activities and exposure to noise while he is away from work. Thus, one must turn to the regulation of sources of noise.

In general, any source with an A-weighted sound level of 70–80 dB has the potential to contribute to a pattern of exposure that might produce temporary threshold shifts (see Fig. 3) and this could lead to permanent hearing impairment. Therefore, it seems desirable to have as few sources as possible that expose people to A-weighted sound levels in excess of 70–80 dB. But people can tolerate many brief exposures in excess of 70–80 dB if they are widely spaced in time. For example, a shower bath may have an A-weighted sound level of about 74 dB, but one would have to shower for over an hour before a temporary threshold shift would appear (see Fig. 3). Clearly, it is impractical to regulate against sources of noise with A-weighted sound levels in excess of 70–80 dB. On the other hand, if such sources are allowed to proliferate without bound, then vast numbers of persons will suffer chronic threshold shifts.

Sources with A-weighted sound levels in excess of 80 dB have the potential to contribute to the incidence of hearing handicap. The argument about regulation of such sources runs exactly parallel to that of the previous paragraph.

Finally, from studies of hearing loss from occupational exposures to noise, one can identify exposures that, in and of themselves, increase the incidence of hearing handicap (Kryter et al., 1966; Radcliff, 1970). Sources that provide exposures as severe as these should be avoided, eliminated, or controlled.

Part of the problem of the evaluation of hearing hazard from various sources of noise is this. While knowledge has accumulated about the effects of schedules of noise exposure such as those encountered in the occupational setting, very much less is known about the effects of other irregular schedules such as those associated with occasional use of home tools and recreational devices (snowmobiles, for example). Here, much more research is needed.

Another approach to the protection of hearing from noise is the use of ear plugs and earmuffs when hazardous noises are encountered. Effective devices are available for this purpose, but they must be carefully selected and properly used. In spite of the effectiveness of earplugs and earmuffs, people will often refuse or neglect to use them for reasons of appearance, discomfort, and bother.

B. Masking and Interference with Speech Communication

Man has a formidable ability to "hear out" one sound from a background of other sounds. For example, one can often hear the doorbell over a background of music and conversation. But there are very definite limits to this ability. Unwanted sounds, noises, can interfere with the perception of wanted sounds, signals. This is called *masking*. By masking, an auditory signal can be made inaudible or the signal can be changed in quality, apparent location, or distinctiveness. Masking has been studied extensively in the laboratory, and, consequently, the effects of noise on the perception of auditory signals can be calculated for many environmental conditions. Descriptions of the masking of auditory signals by noise can be found elsewhere (Hirsh, 1952; Jeffress, 1970; Kryter, 1970; Scharf, 1970; Ward, 1963).

Much of the research on auditory masking has been motivated by auditory theory. From this research, one hopes to learn the basic laws of hearing. The study of the masking of speech by noise has been undertaken to meet both practical and theoretical goals. While it is important for everyday life to be able to understand generally the perceptibility of auditory signals, most would agree that the understanding specifically of the problem of speech perception has great significance for the quality of human life. If speech is totally drowned out by a masker, the speech is said to be inaudible or below the threshold of detectability. If the presence of the speech can be detected, but it is indistinct or difficult to understand, the speech is said to be above the threshold of detectability and to have poor intelligibility or discriminability. Intelligibility or discriminability refers to the clarity or distinctness with which speech can be heard over a background noise and it is usually measured in the percentage of messages that a listener can understand.

1. INTERFERENCE WITH SPEECH COMMUNICATION

a. SPEECH AND UNDERSTANDING SPEECH. A talker generates a complicated series of sound waves. This series is called the speech stream. It is not possible to assign a particular acoustic pattern to each of the "sounds" of the English language in a one-to-one fashion. Rather, the "speech stream" carries the cues for the "sounds" of English, and the listener decodes the "speech stream" by a complicated, synthetic process that not only relies on the acoustic cues carried by the "speech stream," but also relies on the listener's knowledge of the language and the facts of the situation. Not all of the cues carried by the "speech stream" are known. Also, the synthetic processes by which the "speech stream" is decoded and "heard as speech" are not fully understood. Nonetheless, much is known about which regions of the audible range of frequencies carry the cues for the intelligibility of speech.

Cues in the speech stream can be found at frequencies as low as about 100 Hz, to as high as about 8000 Hz. Most of the acoustical energy of the speech stream is concentrated between 100 and 6000 Hz. But the most important cue-bearing energy falls between about 300 and 3000 Hz. The speech stream carries much extra information. It is redundant. Therefore, speech can be heard with high intelligibility even when some of the cues have been removed.

b. HOW SPEECH RECEPTION IN NOISE IS STUDIED. There are many variables that influence the accuracy of speech communication from talker to listener in an experiment. The characteristics of the talker; the test materials; the transmission path from talker to listener; the background noise; the spatial locations of the talker, noise source, and listener; and the integrity of the listener's auditory system all can be important. The outcome of such an experiment is usually measured in the percentage of messages understood, and this percentage is taken as a measure of intelligibility or discriminability of the speech. Other measures are sometimes used. Among these are response times, the time taken to transmit a message, ratings of the quality or the naturalness of speech, recognition of the talker, or recognition of the personality or psychological state of the talker.

In no one experiment are all of the variables studied. Rather, most are held constant and the effects of a few are evaluated. The experiments of Miller *et al.* (1951) provide a good illustration. Only two subjects were used, and they alternated roles as talker and listener. The subjects were located in different rooms and could only communicate via a microphone–amplifier–earphone system which passed only frequencies between 200 and 3000 Hz. Noise could be added into this communication link and the ratio of speech-to-noise power could be controlled. In one experiment, the test materials were one-syllable words. The talker always said, "You will write __," with the test item read at the blank. He monitored his voice level with an appropriate meter and, thus, the speech intensity at the microphone was held constant. The level of the speech and noise at the listener's ear was controlled by the experimenter through appropriate adjustments of the electronic equipment. Of major interest in this experiment were the relations between the speech power and noise power, the number of possible messages (one-syllable words), and the percentage of messages understood. For some tests, the message could be one of two alternatives known to the listener; for other tests the message could be one of 4, 8, 16, 32, 256, or any of 1000 possible one-syllable words. The results are shown in Fig. 13.

It can be seen clearly that the more intense the speech in relation to the noise, the greater the percentage of messages correctly understood. Also, the fewer the number of alternative messages, the greater the percentage of correctly understood messages. It is important to realize that the absolute percentage of correct messages transmitted for each speech-to-noise ratio will depend on the talker, the exact nature of the noise, its spectrum and intensity, and on the way in which the speech and noise intensities are measured.

c. THE EFFECTS OF STEADY BACKGROUND NOISE ON SPEECH COMMUNICATION. An important effect of background noise on speech communication is that the distances over which speech can be understood are greatly reduced. Even when speech can be accurately understood, the presence of noise may require greater pains on the part of the talker and listener than otherwise would be needed. Graphical summaries of these effects are given in Fig. 14 and in simplified form in Fig. 15. The vertical axis is the

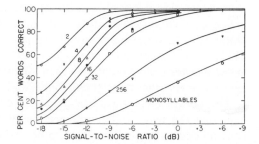

FIG. 13. The dependence of the accuracy of speech communication on the relations between the intensity level of the speech in relation to the intensity level of the noise. The several curves are for various numbers of possible messages. When the message could be one of two possible words, the scores were high. When the message could be one of approximately 1000 one-syllable words, the scores were low. [From Miller *et al.* (1951). Copyright 1951 by the American Psychological Association. Reprinted by permission.]

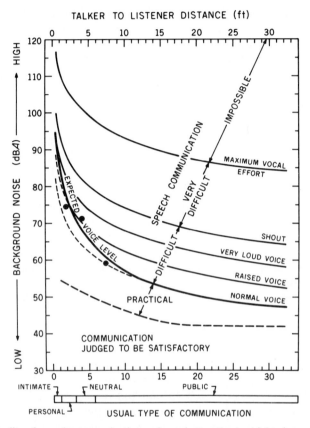

FIG. 14. Quality of speech communication as dependent on the *A*-weighted sound level (dB*A*) of the background noise and the distance between the talker and listener. The heavy data points represent scores of 90% correct with tests done with phonetically balanced lists of one-syllable words (Waltzman & Levitt, 1971). The dashed contour is extrapolated from Beranek (1960, pp. 515–518). The types of speech communication typical of various talker–listener distances are based on observation (Hall, 1959). [Modified from Webster (1969), SIL—Past, present, and future, *Journal of Sound and Vibration*, **3**, 22–26.]

A-weighted sound level of the background noise in decibels. The horizontal axis is the distance between talker and listener in feet. Accurate and useful communication is possible in the region below each solid contour when the talker uses the indicated degree of vocal effort. However, such communication seems to require additional exertion on the part of talker and listener. When frequent speech communication is demanded, as is the case for many office workers and executives, then an environment will not be judged satisfactory unless the *A*-weighted sound levels fall below the dashed contour.

The heaviest contour, labeled with "expected voice level," reflects the fact that the usual talker unconsciously raises his voice level when he is surrounded by noise. Therefore, practical (accurate and useful) speech communication is possible in the region falling under this heaviest contour without a conscious increase in vocal effort.

Consider the example of a talker in the quiet who wishes to speak to a listener near a running faucet. The A-weighted sound level of the background noise may be about 74 dB for the listener. If the talker is 20 ft away, it is clear from Figs. 14 and 15, as well as from everyday experience, that communication would be difficult even if the talker were to shout. But, if the talker were to move within 1 ft of the listener, communication would be practical even when a normal voice is used. It can be seen that at 15–20 ft, distances not uncommon to many living rooms or classrooms, A-weighted sound levels of the background noise must be below 50 dB if speech communication is to be nearly normal.

People vary their voice levels and distances not only in accordance with the level of background noise and physical convenience, but also in accordance with cultural standards (Hall, 1959). Distances less than about $4\frac{1}{2}$ ft tend to be reserved for confidential or personal exchanges usually with a lowered voice. Distances greater than about 5 ft are usually associated with a slightly raised voice and reserved for messages that others are welcome to hear. Thus, levels of background noise that require the talker and listener to

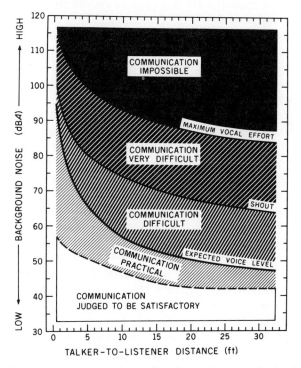

FIG. 15. Simplified chart that shows the quality of speech communication in relation to the A-weighted sound level of noise (dBA) and the distance between the talker and the listener.

move within less than 4 ft may be upsetting to persons who do not normally have an intimate association. When the content of the message is personal, there will be reluctance to raise the voice level even if the background noise demands it for intelligibility.

In face-to-face personal conversations, the distance from talker to listener is usually of the order of 5 ft and practical speech communication can proceed in A-weighted noise levels as high as 66 dB. Many conversations involve groups, and for this situation distances of 5–12 ft are common and the intensity level of the background noise should be less than 50–60 dB. At public meetings or outdoors in yards, parks, or playgrounds distances between talker and listener are often of the order of 12–30 ft, and the A-weighted sound level of the background noise must be kept below 45–55 dB if practical speech communication is to be possible.

d. CHARACTERISTICS OF PEOPLE (SPEECH, AGE, AND HEARING) AND SPEECH INTERFERENCE BY NOISE. The contours of Figs. 14 and 15 represent conditions for young adults who speak the same dialect when they are in a diffuse noise field. The location of these contours would shift in accordance with many variables. Lower noise levels would be required if the talker has imprecise speech (poor articulation) or if the talker and the listener speak different dialects. Children have less precise speech than do adults (Eguchi & Hirsh, 1969), and also their lack of vocabulary or different concepts of the rules of language may render speech unintelligible when some of the cues in the speech stream are lost. Thus, adequate speech communication with children under about 13 years of age probably requires lower noise levels than are required for adults. One's ability to understand partially masked or distorted speech seems to begin to deteriorate at about age 30, and declines steadily thereafter (Palva & Jodinen, 1970). Generally, the older the listener, the lower the background noise must be for practical or satisfactory communication. It is well known that persons with hearing losses require more favorable speech-to-noise ratios than do those with normal hearing. This group again requires lower noise levels for practical speech communication than do young adults with normal hearing.

e. SITUATIONAL FACTORS (MESSAGE PREDICTABILITY, OPPORTUNITY FOR LIP READING, SPATIAL ARRANGEMENTS AND REVERBERATION, AND KINDS OF NOISE) AND SPEECH INTERFERENCE BY NOISE. Of course, adequate communication in higher noise levels than those indicated in Figs. 14 and 15 can occur if the possible messages are predictable. Thus, at ball games, we may be able to discriminate the umpire's "ball" and "strike" at much greater distances and in more intense levels of noise than indicated on the chart. This factor accounts for the success of communication in many industrial situations with high levels of noise. Success may give way to failure, however, when an important but *unpredictable* message must be communicated. For example, firemen in a high-level noise may have little difficulty with standard communications about the use of equipment, but may encounter grave difficulty communicating about unexpected events that occur at the scene of the fire.

The opportunity to lip-read or use facial or bodily gestures in support of hearing will improve the success of communication in background noise. Almost everyone has some small amount of lip-reading skill which they often use without awareness of its contribution to intelligibility.

Spatial variables also may facilitate speech communication in noise. If the source of noise is clearly localized in a position different from that of the talker, speech communication may be possible under noise conditions less favorable than those indicated in Figs. 14 and 15. On the other hand, spatial factors can sometimes reduce the intelligibility of speech. If a space produces many reflections of sound, it is said to be reverberant or lively. Noise interferes with speech communication more in a very reverberant space than in one that is not.

Sometimes unusual acoustic conditions can make our voices clearly audible at great distances. If one raises his voice to talk to a nearby person over the sound of a power lawnmower or outboard motor, he can sometimes be heard more clearly by a distant accidental spectator than by the nearby friend.

The exact characteristics of the noise are also important for predicting speech communication. While the A-weighted noise level is an adequate measure of many noises, some situations and noises demand a more complicated analysis of the noise. A discussion of the use of the various methods of measuring noise to predict speech interference can be found elsewhere (Kryter, 1970, pp. 70–91).

2. Implications of Masking and Interference with Speech Communication

a. Masking of auditory signals. Many auditory signals serve important functions in our lives, and these functions may be lost in noise. While the masking of a doorbell because of noise may only be a source of inconvenience and annoyance, other times masking can interfere with the performance of important tasks. In the extreme, the masking of a signal such as that of an approaching vehicle can lead to property damage, personal injury, or even death.

b. Interference with speech communication. The implications of reduced opportunity for nearly normal speech communication are considerable.

Those who must work in high levels of background noise claim that they "get used to it." There is evidence, however, that they adopt a "noncommunicating life style" and increase their use of nonverbal communication through gestures, posture, and facial expression (Kryter, 1970, p. 459). Even though nonverbal communication is important, it is unlikely that it is nearly as important as verbal communication. Many subtleties of life are lost when verbal communication is restricted.

Among adults, free and easy speech communication is probably essential for full development of social relations and self.

For very young children, there may be an additional problem. They gradually induce their knowledge of language and its subtleties from the speech to which they are exposed. Also, previously stated, because their knowledge of language is still developing, children probably have more difficulty understanding speech in noise than do adults. Because noise can reduce the amount of speech used at home, in the yard, or on the playground—and because noise can make speech difficult to understand—it is possible, though unproven, that the language development of early childhood might be adversely affected. From this, difficulty in learning language and learning to read may ensue. One can only guess at how severe the noise must be to produce such effects; nearly continuous A-weighted sound levels in excess of 70 dB might be required. Such conditions do exist at some residences in urban areas near freeways. When contemplating possible increases in general levels of community noise, one should give consideration to these possible effects on the linguistic development of children.

Later, school-age children probably encounter more difficulty in noisy classrooms than, for example, do sailors in noisy engine rooms who exchange a limited number of prescribed technical messages. With regard to the impact of noise on formal education, the Jamaica Bay Environmental Study Group of the National Academy of Sciences summarized their findings as follows:

> Within the present impacted area (NEF 30 or greater) there are 220 schools attended by 280,000 pupils. With normal school-room usage, this implies about an hour's interruption of classroom teaching each day and the development by the teachers of the "jet pause" teaching technique to accommodate the impossibility of communicating with the pupils as an aircraft passes overhead. The noise interference goes beyond the periods of enforced noncommunication, for it destroys the spontaneity of the educational process and subjects it to the rhythm of the aeronautical control system. Given the advanced age of many of these schools, noise-proofing (where possible) would cost an appreciable fraction of their replacement cost.

Any casual observer of intimate family life is aware of the irritation and confusion that can arise when simple, everyday messages need frequent repetition in order to be understood. Noise does not cause all of these occurrences, but surely it causes some.

The enjoyment of retirement and later life can be hampered by masking noises. It is well known that speech reception abilities deteriorate with age and clinical observations clearly indicate that older persons are more susceptible to the masking of speech by noise than are young adults.

It is likely that one must somehow "work harder" to maintain speech reception in noise than in quiet. Thus, successful speech communication in noise probably has its cost. If the cost is too high, the number of verbal exchanges declines.

In a highly intellectual, technical society, speech communication plays an extremely important role. Background noise can influence the accuracy, frequency, and quality of verbal exchange. In excessive background noise, formal education in schools, occupational efficiency, family life styles, and the quality of relaxation can all be adversely affected.

References

Beranek, L. L. (Ed.) *Noise reduction.* New York: McGraw-Hill, 1960. P. 732.

Botsford, J. H. Theory of temporary threshold shift. *Journal of the Acoustical Society of America,* 1971, **49**, 440–446.

Bredberg, G. Cellular pattern and supply of the human organ of corti. *Acta Oto-Laryngologica,* 1968, Suppl. 236, 135.

Butterfield, E. C., & Siperstein, G. N. Influence of contingent auditory stimulation upon non-nutritional suckle. Paper presented at the Third Symposium on Oral Sensation and Perception: The Mouth of the Infant, 1970. [Proceedings to be published by Charles C Thomas, Springfield, Illinois.]

Carder, H. M., & Miller, J. D. Temporary threshold shifts produced by noise exposures of long duration. *Journal of Speech and Hearing Research,* 1972, **15**, 603–623.

Cohen, A., Anticaglia, J., & Jones, H. H. Sociocusis'—Hearing loss from non-occupational noise exposure. *Journal of Sound and Vibration,* 1970, **4**, 12–20.

Davis, H. Guide for the classification and evaluation of hearing handicap in relation to the international audiometric zero. *Transactions of the American Academy of Ophthalmology and Otolaryngology,* 1965, **69**, 740–751.

Davis, H., Morgan, C. T., Hawkins, J. E., Galambos, R., & Smith, F. Temporary deafness following exposure to loud tones and noise. *Acta Oto-Laryngologica,* 1950, **88**.

Eguchi, S., & Hirsh, I. J. Development of speech sounds in children. *Acta Oto-Laryngologica,* 1969, Suppl. 257, 51.

Glorig, A., & Davis, H. Age, noise, and hearing loss. *Annales d'Otologie, Rhinologie et Laryngologie,* 1961, **70**, 556–571.

Hall, E. T. *The silent language.* New York: Doubleday, 1959.

Hirsh, I. J. *The measurement of hearing.* New York: McGraw-Hill, 1952.

Jeffress, L. A. Masking. In J. V. Tobias (Ed.), *Foundations of modern auditory theory.* Vol. 1. New York: Academic Press, 1970. Pp. 85–114.

Kryter, K. *The effects of noise on man.* New York: Academic Press, 1970.

Kryter, K. D., Ward, W. D., Miller, J. D., & Eldredge, D. H. Hazardous exposure to intermittent and steady-state noise. *Journal of the Acoustical Society of America,* 1966, **39**, 451–464.

Miller, G. A., Heise, G. A., & Lichten, W. The intelligibility of speech as a function of the context of the test materials. *Journal of Experimental Psychology,* 1951, **41**, 329–335.

Miller, J. D., Rothenberg, S. J., & Eldredge, D. H. Preliminary observations on the effects of exposure to noise for seven days on the hearing and inner ear of the chinchilla. *Journal of the Acoustical Society of America,* 1971, **50**, 1199–1203.

Miller, J. D., Watson, C. S., & Covell, W. P. Deafening effects of noise on the cat. *Acta Oto-Laryngologica,* 1963, Suppl. 176, 91.

Mills, J. H., Gengel, R. W., Watson, C. S., & Miller, J. D. Temporary changes of the auditory system due to exposure to noise for one or two days. *Journal of the Acoustical Society of America,* 1970, **48**, 524–530.

Mosko, J. D., Fletcher, J. L., & Luz, G. A. Growth and recovery of temporary threshold shifts following extended exposure to high-level, continuous noise (U.S. AMRL Rep. No. 911). Fort Knox, Kentucky: U.S. AMRL, 1970.

Niemeyer, W. Speech discrimination in noise-induced deafness. *Internal Audiology*, 1967, **6**, 42–47.

Nixon, J. C., & Glorig, A. Noise-induced permanent threshold shift at 2000 cps and 4000 cps. *Journal of the Acoustical Society of America*, 1961, **33**, 904–908.

Palva, A., & Jodinen, K. Presbyacusis. V. Filtered speech test. *Acta Oto-Laryngologica*, 1970, **70**, 232–241.

Radcliffe, J. C., *et al.* Guidelines for noise exposure control. *Journal of Sound and Vibration*, 1970, **4**, 21–24.

Scharf, B. Critical bands. In J. V. Tobias (Ed.), *Foundations of modern auditory theory.* Vol. 1. New York: Academic Press, 1970. Pp. 157–202.

Taylor, G. D., & Williams, E. Acoustic trauma in the sports hunter. *Laryngoscope*, 1966, **76**, 863–879.

Taylor, W., Pearson, J., Mair, A., & Burns, W. Study of noise and hearing in jute weaving. *Journal of the Acoustical Society of America*, 1965, **38**, 113–120.

von Gierke, H. E. On noise and vibration exposure criteria. *Archives of Environmental Health*, 1965, **2**, 327–339.

Waltzman, S., & Levitt, H. Personal communication, 1971.

Ward, W. D. Recovery from high values of temporary threshold shift. *Journal of the Acoustical Society of America*, 1960, **32**, 497–500.

Ward, W. D. Auditory fatigue and masking. In J. Jerger (Ed.), *Modern developments in audiology.* New York: Academic Press, 1963. Pp. 240–286.

Ward, W. D. Temporary threshold shift in males and females. *Journal of the Acoustical Society of America*, 1966, **40**, 478–485.

Ward, W. D. Susceptibility to auditory fatigue. In W. D. Neff (Ed.), *Contributions to sensory physiology.* Vol. 3. New York: Academic Press, 1968. Pp. 192–225. (a)

Ward, W. D., (Ed.) Proposed damage-risk criterion for impulse noise (gunfire) (U) (Rep. WG-57). Washington, D.C.: NAS–NRC Committee on Hearing and Bioacoustical Biomechanics, 1968. (b)

Ward, W. D. Hearing loss and audio engineering. *Sound Engineering Magazine*, 1970, **4**, 21–23. (a)

Ward, W. D. Temporary threshold shift and damage-risk criteria for intermittent noise exposures. *Journal of the Acoustical Society of America*, 1970, **48**, 571–574(b)

Ward, W. D., & Glorig, A. A case of firecracker-induced hearing loss. *Laryngoscope*, 1961, **71**, 1590–1596.

Ward, W. D., Glorig, A., & Sklar, D. L. Temporary threshold shift from octave-band noise: Applications to damage-risk criteria. *Journal of the Acoustical Society of America*, 1959, **31**, 522–528. (a)

Ward, W. D., Glorig, A., & Sklar, D. L. Relation between recovery from temporary threshold shift and duration of exposure. *Journal of the Acoustical Society of America*, 1959, **31**, 600–602. (b)

Webster, J. C. SIL—Past, present, and future. *Journal of Sound and Vibration*, 1969, **3**, 22–26.

Yoshii, U. Expirementelle Untersuchungen über die Schadigung des Gehörorgans durch Schalleinwirkung. *Zeitschrift für Ohrenheilkunde*, 1909, **58**, 201–251.

Chapter 15

GENERAL PSYCHOLOGICAL AND SOCIOLOGICAL EFFECTS OF NOISE*

J. D. MILLER

I. INTRODUCTION

Noise not only has direct effects on auditory function as previously described, but it also produces other behavioral effects of a more general nature. Included among these effects are "interference with sleep"; the general evaluation of auditory experience included under "loudness, preceived noisiness, and unacceptability"; and "annoyance and community response." All of these areas have been investigated and certain clear-cut patterns have emerged. Plausible, but less thoroughly studied behavioral

* Chapters 14, 15, and 16 originally appeared in the *Journal of the Acoustical Society of America*, Vol. 56, No. 3, September 1974, pp. 729–764. © 1974 Acoustical Society of America. Reprinted by permission of the Acoustical Society of America.

effects of noise are discussed under "other possible psychological and sociological effects."

Many of the psychological and sociological effects of noise can be traced to the role of hearing in man's evolutionary development as described in Chapter 14. Others may be linked more specifically to the auditory effects described in Chapter 14, Section II, or to the general physiological responses to be described in Chapter 16. Because of these interrelations among the effects of noise on people, the organization of topics is necessarily somewhat arbitrary.

II. INTERFERENCE WITH SLEEP

The effects of noise on sleep are discussed at greater length in this chapter than are other effects of equal or greater importance. This was done because other reviews of the effects of noise on people have given relatively less attention to the subject of sleep disturbance.

From everyday experience it is evident that sound can interfere with sleep. Almost all have been wakened or kept from falling to sleep by loud, strange, frightening, or annoying sounds, and it is commonplace to be waked by an alarm clock or clock radio. But it also appears that one can "get used to" sounds and sleep through them. Possibly, environmental sounds only disturb sleep when they are unfamiliar. If so, disturbance of sleep would depend only on the frequency of unusual or novel sounds. Everyday experience also suggests that sound can help to induce sleep and, perhaps, to maintain it. The soothing lullaby, the steady hum of a fan, or the rhythmic sound of the surf can serve to induce relaxation. Perhaps certain steady sounds can serve as an acoustical eyeshade and mask possibly disturbing transient sounds.

Common anecdotes about sleep disturbance suggest an even greater complexity. A rural person may have difficult sleeping in a noisy urban area. An urban person may be disturbed by the quiet, the sounds of animals, and so on when sleeping in a rural area. And how is it that a mother may wake to a slight stirring of her child, yet sleep through a thunderstorm? These observations all suggest that the relations between exposure to sound and the quality of a night's sleep are complicated. They are. Nonetheless, research is beginning to untangle the story.

Before these studies are described, it will be necessary to consider the problem of the nature of sleep. There has been significant headway in the description of a night of sleep. Sleep is a complicated series of states rather than a single, uniform state. Experiments verify the common belief that sleep is essential for normal functions while awake. But the "hows" and "whys" are unknown, and therefore, it is difficult to state flatly that this or that alteration in sleep is harmful. One must rely on everyday wisdom for these judgments.

A. Methods for Studying Sleep Disturbance by Noise

a. FIELD STUDIES. One of the most obvious and direct methods is to interview people who live in areas that receive various exposures to noise. People can be asked whether the noise prevents them from falling asleep or whether it wakes them from sleep. Of course, if such direct questions are embedded in a series of questions concerning noise and sound, the answers may be biased by the person's attitude toward the source of sound. It may be better to ask about the quality of sleep, the number of hours slept, judgments about well-being upon arising, and so on in the context of a survey unrelated to noise.

b. LABORATORY STUDIES. Typically, a subject sleeps in a special laboratory bedroom where his physiological state can be monitored from electrodes attached to his body, and calibrated sounds can be presented by loudspeakers or by other sound-making instruments. By these techniques subtle responses to sounds or subtle changes in the pattern of sleep can be recorded and measured. Furthermore, a variety of instructions and adaptation procedures can be tested. However, such research is very slow, hard work; the required apparatus is expensive; usually only a few subjects can be studied; and the routine is demanding on the experimenter. Furthermore, even though the subjects are adapted to the routine, they are not at home and they are constrained by electrodes and wires. In spite of these difficulties, however, some rather clear trends have emerged.

B. General Properties of Sleep

a. SLEEP STAGES AND A NIGHT OF SLEEP. Examination of brain waves, other physiological measures, responsiveness, behavior, and the sequence of events during a night's sleep have led to the concept of sleep stages or states. There are recognizably different patterns that occur during a period of sleep. Since these patterns blend from one to another, there are several schemes for categorizing them into sleep stages or states. A popular set of categories is labeled I, II, III, IV, and I-REM. Another set of stages is defined in a slightly different manner. They are labeled A, B, C, D, and E. Some authors even combine the two sets of definitions.

Perhaps the easiest approach to these stages is to follow an idealized progression as one falls asleep. As one relaxes and enters a stage of drowsiness, the pattern of the electroencephalogram (EEG) changes from a jumble of rapid, irregular waves to the regular 9–12 Hz pattern known as the alpha rhythm. One is relaxed, but not asleep. Later, the alpha rhythm diminishes in amplitude and intermittently disappears. This is sleep stage A. As time progresses, the alpha rhythm is present less and less often until it disappears and is replaced by a low-voltage, fast, irregular pattern in the EEG; this is stage B. In the roman numeral system, stage I corresponds to the late portions of stage A and all of stage B.

Next, there appear quick bursts of larger amplitude waves known as spindles or the spindles of sleep. Mixed with these spindles there will appear small-amplitude, low-frequency (1.5–3 Hz) waves known as delta waves. This stage is known as stage C or stage II. In the next stage of sleep, the spindles disappear and the delta waves become more regular and grow in amplitude. This is known as stage D. Later, the delta waves become even larger and of lower frequency (.61–1 Hz). This is stage E. The roman numeral system III and IV include stages D and E but the criterion for division is different. Stages D and E or III and IV are often referred to as deep or delta sleep.

The purpose is not to confuse the reader with two sets of sleep stages, but rather to communicate the idea that there is a progression of sleep stages. One can reasonably divide this progression by various criteria. Generally, in stage A or early I, man is drowsy, but awake. In stage B, or late I, one drifts or "floats" back and forth between waking and sleeping. When awakened at this stage of sleep, one is not quite sure whether he has been asleep. Stages C, D, and E or II, III, and IV represent definite sleep.

The remaining stage, which has been of great interest, is the so-called *R*apid *E*ye *M*ovement (REM) stage of sleep. In REM sleep, the sleeper exhibits characteristics of stage I (late A and B). These are fast, low-voltage brain waves; other evidence of variable but definite physiological activation; and rapid eye movements. Consequently, this stage is usually tagged I-REM. While dreaming and mental activity can take place in all sleep stages, it is during I-REM that most dreams occur.

A typical night's sleep initially follows a progression, with occasional reversals, from stages A(I) to stages D and E(IV). This progression usually occurs within the first 80 min of sleep. After about 90 min of sleep, one has left stage IV and has had a period of I-REM. A 90-min cycle from I-REM to I-REM tends to recur throughout the period of sleep. There are, however, some irregularities and some systematic changes.

Roughly equal amounts of time are spent in I-REM and in IV. Early in the sleep period more time is spent in IV than in I-REM, and later in the sleep period more time is spent in I-REM than in IV. Generally, after the first 80–90 min of sleep, more and more time is spent in the "lighter" stages of sleep. These facts are summarized in Fig. 1. Overall, sleeping young adults distribute sleep as follows: Stage I—5%, Stage I-REM—20–25%; Stage II—50%; and Stages III and IV—20% (Berger, 1969).

Even after falling asleep, one wakes up during the night. Roughly, 5% of the total period of "sleep" is spent awake from adolescence to about age 40. From ages 40 to 90 the time awake during "sleep" increases to nearly 20% (Feinberg, 1969). The number of times one wakes up after falling asleep increases from an average of about two at age 6 to six at age 90 (Feinberg, 1969).

   b. SENSORY RESPONSES TO STIMULATION DURING SLEEP. The sense organs

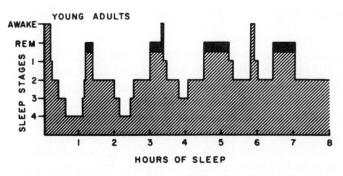

FIG. 1. The nocturnal sleep pattern of young adults is shown. During the latter part of the sleep period stage IV is absent and more time is spent in Stage II and in REM. Notice the two brief periods that the sleeper spontaneously awoke. [From Berger (1969) in *Sleep Physiology and Pathology*, A. Kales, Ed., by permission of J. B. Lippincott Company.]

are just as sensitive to their appropriate physical stimuli during sleep as they are during wakefulness. One may wonder whether mechanisms near the periphery of the nervous system somehow "block" the sensory pathways during sleep. Such mechanisms would prevent the neural messages from the sense organs from reaching the higher centers of the brain. Available research (Koella, 1967) does not support this view. Rather, one can state quite strongly that information from the sense organs does reach the highest centers of the brain even during deepest sleep. This conclusion is based on the fact that electrical responses to stimuli can be recorded in the highest center of the brains of sleeping or anesthetized men and animals. These responses usually are of brief duration and have latencies of .01–.8 sec.

Therefore, the apparent indifference to stimulation during sleep is not a simple "shutting out" of the neural messages at or near the periphery of the nervous system close to the sense organ. Rather, this apparent indifference to external stimulation is due to a complicated reorganization of brain processes during sleeping as opposed to waking states.

c. AROUSAL. Sensory messages reach the highest centers of the brain, but whether or not they influence the sleeper will depend on a complicated set of circumstances. Many theorists believe that mechanisms in the brain busily carry out "sleep work" throughout the sleeping period. These mechanisms assess the significance of incoming sensory messages and adjust the state of the brain in accordance with the sensory message and the whole situational complex. This view is supported by everyday experience as well as by scientific investigation.

Arousal from sleep can be recognized by brief changes in physiological function; by shifts from deeper to lighter stages of sleep; or by behavioral evidence of awakening. Some of the properties of arousal mechanisms will become apparent as the effects of noise on sleep are discussed.

C. Noise and Sleep

a. EFFECTS OF BRIEF NOISES. In the area of sleep disturbance by noise it is the effects of relatively brief noises (about 3 min or less) on a person sleeping in a quiet environment that have been studied most thoroughly. Typically, presentations of the sounds are widely spaced throughout a sleep period of 5–7 hours.

A summary of some of these observations is presented on Fig. 2. The heavy dashed lines are hypothetical curves which represent the percent wakings under conditions in which the subject *(1)* is a normally rested young adult male who has been adapted for several nights to the procedures of a quiet sleep laboratory, *(2)* has been instructed to press an easily reached button to indicate that he has waked, and *(3)* has been moderately motivated to wake and respond to the noise (such motivation can be established by instructions which imply that somehow the subject's ability is being tested). A datum for sleep stage II is indicated by an arabic two (2). A datum for sleep stages III and IV is indicated by a Greek delta (Δ). While in stage II, subjects can wake to sounds that are about 30–40 dB above the level at which they can be detected when subjects are conscious, alert, and attentive. While in deep sleep, stages III or IV, the stimulus may have to be 50–80 dB above the level at which they can be detected by conscious, alert, attentive subjects before they will wake the sleeping subject.

The solid lines in Fig. 2 are data from questionnaire studies of persons who live near airports. The percentage of respondents who claim that flyovers wake them or keep them from falling asleep is plotted against the A-weighted sound level of a single flyover (Wyle Staff, 1971). These curves are for the case of approximately 30 flyovers spaced over the normal sleep period of 6–8 hours. The filled circles represent the percentage of sleepers that wake to a 3-min sound at each A-weighted sound level (dBA) or lower. This curve is based on data from 350 persons, each tested in his own bedroom (Steinicke, 1957). These measures were made between 2:00 and 7:00 a.m., and it is reasonable to assume that most of the subjects were roused from stages II or I-REM.

b. MOTIVATION TO WAKE AND INTENSITY LEVEL OF THE NOISE. There is clear evidence that motivation to wake can influence the probability of waking to noise (Williams *et al.*, 1965; Watson & Rechtschaffen, 1969; Wilson & Zung, 1966). The effects of motivation, however, depend on the stage of sleep and the intensity level of the noise. For weak stimuli, motivation may have a strong influence on arousal only during light sleep (Williams *et al.*, 1965). For moderately strong stimuli, motivation to wake may have a powerful effect on the probability of an upward shift in sleep stage (probably awakening also) from all depths of sleep (Wilson & Zung, 1966). With very intense stimuli it is likely that motivation would have little influence; for example, brief noises with A-weighted sound levels of 100–120 dB wake nearly everyone from any stage of sleep.

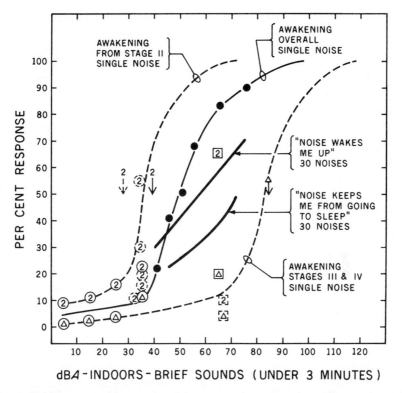

FIG. 2. Wakings to sound from various laboratory and questionnaire studies are shown. The horizontal axis gives the approximate A-weighted sound level (dBA) of the noise. The curves labeled "wakings" are from normally rested young adults who were sleeping in a laboratory and were moderately motivated to awake in response to sound. The percentage of responses will depend not only on the intensity of the sound but also on the definition of "waking," the motivation of the subject to wake in response to sound, and the sleep stages I, II, III, IV, or I-REM) when the stimulus is presented. The questionnaire results, "Noise wakes me up," and "Noise keeps me from going to sleep," are derived from the Wilson Report (1963) for the case of 30 brief noises distributed throughout the night. The laboratory results are from various studies. The filed circles were gathered throughout the night without regard to sleep stage (Steinicke, 1957). Data from sleep stage II are represented by 2's; those from sleep stages III and IV by deltas (Δ). The circles with unbroken borders are from Williams *et al.* (1964). The circles with broken borders are from Williams *et al.* (1965). The boxes with solid borders are from Rechtschaffen *et al.* (1966). The boxes with broken borders are from Lukas and Kryter (1970). The broken arrow is from Watson and Rechtschaffen (1969). The solid arrows are from Kryter and Williams (1970).

The effects of motivation are illustrated indirectly on Fig. 2. The results of Lukas and Kryter (1970) are the boxes with broken borders that lie toward the lower right of the graph. Here, waking is defined in the experimental setting by instructions that imply "if you happen to wake up, push the button." The button is located on the headboard of the bed and requires that the subject find it (often having to turn over to do so) and press it. This definition of waking is similar, perhaps, to a spontaneous nocturnal waking.

The ascending series of stage 2 wakings for stimuli of 30–40 dB (encircled by broken lines on Fig. 2) are from Williams *et al.* (1965). The ascending percentage of waking is correlated with the sleeper's motivation, as controlled by instructions and punishments for failure to respond by pushing a convenient button. As the motivation to wake was increased, the percentage of wakings showed a fivefold increase from less than 11% to about 55% of the presentations of the same noise at the same stage of sleep.

c. FLUCTUATING NOISE LEVEL. A very important and extensive study of the effects of noise on sleep was done at the Centre d'Etudes Bioclimatiques du CNRS in Strasbourg, France (Schieber, Mery, & Muzet, 1968). Several measures of the quality of sleep were used. These included the amount of time in each of the sleep stages; the numbers of brief wakings as evidenced by the appearance of alpha waves in the electroencephalogram; the number of bodily movements; the degree of muscular tension; the occurrence of perturbations in heart rate; the presence of eye movements; and the occurrence of various components of the electroencephalogram such as K-complexes, sleep spindles, alpha waves, theta waves, and delta waves. Artificial sounds (crescendos of white noise that rose to about 80 dB in 10 sec and were terminated abruptly), sounds of air-craft flyovers with peak values of 72 and 89 dB (either 16 or 33 per night), or traffic noises were used in various experiments. The time required to fall asleep was longer for noise than control conditions. Under control conditions, about 26 min elapsed between going to bed and the first occurrence of stage IV. Under traffic noise, the delay between going to bed and the first occurrence of stage IV was 33 or 53 min, depending on the type of noise. When noises were presented, there was a tendency for sleep to be much lighter than normal for the first half of the night and slightly deeper than normal for the second half of the night. Thus, there was a tendency to compensate for the loss of deep sleep in the early part of the night by an increase in deep sleep in the later part of the night. Nonetheless, almost all measures of sleep disturbance indicated that sleep was disturbed overall and throughout the sleep period.

The results with traffic noise were of particular interest. These sounds were actually recorded in a bedroom near a busy street. One set of recordings was made between 10:00 p.m. and midnight. Another was made between midnight and 4:00 a.m. The 10:00 p.m. to midnight sample represented about 4.3 vehicles passing per minute, while the midnight to 4:00 a.m. sample had only about 1.8 vehicles per minute. The peaks in both samples reached A-weighted sound levels of nearly 80 dB, but the long-term averages were 70 dB for the high-density traffic and only 61 dB for the low-density traffic. The control night had steady ventilation noise with a median A-weighted sound level of 48 dB. The interesting fact was that the low-density traffic pattern was more disruptive of sleep than was the high-density pattern. However, both traffic patterns were more disruptive than the control noise.

These results strongly suggest that fluctuations in the noise levels and degree of fluctuation are important factors in determining sleep disturbance by sound.

d. STEADY AND RHYTHMIC SOUNDS. It seems plausible that steady or rhythmic sounds might improve the quality of sleep. Certainly, anecdotal evidence suggests that steady sounds can mask out brief disturbing sounds and that some periodic or rhythmic sounds have certain soothing qualities. Investigations along these lines are badly needed. Pertinent questions are

(1) At what levels do steady sounds begin to adversely influence sleep patterns?

(2) Can a moderate amount of masking noise reduce the influence of brief sounds on sleep, or are brief sounds that suddenly emerge above a masking noise more disturbing than those that simply join the usual rise and fall of community noise?

(3) Can sleep be induced and maintained by particular rhythms of sound?

One investigation of complaints about noises produced by air-conditioning and heating equipment may be relevant to the effects of steady noise on sleep (Blazier, 1959). From complaint files, conversations with dealers and distributers, and field trips to problem sites, the investigator found what types of noises in bedrooms resulted in adverse responses. He also noted that the fewer the complaints, the greater the customer's acceptance of the product.

It was found that people especially objected to noises that included "tones" and "throbbing" or "beats." Blazier summarized the frequency of complaints in relation to A-weighted sound levels of noises in sleeping quarters as follows: Below about 33 dB, no complaints; 33–38 dB, occasional complaints, 38–48 dB, frequent complaints; and over about 48 dB, unlimited complaints. While it is not known whether these complaints are due to sleep disturbance or other factors, these results do appear to be in remarkable agreement with the trends for sleep disturbance by brief noises shown in Fig. 2.

e. SOUND QUALITY AND SLEEP DISTURBANCE. As yet we have no evidence on the role that pitch, timbre, and temporal structure play in sleep disturbance or enhancement. Until such data are forthcoming, it may be useful to assume that those variables that influence perceived noisiness would similarly influence sleep disturbance.

f. SLEEP DEPRIVATION AND SLEEP DISTURBANCE. Subjects who have been deprived of sleep require more intense noises for waking than do normally rested subjects (Williams et al., 1965).

g. DIFFERENCE BETWEEN MEN AND WOMEN. One study found that women tended to wake to noises of lower levels than did men (Steinicke, 1957). Another study (Wilson & Zung, 1966) found a clear difference in arousal as defined by upward shifts in sleep stage. In response to noise, women shifted toward lighter stages of sleep much more frequently than did men. Lukas (1971) finds that sleep disturbance from subsonic-aircraft noise or sonic booms is greater for middle-aged women than for middle-aged men. Thus, it appears that women's sleep is more easily disturbed by noise than is men's, even when other variables such as motivation and stage of sleep are equated.

h. AGE AND SLEEP DISTURBANCE BY NOISE. There is clear evidence that persons over about 60 years of age are much more easily waked or shifted towards lighter sleep stages than are middle-aged adults or children (Lukas & Kryter, 1970). This effect is large and dramatic. More specifically, simulated sonic booms that wake middle-aged adults and 7- and 8-year-old children on less than 5% of their occurrences will wake 69- to 72-year-old adults on nearly 70% of their occurrences. These dramatic differences hold over all stages of sleep. Also, once awake, an older person has more difficulty in returning to sleep than does a middle-aged adult or a child. There is no evidence that children are especially sensitive to sleep disturbance by noise. On the contrary, Lukas et al. (1971) found that 7- and 8-year-old children are slightly less sensitive to noise during sleep than are middle-aged adults. However, since general sleep disturbance in children (enuresis, somnambulism, night terrors, and nightmares) seems to peak between 4 and 6 years of age (Broughton, 1968; Feinberg, 1969; Jacobson et al., 1969; Kessler, 1966), one suspects that sleep disturbance by noise may have a special impact on children in this age range. It is well known, for instance, that thunderstorms can wake and frighten children of these ages. Children in the age group of 4 to 6 years seem to be particularly disturbed by sudden arousal from stage IV of sleep (Broughton, 1968).

i. SLEEP STAGE AND ACCUMULATED SLEEP. In terms of either behavioral waking or an upward shift in sleep stage as indicated by the electroencephalogram, sleep can be influenced most easily in stages I and II and least easily in stages III and IV. Sometimes I-REM seems to be more like III and IV in this regard; other times it is more like stages I and II. A person can be aroused from sleep more easily the longer he has slept no matter what the stage of sleep (Lukas & Kryter, 1970; Rechtschaffen et al., 1966; Williams et al., 1964).

j. STIMULUS MEANING AND FAMILIARITY. The effects of stimulus meaning and familiarity are closely bound to those of motivation and stimulus intensity. There is considerable evidence that people can discriminate among stimuli while asleep if the differences were learned and the discrimination was established while they were awake (Williams et al., 1965; Wilson & Zung, 1966). In a classic experiment, Oswald et al. (1960) demonstrated that sleeping subjects will respond when their own names are spoken but show few responses to other names. Generally, when auditory stimuli are faint and similar, discriminations are probably performed better in light sleep (I, II, and I-REM) than during deep sleep (III and IV). The effect of stimulus familiarity on arousal from sleep has not been studied extensively. In one experiment, small but consistent differences were found between familiar and unfamiliar sounds. "Familiar" sounds shifted sleep stages less frequently than "unfamiliar" sounds (Zung & Wilson, 1961).

k. ADAPTATION TO SLEEP DISTURBANCE BY NOISE. Whether adaptation takes place is the subject of considerable debate. A reasonable guess at this story is as follows. The stronger the stimulus, the less likely it is that total adaptation will take place. Behavioral waking and time awake after arousal will probably show the most adaptation. Upward shifts in sleep stage are likely to show some adaptation, but less than behavioral waking. Brief responses in the electroencephalogram and autonomic responses such as changes in heart rate, blood flow, skin resistance, and so on appear to show very little adaptation. The most significant and surprising finding has been that adaptation, even in behavioral waking, has been absent (Thiessen, 1970) or slight (Lukas & Kryter, 1970). The adaptation that seems apparent from everyday experience may be the result of *(1)* changes in the motivation to wake; and *(2)* amnesia for having been awake. The last point is supported by the observation of sleep researchers that subjects in their laboratories often cannot remember and often underestimate the number of times that they awake during a sleep period.

There is clear evidence for adaptation to the total sleeping environment. Sleep researchers talk of the "first night" effect. Normal sleep is rarely, if ever, observed during the first night in the laboratory. It is likely then that some of the disturbance reported by the rural person trying to sleep in an urban area and the urban person trying to sleep in a rural area is but the "first night" effect. It is commonplace that when we cannot sleep, for whatever reasons, we "hear" many sounds.

l. OTHER FACTORS. There are, of course, a host of other factors related to sleep and arousal from sleep (Kales, 1969). These include mental and physical disease states, drug usage, general stress, and so on. Most of these have not been studied in relation to the problem of sleep disturbance by noise. There is, however, clear evidence that male patients suffering from depression are more easily shifted from deeper to lighter stages of sleep by sounds than are normal males (Wilson & Zung, 1966). Generally, it seems probable that persons with disorders which result in light, restless sleep or frequent wakings will be more frequently aroused by sounds than will normal persons or persons with disorders that produce unusually deep and prolonged sleep. Also, it has been demonstrated that sleep deprivation has more adverse effects on "poor" than on "good" sleepers (Williams & Williams, 1966).

D. Noise, Sleep Disturbance, Health, and Quality of Life

Brief sounds of sufficient intensity and fluctuating noise levels definitely can alter the normal sleep pattern. These changes in sleep pattern are in the direction of lighter sleep. The effects of noises are to produce sleep patterns that are more like those of "poor sleepers" than "good sleepers" (Luce, 1966, pp. 105–108; Williams & Williams, 1966).

Whether such sleep disturbance constitutes a health hazard is debatable. While good sleep is necessary for physical and mental health, normal persons who lose sleep compensate by spending more time in deep sleep, by becoming less responsive to external stimuli, and by napping. Thus, it may be very difficult to deprive a normal person of sufficient sleep to produce adverse health effects.

On the other hand, the data presented here amply support the notion that people exposed to sufficient noise will complain of sleep loss. Everyday experience strongly supports the notion that a "good" sleep is important to one's feeling of well-being.

All factors considered, one must tentatively assume that sleep disturbance by excessive noise will reduce one's feelings of well-being. Furthermore, when noise conditions are so severe as to disturb sleep on a regular, unrelenting basis, then such sleep disturbance may constitute a hazard to one's physical and mental health.

III. LOUDNESS, PERCEIVED NOISINESS, AND THE QUALITY OF AUDITORY EXPERIENCE

Whether a sound is classed as noise depends in part on the quality of auditory experience it produces. If there were a comprehensive system to describe the quality of auditory experience produced by complex sounds, one could imagine a model that would relate auditory experience to physical measurements of the sounds and another model which would in turn relate the quality of the auditory experience to the annoyance produced by the sound. Unfortunately, our knowledge is not so extensive as to allow a model of this kind.

One dimension of auditory experience that has received intensive study is the judged loudness of sounds. This dimension is particularly important to problems of noise pollution and control. The adverse effects of sounds often occur because the sound is too loud, and therefore design engineers often strive to reduce the loudness of sounds generated by machines.

Another strategy has led to the development of the concept of perceived noisiness. In the absence of the model outlined in the first paragraph above, people are asked directly to judge the apparent unwantedness or noisiness of sounds. Presumably, these judgments are not only based on the quality of the auditory experience produced by the sound but also on the listener's predictions of the other adverse effects that the sound might produce.

Knowledge of loudness and perceived noisiness and their relations to the physical characteristics of sounds as well as other dimensions of auditory experience provide one class of evaluation of the auditory environment. This knowledge also provides part of the foundation for the description of annoyance and community response.

A. Measurement of Auditory Dimensions

a. FIELD STUDIES. One approach to the relations between the physical properties of sounds and judgments of loudness or noisiness is the field study and questionnaire. By this technique, people are asked either directly or indirectly to what degree they judge various sounds to be loud, noisy, or unacceptable. The characteristics of the sounds are then measured, and one attempts to find the relations between the characteristics of the sounds and the responses to them. These methods and their results are discussed in the next section, because they are most often applied to the annoyance and disturbance of activities produced by noise.

b. LABORATORY METHODS. Another approach is to bring subjects to the laboratory and ask them to judge a variety of sounds which are often artificial sounds with well-specified properties. In this way the underlying relations between the physical properties of sounds and their judged quality can be determined. Three types of procedures are often used.

Category scaling is a very simple procedure. One asks the subject to place a sound into one of several categories that seem to fall along a single dimension. For example, a subject may be asked to categorize each of a series of sounds as not noisy, slightly noisy, moderately noisy, very noisy, or intolerably noisy. Category scaling is the familiar everyday process of judgment that we all use many times in many different situations. It has the advantage of simplicity. Among its disadvantages are the following: People tend to use the middle categories; the way people categorize one stimulus strongly depends on the other stimuli included in the set being judged; and people are often strongly influenced by seemingly irrelevant aspects of the stimuli or the judgmental situations (for example, judgments of the loudness of sounds may be influenced by their esthetic quality).

Another method is that of *magnitude scaling*. People can and will judge in quantitative terms the apparent "somethingness" of a stimulus. These judgments can be obtained in a variety of ways. For example subjects can be asked to estimate the apparent magnitude along a specified dimension of each stimulus presented to him. This procedure is called magnitude estimation. Or, subjects can be asked to judge the ratio of one stimulus to another along the dimension of interest. Another variant is to have the subject adjust one stimulus until it seems to stand in some ratio relation to another stimulus such as one-half or twice as loud. Magnitude scaling allows description of the apparent "somethingness" of a stimulus in quantitative but subjective terms.

A third method is that of *paired comparisons*. People are presented with a pair of stimuli. They are then asked to judge which is louder, more pleasant, noisier, and so on. By many such comparisons the stimuli can be ordered along so-called "psychological dimensions."

"Psychological dimensions" measured by scaling procedures such as these may seem formidable or mysterious to the uninitiated, but they are neither. Rather, they are orderly descriptions of the kinds of judgments we all make in our everyday lives.

B. Loudness, Perceived Noisiness, and the Physical Characteristics of Sounds

a. LOUDNESS. Loudness is an attribute of auditory experience. As a rule of thumb, people agree that when moderately intense single-component sound such as a tone or a band of noise is raised in intensity by about 10 dB, it sounds twice as loud. While this basic and simple rule is of great importance, the complete story of loudness is much more complicated. Loudness depends on the frequency of a sound as well as its intensity level. At moderate levels, low-frequency sounds (those below 900 Hz) are judged to be less loud than high-frequency sounds (those between about 900 and 5000 Hz) when both sounds are of equal physical intensity (sound pressure level). The sound-level meter is so designed that tones or narrow bands of noise will all sound equally loud if their A-weighted sound levels are about 40 dB. These relations change with intensity, however.

If a complex sound is made by simultaneous presentation of components that are widely spaced in frequency and about equally loud, then the total loudness of the complex sound is the sum of the loudnesses of the individual components. When the components are not widely spaced or are greatly unequal in loudness, then there is mutual inhibition and interference resulting in the total loudness being less than the sum of the loudnesses of the components. Fortunately, methods are available to measure the loudness of combinations of sounds (Stevens, 1961; Zwicker & Scharf, 1965).

The growth of loudness near the threshold of detectability is more rapid than the growth of loudness implied by the general rule that a change of 10 dB of intensity level equals double the loudness. Indeed, as a sound emerges from inaudibility, a 10-dB change of intensity level may increase the judged loudness by a factor of 10 instead of 2. Also, rapid growth of loudness may occur as sounds become audible over a masking noise. Thus, masking sometimes may be an ineffective way of reducing the loudness of unwanted sounds. Once audible, the unwanted sounds may seem nearly as loud as without the masking noise.

b. PERCEIVED NOISINESS. If one assumes that people do not like loud noise, it would seem that the goal of acoustical engineers should be to reduce the loudness of noise. If this were the case, design objectives could be specified in terms of loudness and the appropriate measurements of noise would then be measurements of loudness.

It has been proposed that another dimension of human response to noise, perceived noisiness, is similar to, but distinct from, loudness, and that perceived noisiness may be a better preditor than loudness of the adverse reactions to sound. The notion is that people can judge their impression of the unwantedness of a sound. These judgments are made of sounds that are expected and that do not provoke pain or fear. The developer of the concept explains it as follows (Kryter, 1970, pp. 270–277).

Perceived Noisiness. The subjective impression of the unwantedness of a not unexpected, nonpain or fear-provoking sound as part of one's environment is defined as the attribute of perceived noisiness. . . .

Confusion sometimes results in the use of the word noise as a name for unwanted sound because there are two general classes of "unwantedness." The first category is that in which the sound signifies or carries information about the source of the sound that the listener has learned to associate with some unpleasantness not due to the sound *per se,* but due to some other attribute of the source. . . . In these cases, it is not the sound that is unwanted (although for other reasons it may also be unwanted), but the information it conveys to the listener that is unwanted. This information is strongly influenced by the past experiences of each individual; because these effects cannot be quantitatively related to the physical characteristics of the sounds, they are rejected from the concept of perceived noisiness. After all, the engineer, attempting to control the noise from a given source, must shape the characteristics of the noise in as effective a way as possible for the majority of the people and the most typical of circumstances; those legislating or adjudicating the amounts of noise to be considered tolerable must also have a quantitative yardstick that is relatable to groups of people and typical circumstances.

Psychological judgment tests have demonstrated that people will fairly consistently judge among themselves the "unwantedness," "unacceptableness," "objectionableness," or "noisiness" of sounds that vary in their spectral and temporal nature, provided that the sounds do not differ significantly in their emotional meaning and are equally expected. Presumably this consistency is present because men learn through normal experience the relations between the characteristics of sounds and their basic perceptual effects; masking, loudness, noisiness, and, for impulses, startle. This is a basic premise of the concept of perceived noisiness and of the word noise as unwanted sound. . . .

Loudness versus Noisiness. Loudness of sounds is often assumed to be an adequate indicator of the unwantedness, for general noise control purposes, of sounds. Experiments have shown, however, that for many sounds there are differences between some physical aspects of sounds, and judgments of loudness compared to judgments of perceived noisiness. The difference between loudness and perceived noisiness in terms of spectral content *per se* (the equal loudness versus equal noisiness contours) is insignificantly small for broad-band sounds. . . . On the other hand, the differential effects of duration and spectral complexity upon these two attributes . . . are rather large.

The fact that loudness is apparently not influenced by duration and spectral complexity features of a sound would seem to disqualify loudness as an appropriate attribute for the estimation of the unacceptability of environmental noises. Although loudness and perceived noisiness differ in some respects, an assumption of the concept of the perceived noisiness of nonimpulsive noises is that, as the intensity of a noise changes, keeping other factors constant, the subjective magnitude of loudness and noisiness change to a like degree; e.g., a 10-dB increase in the physical intensity of nonimpulsive sounds causes a doubling of the subjective magnitude of its loudness and its noisiness. There is some experimental proof of this common relation between this subjective scale of noisiness and loudness, but, as with loudness, the scale found is somewhat dependent on the experimental methods used and sounds judged.

Instructions to Subjects. The words used in the instructions to the subjects for judgment tests of the acceptability of sounds have some influence upon their rating of sounds. . . . It is difficult and probably academic to fathom what is the basis for the range of differences [usually small], . . . such as whether the words used really mean different things to different people. In any event, there is no apparent reason why listeners should not be asked to rate directly sounds in terms of their unwantedness, unacceptability, annoyance, or noisiness, as synonyms, rather than to rate their loudness in the expectation that the latter is an indirect clue to the noisiness or unwantedness of the sounds.

Following are parts of the instructions that have been given to subjects who were asked to make subjective judgment tests of the noisiness of sounds. *"Instructions, Method of Paired-Comparison, for Judgments of Noisiness*. You will hear one sound followed immediately by a second sound. You are to judge which of the two sounds you think would be the most disturbing or unacceptable if heard regularly, as a matter of course 20 to 30 times per day in your home. Remember, your job is to judge the second of each pair of sounds with respect to the first sound of that pair. You may think that neither of the two sounds is objectionable or that both are objectionable; what we would like you to do is judge whether the second sound would be more disturbing or less disturbing than the first sound if heard in your home periodically 20 to 30 times during the day and night." The purpose of including in the instructions to the listeners a number of terms in rating the noisiness or unwantedness of expected sounds is to try to reduce possible differences in how different subjects might interpret the purpose or intent of the judgments when only one term such as "disturbing" or "annoyance" is used. . . .

Five Physical Aspects. So much for the general concept of the perceived noisiness of individual sounds. For practical purposes the measurable physical aspects of a sound that are most likely to control its perceived noisiness must be determined. To date, five significant features have been identified or suggested *(1)* spectrum content and level; *(2)* spectrum complexity (concentration of energy in pure-tone or narrow frequency bands within a broad-band spectrum); *(3)* duration of the total sound; *(4)* duration of the increase in level prior to the maximum level of nonimpulsive sounds; and *(5)* the increase in level, within an interval of .5 sec, of impulsive sounds. Some physical aspects that might seem important—for example Doppler shift (the change in the frequency and sometimes noted pitch of a sound as a sound source moves towards and away from the listener) and modulation of pure tones—appear to be very secondary in their effects on people compared to the five physical characteristics mentioned.

The five physical factors mentioned by Kryter operate approximately as follows: *(1) Intensity and frequency content*—noisiness increases with SL approximately as does loudness, that is a 10-dB increase in the level of moderately intense sounds results in a doubling of judged noisiness. Sounds with energy concentrations between 2000 and 8000 Hz are judged to be more noisy than sounds of equal SPL outside this range. This effect can be equivalent to a 10–20 dB increase in level or a factor of 2–4 in judged noisiness. *(2)* A *concentration of energy* or *spectrum complexity*—this may have an effect which increases the noisiness by 2–3 times or the equivalent of 10–15 dB over that noisiness that would be otherwise predicted. *(3) Duration*—the noisiness of a sound increases with its duration. The relation in logarithmic, and over a range from a few seconds to a few minutes, an increase in duration by a factor of ten results in a change that is roughly equal to a 10-dB increase in level, in other words, an increase in noisiness by a factor of two. Detailed study indicates that the growth of noisiness with duration is more rapid in the range of 1–4 sec and less rapid beyond 15 sec than predicted by a single logarithmic relation. *(4) Duration of the period of rising SPL*—sounds that are increasing in level are judged to be of greater noisiness than those decreasing in level. A sound that takes 10 sec to reach a maximum level may be judged more noisy than one of equal energy that reaches its maximum level in 3 sec. This difference can be the equivalent of about 3 dB or a factor of 1.2 in noisiness. *(5) Sudden increases in level*—in contrast, impulsive sounds that reach a high peak very abruptly, i.e., in a fraction of a second, may be judged to be very noisy. While this effect depends on the magnitude of the impulse, it can be very large. People judge impulsive sounds to be very noisy even when these sounds are familiar and expected.

Physical measurements of sounds can be weighted in such a manner as to enable one to predict judgments of noisiness. The resulting decibel values are said to be perceived noisiness levels (PNLs) and they are expressed as PNdB.

There has been great debate among students of loudness and noisiness concerning *(1)* whether these two attributes are the same or different; *(2)* the relative importance of the various temporal and spectral attributes of sound for loudness and noisiness; and *(3)* the relative merits of various schemes for predicting loudness and noisiness from physical measurements of sound. These debates are of great significance to the practical problems of noise control. For example it is important to be able to predict the loudness or perceived noisiness of a potential source of sound, such as a new machine, early in the design stage so as to minimize production costs. Since different sources of noise such as a high-frequency whine or a wide-spectrum random vibration may require interdependent design changes, it is important to know in quantitative terms how these noises combine perceptually.

No doubt these debates will continue and as a result our knowledge will become more refined. Despite the apparent conflict and confusion, numerous reports indicate that many of the major variables have been identified and their effects are known, at least qualitatively.

C. Verbal Descriptions of Sound and Auditory Experience

Auditory experience has a richness and variety that far exceeds those aspects represented by loudness or noisiness. Even sustained pure tones have the attributes of loudness, pitch, and volume. Tones appear to be of low or high loudness, low or high pitch, and of small or large volume (Stevens & Davis, 1938). Volume refers to the fact that some tones seem to be large and diffuse, while other tones seem to be thin and compact. Complex tones, being mixtures of pure tones, vary in quality or timbre and seem to have at least three qualities in addition to loudness, pitch, and volume. These are brightness, roughness, and fullness (Lichte, 1940). Everyday sounds and music grow in dimensionality and variety as they are extended in time. The full richness of sound only emerges when sounds form a sequence spread over time. While an extremely rich visual scene can be "taken in" at a glance, the auditory scene must be "taken in" over a period of time. Psychologists have only begun to study the richness and variety of auditory experience. A few studies (Solomon, 1958, 1959a,b) have been done. Even though only limited sets of sounds have been used, the results suggest that people can meaningfully evaluate sounds on a magnitude dimension (heavy–light); on an esthetic-evaluative dimension (good–bad, beautiful–ugly); a clarity dimension (clear–hazy); a security dimension (gentle–violent, safe–dangerous); a relaxation dimension (relaxed–tense); a famliarity dimension (familiar–strange); and a mood dimension (colorful–colorless). These dimensions relate to the overall spectral patterns of the sounds, their temporal pattern of spectral changes, and their rhythmic structure. These examples of possible dimensions are not meant to be taken as *the* dimensions of auditory experience. Rather, these results are mentioned only to suggest the diversity of auditory experience and its description.

Another approach to the verbal description of objects, events, and perceptions is that of Osgood (1952). Subjects are allowed to rate objects, events, or stimuli along many dimensions as defined by pairs of adjectives in opposition. After statistical treatment, it is found that many of these dimensions are highly correlated. In general, an intensity dimension (weak–strong), an activity dimension (active–inactive), and an evaluative dimension (good–bad) emerge whether people are judging pictures, sounds, political ideals, or whatever. In addition, several special dimensions are usually isolated that are specific to the situation and the set of stimuli being judged.

Loudness is the intensive dimension of auditory experience. Noisiness is probably a correlated but distinct dimension which includes evaluation along with judgment of intensity. Loudness and noisiness are in turn correlated with many of the adverse effects of excess and unwanted sound.

Perhaps other dimensions—as, for example, apparent extent in space—will be found to correlate with adverse reactions to noise. But it is also necessary to learn much more about the desirable aspects of sound if we are to reach a stage where we wish to speak of an optimal acoustical environment. Perhaps the techniques of Osgood and Solomon will lead to a better understanding of auditory experience and allow improved acoustical design. For example, it may be possible to design a vacuum cleaner that sounds "busy" and "active" without excessive loudness.

IV. ANNOYANCE AND COMMUNITY RESPONSE

Annoyance by noise is a response to auditory experience. Annoyance has its base in the unpleasant nature of some sounds, in the activities that are disturbed or disrupted by noise, in the physiological reactions to noise, and in the responses to the meaning or "messages" carried by the noise.

The degree of annoyance and whether that annoyance leads to complaints, product rejection, or action against an existing or anticipated noise source are dependent upon many factors. Some of these factors have been identified and their relative importance has been assessed. Responses to aircraft noise have received the greatest attention. There is less information available concerning responses to other noises such as those of surface transportation and industry and those from recreational activities. Nonetheless, the principal factors controlling annoyance appear to be understood. Action by individuals or communities against noise sources or those responsible for the regulation of noise is not as well understood; but even in this difficult area there seem to be sufficient data to allow prediction of major trends.

A. How Annoyance and Community Response to Noise Are Studied

a. CASE HISTORIES. Case history data are usually collected when there are complaints about particular noise sources. Often an acoustical consultant analyzes the problem. The consultant usually obtains the following kinds of information: *(1)* He measures the sound and tries to analyze how it is being generated by the source. *(2)* He interviews the involved people. *(3)* He establishes hypotheses concerning the "noise problem." *(4)* He suggests corrective action. If the corrective action is taken and the "problem" is eliminated or significantly reduced, he feels that the hypotheses were probably correct. Such case history data have contributed greatly to our understanding of the problem of noise.

b. SOCIAL SURVEYS. The social survey is a more elaborate version of the case history. There are two kinds of social surveys. One can either study areas that are experiencing high levels of noise, or one can deliberately introduce a new source of noise, such as a sonic boom, and evaluate its effects on the community.

The tools of the field study are *(1)* instruments for the measurement of the noise, *(2)* interviews and questionnaires, *(3)* records of complaints, and *(4)* statistical description of the measurements, whether they be of the noise or of the responses to it.

The appropriateness of social surveys has been discussed elsewhere (Borsky, 1970), and there are many difficulties. The mere presence of observers in a community as well as the way in which they present themselves can influence the response. The exact method of an interview and the construction of a questionnaire are also important. The measurement of the irregularly fluctuating noise levels within a community is also difficult. The measurement of both the noise and the responses to it require careful sampling methods and adequate statistical treatment of the resulting data.

Despite these difficulties, the results of case histories and more formal social surveys appear to be in overall agreement concerning the major facts of annoyance and community response to noise.

B. Acoustical and Situational Factors

a. ACOUSTICAL FACTORS. Annoyance from sound depends, in part, on the properties of the acoustical environment, and some of these properties were discussed in the previous section. Included among these are the intensity level and frequency content of the noise, the concentrations of energy in narrow regions of frequency, the duration of a noise, the period of initial rising intensity level, and the presence of impulses (such as those associated with gunfire, automobile backfires, hammering, and so on). These variables have been isolated in laboratory studies of judgments of single noise events in relatively controlled and quiet environments.

Other variables become obvious in social surveys or case histories where attention is usually focused on one kind of noise such as aircraft noise, and other noises are considered as part of the background noise. The definitions of the terms "noise" and "background noise" shift with the intent of the discussion. For example, if interest is focused on aircraft noise, then the noises of flyovers will be called "intruding noise" or "the noise" while other noises, such as those of surface transportation, household devices, and so on, would be grouped together as "background noise." It is interesting that when the "background noise" is great, then the annoyance attributed to a particular "intruding noise" may be less than when the same intruding noise appears against a lesser background noise. Field studies of annoyance and community responses to particular types of noises must include, therefore, direct or indirect measures of the number of repetitions of the "intruding noise," the level of the "background noise" from all other sources, and in one way or another the variability in the noise exposure from the combination of "intruding noises" and "background noises."

Further complications arise in field studies because the exposure that each individual receives is not measured. Rather, the noise is usually measured at some rationally selected monitoring point. For this reason, there are two other sets of acoustical variables that are crucial for an individual's response to sound. One set concerns the transmission path between the point where the sound is measured and the location of the exposed person. The other set of acoustical variables has to do with the acoustical characteristics of the exposed person's immediate environment.

Propagation of sound along a transmission path depends on many factors. The nature of the terrain, such as the sound-absorbing properties of its surface and whether it includes barriers which produce "sound shadows" are important. Weather conditions such as wind, temperature gradients, and humidity also influence the transmission of sound. Thus, an individual's exposure can only be predicted on a statistical basis from noise-monitoring stations. An individual's exposure will depend on whether there is a building between him and the sound source, whether he is outside or inside, in which part of his dwelling he spends most of his time, whether windows are open or closed, the construction of his dwelling, and so on.

The acoustical properties of an individual's immediate environment are also important. In the exposed person's immediate environment, it is the intensity level of the background noise and the reverberant characteristics of the space that are crucial. For example, background noise can mask an intruding noise, also an intruding noise may have a greater impact in a space that is acoustically lively than in one that is acoustically dead.

It is not surprising, therefore, that measures of acoustical variables at the monitoring points are not successful in predicting each exposed individual's degree of annoyance or disturbance. However, as will be shown, measurements from monitoring points have been successful in predicting *average* levels of annoyance and disturbance among persons located near the point where the measurements are made.

b. RELATIONS BETWEEN SITUATIONAL AND ACOUSTICAL VARIABLES. It has been found that evaluation of intruding noises should include situational variables if annoyance, disturbance, and community responses are to be predicted. For example, the type of neighborhood makes a difference. For a fixed exposure, instances of annoyance, disturbance, and complaint will be greatest in number for rural areas, followed by suburban, urban, residential, commercial, and industrial areas, in decreasing order. Similarly, a given noise usually will be more disturbing at night than during the day. Seasonal variations have also been noted; noise is more disturbing in summer than in winter.

Some of the situational factors that are correlated with annoyance by noise may be related to the attitudes and activities of people in these various locations and at different times of the day or year. But it is also plausible that these situational variables directly influence the noise exposures that people actually receive. Background noise levels vary in an appropriate manner with type of neighborhood and with the time of day that is, it is generally quieter in a rural than in an industrial area, and it is often quieter at night than during the day. Also, there are fewer acoustical barriers in rural than urban areas. There are fewer acoustical barriers between the people and the point of measurement in summer than in winter. This is true because in summer, more often than in winter, people are likely to be outdoors or, when indoors, to have their windows open.

c. PHYSICAL MEASUREMENTS OF NOISE EXPOSURE. From the previous discussion, it should be obvious that annoyance, disturbance, and complaints cannot be predicted simply by measurement of the sound emitted by a single source. Furthermore, it should be obvious that measurements from noise-monitoring stations cannot be expected to predict the responses of particular individuals.

A variety of methods have been proposed for the measurement of community noise or noise due to particular sources, such as aircraft, traffic, and so on. The array of methods and their names, usually given by initials, is bewildering to the uninitiated and the experienced specialist alike. There are CNR, NNI, NEF, TNI, NPL, CNEL, and even more. However, in general, these measurement schemes are more alike than they are different. Each includes several of the following factors: *(1)* a scheme for the identification of single noise "events"; *(2)* allowance for the intensity levels and durations of the noise events; *(3)* allowance for the number of noise events; *(4)* allowance, either direct or indirect, for the intensity levels of the background noise; *(5)* allowance for the variability of the intensity levels of the noises; and *(6)* allowance for one or more special factors related to the loudness or perceived noisiness of the noises. As previously discussed, situational factors such as season, time of day, and type of area often are included as corrections on the acoustical measurements.

A measure has been proposed which does not require the identification of specific noise sources (Robinson, 1971). This measure is called the noise pollution level (NPL), and the author's intention was to provide an overall estimation of a community's acoustical environment. The measure weights both the long-term average noise level as well as the variation in these noise levels. The notion has merit, but measurements (Wyle, 1971) suggest that the noise pollution level as proposed gives too high a weighting to the variance the sound levels in relation to their average level.

C. Annoyance, Attitudes, and Disruption of Activities

a. ANNOYANCE AND NOISE. Annoyance as measured in field studies is distinct from judgments of loudness and perceived noisiness. Annoyance, as described at the beginning of this section, is a response to noise rather than a dimension of auditory experience. A variety of techniques have been used to measure the *annoyance* that results from noise. The most direct is simply to ask a person to categorize his degree of annoyance. "Rate your annoyance from one to seven where one is 'no annoyance' and seven is 'extremely annoyed.' " While such direct ratings have been found generally to be subject to a great many biasing influences, in the case of annoyance by noise such direct ratings correlate very highly with more subtle and indirect measures. The complicated procedures developed for the study of general attitudes may not be necessary for investigations of annoyance by noise (McKennel, 1970).

Indirect measures are obtained by asking a person about the kinds of activities that are disturbed by noise and about the degree of the disturbance. Total annoyance is calculated from a combination of the number of activities disturbed and the degree to which they are disturbed (Tracor Staff, 1971). For example, persons may be asked to rate the degree of disturbance by noise for TV/radio reception, conversation, telephone use, relaxing outside, relaxing inside, listening to records or tapes, sleeping, reading, and eating. The degree of annoyance might then be taken as the sum of the ratings of the degree of disturbance (Tracor Staff, 1971).

Annoyance by noise depends in part on the characteristics of the noise itself, and typical results are illustrated in Figs. 3 and 4. These graphs support the contention that the *average* degree of annoyance among people in an

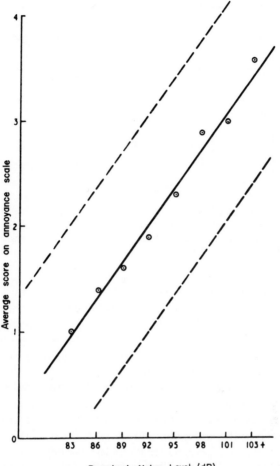

FIG. 3. Average scores on an annoyance scale for persons exposed to various levels of aircraft noise are shown. The dashed lines include two-thirds of the persons interviewed. [From McKennel (1970), Noise complaints and community action. In J. D. Chalupnik (Ed.), *Transportation Noises*, pp. 228–244. Copyright 1970 by the University of Washington Press.]

area can be predicted from the characteristics of the noise measured at an appropriately selected monitoring point. Nonetheless, reported annoyance also depends on other attitudinal–psychological factors.

b. ANNOYANCE AND ATTITUDES. There are several attitudinal–psychological factors which correlate with the degree of scaled annoyance. These can be classified under: *(1)* general attitudes toward noise including differences among individuals in their sensitivity; *(2)* attitudes of the exposed person toward the source of noise, such as whether they consider the noise-producing activity to be important for their social and economic well-being

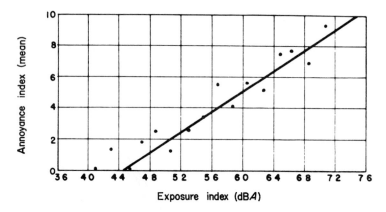

F<small>IG</small>. 4. Average annoyance scores for persons exposed to various levels of traffic noise are shown. Notice that the scales of Figs. 3 and 4 cannot be compared for absolute magnitudes. [From Kajland (1970), Traffic noise investigation. In J. D. Chalupnik (Ed.), *Transportation Noises,* pp. 327–330. Copyright 1970 by the University of Washington Press.]

and whether they believe that the noise is a necessary by product of the activity that produces it; *(3)* whether they believe that those persons responsible for the operation and regulation of the noise-producing activity are concerned about their (the exposed population's) welfare; and *(4)* factors specific to particular noise sources, such as fear of aircraft crashes or the belief that sonic booms cause property damage.

For example, highly annoyed persons are likely to believe that those responsible for the noise are not concerned about those being exposed to the noise, and they are also likely to believe that the source of noise is not of great importance to the economic and social success of the community. In addition, highly annoyed persons are likely to have negative attitudes toward many kinds of noise; to be generally sensitive to irritation produced by noise; to believe that their neighbors share their annoyance; to say that they would be unwilling to accept further increases in noise levels; and to believe that noise is a health hazard. People highly annoyed by the noise of subsonic aircraft are likely to express a fear of a crash in their neighborhood, whereas people highly annoyed by sonic booms are likely to believe that these booms cause property damage. Such statements are based on statistical relations and many highly annoyed people do *not* conform to the profile given above.

The examples of characteristics of highly annoyed persons were abstracted from several sources (Borsky, 1970; Kryter, 1970; McKennel, 1970; Tracor Staff, 1971; and references cited therein). Unfortunately, when one tries to compare social surveys, he finds that the exact attitudinal–psychological variables that emerge as most prominent vary from study to study. Such variation is to be expected because of differences in the methods, the sample populations, and the noises.

A published survey of responses to the noise of subsonic aircraft (Tracor Staff, 1971) reports that an *individual's* level of annoyance as measured by interview–questionnaire techniques can be fairly accurately predicted if one knows the noise exposure (measured at a community monitoring point) and the weights to assign to seven attitudinal–psychological factors. These factors, ranked in order of predictive power, are *(1)* the fear of aircraft crashes, *(2)* the susceptibility of the individuals to other noises, such as banging doors, dripping water, and so on, *(3)* the distance from the airport, *(4)* the willingness of the individual to accept additional increases in noise exposure from aircraft, *(5)* city of residence, *(6)* the extent to which residents of the community believe that they are being treated unfairly, and *(7)* the attitudes of the residents with respect to the importance of the airport and air transportation. Most of these factors can be placed into the four general classes described at the beginning of this subsection. However, exactly why "distance from the airport" and "city of residence" should be important is unexplained.

It is also interesting to contrast responses to sonic booms with responses to the noise of subsonic aircraft. There is some indication that annoyance from sonic booms may be most related to the physiological and psychological responses to the suddenness of the booms, whereas annoyance from the noise of subsonic aircraft may be more strongly related to the activities disturbed by the noise (Tracor Staff, 1971). The major attitudinal factor that contributes to annoyance by sonic booms is the belief held by many people that booms cause property damage, while the major attitudinal factor that contributes to annoyance by the noise of subsonic aircraft is the fear of aircraft crashes.

All of the above is convincing evidence that people's responses to noise depend on their values, beliefs, and attitudes. This is not surprising, for the definition of noise as an unwanted sound is a statement of an attitude and a value judgment. Some researchers have gone so far as to state that the attitudinal–psychological factors are more important for predicting annoyance (by noise) than are the properties of the noise itself. But individuals' exposures to noise, as opposed to community exposure measured at a monitoring point, have never been measured in these social surveys. Also, if the noise were not present, then the attitudinal–psychological factors could not operate. Thus, one must return to the sound itself as the fundamental stimulus for the annoyance from noise.

c. EXAMPLES OF ACTIVITIES DISTURBED BY AIRCRAFT AND TRAFFIC NOISES AS MEASURED IN SOCIAL SURVEYS. Two studies (Tracor Staff, 1971; Griffiths & Langdon, 1968) report activities disturbed by subsonic-aircraft and traffic noise. In the Tracor study (Phase I) people were interviewed in an area with a radius of 12 miles and within an angle of 40° to the right and left of the end of a runway. These runways were in the major airports near Chicago, Dallas, Denver, and Los Angeles. Of 4153 persons interviewed, 98.6% reported one or more disturbances of daily activities by aircraft noise and, correspondingly, at least some degree of bother. The percentage who rated an activity as *extremely* disturbed were as follows: TV/radio reception, 21%; conversation, 15%; telephone use, 14%; relaxing outside, 13%; relaxing inside, 11%; listening to records or tapes, 9%; sleep, 8%; reading, 6%; and eating, 4%. In the study of Griffiths and Langdon, people indicated that traffic noise disturbed sleep, conversation with visitors, conversation at mealtimes, TV and radio reception, and increased the time for children to fall asleep.

Of course, these examples of disturbed activities are based on responses to interviews and questionnaires. These lists are neither complete nor do they necessarily reflect the true ranking of activities disturbed by noise. For example, the interference with formal education in schools does not appear on these lists probably because only adult residents of an area were interviewed. Also, the person being interviewed is not necessarily aware of all the ways in which noise may disturb his activities.

d. ADAPTATION TO NOISE. There is little evidence that annoyance due to community noise decreases with continued exposure. Rather, under some circumstances, annoyance may increase the longer one is exposed to it (Borsky, 1970).

D. Community Response

There are ample data to show that community responses to aircraft noise are related to measures of the exposures. Typical results are shown in Figs. 5 and 6. These graphs speak for themselves and clearly show that community response can vary from indifference and mild annoyance to highly organized community action. Complaints such as letters or telephone calls to relevant officials and community action are determined by much more complicated sets of circumstances than are annoyance and disturbance of activities. It has been shown, however, that those who complain are not necessarily highly annoyed by noise. In spite of intensive efforts (one study included as many as 17 sociological variables such as age, socioeconomic status, and so on), there has been little success in identifying and characterizing those who complain as opposed to those who do not.

It is clear, however, that only a small percentage of those who are highly annoyed or disturbed actually register a formal complaint to some authority in the form of a letter or a telephone call. For example, it was found (Tracor Staff, 1971) that in an area with high noise levels, the number of highly annoyed households per thousand (h) can be predicted from the number of complaints per thousand (c) in the area by the simple equation,

$$h = 196 + 2c.$$

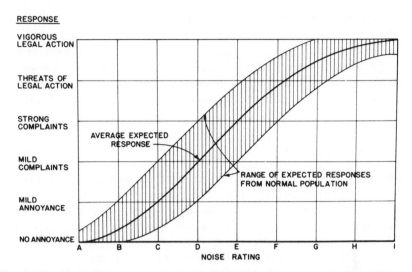

FIG. 5. The relation between community response and noise exposure is shown. The noise exposure increases from A to I. [From Rosenblith *et al.* (1953).]

By simple calculation, if there are 200 persons who complain in a tract of 1000 households, there will be nearly 600 highly annoyed households! This equation, however, probably holds only for a given set of sociological and political circumstances. Annoyance is probably a good measure of the po-

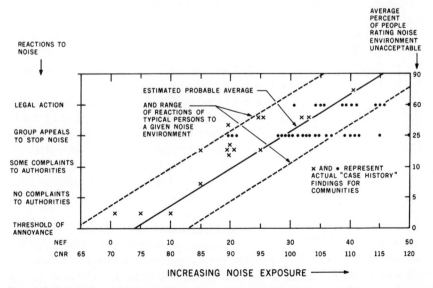

FIG. 6. Relations between community noise levels (measured in CNR or NEF), judgments of unacceptability, and community responses are shown. [After Kryter *et al.* (1971), *Non-auditory Effects of Noise* (Rep. WG-63). Copyright 1971 by the NAS–NRC Committee on Hearing and Bioacoustical Biomechanics.]

tential for complaint and action. Whether complaints or antinoise actions actually develop will depend on social and political factors such as the presence of antinoise leadership, attitudes toward the source of noise or regulatory agents, and so on. These last-mentioned factors are only a few of the factors that make up the whole of community dynamics. These community dynamics, which are poorly understood, very strongly control antinoise actions.

E. Concluding Statement

Community noise exposure can be measured and summarized. There are a variety of competing methods that take into account at least some of the following, not necessarily independent, factors: *(1)* a scheme for identification of noises; *(2)* the intensity levels and durations of identifiable noise events; *(3)* number of occurrences of the noise events; *(4)* the background noise level; *(5)* the variability of the noise levels; *(6)* one or more special factors related to the perceived noisiness or loudness of the sounds; and *(7)* the time of day and type of area, whether urban, suburban, rural, and so on. While efforts to standardize and refine these measurements will and should continue, many of the important variables have been identified and methods for their measurement have been developed. Of course, these methods cannot accurately measure any single person's exposure to noise.

The degree of annoyance averaged over a large number of individuals near a noise-monitoring station can be predicted, in a statistical sense, from the physical characteristics of the noise. Each individual's degree of annoyance cannot be as accurately predicted as can the average annoyance. This is true because individuals differ considerably in the exact noise exposure they receive (due to variations in environmental acoustics), because individuals differ in their sensitivity to disturbance by noise, and because individuals differ in other relevant psychological and social attitudes.

Community responses to noise can range from indifference and mild annoyance to highly organized group action. Those who complain about aircraft noise cannot be identified as having a special set of psychological and sociological characteristics. Those who complain about aircraft noise, contrary to the beliefs of some, are not necessarily highly sensitive to noise. They do not seem to be, in general, unusual citizens. Nevertheless, total number of complaints and commmunity antinoise action are correlated with measures of the severity of the noise exposure.

While community responses to aircraft noises have been more thoroughly studied than the responses to other noises, such as those of traffic and construction, case histories reveal that people become annoyed and they complain about a wide variety of noises. In addition to noise exposure, psychological and sociological considerations modify the extent of the annoyance and the inclination to complain. Case histories also reveal that, regardless of whether the noise is produced by traffic, aircraft, construction, and so on, the probability of overt action against the noise producers or regulators can be estimated from knowledge of the noise exposure. However, these estimates are fallible and numerous exceptions can be cited.

One fact about the relations among perceived noisiness, annoyance from noise, disturbance of activities by noise, complaints about noise, and community actions against noise is especially significant. It is that noisiness, annoyance, and disturbance of activities are more closely tied to the physical characteristics of the noises than are the rates of formally placed complaints or the probabilities of group antinoise action. Thus, whether or not one files a formal complaint or participates in group antinoise action, the quality of one's life is influenced by unwanted sound.

V. OTHER POSSIBLE PSYCHOLOGICAL AND SOCIOLOGICAL EFFECTS

There have been numerous claims of many kinds of deleterious psychological and sociological effects of noise on man. Many of these are difficult to evaluate because of conflicting information or because of lack of information. Often firm conclusions cannot be drawn and one must rely on one's experience, intuition, and judgment, as well as upon published data in order to reach a tentative conclusion.

Even the selection of the claims to be discussed requires a considerable degree of arbitrary judgment. The areas discussed in this section were selected on the basis of the amount of available information and on the basis of judgments concerning plausibility, importance, and interest. No more could be done.

A. Noise and Performance

The action of noise on the performance of tasks has been studied extensively in the laboratory and in actual work situations. Excellent summaries and reviews of these studies are available (Broadbent, 1957; Burns, 1968; Cohen, 1969; Kryter, 1970; Kryter et al., 1971).

When a task requires the use of auditory signals, speech or nonspeech, then noise at any intensity level sufficient to mask or interfere with the perception of these signals will interfere with the performance of the task.

When mental or motor tasks do *not* involve auditory signals, the effects of noise on their performance have been difficult to assess. Human behavior is complicated and it has been difficult to discover exactly how different kinds of noises might influence different kinds of people doing different kinds of tasks. Nonetheless, certain general conclusions have emerged. *(1)* Steady noises without special meaning do not seem to interfere with human performance that does not include auditory components, unless the A-weighted noise level exceeds about 90 dB. *(2)* Irregular bursts of noise are more disruptive than steady noises. Even when the A-weighted sound levels of irregular bursts are below 90 dB, they may sometimes interfere with performance of a task. *(3)* High-frequency components of noise, above about 1000–2000 Hz, may produce more interference with performance than low-frequency components of noise. *(4)* Noise does not seem to influence the overall rate of work, but high levels of noise may increase the variability of the rate of work. There may be "noise pauses" followed by compensating increases in work rate. *(5)* Noise is more likely to reduce the accuracy of work than to reduce the total quantity of work. *(6)* Complex tasks are more likely to be adversely influenced by noise than are simple tasks.

It has been and will continue to be difficult to assess the effects of noise on human performance. Laboratory studies are usually of short duration and the subjects are usually well-motivated young adults. These subjects may be able to perform without decrement in noises that might influence performance under more "everyday" conditions. Studies of the effects of noise in actual work conditions are difficult because factors other than the noise itself are difficult to control.

Even when a person maintains high performance in noise as opposed to quiet, there may be a cost. This cost might include reduced psychological of physiological capacity to react to additional demands and increased fatigue after completion of the task (Finkelman & Glass, 1970; Glass *et al.*, 1969).

The effects of noise on human performance are often conceptualized in terms of three classes of effects: *(1)* arousal, *(2)* distraction, and *(3)* specific effects. *Arousal* of bodily systems including the musculature can result in either detrimental or beneficial effects on human performance. The direction of the effect will depend on the nature of the task and on the person's state prior to exposure. For example, noise might induce muscular tension that could interfere with delicate movements. On the other hand, a sleepy person might be aroused by noise and, therefore, may perform more effectively in noise than in quiet. *Distraction* can be thought of as a lapse in attention or a diversion of attention from the task at hand. Often distraction is due to the aversive or annoying characteristics of the noise. Distraction can sometimes be related to the physiological responses to noise or to the responses to messages carried by the noise. Also, it has been proposed (Broadbent, 1957) that if the noise is sufficiently intense, it may somehow "overload" the mental capacities and result in a momentary lapse in attention or "mental blink." *Specific effects* include auditory masking, muscular activation such as startle responses to brief intense noises (sonic booms, backfires, etc.), and the like.

Many physiological and psychological responses to sound diminish or disappear when noises are regular or predictable. Sometimes strategies can be learned so that the detrimental effects of noise on performance can be avoided. Under certain conditions noise may even result in better concentration due to auditory isolation provided by the noise's masking of other sounds, greater activation and alertness of the worker, or pace performance when the noise is regular or rhythmic. For these reasons, people sometimes achieve excellent performance or even exceed their normal performance in spite of noise.

Noises, however, often are not regular and predictable, adaptation of responses to noise is not always complete, and strategies to eliminate the effects of noise are not always learned. Furthermore, the fact that distraction or disturbance can be the result of the "message" carried by the noise rather than a result of the noise, *per se,* may not seem important to the average person. An ideal acoustical environment is one that does not disturb human performance either because of the properties of the noise itself or because of irrelevant messages carried by the noise. The trick, of course, is to eliminate disturbing noises while maximizing the chances that important, relevant messages carried by sound will reach the appropriate party.

B. Acoustical Privacy

Without opportunity for privacy, either everyone must conform strictly to an elaborate social code, or everyone must adopt highly permissive attitudes. Opportunity for privacy avoids the necessity for either extreme. In particular, without opportunity for acoustical privacy one may experience all of the effects of noise previously described and, in addition, one is constrained because his own activities may disturb others (Cohen, 1969).

It would be helpful for owner and renter and for seller and buyer if standardized acoustical ratings were developed for dwellings. These ratings might include measures of acoustical privacy as well as other measures of acoustical quality. Such ratings would be particularly useful because the acoustical properties of a dwelling are not immediately obvious to the nonspecialist. If such ratings were available, the parties involved could balance the acoustical value of a dwelling in relation to those of appearance, size, convenience, cost, and so on.

C. Time Judgments

Steady noise with an *A*-weighted sound level up to about 90 dB seems to expand the subjective time scales; that is, less time has been judged to pass than actually has (Hirsh *et al.,* 1956).

Steady noise more intense than about 90 dB seems to contract subjective time; that is, more time is judged to pass than actually has (Jerison & Arginteanu, 1958).

D. Effects on Other Senses

A variety of effects of auditory stimulation on the other senses have been reported. These are called intersensory effects. Subtle intersensory effects may occur as part of normal psychological and physiological function. At very high noise levels, more dramatic intersensory effects have been reported. For example, there can be disturbances of equilibrium at levels of about 130–150 dB (Anticaglia, 1970; Kryter, 1970; von Gierke, 1965). Dramatic intersensory effects would not occur in response to current levels of community noise.

E. Mental Disorders

There is no definitive evidence that noise can induce either neurotic or psychotic illness. There is evidence that the rate of admissions to mental hospitals is higher from areas experiencing high levels of noise from aircraft operations than in similar areas with lower levels of noise. The type of person most affected appears to be the older woman who is not living with her husband and who suffers from neurotic or organic mental illness (Abey-Wickrama et al., 1969). These authors did not believe that aircraft noise *caused* mental illness, but their tentative conclusion is that such noise could be a factor that increases admissions to psychiatric hospitals.

F. Anxiety and Distress

Nausea, headaches, instability, argumentativeness, sexual impotency, changes in general mood, general anxiety, and other effects have all been associated with exposure to noise (Andriukin, 1961; Cohen, 1969; Davis, 1958; Jansen, 1959; Shatalov et al., 1962).

These effects are difficult to assess because intense noises are often associated with situations that in and of themselves, even without noise, might involve fear and stress. Whether the noise, purely as noise, contributes significantly to the stress of life (see Chapter 16) is difficult to assess at this time. But all of the facts of speech interference, hearing loss, noisiness, annoyance, and arousal and distraction previously recited clearly support the contention that noises can act as a source of psychological distress, either because of responses directly to the noise itself or because of responses to irrelevant "messages" carried by the sound. Psychological distress in turn can contribute to the unpleasant symptoms listed above.

References

Abey-Wickrama, I., A'Brook, M. F., Gattoni, F. E. G., & Herridge, C. F. Mental-hospital admissions and aircraft noise. *The Lancet,* 1969, 1275–1278.

Andriukin, A. Influence of sound stimulation on the development of hypertension. Coret Vasa, 1961, 3, 285–293. (Cited in Kryter, 1970.)

Anticaglia, J. R. Extra-auditory effects on the special senses. In B. L. Welch & A. S. Welch (Eds.), *Physiological effects of noise.* New York: Plenum, 1970. Pp. 143–150.

Berger, R. J. The sleep and dream cycle. In A. Kales (Ed.), *Sleep physiology and pathology—A symposium.* Philadelphia: Lippincott, 1969. Pp. 15–32.

Blazier, W. F., Jr. Criteria for residential heating and air-conditioning systems. *Noise Control,* 1959, **5,** 48–53.

Borsky, P. N. The use of social surveys for measuring community response to noise environments. In J. D. Chalupnik (Ed.), *Transportation noises.* Seattle: University of Washington Press, 1970. Pp. 219–227.

Broadbent, D. E. Effects of noise on behavior. In C. M. Harris (Ed.), *Handbook of noise control.* New York: McGraw-Hill, 1957. Chap. 10.

Broughton, R. J. Sleep disorders: Disorders of arousal? *Science,* 1968, **159,** 1070–1078.

Burns, W. *Noise and man.* London: John Murray, 1968.

Cohen, A. Effects of noise on psychological state. In W. Ward & J. Fricke (Eds.), *Noise as a public health hazard* (ASHA Rep. 4). Washington, D.C.: American Speech and Hearing Association, 1969. Pp. 74–88.

Davis, H. (Ed.) Auditory and non-auditory effects of high intensity noise (Final Report, Joint Project NM 1301 99, Subtask 1, Rep. 7). Pensacola, Florida: Central Institute for the Deaf and Naval School of Medicine, 1958.

Feinberg, I. Effects of age on human sleep patterns. In A. Kales (Ed.), *Sleep physiology and pathology—A symposium.* Philadelphia: Lippincott, 1969. Pp. 39–52.

Finkelman, J. M., & Glass, D. C. Reappraisal of the relationship between noise and human performance by means of a subsidiary task measure. *Journal of Applied Psychology,* 1970, **54,** 211–213.

Glass, D. C., Singer, J. E., & Friedman, L. N. Psychic cost of adaptation to an environmental stressor. *Journal of Personality and Social Psychology,* 1969, **12,** 200–210.

Griffiths, I. D., & Langdon, F. J. Subjective response to road traffic noise. *Journal of Sound and Vibration,* 1968, **8,** 16–32.

Helson, H. *Adaptation-level theory.* New York: Harper & Row, 1964.

Hirsh, I. J., Bilger, R. C., & Deatherage, B. H. The effect of auditory and visual background on apparent duration. *American Journal of Psychology,* 1956, **69,** 561–574.

Jacobson, A., Kales, J. D., & Kales, A. Clinical and electrophysiological correlates of sleep disorders in children. In A. Kales (Ed.), *Sleep physiology and pathology—A symposium.* Philadelphia: Lippincott, 1969. Pp. 109–118.

Jansen, G. On the origination of vegetative functional disturbances due to noise effect. *Archiv für Gewerbepathologie und Gewerbehygiene,* 1959, **17,** 238–261.

Jerison, J. J., & Arginteanu, J. Time judgments, acoustic noise, and judgment drift (Rep. No. WADC-TR-57-454, AD130963). Dayton, Ohio: Wright Air Development Center, Wright–Paterson AFB, 1958.

Kajland, A. Traffic noise investigation. In J. D. Chalupnik (Ed.), *Transportation noises.* Seattle: University of Washington Press, 1970. Pp. 327–330.

Kales, A. (Ed.) *Sleep physiology and pathology—A symposium.* Philadelphia: Lippincott, 1969.

Kessler, J. W. *Psychopathology of childhood.* Englewood Cliffs, New Jersey: Prentice-Hall, 1966.

Koella, W. P. *Sleep: Its nature and physiological organization.* Springfield, Illinois: Charles C Thomas, 1967.

Kryter, K. D., Jansen, G., Parker, D., Parrack, H. O., Thiessen, G., & Williams, H. L. Non-auditory effects of noise (Rep. WG-63). Washington, D.C.: NAS–NRC Committee on Hearing and Bioacoustical Biomechanics, 1971.

Kryter, K. D., & Williams, C. E. Cited in Kryter, K. D. *The effects of noise on man.* New York: Academic Press, 1970. P. 518.

Lichte, W. H. Attributes of complex tones. *Journal of Experimental Psychology,* 1940, **28,** 455–480.

Luce, G. G. Current research on sleep and dreams (PHS Pub. No. 1389). Washington, D.C.: U.S. Government Printing Office, 1966.

Lukas, J. S. Personal communication, 1971.

Lukas, J. S., Dobbs, M. E., & Kryter, K. D. Disturbance of human sleep by subsonic jet aircraft noise and simulated sonic booms (NASA Rep. No. CR-1780). Washington, D.C.: National Aeronautics and Space Administration, 1971.

Lukas, J. S., & Kryter, K. D. Awakening effects of simulated sonic booms and subsonic aircraft noise. In B. L. Welch & A. S. Welch (Eds.), *Physiological effects of noise*. New York: Plenum, 1970. Pp. 283–293.

McKennel, A. C. Noise complaints and community action. In J. D. Chalupnik (Ed.), *Transportation noises*. Seattle: University of Washington Press, 1970. Pp. 228–244.

Mills, J. H., & Talo, S. J. Temporary threshold shifts produced by prolonged exposure to high-frequency noise. *Journal of Speech and Hearing Research*, 1971, **15**, 624–631.

Osgood, C. E. The nature and measurement of meaning. *Psychological Bulletin*, 1952, **49**, 197–237.

Oswald, I., Taylor, A. M., & Treisman, M. Discriminative responses to stimulation during human sleep. *Brain*, 1960, **83**, 440–453.

Rechtschaffen, A., Hauri, P., & Zeitlin, M. Auditory awakening thresholds in REM and NREM sleep stages. *Perceptual and Motor Skills*, 1966, **22**, 927–942.

Robinson, D. W. Towards a unified system of noise assessment. *Journal of Sound and Vibration*, 1971, **14**, 279–298.

Rosenblith, W. A., Stevens, K. N., & the Staff of Bolt Beranek and Newman. Handbook of acoustic noise control—Noise and man (WADC Tech. Rep. 52-204, Vol. II). Dayton, Ohio: Wright Air Development Center, 1953. Pp. 181–200.

Schieber, J. P., Mery, J., & Muzet, A. Etude analytique en laboratoire de l'influence due bruit sur le sommeil. Strasbourg, France: Report of the Centre d'Etudes Bioclimatique du CNRS, 1968.

Shatalov, N. N., Saitanov, A. O., & Glotova, K. V. On the state of the cardiovascular system under conditions of exposure to continuous noise (Rep. T-411-R, N65-15577). Toronto, Canada: Defense Research Board, 1962.

Solomon, L. N. Semantic approach to the perception of complex sounds. *Journal of the Acoustical Society of America*, 1958, **30**, 421–425.

Solomon, L. N. Search for physical correlates to psychological dimensions of sound. *Journal of the Acoustical Society of America*, 1959, **31**, 492–497. (a)

Solomon, L. N. Semantic reactions to systematically varied sounds. *Journal of the Acoustical Society of America*, 1959, **31**, 986–990. (b)

Steinicke, G. Die Wirkungen von Lärm auf den Schlaf des Menschen. In Forschungsberichte des Wirtschafts- und Verkehrsministriums Nordrhein-Westfalen (No. 416). Köln: Westdeutscher Verlag, 1957.

Stevens, S. S. Procedure for calculating loudness: Mark VI. *Journal of the Acoustical Society of America*, 1961, **33**, 1577–1585.

Stevens, S. S., & Davis, H. *Hearing: Its psychology and physiology*. New York: Wiley, 1938.

Stevens, S. S., & Warshofsky, F. (Eds.) *Sound and hearing*. New York: Life Science Library, Time, Inc., 1965.

Thiessen, G. Effects of noise during sleep. In B. L. Welch & A. S. Welch (Eds.), *Physiological effects of noise*. New York: Plenum, 1970. Pp. 271–275.

Tracor Staff. Community reaction to airport noise (NASA CR-1761, Vol. 1). Washington, D.C.: National Aeronautics and Space Administration, 1971.

von Gierke, H. E. On noise and vibration exposure criteria. *Archives of Environmental Health*, 1965, **2**, 327–339.

Watson, R., & Rechtschaffen, A. Auditory awakening thresholds and dream recall in NREM sleep. *Perceptual and Motor Skills*, 1969, **29**, 635–644.

Williams, H. L., Hammack, J. T., Daly, R. L., Dement, W. C., & Lubin, A. Responses to auditory stimulation, sleep loss, and the EEG stages of sleep. *Electroencephalography and Clinical Neurophysiology*, 1964, **16**, 269–279.

Williams, H. L., Morlock, H. C., & Morlock, J. V. Instrumental behavior during sleep. *Psychophysiology,* 1965, **2,** 208–216.

Williams, H. L., & Williams, C. L. Nocturnal EEG profiles and performance. *Psychophysiology,* 1966, **3,** 164–175.

Wilson, A., *et al.* Noise—Final report. London: Her Majesty's Stationery Office, 1963.

Wilson, W. P., & Zung, W. W. K. Attention, discrimination, and arousal during sleep. *Archives of General Psychiatry,* 1966, **15,** 523–528.

Wyle Staff. Supporting information for the adopted noise regulations for California airports: Final report to the California department of aeronautics [Rep. No. WCR 70-3 (R)]. El Segundo, California: Wyle Laboratories, 1971.

Zung, W. W. K., & Wilson, W. P. Response to auditory stimulation during sleep. *Archives of General Psychiatry,* 1961, **4,** 548–552.

Zwicker, E., & Scharf, B. A model of loudness summation. *Psychological Review,* 1965, **72,** 3–26.

Chapter 16

GENERAL PHYSIOLOGICAL EFFECTS OF NOISE*

J. D. MILLER

I. INTRODUCTION

There are three classes of *transient* general physiological responses to sound: *(1)* the fast responses of the voluntary musculature mediated by the somatic nervous system; *(2)* the slightly slower responses of the smooth muscles and glands mediated by the visceral nervous system; and *(3)* the even slower responses of the neuroendocrine system.

It has been proposed that frequent repetition of these responses might lead to *persistent* pathological changes in nonauditory bodily functions (Jansen, 1959, 1969). Also, it has been proposed that frequent repetition of these transient physiological responses might aggravate known disease conditions, and evidence consistent with this proposal has been gathered (Kryter *et al.,* 1971; von Gierke, 1965).

The transient physiological responses to sound, the possible persistent physiological responses to sound, and the possible relation of noise to stress theory are each discussed in the sections that follow.

II. TRANSIENT AND POSSIBLE PERSISTENT PHYSIOLOGICAL RESPONSES TO NOISE

A. Transient Physiological Responses to Noise

a. RESPONSES OF THE VOLUNTARY MUSCULATURE. Man is equipped with an elaborate set of auditory–muscular reflexes. These serve the basic func-

---

* Chapters 14, 15, and 16 originally appeared in the *Journal of the Acoustical Society of America,* Vol. 56, No. 3, September 1974, pp. 729–764. © 1974 Acoustical Society of America. Reprinted by permission of the Acoustical Society of America.

tions of orienting the head and eyes toward a sound source and of preparing for action appropriate to an object whose presence is signalled by a sound. These reflexes operate even at low levels of sound (Bickford *et al.*, 1964; Davis, 1950; Mast, 1965), and they can often be detected by suitable electrical recording and averaging even after bodily movements have habituated and are no longer detectable. Auditory–muscular reflexes undoubtedly play a part in all muscular responses to sound. These may range from rhythmic movement and dance to the body's startle responses to impulsive sounds such as those produced by gunshots or sonic booms.

These muscular responses to sound can be measured by direct observation of bodily movements (sometimes with the aid of amplifying levers or high-speed motion pictures) or by measurements of the electrical activity of the musculature.

The startle response has been studied in detail (Landis & Hunt, 1939). It includes an eyeblink, a typical facial grimace, bending of the knees, and, in general, flexion (inward and forward) as opposed to extension of the bodily parts. The startle response to the sound of a nearby gunshot, even when expected, may undergo various degree of diminution with repetition of the sound. The amount of diminution of the response depends on the individual, the rate of repetition, and the predictability of the impulse sound. Some individuals show little diminution of the startle response with repetition while others show a marked reduction of this response. The eyeblink and head movement aspects of the startle response may never habituate completely. Even experienced marksmen exhibit these responses each time they fire a gun.

All of the observations described in the preceding paragraph were made with the aid of high-speed motion pictures. Using the electrical devices available to them, Davis and Van Liere (1949) found that muscular responses to the sound of a gunshot did not disappear with repetition. An early response (the *a* response with a latency of about .1 sec) showed little reduction with repetition of the sound. A later response (the *b* response with a latency of about .8 sec) showed more reduction with repetition.

A series of experiments, done by R. C. Davis and his colleagues at Indiana University, demonstrated that the particular muscular responses to sound and the way in which these responses will influence the performance of a motor task depend in detail on *(1)* the pattern of muscular tension, or posture, prior to the sound, *(2)* the movements required by the task, and *(3)* the auditory–muscular reflexes (Davis, 1935, 1942, 1948a,b, 1956a–e; Patton, 1953).

Among the important findings was that the magnitude of the muscle-tension reflex in response to sound increased with increasing resting tension in the muscle. (This generalization, of course, would not hold as a muscle approaches its maximum level of tension.) Thus, if the subject was required to make a movement that required flexion and if the subject's posture heightened tension in the appropriate flexor muscle, then a burst of sound, which ordinarily produces the reflex action of flexion, would speed the performance of the movement. Under other conditions, however, the burst of sound could greatly interfere with the required movement. For example, suppose that, as before, the required movement was that of flexion but that the subject's posture heightened the resting tension in the opposing extensor. In this case, the burst of sound would result in a greater response in the extensor (because of the higher resting tension) than in the flexor, and consequently, the required flexion response would be interfered with and delayed.

R. C. Davis (1956a,c) also found that steady noise of 90 dB increased tension in all muscles and influenced the response time in a simple choice task.

In summary, the ebb and flow of muscular activity is closely linked to and influenced by the rise and fall of sound. The relations are complicated. Gross bodily orientation toward an unexpected source of sound will diminish as the sound becomes familiar and predictable. Some components of the startle response to impulse sounds, for instance, will diminish with the repetition of the stimulus. The exact amount of reduction, however, depends on the individual person, his state of muscular tension as defined by posture or activity, and the characteristics of the impulse sound. Subtle changes in the musculature in response to sound may persist and their effects will depend in a complicated way on posture, activity, and the characteristics of the sound.

b. RESPONSES OF THE SMOOTH MUSCLES AND GLANDS. In response to brief sounds there is general constriction in the peripheral blood vessels with a reduction in peripheral blood flow. There may be acceleration or deceleration of heart rate, reduction in the resistance of the skin to electrical current (an indication of activation of the peripheral visceral nervous system), changes in breathing pattern, changes in the motility of the gastrointestinal tract, changes in the size of the pupils of the eyes, and changes in the secretion of saliva and gastric secretions (Davis et al., 1955; Jansen, 1969). These responses to brief sounds are obvious for A-weighted sound levels over about 70 dB. For sound levels below 70 dB, it is doubtful whether the recording techniques have been sufficiently sensitive to detect whether these responses occur. In any case, they are either small or nonexistent.

Some aspects of these responses diminish and seem to disappear with predictable repetition of the sounds. Others may not disappear (Davis et al., 1955). Jansen (cited by von Gierke, 1965), for example, found these responses persisted in industrial workers when they were exposed to the same noises in which they had worked for many years.

c. ORIENTING AND DEFENSE REFLEXES. Some of the responses of the smooth muscles and glands to sound are part of a pattern of response known as the orienting reflex. The orienting reflex is a "What is it?" response, and this reflex diminishes rapidly as a stimulus becomes familiar and predictable.

Some of the responses of the smooth muscles and glands in response to sound are part of a pattern of response known as the defense reflex. A defense reflex prepares the organism to escape or accept injury and discomfort. Responses that are part of a defense reflex disappear more slowly with stimulus repetition than do those that are part of the orienting reflex. Sometimes they may never completely disappear. Defense reflexes occur in response to warnings of painful stimuli, to painful stimuli themselves, or in response to very intense stimuli to any sense organ. Informative discussions of the orienting and defense reflexes can be found elsewhere (Sokolov, 1963a,b; Voronin et al., 1965).

d. NEUROENDOCRINE RESPONSES. Loud sounds as well as other intense stimuli such as cold, forced immobilization, forced exercise, pain, injuries, and so on can activate a complicated series of changes in the endocrine system with resulting changes in hormone levels, blood composition, and a whole complex of other biochemical and functional physiological changes (Lockett, 1970; Welch & Welch, 1970). Some of these changes and their implications will be mentioned in the sections to follow.

B. Possible Persistent Physiological Responses to Noise

It has been claimed that steady noise of approximately 110 dB can cause some changes in the size of the visual field after years of chronic exposure, but there is very little evidence to support this contention. Noise of about 130 dB can cause nystagmus and vertigo. However, these noise conditions are rarely encountered in the present environment (Kryter et al., 1971).

Evidence from animals exposed to very high noise levels suggests that exposure to these noises can interfere with sexual-reproductive functions, can interfere with resistance to viral disease, and can also produce other pathological effects (Kryter et al., 1971; Welch & Welch, 1970). Among these other effects are hypertrophy of the adrenal glands, developmental abnormalities of the fetus, and brain injury (Welch & Welch, 1970). These experiments often have not been so well reported that one can be sure that variables such as fear, handling, etc., have always been equated for noise-exposed animals and non-noise-exposed animals. Also, rodents have often been used as subjects, and these animals seem to have special susceptibility to the effects of certain sounds. Furthermore, the sound levels used in these experiments have usually been well above those normally encountered in our present environment.

There is evidence that workers exposed to high levels of noise have a higher incidence of cardiovascular disorders; ear, nose, and throat problems; and equilibrium disorders than do workers exposed to lower levels of noise (Andriukin, 1961; Jansen, 1959, 1969; Kryter et al., 1971). The results of one of these studies are summarized in Fig. 1.

The fact that those who work in high noise levels show greater evidence of

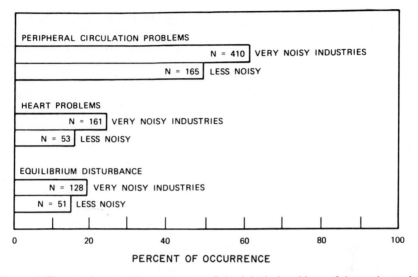

FIG. 1. Differences between the percentages of physiological problems of those who work in two different levels of noise. These data are from 1005 German industrial workers. Peripheral circulation problems include pale and taut skin, mouth and pharynx symptoms, abnormal sensations in the extremities, paleness of the mucous membranes, and other vascular disturbances. [From Kryter *et al.* (1971), *Non-auditory Effects of Noise* (Rep. WG-63). Copyright 1971 by the NAS–NRC Committee on Hearing and Bioacoustical Biomechanics.]

medical problems than those who work in lower noise levels is not conclusive evidence that noise is the crucial factor. In each case it is possible that the observed effects can be explained by other factors such as age, dust levels, occupational danger, life habits, and other nonnoise hazards. However, much more research of this type should be undertaken with attempts to rule out the effects of nonnoise factors.

From the facts presented about transient physiological responses to noise, one can argue that chronic arousal by sound might lead to some of the medical problems just described. The crux of the problem is whether one adapts to sufficiently loud or abrupt sounds and whether the modern environment presents such ever-changing auditory stimulation that arousal responses are chronically maintained.

III. STRESS THEORY, HEALTH, AND NOISE

A. Stress Theory

The neuroendocrine responses to intense sound are similar to the responses to stress. The response to stress is called the general adaptation syndrome (Selye, 1956). It consists of three stages: an alarm reaction, a stage of resistance, and a stage of exhaustion. If a stressor is very severe and is maintained for prolonged periods of time, an organism passes in succession through the stages of the alarm reaction, resistance, and exhaustion. In the extreme case, the end result is a breakdown of bodily function and death. In a less severe case, there may be a price to be paid in the stage of resistance. This price may include lowered resistance to infection, and perhaps, specific diseases known as the diseases of adaptation. These *may* include, among others, some types of gastrointestinal ulcers, some types of high blood pressure, and some types of arthritis. Many medical authorities do not accept the theory that there are diseases of adaptation. Rather, they theorize that each disease has its own special set of causes.

Stress theory, even as presented by its strongest advocates, is complicated. These advocates speak of complicated interactions between conditioning factors that set the scene for disease, specific reactions to particular stressors, and general reactions to nonspecific stressors.

It is nearly certain that noise of extremely high level can act as a stressor and, at least for some animals, can lead to some of the physiological changes associated with the general adaptation syndrome. Also, it is plausible that some of the more intense noises encountered in our present environment can act as stressors for people. However, the details of how such noises might act as stressors for people are unknown. The intensity level of the noise, the amount of fear and annoyance produced by the noise, and the susceptibility of the individual are probably examples of important factors. While certain pathways in the central nervous system and the hormonal system are probably important, these have not yet been established for the case of noise. For example, it could be necessary for the noise to produce ear damage, evoke annoyance and negative emotional reactions, or disturb sleep before elements of the general adaptation syndrome would appear. The picture is further complicated by the fact that a mild amount of stress at the right time of life may be beneficial. Therefore, while it is plausible that noise can be a detrimental stressor for people, it appears to be impossible to make firm statements about noise stress at this time.

B. Noise and General Health

While physiological arousal in response to sound can be of great benefit in the maintenance of response to possibly dangerous events, unnecessary arousal to irrelevant sounds can provide a basis for annoyance and for interference with performance of tasks. Chronic arousal from noises of sufficiently high levels or from noises that are sufficiently varied may, although it is unproven, contribute to the incidence of nonauditory disease. However, the evidence does suggest that, if noise control sufficient to protect persons from ear damage and hearing loss were instituted, then most of the noises of lower level and duration resulting from this effort would not directly induce nonauditory disease. Even so, perhaps certain patterns of exposure to irregular, brief sounds may be able to produce significant effects, such as sleep disturbance and psychological distress.

As mentioned earlier, general psychological distress produced by noise can add to the overall stress of life and in this way may contribute to the incidence of nonauditory disease. At this time, however, one cannot evaluate the contribution of noise-induced distress in relation to those other sources of stress we all encounter in our daily activities.

IV. CONCLUSIONS

It has not been demonstrated that many people have had their lives shortened by noise. While undoubtedly there have been accidental injuries and deaths when auditory warning signals were misunderstood or not heard because of the effects of noise, the prevalence of these has not been evaluated. Perhaps the stress of continued exposure to high levels of noise can produce disease or make one more susceptible to disease, but the evidence is not conclusive. While there are suggestions of relations between exposure to noise and the incidence of disease, the effects of noise on people have not been successfully measured in terms of "excess deaths" or "shortened lifespan" or "days of incapacitating illness." The only conclusively established effect of noise on health is that of noise-induced hearing loss.

There is clear evidence to support the following statements about the effects on people of exposure to noise of sufficient intensity and duration.

(1) Noise can permanently damage the inner ear with resulting permanent hearing losses that can range from slight impairment to nearly total deafness.
(2) Noise can result in temporary hearing losses and repeated exposures to noise can lead to chronic hearing losses.
(3) Noise can interfere with speech communication and the perception of other auditory signals.
(4) Noise can disturb sleep.
(5) Noise can be a source of annoyance.
(6) Noise can interfere with the performance of complicated tasks, and, of course, can especially disturb performance when speech communication or response to auditory signals is demanded.
(7) Noise and other acoustical considerations can reduce the opportunity for privacy.
(8) Noise can adversely influence mood and disturb relaxation.

In all of these ways noise can effect the essential nature of human life—its quality.

Acknowledgments

The preparation of Chapters 14–16 was supported by a contract between the Office of Noise Abatement and Control of the Environmental Protection Agency and the Central Institute for the Deaf and by a Public Health Service Grant from the National Institute of Neurological Diseases and Stroke to the Central Institute for the Deaf.

The author gratefully acknowledges the part-time assistance of several members of the staff of the Central Institute for the Deaf. The original manuscript has been distributed by the Environmental Protection Agency (NTID 300.7).

The original manuscript was reviewed by the following members of the NAS–NRC Committee on Hearing Bioacoustics, and Biomechanics: Hallowell Davis, Karl D. Kryter, William D. Neff, Wayne Rudmose, W. Dixon Ward, Harold L. Williams, and Jozef J. Zwislocki. Later members of the Coordinating Committee on Environmental Acoustics of The Acoustical Society of America reviewed the manuscript as published here. These members were Barry H. Leshowitz, Harry Levitt, Edgar A. G. Shaw, and John C. Webster. The reviewers have approved this paper for publication in the limited sense that they believe that most of the major issues have been accurately presented and identified as they stood in the Fall of 1971. A reviewer's approval does *not* imply that he agrees with each statement or graph presented in the text.

References

Andriukin, A. Influence of sound stimulation on the development of hypertension. *Coret Vasa,* 1961, **3**, 285–293. (Cited in Kryter, 1970.)

Bickford, R. G., Jacobson, J. L., Cody, D. T., & Lambert, E. H. Fast motor systems in man—Physiopathology of the sonomotor response. *Transactions of the American Neurological Association,* 1964, **89**, 56–58.

Davis, R. C. The muscular tension reflex and two of its modifying conditions. *Indiana University Public Science Series,* 1935, **3**, 22 pp.

Davis, R. C. The pattern of muscular action in simple voluntary movement. *Journal of Experimental Psychology,* 1942, **31**, 347–366.

Davis, R. C. Motor effects of strong auditory stimuli. *Journal of Experimental Psychology,* 1948, **38**, 257–275. (a)

Davis, R. C. Responses to meaningful and meaningless sounds. *Journal of Experimental Psychology,* 1948, **38**, 744–756. (b)

Davis, R. C. Motor responses to auditory stimuli above and below threshold. *Journal of Experimental Psychology,* 1950, **40**, 107–120.

Davis, R. C. Electromyographic factors in aircraft control: Muscular activity during steady noise and its relation to instructed responses evoked by auditory signals (USAF Rep. No. 55-124). Randolph Field, Texas: School of Aviation Medicine, 1956. (a)

Davis, R. C. Electromyographic factors in aircraft control: A muscular action potential study of 'conflict' (USAF Rep. 55-125). Randolph Field, Texas: School of Aviation Medicine, 1956. (b)

Davis, R. C. Electromyographic factors in aircraft control: Muscular activity during steady noise and its relation to instructed responses evoked by visual signals (USAF Rep. No. 55-126). Randolph Field, Texas: School of Aviation Medicine, 1956. (c)

Davis, R. C. Electromyographic factors in aircraft control: Response and adaptation to brief noises of high intensity (USAF Rep. No. 55-127). Randolph Field, Texas: School of Aviation Medicine, 1956. (d)

Davis, R. C. Muscular tension and performance. In Muscle action potentials in relation to task performance (USAF Rep. No. 55-122). Randolph Field, Texas: School of Aviation Medicine, 1956. (e)

Davis, R. C., Buchwald, A. M., & Frankmann, R. W. Autonomic and muscular responses and their relation to simple stimuli. *Psychological Monographs,* 1955, **69,** 1–71.

Davis, R. C., & Van Liere, D. W. Adaptation of the muscular tension to gunfire. *Journal of Experimental Psychology,* 1949, **39,** 114–117.

Jansen, G. On the origination of vegetative functional disturbances due to noise effect. *Archiv für Gewerbepathologie und Gewerbehygiene,* 1959, **17,** 238–261.

Jansen, G. Effects of noise on physiological state. In W. Ward & J. Fricke (Eds.), *Noise as a public health hazard* (Rep. 4). Washington, D.C.: American Speech and Hearing Association, 1969.

Kryter, K. D., Jansen, G., Parker, D., Parrack, H. O., Thiessen, G., & Williams, H. L. Non-auditory effects of noise (Rep. WG-63). Washington, D.C.: NAS–NRC Committee on Hearing and Bioacoustical Biomechanics, 1971.

Landis, C., & Hunt, W. A. *The startle pattern.* New York: Farrar and Rinehart, 1939.

Lockett, M. F. Effects of sound on endocrine function and electrolyte excretion. In B. L. Welch & A. S. Welch (Eds.), *Physiological effects of noise.* New York: Plenum, 1970. Pp. 21–41.

Mast, T. E. Short-latency human evoked responses to clicks. *Journal of Applied Physiology,* 1965, **20,** 725–730.

Patton, R. M. The effect of induced tension upon muscular activity during simple voluntary movement. Unpublished doctoral dissertation, Indiana University, Bloomington, 1953.

Selye, H. *The stress of life.* New York: McGraw-Hill, 1956.

Sokolov, Ye. N. *Perception and the conditioned reflex.* New York: Macmillan, 1963. (a)

Sokolov, Ye. N. Higher nervous functions: The orienting reflex. *Physiological Review,* 1963, **25,** 545–580. (b)

von Gierke, H. E. On noise and vibration exposure criteria. *Archives of Environmental Health,* 1965, **2,** 327–339.

Voronin, L. G., Leontiev, A. N., Luria, A. R., Sokolov, E. N., & Vinogradova, O. S. (Eds.) *Orienting reflex and exploratory behavior.* Washington, D.C.: American Institute of Biological Sciences, 1965.

Welch, B. L., & Welch, A. S. (Eds.) *Physiological effects of noise.* New York: Plenum, 1970.

AUTHOR INDEX

Numbers in italics refer to the pages on which the complete references are listed.

A

Abey-Wickrama, I., *672*
A'Brook, M. F., *672*
Ades, H. W., 146, *161*
Adrian, E. D., 17, *34*
Aggazzotti, A., 12, *34*
Agren, C. H., 540, *554*
Albert, K., 256, *278*
Allaire, P., 138, *160*
Allanson, J. T., 256, *278*
Allen, D., 232, *234*, 528, 531, *554*
Allen, J. D., 529, *559*
Alles, H. G., 553, *554*
Anderson, C. M. B., 191, 197, *234*
Anderson, D. J., 255, 257, 277, *278, 281*
Andriukin, A., *672, 672*, 680, *684*
Angel, A., 212, *234*
Angell, J. R., 377, *455, 456*
Alonso, S., 553, *554*
Anticaglia, J., 630, *639, 672*
Antonelli, A., 594, *604*
Appleton, J. H., 553, *554*
Aran, J.-M., 233, *234*
Arfib, D., *554*
Arginteanu, J., 671, *673*
Aristotle, 5, *34*
Atal, B. S., 33, *34*
Atkinson, J. W., 536, *560*
Attneave, F., 524, *554*

B

Babbitt, M., *554*
Babkoff, H., 384, 385, 388, 402, 409, 421, 422, 423, *456*
Bachem, A., 529, 530, 531, *554*
Backhaus, W., 543, *554*
Backus, J., 524, 528, 532, 539, 541, *554*
Baird, J. W., 529, 530, *554*

Banks, M. S., 416, *456*
Bannister, H., 390, *456*
Barany, E., 574, *604*
Barbaud, P., 551, *554*
Barbour, J. M., 524, *554*
Barkhausen, H., 188, *234*
Barris, M., 422, 423, *456*
Barron, B., 551, *554*
Barron, L., 551, *554*
Barry, S. H., 396, 397, 416, *462*
Bassett, I. G., 65, *75*
Batteau, D. W., 44, *75*, 378, *456*
Bauch, H., 201, *234*
Bauer, B. B., *554*
Bauer, J. W., 211, 233, *234, 236*
Bauhin, Caspar, 21, *34*
Bauman, V. H., 539, *554*
Bean, C., 536, *558*
Beatty, R. T., 50, *75*
Beauchamp, J. W., 526, 544, 545, 552, *554, 557*
Beauregard, H., 16, *35*
Beck, A., 16, *35*
Békésy, G. von, 24, 25, 26, 27, *35,* 48, 53, 55, *75,* 131, 132, 133, 134, 135, 140, 146, 151, 156, *160, 234,* 245, 248, 250, *278,* 298, 299, *333,* 373, 375, 379, 380, 381, 384, 398, 409, 420, *456,* 468, *515,* 571, 574, 586, *604*
Benade, A. H., 539, 541, 545, *554*
Benson, W., 451, 453, *458*
Beranek, L. L., 549, *554, 555*
Berger, K., 544, *555,* 603, *604*
Berger, R. J., 645, *673*
Berglund, B., 201, 206, 208, *234, 235*
Berglund, U., 201, 206, 208, *234, 235*
Berlyne, D. E., 535, 536, *555*
Bernstein, S., 396, 397, *465*
Bertrand, M. P., 387, *456*
Bess, F., 590, *604*
Bever, T., 527, *555*
Bickford, R. G., 678, *684*

SUBJECT INDEX

C

Cell, left and right ``tuning'' of, 468–480

Center frequency, critical base width as function of, 289–290

Central auditory nervous system disorders, 593

Central deafness, 592

Central masking, 319–324, *see also* Masking
 defined, 446
 fast decay of, 319
 hearing mechanisms and, 328
 masker intensity and, 323–324
 sensation level and, 324
 signal-to-noise ratio in, 329
 slow decay of, 320–322

Central pitch, 410

Centrifugal influence, 175

Chhi, Chinese concept of, 4

Claudius cells, 128

Cleveland Symphony Orchestra, 61

Click(s)
 in binaural loudness studies, 409
 broad-band, 383–386
 centering method for, 387
 in fusion and lateralization phenomena, 405–406
 high-pass vs. low-pass, 387–388
 in image centering, 404
 intensity and spectral content of, 384
 in interaural frequency differences, 397
 multiple, 403–406

Click-image position, schematic of, 389

Click stimuli, in interaural intensity effects, 490

Click trains, 386, 390

Click waveform, in interaural differences, 372

CM, *see* Cochlear microphonic

Cochlea
 acoustic input impedance of, 135
 action potential and, 52
 amplitude distributions in, 298–300
 anatomy of, 125–131
 biophysics of, 125–160
 compressional wave in, 47
 disorders of, *see* Cochlear disorders
 energy consumed by, 129
 first views of, 21
 function of, 50–54
 generator potential and, 148
 gross motion patterns of, 131–144

hair cells of, 128, 144
 mathematical model of, 53
 mechanisms of, *see* Cochlear mechanics
 pitch localization in, 19
 receptor potential and, 148
 resonators in, 245
 schematic drawing of, 25
 signal-to-noise-power ratio in, 354
 sound analysis resonators in, 245
 spiral form of, 21
 spiral reconstruction charts for, 18
 transducer processes in, 144, 146–159
 traveling wave pattern in, 131–135

Cochlear analysis, 53–54

Cochlear artery, 129

Cochlear disorders, 584–590
 intensity change and, 585

Cochlear duct, 126
 outer wall lining of, 128–129
 stria vascularis and, 129

Cochlear dynamics, 19
 fluid mechanics and, 24–26

Cochlear fluid
 pressure wave in, 143
 role of, 131

Cochlear impairment
 recruitment and, 220
 threshold decay and, 586

Cochlear mechanics, 131–146
 Bessel differential equation in, 141

Cochlear microphonic, 17, 51
 as receptor potential, 151–159

Cochlear microphonic potential
 frequency analysis and, 153–155
 hair-cell generation of, 156
 tuning curves for, 155–156

Cochlear partition, 126

Cochlear reserve, 574

Cochlear response, 16–17

Cocktail party effect, 70, 365

Coding periodicity problems, 177

Coincidence network, 475

Combination jnds (just-noticeable differences), 422–426

Combination tones, maximum audibility of, 303

Complex exponential, defined, 101

Complex numbers, 100–102

Complex sounds, *see also* Sound
 mixed, 272–277
 perception of as whole, 271–277

HANDBOOK OF PERCEPTION

EDITORS: *Edward C. Carterette and Morton P. Friedman*

Department of Psychology
University of California, Los Angeles
Los Angeles, California

Volume I: Historical and Philosophical Roots of Perception. 1974

Volume II: Psychophysical Judgment and Measurement. 1974

Volume III: Biology of Perceptual Systems. 1973

Volume IV: Hearing. 1978

Volume V: Seeing. 1975

Volume VIA: Tasting and Smelling. 1978

Volume VIB: Feeling and Hurting. 1978

Volume VII: Language and Speech. 1976

Volume VIII: Perceptual Coding. 1978

Volume IX: Perceptual Processing. 1978

Volume X: Perceptual Ecology. 1978

CONTENTS OF OTHER VOLUMES

A
B
C 8
D 9
E 0
F 1
G 2
H 3
I 4
J 5